Fundamental Biomechanics Sport and Exercise

Fundamental Biomechanics of Sport and Exercise is an engaging and comprehensive introductory textbook that explains biomechanical concepts from first principles, showing clearly how the science relates to real sport and exercise situations.

The book is divided into two parts. The first provides a clear and detailed introduction to the structure and function of the human musculoskeletal system and its structural adaptations, essential for a thorough understanding of human movement. The second part focuses on the biomechanics of movement, describing the forces that act on the human body and the effects of those forces on the movement of the body.

Every chapter includes numerous applied examples from sport and exercise, helping the student to understand how mechanical concepts describe both simple and complex movements, from running and jumping to pole-vaulting or kicking a football. In addition, innovative worksheets for field and laboratory work are included that contain clear objectives, a description of method, data recording sheets, plus a set of exemplary data and worked analyses. Alongside these useful features are definitions of key terms plus review questions to aid student learning, with detailed solutions provided for all numerical questions.

No other textbook offers such a clear, easy-to-understand introduction to the fundamentals of biomechanics. This is an essential textbook for any biomechanics course taken as part of a degree programme in sport and exercise science, kinesiology, physical therapy, sports coaching or athletic training.

James Watkins is a professor of biomechanics in the College of Engineering at Swansea University, UK. His main teaching and research specialisms are musculoskeletal anatomy and biomechanics.

WITHDRAWN

1 5 MAR 2024

York St John University

3 8025 006141199 9

Fundamental Biomechanics of Sport and Exercise

James Watkins

YORK ST. JOHN
LIBRARY & INFORMATION
SERVICES

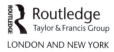
Routledge
Taylor & Francis Group

LONDON AND NEW YORK

First published 2014
by Routledge
2 Park Square, Milton Park, Abingdon, Oxon OX14 4RN

Simultaneously published in the USA and Canada
by Routledge
711 Third Avenue, New York, NY 10017

Routledge is an imprint of the Taylor & Francis Group, an Informa business

© 2014 James Watkins

The right of James Watkins to be identified as author of this work has been asserted by him in accordance with Sections 77 and 78 of the Copyright, Designs and Patents Act 1988.

All rights reserved. No part of this book may be reprinted or reproduced or utilised in any form or by any electronic, mechanical or other means, now known or hereafter invented, including photocopying and recording, or in any information storage or retrieval system, without permission in writing from the publishers.

Trademark notice: Product or corporate names may be trademarks or registered trademarks, and are used only for identification and explanation without intent to infringe.

British Library Cataloguing in Publication Data
A catalogue record for this book is available from the British Library

Library of Congress Cataloging in Publication Data
[CIP data]

ISBN: 978-0-415-81507-9 (hbk)
ISBN: 978-0-415-81508-6 (pbk)
ISBN: 978-0-203-06646-1 (ebk)

Typeset in Perpetua and Bell Gothic by
Servis Filmsetting Ltd, Stockport, Cheshire

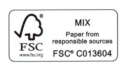

Printed and bound by CPI Group (UK) Ltd, Croydon, CR0 4YY

To Shelagh

Contents

CONTENTS

CONTENTS

Practical worksheets

PRACTICAL WORKSHEET 1   LINEAR KINEMATIC ANALYSIS OF A 15M SPRINT

In this worksheet the students collect distance–time data for a 15m sprint and use the data to plot the corresponding distance–time, speed–time and acceleration–time graphs.

PRACTICAL WORKSHEET 2   THE EFFECT OF INCREASE IN SPEED ON STRIDE LENGTH, STRIDE RATE AND RELATIVE STRIDE LENGTH IN RUNNING

In this worksheet the students collect stride rate, stride length and relative stride length data for running on a treadmill over a speed range of 2.0–4.5m/s and use the data to plot the corresponding stride length–speed, stride rate–speed, and relative stride length–speed graphs.

PRACTICAL WORKSHEET 3   FORCE–TIME ANALYSIS OF THE GROUND REACTION FORCE IN WALKING

In this worksheet the students record the anteroposterior and vertical components of the ground reaction force for a student walking across a force platform and carry out force–time analyses of the two components.

PRACTICAL WORKSHEET 4   FORCE–TIME ANALYSIS OF THE GROUND REACTION FORCE IN RUNNING

In this worksheet the students record the anteroposterior and vertical components of the ground reaction force for a student running across a force platform and carry out force–time analyses of the two components.

PRACTICAL WORKSHEET 5   DETERMINATION OF THE POSITION OF THE WHOLE BODY CENTRE OF GRAVITY BY THE DIRECT METHOD USING A ONE-DIMENSION REACTION BOARD

In this worksheet the students determine the position of the whole body centre of gravity by the direct method and examine the effect of changes in body position on the location of the whole body centre of gravity.

PRACTICAL WORKSHEET 6   COMPARISON OF THE DIRECT AND SEGMENTAL ANALYSIS METHODS OF DETERMINING THE POSITION OF THE WHOLE BODY CENTRE OF GRAVITY OF THE HUMAN BODY

In this worksheet the students compare the direct and segmental methods of determining the position of the whole body centre of gravity.

PRACTICAL WORKSHEET 7   DETERMINATION OF TAKE-OFF DISTANCE, FLIGHT DISTANCE AND LANDING DISTANCE IN A STANDING LONG JUMP

In this worksheet the students record a video of a standing long jump and analyse the video to determine take-off distance, flight distance and landing distance.

PRACTICAL WORKSHEET 8   MEASUREMENT OF THE MOMENT OF INERTIA OF THE HUMAN BODY

In this worksheet the students determine the moment of inertia of the human body about a vertical axis.

PRACTICAL WORKSHEET 9   DETERMINATION OF HUMAN POWER OUTPUT IN STAIR CLIMBING AND RUNNING UP A SLOPE

In this worksheet the students determine and compare the average power output of the human body in climbing stairs and running up a slope.

PRACTICAL WORKSHEET 10   DETERMINATION OF HUMAN POWER OUTPUT IN A COUNTERMOVEMENT VERTICAL JUMP

In this worksheet the students determine peak power output and average power output in a countermovement jump.

Preface

A book resting on a table has two forces acting on it; the weight of the book and the force exerted by the table. The two forces are equal in magnitude and opposite in direction so that the net force or resultant force acting on the book is zero. The book will remain at rest as long as the resultant force acting on it is zero. To lift the book from the table, it is necessary to create a resultant upward force on it by applying an upward force to it that is greater than its weight. Similarly, to lower the book down to the table, it is necessary to create a resultant downward force on it by applying an upward force to it that is less than its weight. It is clear from these examples that the movement of the book is completely determined by the resultant force acting on it. The examples illustrate the fundamental mechanical principle that the movement of any object or living organism (or part of a living organism, such as an arm or leg) is completely determined by the resultant force acting on it and that any change in the way that an object or living organism moves, i.e. any change in its speed or direction of movement, is the direct result of a change in the resultant force acting on it. There are three fundamental types of force: compression, tension and shear. The three types of force occur separately as, for example, when pressing a key on a keyboard (compression force exerted on the key), pulling on a rope (tension force exerted on the rope), and cutting a piece of paper with scissors (shear force exerted on the paper). The three types of force also occur in combination in bending and twisting.

Human movement is brought about by the musculoskeletal system under the control of the nervous system. The skeletal muscles pull on the bones to control the movements of the joints and, in doing so, control the movement of the body as a whole. By coordination of the various muscle groups, the forces generated by our muscles are transmitted by our bones and joints to enable us to apply forces to the external environment, usually by our hands and feet, so that we can adopt upright postures (counteract the constant tendency of body weight to collapse the body), transport the body and manipulate objects, often simultaneously. Consequently, the capacity of the body to move and carry out all of the activities that constitute daily living depends upon the capacity of the musculoskeletal system to generate and transmit forces. The forces generated and transmitted by the musculoskeletal system are referred to as internal forces. Body weight and the forces that we apply to the external environment are referred to as external forces. At any point in time we cannot change body weight and, as such, body weight is a passive external force. The external forces that are actively generated are active external forces. The magnitude, duration and timing of the active external forces are determined by the magnitude, duration and timing of the internal forces. Biomechanics is the study of the forces that act on and within living organisms and the effect of the forces on the size, shape, structure and movement of the organisms. The musculoskeletal components (skeletal muscles, bones, joints) normally continuously adapt their size, shape and structure to more readily withstand the time-averaged internal forces exerted on them in everyday physical activity. For example, skeletal muscles normally adapt to sustained strength training by changes in size, shape and structure that enable the muscles to produce more force, i.e. the muscles become stronger. Similarly, skeletal muscles adapt to a prolonged period of relative inactivity by changes in size, shape and structure that result in the muscles becoming weaker. The adaptation of musculoskeletal components to the time-averaged internal forces exerted on them is called structural adaptation. Structural adaptation is the branch of biomechanics concerned with the effect of internal forces on the size, shape and structure of the components of the musculoskeletal system.

Biomechanics of movement is the branch of biomechanics concerned with the effect of external forces on the movement of the body. In sport and exercise, whenever a physical education teacher or sports coach attempts to improve an individual's technique (the way that the arms, legs, trunk and head move in relation to each other during the performance of a particular movement, such as a forward roll in gymnastics or a jump shot in basketball), s/he is trying to change the magnitude, duration and timing of the internal forces to change the magnitude, duration and timing of the active external forces, which, in turn, determine the quality of performance. Good technique is characterised by effective performance (the purpose of the movement) and decreased risk of injury (distribution of forces in muscles, bones and joints so that no component is excessively overloaded). Poor technique is characterised by increased risk of injury, even though performance may be effective, at least for a while.

Biomechanics, with varying emphasis on structural adaptation and technique, is an essential component in the professional preparation of athletic trainers, physical therapists, physical education teachers and sports coaches. The purpose of this book is to develop knowledge and understanding of the fundamental concepts underlying structural adaptation and biomechanics of movement. The key to understanding structural adaptation is a thorough knowledge of the intimate relationship between the structure and functions of the components of the musculoskeletal system. Part I, Functional anatomy of the musculoskeletal system, describes this intimate relationship. The key to understanding biomechanics of movement is a thorough knowledge of force, Newton's laws of motion, work and energy. Part II, Biomechanics of movement, develops knowledge and understanding of these fundamental concepts through consideration of the biomechanics of a wide range of human movements.

The book is designed primarily as a first-level biomechanics course text for undergraduate students of sport and exercise science, physical education, physical therapy and athletic training. Students of occupational therapy and podiatry will also find the book useful, as an understanding of biomechanics is essential to successful practice in these professions.

No previous knowledge of biomechanics is assumed. All of the biomechanical concepts are explained from first principles. To aid learning, the book features a content overview and objectives at the start of each chapter, key points highlighted within the text, a large number of applied examples with illustrations, review questions with detailed solutions to all numerical questions, practical worksheets with example results, references to guide further reading, and an extensive index.

Acknowledgements

I thank all of the staff at Routledge who have contributed to the commissioning and production of the book. I also thank my academic colleagues and the large number of undergraduate and graduate students who have helped me, directly and indirectly, over many years, to develop and organise the content of the book.

About the author

James Watkins BEd, MA, PhD, FHEA, FBASES, FPEA is a professor of biomechanics in the College of Engineering at Swansea University, Swansea, UK. His main teaching and research specialisms are musculoskeletal anatomy and biomechanics. In addition to this book, he has written four other well-known books (*An Introduction to Mechanics of Human Movement*, 1983; *Structure and Function of the Musculoskeletal System*, 1999; *An Introduction to Biomechanics of Sport and Exercise*, 2007; *Functional Anatomy*, 2009). He is an advisory board member of the *Journal of Sports Sciences* and is a former chair of the Biomechanics Section of the British Association of Sport and Exercise Sciences (BASES). He is a fellow of the Higher Education Academy (HEA), a fellow of the British Association of Sport and Exercise Sciences, a fellow of the Physical Education Association of the United Kingdom (PEA), and an honorary member of the Association for Physical Education (afPE).

Part I

Functional anatomy of the musculoskeletal system

The open-chain arrangement of the bones of the skeleton – two arms and two legs attached independently to the vertebral column – allows us to adopt a wide range of body postures and perform a wide range of movements. However, this movement capability is only possible at the expense of low mechanical advantage of skeletal muscles, such that in most postures and movements other than lying down, the muscles have to exert very large forces, which, in turn, result in very large forces in bones and joints. The musculoskeletal components normally adapt their size, shape and structure, a process referred to as structural adaptation, to more readily withstand the time-averaged forces exerted on them in everyday physical activity. Structural adaptation is continuous throughout life, but the capacity for structural adaptation decreases with age after maturity. Consequently, there is an intimate relationship between the structure and functions of the components of the musculoskeletal system. Part I describes how musculoskeletal function – the generation and transmission of forces to control the movement of the body – is reflected in the structure of the musculoskeletal components.

Chapter 1 – The musculoskeletal system – describes the composition and function of the musculoskeletal system. Chapter 2 – The skeleton – describes the bones of the skeleton and, in particular, the features of the bones associated with force transmission at joints. Chapter 3 – Connective tissues – describes the ordinary connective tissues, in particular, ligaments, tendons and fascia, and the special connective tissues of cartilage and bone. Chapter 4 – The articular system – describes the joints and, in particular, the way joint design reflects a trade-off between stability and flexibility. Chapter 5 – The neuromuscular system – describes the interaction between the nervous and muscular systems in the control of joint movements. Chapter 6 – Mechanical characteristics of musculoskeletal components – describes the response of the musculoskeletal components to the forces exerted on them during everyday activity. Chapter 7 – Structural adaptation – describes how the musculoskeletal components adapt to the time-averaged forces exerted on them.

1

The musculoskeletal system

All living organisms are made up of cells. The human body is made up of billions of cells, which are organised into complex groups that carry out specific functions. These groups include the cardiovascular system, which transports blood around the body, and the musculoskeletal system, which enables us to move. The first part of this chapter describes the four fundamental types of cell in the body and the organisation of the cells within functional groups. The second part of the chapter describes the composition and structure of the musculoskeletal system.

OBJECTIVES

After reading this chapter, you should be able to do the following:

1. Describe the four types of tissue.
2. Describe cellular organisation in multicellular organisms.
3. Describe the composition and function of the musculoskeletal system.

UNICELLULAR AND MULTICELLULAR ORGANISMS

The fundamental structural and functional unit of all living organisms is the cell. The lowest forms of life consist entirely of single cells and are referred to as unicellular organisms. Higher forms of life, like the human body, consist of many cells and are referred to as multicellular organisms.

There are two general categories of cells, prokaryotes and eukaryotes (Alberts *et al.* 2002). A prokaryotic cell consists of an outer cell membrane (comprised of proteins and lipids) that encloses a semitransparent fluid called cytosol (a complex solution of proteins, salts and sugars). The cell membrane, usually referred to as the plasma membrane or plasmalemma, separates and protects the cell from its surrounding environment and allows interchange of substances between the cytosol and the surrounding environment via a system of channels and pumps.

Eukaryotes are similar to prokaryotes in that they have a cell membrane that encloses cytosol. However, whereas the cytosol of a prokaryotic cell is largely featureless, the cytosol of a eukaryotic cell surrounds a number of distinct structures, which differ in size and shape (Figure 1.1). The most distinct of these structures is the nucleus, which contains the cell's genetic material (23 pairs of chromosomes in human beings). The other structures are called organelles; these include lysosomes (involved in digestion of nutrients), mitochondria (production of energy),

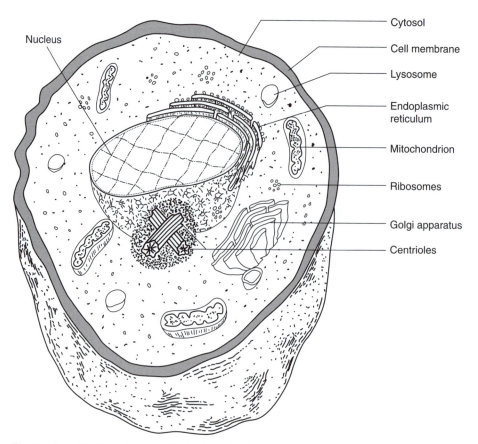

Nucleus

Cytosol

Cell membrane

Lysosome

Endoplasmic reticulum

Mitochondrion

Ribosomes

Golgi apparatus

Centrioles

Figure 1.1 Section through a generalised eukaryotic cell.

ribosomes (assembly of amino acids into proteins), and centrioles (involved in cell division). The nucleus organises and controls, via the organelles, the life processes of the cell. The life processes include growth and development, respiration, circulation, digestion, excretion, reproduction and movement. In prokaryotes the genetic material is distributed throughout the cytosol and the life processes are carried out by indistinct structures in the cell membrane.

All prokaryotic organisms, which include bacteria, are unicellular. Eukaryotic organisms range from unicellular organisms, such as amoeba and euglena, to multicellular organisms, such as the human body. All mammals, birds and fish are multicellular organisms. The number of cells in multicellular organisms varies considerably. For example, the nematode worm *Caenorhabditis elegans* is 1 mm (millimetre) in length and consists of 959 cells (Kenyon 1988). Most multicellular organisms consist of millions of cells; the human body consists of approximately 10^{14} (one hundred million million) cells (Alberts *et al.* 2002).

> The fundamental structural and functional unit of living organisms is the cell. A unicellular organism consists entirely of a single cell. A multicellular organism consists of many cells.

Like cytosol, the cell membrane consists of a viscous fluid, but it is usually much more viscous than the cytosol. The viscous (capacity to change shape in response to an applied force) nature of the cell membrane and cytosol enables a cell to change its shape without losing its integrity. During normal functioning, many cells regularly change shape and the amount of change depends on the type of cell. For example, in muscle cells the ability to change shape is highly specialised and is an essential feature of normal function. Muscle cells are long and thin and may shorten by up to 40% during contraction (production of a pulling force). In contrast, bone cells occupy tiny spaces within a fairly hard bony matrix, such that change in shape of bone cells is minimal during normal everyday activity.

The structure of a cell determines its function. Whereas muscle cells and bone cells are both eukaryotic, they have different functions and, as such, are different in structure. The human body is made up of four fundamental types of eukaryotic cells, called tissues.

CELLULAR ORGANISATION IN MULTICELLULAR ORGANISMS

All living organisms carry out all of the essential life processes. In unicellular organisms the life processes are, in biological terms, relatively simple. However, in multicellular organisms the cells are organised into complex functional groups that carry out the various life processes for the organism as a whole. There are three levels of cellular organisation in each functional group: tissues, organs and systems.

Tissues

In multicellular organisms all of the cells originate from a single cell formed by the fertilisation of a female ovum by a male sperm. This cell undergoes rapid cell division to form a large number of similar cells. Soon after this, the cells differentiate in size, shape and structure, in order to carry out different functions within the developing organism (Wozniak and Chen 2009). This process of cellular differentiation results in the formation of four types of cells called tissues: epithelia, nerve, muscle and connective. A tissue is a group of cells having the same specialised structure, so as to perform a particular function in the body (Freeman and Bracegirdle 1967). The word tissue is also used in a general sense, such as in the description of skin, muscles, tendons, ligaments and fat as soft tissues.

Epithelial tissue

There are two types of epithelial tissue: covering and glandular. Covering epithelia form the surface layers of cells of all the internal and external free surfaces of the body except the surfaces inside synovial joints. For example, the surfaces of the skin and the lining of the alimentary canal, heart chambers and blood vessels are all examples of covering epithelia.

All cells secrete fluid to a certain extent, but glandular epithelial cells are specialised for this purpose and form the two types of glands: exocrine and endocrine. Many of the exocrine glands (glands with ducts that discharge secretions onto a surface), such as the gastric glands in the lining of the stomach, secrete fluids containing enzymes necessary for the digestion of food. Endocrine glands (ductless glands that discharge secretions directly into the blood stream), such as the pituitary gland at the base of the brain and the adrenal glands at the upper end of each kidney, secrete hormones that, in association with the nervous system, regulate and coordinate the various body functions.

Nerve tissue

Nerve cells (neurons) are specialised to conduct electrochemical impulses throughout the body to coordinate the various body functions. The structure and function of nerve tissue is covered in detail in Chapter 5.

Muscle tissue

Muscle cells are specialised to contract, i.e. create a pulling force to stabilise or move parts of the body. There are three types of muscle cells: skeletal, visceral and cardiac.

Skeletal muscle is attached to the skeletal system (skeleton and joint support structures) and, under the control of the nervous system, controls movement in the joints between the bones of the skeleton. Skeletal muscle is also referred to as voluntary muscle because it is normally under the conscious control of the individual. The structure and functions of skeletal muscle are covered in detail in Chapter 5.

Visceral muscle, also referred to as involuntary muscle because it is not normally under conscious control, is found in parts of the body that experience involuntary movement, such as the walls of the larger arteries and the alimentary canal. For example, contraction of visceral muscle in the walls of an artery reduces the diameter of the artery and results in a local increase in blood pressure, which pushes blood around the cardiovascular system. Similarly, contraction of visceral muscle in the walls of the alimentary canal pushes digested food along the canal and eliminates solid waste through the anus.

Cardiac muscle is found only in the heart. It has characteristics of both skeletal muscle and visceral muscle, but differs from them in that it contracts rhythmically throughout life even though the frequency of contractions (heart rate) varies.

Connective tissue

As its name suggests, one of the main functions of connective tissue is to bind other tissues together. The bones of the skeleton and the fibrous structures that hold the bones together at joints are all forms of connective tissue. The structure and functions of connective tissue are covered in detail in Chapter 3.

Cellular differentiation results in the formation of four types of cells called tissues: epithelia, nerve, muscle and connective.

Organs and systems

An organ is a combination of different tissues designed to carry out a specific bodily function. For example, the heart is designed to pump blood around the body. The structure of the heart consists of cardiac muscle cells; connective tissue, which binds the muscle cells together; epithelial tissue, which lines the chambers of the heart; and nerve tissue, which innervates the cardiac muscle cells. Other examples of organs are the brain, the eyes, the lungs, the stomach, the spleen, the kidneys, the liver and each skeletal muscle, together with its tendons, which attach the muscle to the skeletal system.

A system is a combination of different organs working together to carry out a particular bodily function. For example, the function of the cardiovascular system, which consists of the heart and blood vessels, is to transport blood around the body. There are basically 11 separate systems in the human body (Standring 2008):

> *Integumentary system*: The external covering of the body, i.e. the skin and associated structures such as finger and toe nails;
> *Skeletal system*: The bones of the skeleton and the structures that form the joints between the bones;
> *Muscular system*: The skeletal muscles;
> *Nervous system*: The nerves, organised into central (brain and spinal cord) and peripheral (spinal nerves) components;
> *Endocrine system*: The glands that secrete hormones, which regulate and coordinate the various body functions in association with the nervous system;
> *Cardiovascular system*: The heart and blood vessels;
> *Lymphatic system*: The system of vessels and ducts that drains extracellular fluid and returns it to the blood;
> *Respiratory system*: The lungs and associated passageways;
> *Digestive system*: The alimentary canal and associated structures that break down food and eliminate solid waste;
> *Urinary system*: The kidneys, bladder and associated structures that eliminate nitrogenous waste as urine;
> *Reproductive system*: The ovaries and associated structures (female) and testes and associated structures (male) that enable the body to produce offspring.

These systems are responsible for carrying out the body's life processes. Whereas all of the life processes involve a certain degree of integration between different systems, some processes involve closer integration than others. For example, the transport of oxygen from the air to all the cells of the body and the transport of carbon dioxide in the opposite direction is carried out by close integration of the nervous, respiratory and cardiovascular systems. Likewise, movement of the body is brought about by close integration of the nervous, muscular and skeletal systems. Consequently, the systems are often referred to in combination as, for example, the cardiorespiratory, musculoskeletal and neuromuscular systems. Figure 1.2 summarises cellular differentiation and organisation in multicellular organisms.

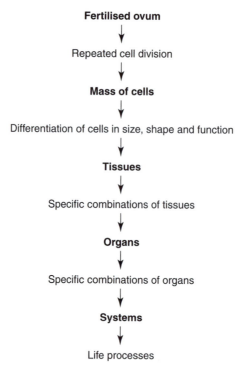

Figure 1.2 Cellular differentiation and organisation in multicellular organisms.

Cellular organisation results in the formation of organs (combinations of different tissues) and systems (combinations of different organs). The systems are responsible for carrying out the body's life processes.

THE MUSCULOSKELETAL SYSTEM

Human movement is brought about by the musculoskeletal system under the control of the nervous system. The musculoskeletal system consists of the skeletal system and the muscular system. The skeletal system consists of the skeleton (the bones) and the fibrous structures that form the joints between the bones. Figure 1.3 shows the skeleton and the muscular system. The skeleton gives the body its shape and provides a very strong, relatively lightweight supporting framework for all the other systems. The adult skeletal system normally has 206 bones and more than 200 joints and accounts for approximately 12% and 15% of total body weight in women and men, respectively (McArdle *et al.* 2007). The structure and function of the skeleton are covered in detail in Chapter 2.

As previously described, there are three types of muscle tissue: visceral, cardiac and skeletal. Visceral muscle is usually considered to be of part the digestive system (in the walls of the alimentary canal) and cardiovascular system (in the walls of arteries), and cardiac muscle is part of the cardiovascular system (Standring 2008). Consequently, the

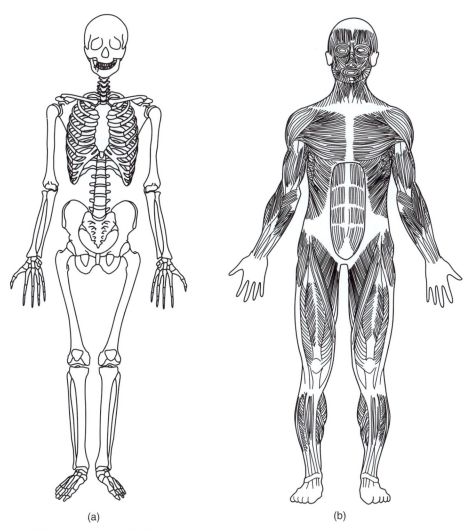

(a) (b)

Figure 1.3 (a) The skeleton. (b) The muscular system.

muscular system refers only to the skeletal muscles. There are approximately 640 skeletal muscles. The skeletal muscles account for an average of approximately 34% and 42% of total body weight in young (18 to 29 years) healthy untrained adult women and men, respectively, and an average of approximately 30% and 34% of total body weight in elderly (70 to 88 years) healthy untrained adult women and men, respectively (Janssen *et al.* 2000).

The musculoskeletal system consists of the skeletal system (the bones and the fibrous structures that form the joints between the bones) and the muscular system (the skeletal muscles).

Musculotendinous units

The most important property of all types of muscle tissue is contractility, i.e. the ability to create a pulling force and, if necessary, change in length (increase or decrease) while maintaining a pulling force. Each complete skeletal muscle consists of a large number of long, thin muscle cells (also referred to as muscle fibres) bound together by various layers of connective tissues. The length of the cells varies from a few millimetres (in the muscles that move the eyes) to about 30 centimetres (in the sartorius muscle in the anterior thigh). In most skeletal muscles the muscle cells occupy the main belly of the muscle, but the ends of the muscle consist entirely of thickened cords or bands of virtually inextensible connective tissue that anchor the muscle onto the skeleton (Figure 1.4). The shape of these connective tissue attachments depends on the shape of the muscle and the attachment areas available on the skeleton. In general, there are two basic shapes: a cord or narrow band called a tendon and a broad

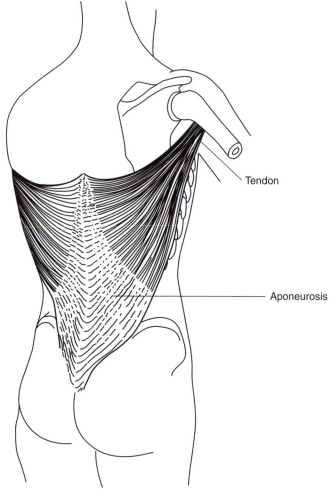

Figure 1.4 Tendon and aponeurosis. The latissimus dorsi muscle on each side of the body originates from a broad aponeurosis and inserts onto the humerus via a narrow-band tendon.

sheet called an aponeurosis (Figure 1.4). A skeletal muscle and its tendons and aponeuroses are usually referred to as a musculotendinous unit or muscle–tendon unit (Taylor *et al.* 1990).

As a muscle can only pull in one direction, the movement of each joint is controlled by opposing pairs of muscle groups, referred to as antagonistic pairs. The muscles in each group cross over one or more joints. For example, the quadriceps muscle group consists of four muscles: vastus lateralis, vastus intermedius, vastus medialis and rectus femoris (Figure 1.5). The rectus femoris originates from the front of the pelvis and the vasti muscles originate from the shaft of the femur. The four muscles join together to form the quadriceps tendon, which covers the anterior aspect of the patella and continues as the patellar ligament to attach onto the tibial tuberosity of the tibia. Consequently, all four muscles cross the front of the knee joint and tend to extend the knee when the quadriceps contract. However, the rectus femoris also crosses the front of the hip joint and tends to flex the hip when the quadriceps contract. The rectus femoris is a two-joint muscle and the vasti muscles are one-joint muscles. The hamstring muscle group is antagonistic to the quadriceps and consists of three muscles: semi-membranosus, semitendinosus and biceps femoris. The semimembranosus, semitendinosus and part of the biceps femoris all originate from the ischial tuberosity and insert onto the tibia, i.e. they are two-joint muscles that tend to extend the hip and flex the knee. Part of the

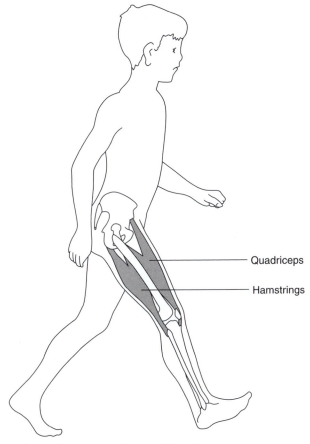

Quadriceps

Hamstrings

Figure 1.5 Antagonistic muscle groups: quadriceps and hamstrings.

11

biceps femoris originates from the shaft of the femur, i.e. part of the biceps femoris is a one-joint muscle (that tends to flex the knee) and the other part is a two-joint muscle.

By coordinated activity between the groups of muscles that cross a joint, the amount and rate of movement in the joint can be carefully controlled. The number of pairs of muscles required to control a particular joint depends on the number of directions in which the joint is free to move. For example, the knee joint is designed to rotate in one plane about a transverse (side-to-side) axis (knee flexion, or extension). However, other joints, such as the hip and shoulder, are designed to move in more than one plane (see Chapter 4). Consequently, two or more antagonistic pairs of muscle groups are required to control movement in these joints.

Each skeletal muscle is attached to the skeleton such that it crosses one or more joints. When a muscle contracts it tends to bring about movement in the joints that it crosses. The muscles are arranged in antagonistic pairs that coordinate action to control the amount and rate of movement in each joint.

Force, mechanics and biomechanics

All movements and changes in the movement of bodies, animate and inanimate, are brought about by the action of forces. The two most common types of force are pulling and pushing. A force can be defined as that which tends to deform a body or that which tends to move a body from rest or change the way that the body is moving. Mechanics is the study of the forces that act on bodies and the effects of the forces on the size, shape, structure and movement of the bodies. Biomechanics is the study of the forces that act on and within living organisms and the effect of the forces on the size, shape, structure and movement of the organisms.

Load, strain and stress

A load is any force or combination of forces that is applied to an object. There are three types of load: tension, compression and shear (Figure 1.6). Loads tend to deform the objects on which they act. Tension is a pulling (stretching) load that tends to make an object longer and thinner along the line of the force (Figure 1.6a,b). Compression is a pushing or pressing load that tends to make an object shorter and thicker along the line of the force (Figure 1.6a,c). A shear load is comprised of two equal (in magnitude), opposite (in direction), parallel forces that tend to displace one part of an object with respect to an adjacent part along a plane parallel to and between the lines of force (Figure 1.6a,d). The cutting load produced by scissors and garden shears is a shear load, while the cutting load produced by a knife is a compression load. It is also a shear load, which forces one object to slide on another (Figure 1.6e). The sliding or tendency to slide is resisted by a force called friction, which is exerted between and parallel to the two contacting surfaces.

The three types of load frequently occur in combination, especially in bending (Figure 1.6a,f) and torsion (Figure 1.6a,g). An object subjected to bending experiences tension on one side and compression on the other. An object subjected to torsion (twisting) simultaneously experiences tension, compression and shear.

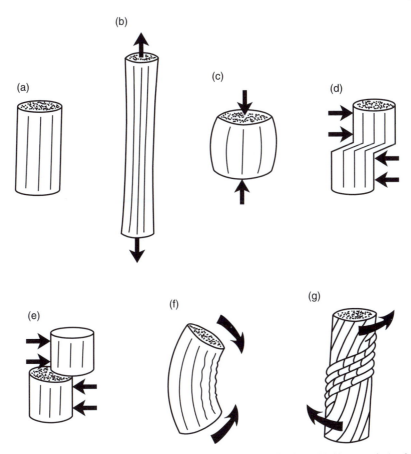

Figure 1.6 Types of load. (a) Unloaded. (b) Tension. (c) Compression. (d) Shear. (e) Shear producing friction. (f) Bending. (g) Torsion.

In mechanics, the deformation of an object that occurs in response to a load is referred to as strain. For example, when a muscle contracts it exerts a tension load on the tendons at each end of the muscle and, consequently, the tendons experience tension strain, i.e. they are very slightly stretched. Similarly, an object subjected to a compression load experiences compression strain and an object subjected to a shear load experiences shear strain. Strain denotes deformation of the intermolecular bonds that comprise the structure of an object.

When an object experiences strain, the intermolecular bonds exert forces that tend to restore the original (unloaded) size and shape of the object. The forces exerted by the inter-molecular bonds of an object under strain are referred to as stress. Stress is the resistance of the intermolecular bonds to the strain caused by the load.

The stress on an object resulting from a particular load is distributed throughout the whole of the material sustaining the load. However, the level of stress in different regions of the material varies depending upon the amount of material sustaining the load in the different regions; the more material sustaining the load, the lower the stress. Consequently, stress is measured in terms of the average load on the plane of material sustaining the load at the point of interest.

A load is any force or combination of forces applied to an object. Strain is the deformation of an object that occurs in response to a load. Stress is the resistance of the intermolecular bonds of an object to the strain caused by a load.

Tension stress

Figure 1.7a shows a person standing upright with the line of action of body weight slightly in front of the ankle joints. In this posture, stability is maintained by isometric (static) contraction of the ankle plantar flexors, as shown in the simple two-segment model in Figure 1.7b. If the force exerted by the ankle plantar flexors in each leg is 38 kgf (kgf = kilogram force; 1 kgf is the weight of a mass of 1 kilogram) and the cross-sectional area of the Achilles tendon at P in Figure 1.7b, perpendicular to the tension load, is 1.8 cm^2 (square centimetres), then the tension stress on the tendon at P is 21.1 kgf/cm^2 (kilograms force per square centimetre), i.e.

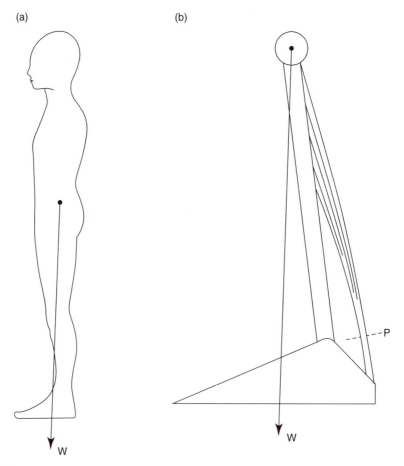

Figure 1.7 Tension load on the Achilles tendon.

$$\text{tension stress at } P = \frac{38\text{kgf}}{1.8\,\text{cm}^2}$$

$$= 21.1\text{kgf/cm}^2.$$

Compression stress

When standing upright and barefoot, as in Figure 1.7a, the ground reaction force (the upward force exerted by the ground on the feet) exerts a compression load on the contact area of the feet (Figure 1.8a). In an adult, the contact area is approximately 260 cm^2 (both feet) (Hennig *et al.* 1994). For a person weighing 70 kgf, the compression stress on the contact area of the feet (on a level floor, contact area perpendicular to the compression load) is 0.27 kgf/cm^2, i.e.

$$\text{compression stress} = \frac{70\text{ kgf}}{260\text{ cm}^2}$$

$$= 0.27\,\text{kgf/cm}^2.$$

By raising the heels off the ground the contact area is approximately halved (Figure 1.8b). Since the compression load (body weight) is the same as before, it follows that the compression stress on the reduced contact area is approximately doubled. Compression stress is usually referred to as pressure.

(a)   (b)

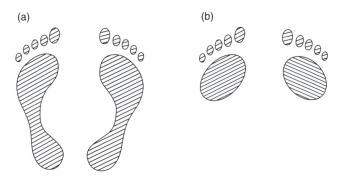

Figure 1.8 Supporting area of the feet. (a) Normal upright standing posture. (b) Standing upright with the heels off the floor.

Shear stress

Many of the joints, especially those in the lower back and pelvis, are subjected to shear load during normal everyday activities, such as standing and walking. For example, in walking, there is a phase when one leg supports the body while the other leg swings forward (Figure 1.9a). In this situation the unsupported side of the body tends to move downward relative to the supported side, subjecting the pubic symphysis joint to shear load. In an adult man, the area

15

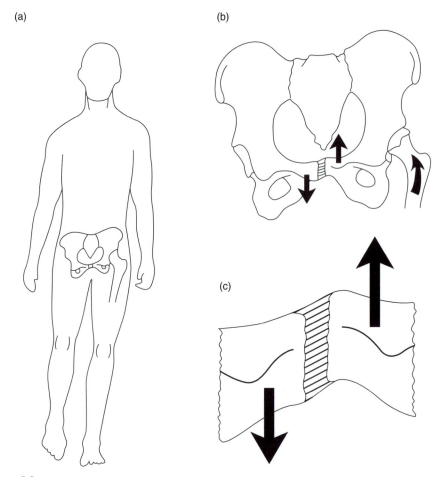

Figure 1.9 Shear load on the pubic symphysis resulting from single-leg support while walking.

of the pubic symphysis in the plane of the shear load is approximately 5 cm². If the shear load at the instant shown in Figure 1.9a is, for example, 2 kgf, then the shear stress on the joint is 0.4 kgf/cm², i.e.

$$\text{shear stress} = \frac{2\text{kgf}}{5\text{cm}^2}$$

$$= 0.4\text{kgf/cm}^2.$$

Musculoskeletal system function

Posture refers to the orientation of the body segments to each other and is usually applied to static or quasi-static positions, such as sitting and standing. When standing upright, there are two forces acting on the body; body weight and the ground reaction force (Figure 1.10a). The combined effect of body weight and the ground reaction force is a compression load (experi-

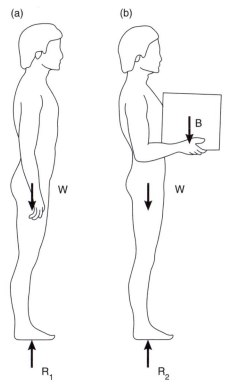

Figure 1.10 Forces acting on the body when standing. (a) Standing upright. (b) Standing upright with additional load. W = body weight, R_1 and R_2 = ground reaction forces, B = additional weight.

enced at the feet) that tends to collapse the body in a heap on the ground. This compression load increases with any additional weight carried by the body (Figure 1.10b). To prevent the body from collapsing while simultaneously bringing about desired movements, the movements of the various joints need to be carefully controlled by coordinated activity between the various muscle groups. For example, when standing upright, the joints of the neck, trunk and legs must be stabilised by the muscles that control them, otherwise the body would collapse (Figure 1.11). Consequently, the weight of the whole body is transmitted to the floor by the feet, but the weight of individual body segments above the feet (head, arms, trunk and legs) is transmitted indirectly to the floor by the skeletal chain formed by the bones and joints of the neck, trunk and legs.

The transmission of body weight to the ground while maintaining an upright body posture illustrates the essential feature of musculoskeletal function, i.e. generation (by the muscles) and transmission (by the bones and joints) of forces that, in turn, enable us to exert forces on our physical environment so that we can maintain upright posture, transport the body and manipulate objects, often simultaneously. The forces generated and transmitted by the musculoskeletal system are referred to as internal forces. Forces that act on the body, such as body weight (the effect of gravity), ground reaction force, water resistance, air resistance, and forces that act on our hands (e.g. when holding or throwing a ball) and feet (e.g. kicking a ball) as we manipulate objects, are referred to as external forces.

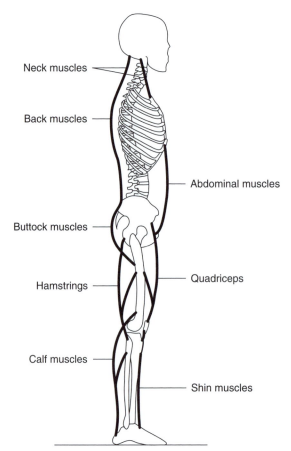

Neck muscles

Back muscles

Abdominal muscles

Buttock muscles

Hamstrings

Quadriceps

Calf muscles

Shin muscles

Figure 1.11 Location of the main muscle groups responsible for maintaining standing posture.

The musculoskeletal system generates and transmits internal forces to enable us to generate external forces to maintain upright posture, transport the body and manipulate objects, often simultaneously.

Maintaining upright posture

Movements in this category involve fairly static postures in which the weight of one or more body segments is transmitted indirectly to the floor or other support surface, such as a chair, by other segments. These postures include standing (Figure 1.12a), sitting (Figure 1.12b–d) and balancing activities (Figure 1.13b). Some upright postures may involve more than one support surface. For example, Figure 1.12c shows a person sitting in an armchair; his arms are supported by the armrests and his feet rest on the floor. In this case, his weight is distributed over four support areas: the backrest, seat, armrests and floor. Similarly, Figure 1.12e shows a person leaning on a table. In this case, his weight is supported partly by the table and partly by the floor.

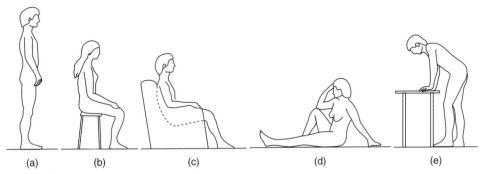

(a)   (b)   (c)   (d)   (e)

Figure 1.12 Standing and sitting postures.

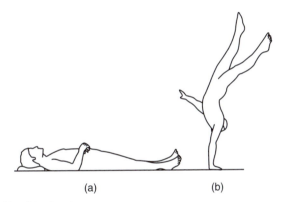

(a)   (b)

Figure 1.13 Lying and handstand postures.

The degree of muscular activity required to maintain a particular body posture depends on the number and size of the support surfaces. Consequently, muscular activity is minimal in the recumbent posture since all of the body segments are supported directly by the support surface (Figure 1.13a). In contrast, balancing on one hand involves a considerable amount of muscular activity to transmit the entire body weight through the small area beneath the hand (Figure 1.13b). In this case, the weight of each body segment above the grounded hand is transmitted indirectly to the floor, from segment to segment down through the skeletal chain.

Body transport

To move from one place to another, the body must push or pull against something to provide the necessary force to drive it in the required direction. In walking and running, forward movement is combined with an upright body posture and movement is achieved by pushing a foot obliquely downward and backward against the ground. Provided that the foot does not slip, the leg thrust results in a ground reaction force directed obliquely upward and forward. The effect of the ground reaction force is that the body moves forward with an upright posture (Figure 1.14).

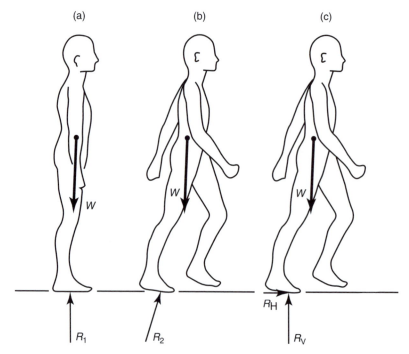

(a)　　　　　　　　　(b)　　　　　　　　　(c)

Figure 1.14 The ground reaction force in standing and walking. (a) Standing. (b) Push-off in walking. W = body weight, R_1 = ground reaction force when standing. R_2 = ground reaction force during push-off. R_H = horizontal component of R_2. R_V = vertical component of R_2

When swimming, the water largely supports body weight (buoyancy force). Consequently, the main function of the musculoskeletal system is to enable the arms and legs to pull and push backward against the water to move the body forward. Since the musculoskeletal system does not have to support the weight of the body in the water, the muscle forces and joint reaction forces (the forces exerted between the articular surfaces in joints) that occur during swimming tend to be considerably less than in land-based activities. For this reason, swimming is often prescribed as part of a rehabilitation program to restore normal muscle function and joint flexibility following injury.

Manipulating objects

Many movements involve manipulating objects with the hands or the feet. These manipulations may involve fairly forceful pushes and pulls or fine manual dexterity. For example, forceful pushes and pulls are required to push a wheelbarrow, pull on an upright post, carry a heavy suitcase, and throw or kick a ball. Activities involving manual dexterity are usually associated with a fairly static body posture (a stable base of support). Such activities include, for example, driving a car, writing or typing at a desk, turning a door handle, and taking a book off a shelf.

The human machine

The skeletal system basically consists of a number of fairly rigid components (bones) that are joined together in ways that allow a certain amount of movement in each joint. The muscular system, under the control of the nervous system, controls the movement of the joints and, thereby, enables the body to apply forces on other objects. Consequently, the musculoskeletal system operates like a machine, i.e. a powered mechanism that is capable of applying forces to other objects (Dempster 1965). Figure 1.15 shows a simple machine that can be made to apply a gripping force at one end by applying a compression load at the other end.

The number of components in a machine, animate or inanimate, tends to reflect the functional complexity of the machine. For example, a pair of scissors, a stapler and a paper punch all have very few components in comparison with a car engine. However, the components of an inanimate machine are usually joined together in a closed-chain arrangement that produces simultaneous and predictable movements of the joints between the components; the movement of one joint determines the movement in all the other joints (as in the simple machine in Figure 1.15). This is not the case with the human musculoskeletal system. The human machine enables the individual to adopt the most suitable posture for applying forces in any given situation. The body's ability to adopt a wide range of postures is due to the skeleton's open-chain arrangement of bones. The arms and legs form four peripheral chains, free at their extremities, which attach onto a central chain (see Figure 1.3a). This open-chain arrangement allows any part of the body to move more or less independently of the rest; movement of one part of the body does not necessarily result in movement in the rest of the body. For example, movements of the arms can accomplish a variety of tasks such as eating, writing and typing while the rest of the body is in a more or less stationary sitting position.

The human machine has a large number of force-producing components (muscles). Muscle activity is carefully coordinated to utilise the muscles most efficiently. For example, in a throwing action, such as pitching a baseball, the speed of the ball as it leaves the pitcher's hand is due to the impulse of the force (the magnitude of the force and the duration of force) exerted on the ball during the pitching action (Figure 1.16). The muscles generate the force;

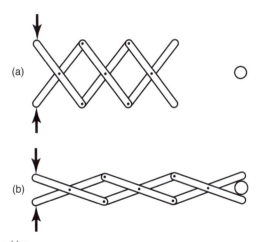

(a)

(b)

Figure 1.15 A simple machine.

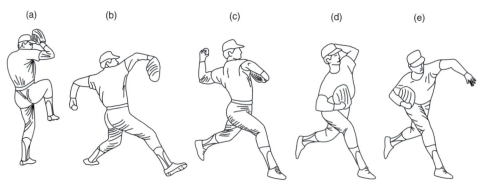

Figure 1.16 Pitching a baseball.

the more muscles that are recruited during the pitching action, and the greater the length of time that the forces act on the ball, the greater the ball speed. In a well-coordinated pitching action, the forces produced by the individual muscle groups are summated to maximise the impulse of the force exerted on the ball during the pitch (Fleisig *et al.* 1996). The pitching action starts with the rear leg driving the body forward into the step (Figure 1.16a,b). The next stage involves foot placement of the lead leg, which provides a firm base for the muscles of the legs and hips to drive the rear hip and, therefore, the trunk forward (Figure 1.16b,c). The muscles of the trunk then drive the throwing arm forward (Figure 1.16c,d). Finally, the shoulder, elbow and wrist of the throwing arm drive the ball forward until release (Figure 1.16d,e).

In propulsive movements like throwing, the amount of force applied to the implement is limited by the number of muscle groups recruited to drive the body and, therefore, the implement in the intended direction. If all of an adult's skeletal muscles could contract simultaneously in the same direction, they would exert a force in the region of 22 tons (Elftman 1966). However, the arrangement of the muscles does not permit this theoretical maximum to be achieved. Even in a highly trained and highly motivated athlete, the amount of force generated in propulsive whole body movements, such as jumping and throwing, is usually a small fraction of the theoretical maximum. Furthermore, injury to any part of the musculoskeletal system used in the movement reduces this force even further. For example, injury to an ankle severely affects a pitcher's performance, since he is unable to provide a strong, stable base of support for upper body action (Figure 1.16). It has been shown that without the initial step, the speed of a baseball pitch is reduced to approximately 80% of normal, and without hip and trunk rotation, the speed of the pitch is reduced to about 50% of normal (Miller 1980).

> If all of an adult's skeletal muscles could contract simultaneously in the same direction, they would exert a force in the region of 22 tons. However, the arrangement of the muscles is such that the amount of force generated in propulsive whole body movements is usually a small fraction of the theoretical maximum.

Loading on the musculoskeletal system

The open-chain arrangement of the bones of the skeleton and the arrangement of the muscles on the skeleton maximises the range of possible body postures. However, the body pays a price for this movement capability; many of the muscles have very low mechanical advantages (see Chapter 10) and, as such, usually have to exert much larger forces than the weights of the body segments they control. Furthermore, the sizes of the joint reaction forces are determined by the size of the muscle forces; the larger the muscle forces, the larger the joint reaction forces. For example, in walking, the peak hip, knee and ankle joint reaction forces in an adult are normally in the range of 5–6, 3–8, and 3–5 times body weight, respectively (Nigg 1985). The more dynamic the activity, the greater the muscle forces and, therefore, the greater the joint reaction forces. For example, in fast running (800 m pace), the peak knee and ankle joint reaction forces in an adult are likely to be in the region of 20 and 8 times body weight, respectively (Nigg 1985).

In any body position other than the relaxed recumbent position, the musculoskeletal system is likely to be subjected to considerable loading. In response to the forces exerted on them, the musculoskeletal components experience strain. Under normal circumstances the musculoskeletal components adapt their size, shape and structure to the time-averaged forces exerted on them, in order to more readily withstand the strain (Frost 1990, 2003, see Chapter 7). However, when the degree of strain experienced by a particular component exceeds its strength, that component will be injured. Consequently, there is an intimate relationship between the structure and function of the musculoskeletal system.

> The open-chain arrangement of the skeleton enables a person to adopt a wide range of body postures and perform a wide range of movements. However, the body pays a price for this ability; the muscles, bones and joints are subjected to very high forces in virtually all postures other than lying down.

REVIEW QUESTIONS

1. Differentiate between cellular differentiation and cellular organisation in multicellular organisms.

2. Describe the four basic tissues.

3. With regard to the musculoskeletal system function, describe the relationship between external and internal forces.

4. Briefly describe the three broad categories of movement brought about by the musculoskeletal system.

5. With reference to the recumbent posture and the standing posture, describe how direct and indirect transmission of the weight of body segments to the support surface is likely to affect the degree of activity in the muscles.

6. Describe the main advantage and disadvantage of the open-chain arrangement of the skeleton.

Chapter 2

The skeleton

The skeleton gives the body its distinctive shape and provides a supporting framework for all other parts of the body. The bones are linked at joints that are operated by the skeletal muscles. The joints are designed to transmit forces and allow joint movement, usually simultaneously. The magnitudes and types of forces transmitted at the joints and the types and ranges of movement that occur in the joints are reflected in the size and shape of the bones. The purpose of this chapter is to describe the bones of the skeleton and, in particular, the features of the bones associated with force transmission and joint movement.

OBJECTIVES

After reading this chapter you should be able to do the following:

1. Describe the composition and functions of the skeleton.
2. List the main bones of the skeleton.
3. Identify and describe the main features of the axial skeleton.
4. Distinguish vertebrae from different regions of the vertebral column.
5. Identify and describe the main features of the appendicular skeleton.

COMPOSITION AND FUNCTION OF THE SKELETON

The mature skeleton normally consists of 206 bones. However, variations in this basic number do occur; for example, some adults have 11 or 13 pairs of ribs, whereas most adults have 12 pairs. The skeleton performs three main mechanical functions:

1. It is a supporting framework for the rest of the body.
2. It is a system of levers on which the muscles can pull, in order to stabilise and move the body.
3. It protects certain organs. For example, the skull protects the brain, the vertebral column protects the spinal cord and the rib cage helps protect the heart and lungs.

TERMINOLOGY

For descriptive purposes the bones are usually divided into two main groups: the axial skeleton and the appendicular skeleton (axial = axis, appendicular = appendage). The adult axial skeleton consists of 80 bones that comprise the skull (29 bones), vertebral column (26 bones) and rib cage (25 bones). The adult appendicular skeleton consists of 126 bones that comprise the upper limbs (arms and hands; 2 × 32 bones) and the lower limbs (legs and feet; 2 × 31 bones) (Figure 2.1).

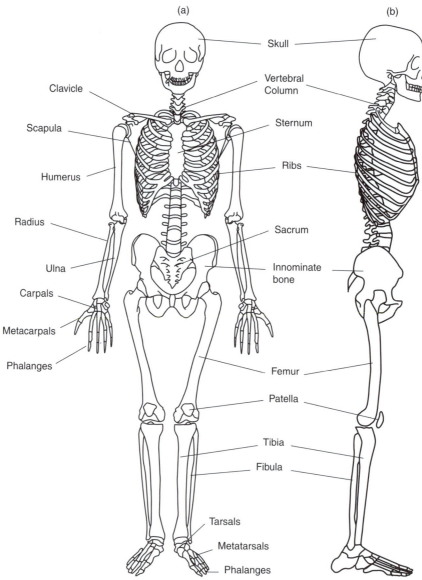

Figure 2.1 The skeleton. (a) Anterior aspect of the skeleton in the anatomical position. (b) Right lateral aspect of the skull, vertebral column and lower limb.

In anatomy, the term aspect refers to appearance from a particular viewpoint. For example, the anterior aspect of the skeleton refers to the anterior (frontal) view (Figure 2.1a). Similarly, lateral aspect (view from the side) (Figure 2.1b), posterior aspect (view from the back), superior aspect (view from above) and inferior aspect (view from below) describe other views.

The bones vary considerably in size and shape. The smallest mature bones are the auditory ossicles. There are three ossicles (malleus, incus, stapes), 5–9 mm in length, in each middle ear. The largest mature bones are the femurs (thigh bones), which may be longer than 45 cm (Standring 2008). There are four general shape categories: long bones, short bones, flat bones and irregular bones. Some bones fit into more than one category; for example, the auditory ossicles and the bones of the wrist are categorised as short and irregular. Whereas there are considerable differences in the size and shape of bones, there are a number of features that are common to many bones.

Common bone features

The common features of bones are illustrated in Figure 2.2.

Articular surface: Part of a bone that forms a joint with another bone;

Concave articular surface: A rounded depression;

Convex articular surface: A rounded elevation;

Facet: A small fairly flat articular surface; a convex facet on one bone usually articulates with a concave facet on an adjacent bone;

Condyle: A rounded projection of bone that provides the base for a rounded articular surface; a convex condyle on one bone usually articulates with a concave condyle on an adjacent bone;

Trochlea: A pulley-shaped condyle;

Fossa: An oval or circular depression or cavity that may also be an articular surface;

Notch: An oval depression that is often an articular surface; a notch may also take the form of a depressed region on the edge of a flat bone;

Groove or sulcus: An elongated depression (like a trench); one or more tendons usually occupy grooves;

Ridge or line: An elongated elevation; a ridge is usually the site of attachment of one or more aponeuroses;

Crest: A broad ridge;

Process: A projection of bone from the main body, usually providing attachment for tendons or ligaments;

Spine: A smooth process that may be slender or flat;

Epicondyle: A small process adjacent to a condyle;

Tubercle: A small roughened process;

Tuberosity: A large roughened process;

Trochanter: Another name for a tuberosity, used specifically in the description of the thigh bone (femur);

Foramen: A hole through a bone for the passage of blood vessels and nerves.

27

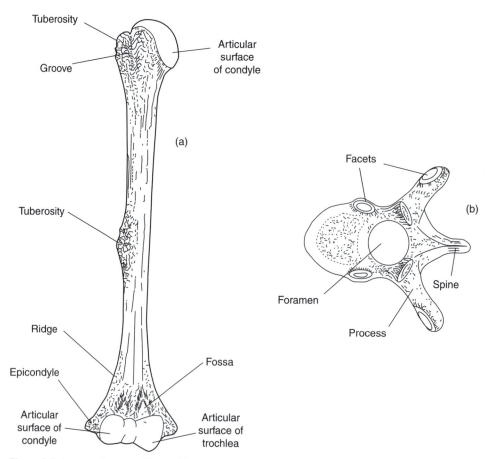

Figure 2.2 Common features of bones. (a) Anterior aspect of the humerus. (b) Superior aspect of a thoracic vertebra.

Those parts of the surface of a bone that do not have any of these specific features are normally fairly smooth. These smooth areas, usually fairly large, are where muscles attach directly to the bone. When a muscle is attached to a bone by a tendon or aponeurosis, the site of attachment to the bone is usually rough and, as such, is likely to be referred to as a tubercle, tuberosity, trochanter, ridge, line or crest.

Anatomical frame of reference and spatial terminology

To describe the spatial orientation of the particular features of a bone, or to describe the position of one bone (or body part) in relation to another, it is necessary to use standard terminology with reference to a standard body posture. In the standard posture, also called the anatomical position (Figure 2.1a), the body is upright with the arms by the sides and the palms of the hands facing forward. In relation to the anatomical position, the generally accepted frame of reference, which is referred to as the anatomical, relative or cardinal frame of reference, describes three principal planes (median, coronal, transverse) and three principal axes

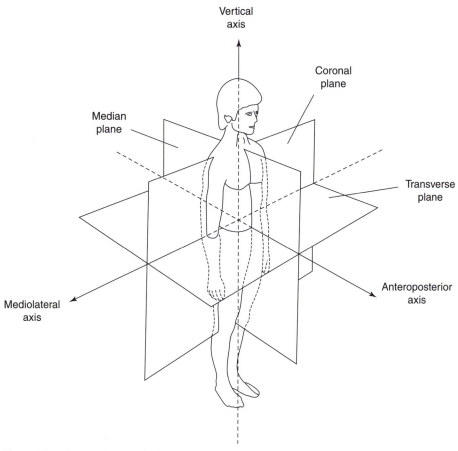

Figure 2.3 Reference planes and reference axes.

(anteroposterior, vertical, mediolateral). The three planes are perpendicular to each other and the three axes are perpendicular to each other (Figure 2.3).

The median plane is a vertical plane that divides the body down the middle into more or less symmetrical left and right portions. The median plane is also frequently referred to as the sagittal plane; the terms sagittal, paramedian and parasagittal (*para* = beside or beyond) are also sometimes used to refer to any plane parallel to the median plane. In this book, the term sagittal is used to refer to any plane parallel to the median plane. The mediolateral axis is perpendicular to the median plane. The terms lateral and medial are used to describe the position of structures with respect to the mediolateral axis. Lateral means farther away from the median plane and medial means closer to the median plane. For example, in the anatomical position, the lateral end of the clavicle (collarbone) articulates with the scapula (shoulder blade) and the medial end of the clavicle articulates with the sternum (breastbone). Similarly, in the anatomical position, the fingers of each hand are medial to the thumbs and the thumbs are lateral to the fingers.

The coronal plane (or frontal plane) is a vertical plane perpendicular to the median plane that divides the body into anterior and posterior portions. The anteroposterior axis is perpendicular to the coronal plane. The terms anterior (in front of) and posterior (behind) are used to describe the position of structures with respect to the anteroposterior axis. For example, the face forms the anterior part of the skull, the sternum is anterior to the vertebral column and the patella (kneecap) is anterior to the lower end of the femur. Similarly, the toes of each foot are anterior to the heels and the heels are posterior to the toes. The terms ventral and dorsal are synonymous with anterior and posterior, respectively.

The transverse plane is a horizontal plane, perpendicular to both the median and coronal planes, that divides the body into upper and lower portions. The vertical axis is perpendicular to the transverse plane. The terms superior (above) and inferior (below) are used to describe the position of structures with respect to the vertical axis. For example, as seen in Figure 2.1, the ribs are superior to the innominate bones (hip bones) and the patellae are inferior to the innominate bones. Similarly, the superior end of the right femur articulates with the right innominate bone to form the right hip joint, and the inferior end of the right femur articulates with the right patella and right tibia to form the right knee joint.

To describe the precise location and orientation of specific features of a particular bone, it is usually necessary to use combinations of the six spatial terms that are applicable to all bones: lateral, medial, anterior, posterior, superior and inferior. For example, a particular feature may be described as being at the anterior-inferior-lateral aspect of a bone; another feature may be described as being at the posterior-superior-medial aspect of the bone. However, there are some spatial terms that apply to some bones but not to others. For example, the terms proximal and distal are normally only used in reference to the long bones of the limbs. Superior features of these bones (with respect to the anatomical position) are referred to as proximal, whereas inferior features of the bone are referred to as distal. For example, in each arm the proximal end of the humerus articulates with its corresponding scapula to form the shoulder joint. The distal end of the humerus articulates with the proximal ends of the radius and ulna to form the elbow joint. The distal ends of the radius and ulna articulate with the carpals to form the wrist joint.

The names of the three reference planes are often used to describe sectional views of bones. For example, Figure 2.4 shows a coronal section through the right elbow joint. The

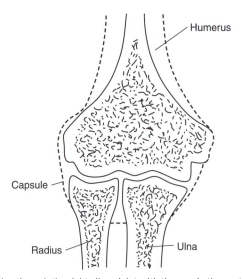

Figure 2.4 Coronal section through the right elbow joint with the arm in the anatomical position.

term longitudinal section normally refers to a vertical section, as in Figure 2.4. A longitudinal section may be in the median plane, a paramedian plane, a coronal plane or some other vertical plane. The term cross section is a general term that may refer to a section in one of the reference planes or to an oblique plane (relative to the reference planes).

THE AXIAL SKELETON

The axial skeleton consists of the skull, the vertebral column and the rib cage. The skull consists of 29 fairly flat or irregular bones that encase the brain, provide bases for the major sense organs and form the upper and lower jaws. The vertebral column consists of 26 irregular bones stacked on top of each other to form a curved structure in the median plane and a linear structure in the coronal plane (Figure 2.1). The vertebral column supports the weight of the head, arms and trunk, and provides protection for the spinal cord. The rib cage consists of 25 bones; the 12 pairs of ribs articulate (form joints) with the vertebral column posteriorly and are linked by cartilage (see Chapter 3) to the sternum anteriorly. The sternum is a fairly flat bone. Even though the ribs are considerably curved, they are fairly flat in cross section. The rib cage is a flexible structure (due largely to the cartilage links to the sternum) which facilitates ventilation of the lungs during breathing. The rib cage also provides protection for the heart and lungs.

The skull

The 29 bones of the skull comprise 8 cranial bones (cranium), 13 facial bones (face), 6 auditory ossicles, the mandible (lower jaw) and the hyoid bone (part of the larynx). The bones of the cranium and face form a single unit that makes up most of the skull (Figure 2.5). The cranium encloses the brain and is made up of eight relatively flat irregular bones.

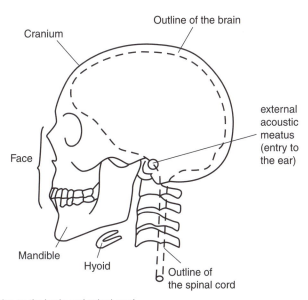

Figure 2.5 The skull in relation to the brain and spinal cord.

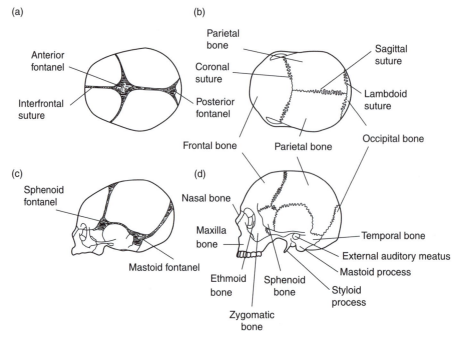

Figure 2.6 Superior and lateral aspects of the cranium and face. (a,c) Infant. (b,d) Adult.

The frontal bone forms the anterior and anterior-superior part of the cranium including the forehead (Figure 2.6). The two parietal bones form a large part of the superior and lateral aspects of the cranium. The two temporal bones form a large part of the superior and lateral aspects of the base and sides of the cranium. The sphenoid bone, together with the ethmoid bone and the inferior aspects of the frontal bone, forms the anterior half of the base of the cranium. The occipital bone forms the posterior-inferior aspect of the cranium and the major portion of the posterior half of the base of the cranium. The occipital bone has a large hole, the foramen magnum, situated anteriorly. The foramen is occupied by the start of the spinal cord, which is continuous with the brain (Figure 2.5).

The 13 bones of the face form the middle third of the anterior aspect of the skull (Figure 2.5). The facial bones form the upper jaw, the anterior part of the nasal cavity and the inferior two-thirds of the eye sockets (orbits). The upper jaw, which provides sockets for the upper teeth, is formed almost entirely by the two maxilla bones that join anteriorly in the median plane.

The mandible, or lower jaw, consists of two L-shaped plates of bone that join anteriorly in the median plane. The upright part of each half of the mandible is called the ramus (branch), and the horizontal part, called the body, provides sockets for the lower teeth. At the posterior-superior aspect of each ramus, there is a convex condyle that articulates with the mandibular fossa on its corresponding temporal bone, to form the corresponding temporomandibular joint (Figure 2.5). These joints enable the mandible to swing up and down, as in closing and opening the mouth, and to move from side to side. Chewing food involves a combination of these two types of movement.

On each side of the skull, the auditory ossicles are located in a chamber, the middle ear, within the corresponding temporal bone. The three ossicles link the lateral and medial walls of the middle ear and transmit sound waves from the outer ear to the sound receptors in the inner ear.

The hyoid bone is not part of the skull, but it is convenient to describe it in relation to the skull. The hyoid is a U-shaped bone suspended in front of the neck (in front of the fourth cervical vertebra) by ligaments from the styloid processes of the temporal bones (see Figure 2.6). The hyoid forms part of the larynx (voice box) and provides attachment for some of the muscles that move the mouth and the tongue.

Sutures and fontanels

In the adult skull, the edges of the bones are serrated so that the bones interlock closely with each other to form immovable joints. The serrated line of the joints is similar in appearance to a line of stitches and, for this reason, each joint is called a suture (see Figure 2.6). In an infant, the joints between the bones of the cranium are also called sutures, even though the bones are joined by sheets of fibrous tissue and, consequently, do not interlock with each other (see Figure 2.6). Fibrous tissue, described in detail in Chapter 4, is flexible, strong and, in an infant, moderately elastic.

At each of the angles (or corners) of the parietal bones, the fibrous tissue is in the form of a small sheet, called a fontanel (Standring 2008). Since each parietal bone has four angles and the parietal bones join each other superiorly in the median plane, there are six fontanels. The anterior fontanel, which normally closes within the first 18 months after birth, is at the junction of the parietal and frontal bones. At birth, the frontal bone is in two halves, joined by the interfrontal or metopic suture; these halves normally fuse together during the first two years after birth. The posterior fontanel is at the junction of the parietal and occipital bones and normally closes during the first two months after birth. There are two sphenoid fontanels, one on each side of the skull at the junction of the parietal, frontal, sphenoid and temporal bones. The sphenoid fontanels normally close during the first three months after birth. There are also two mastoid fontanels, one on each side of the skull at the junction of the parietal, occipital and temporal bones. The mastoid fontanels normally close during the first two years after birth.

The skull consists of 29 fairly flat or irregular bones. The bones of the cranium (8 bones), the face (13 bones) and the auditory ossicles (3 in each middle ear) form a single unit that makes up most of the skull. The other two bones are the mandible and the hyoid.

The vertebral column

Prior to maturity, the vertebral column consists of 33 or 34 irregular bones called vertebrae. The vertebrae are divided into five fairly distinct groups: cervical, thoracic, lumbar, sacral and coccygeal (Figure 2.7). The neck consists of seven cervical vertebrae. The thoracic or chest region consists of 12 thoracic vertebrae that provide articulation for the 12 pairs of ribs. The lower back consists of five lumbar vertebrae. The five sacral vertebrae form the posterior part of the pelvis; at maturity the sacral vertebrae fuse together to form the sacrum. The four or

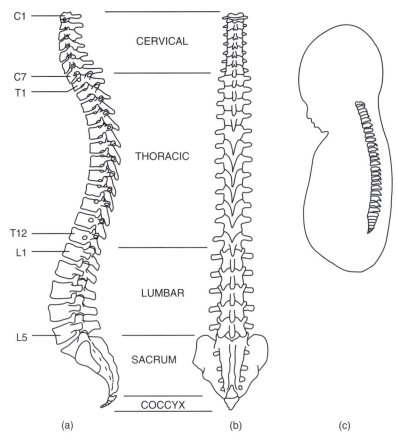

C1

CERVICAL

C7
T1

THORACIC

T12
L1

LUMBAR

L5

SACRUM

COCCYX

(a) (b) (c)

Figure 2.7 The vertebral column. (a) Left lateral aspect in an adult. (b) Posterior aspect in an adult. (c) Left lateral aspect in an infant.

five coccygeal vertebrae are small and represent a vestigial tail. The coccygeal vertebrae normally fuse together at maturity to form the coccyx, or tail bone, which is approximately 3 cm long and is attached to the sacrum by ligaments.

When viewed from the side, the whole of the vertebral column of a newborn infant is concave anteriorly (Figure 2.7c). Between 3 and 6 months of age, the child learns to crawl with the head upright, and, as a result, the shape of the cervical region changes from concave anteriorly to convex anteriorly. Similarly, as the child learns to stand and walk, between 10 and 18 months, the shape of the lumbar region also changes from concave anteriorly to convex anteriorly. The cervical and lumbar curves are referred to as secondary curves, as they develop as the child adopts an upright posture. The thoracic and sacrococcygeal curves are called primary curves, as they are concave anteriorly throughout life (Figure 2.7).

Structure of a vertebra

At birth, each vertebra, with the exception of the first two cervical vertebrae, consists of three bony elements united by cartilage (Standring 2008) (Figure 2.8a). The anterior element, the

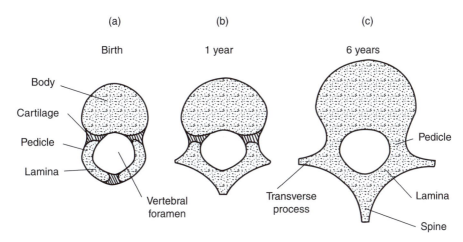

Figure 2.8 Early stages in the development of a vertebra (superior aspect).

centrum or body, is simply a block of bone with slightly concave (waisted) sides and fairly flat kidney-shaped superior and inferior surfaces. The bodies of the vertebrae are mainly responsible for transmitting loads, especially the weight of the head, arms and trunk. The posterior elements are curved struts that form the two halves of an arch called the vertebral or neural arch. Each half of the arch consists of an anterior portion called the pedicle and a posterior portion called the lamina. The two laminae normally fuse together posteriorly during the first year (Figure 2.8b). The pedicles normally fuse with the lateral-superior-posterior aspects of the body of the vertebra between the third and sixth years (Figure 2.8c). The hole formed by the arch and the posterior aspect of the body is called the vertebral foramen. In the vertebral column the spinal cord passes through all of the vertebral foramina.

After fusion of the laminae, seven processes arise from the arch. The spine of the vertebra extends backward from the point of fusion of the laminae. On each side of the arch, three processes arise from the junction of the pedicle and lamina. A transverse process extends laterally, a superior articular process extends upward and an inferior articular process extends downward (Figure 2.9). The spine and transverse processes are levers that provide areas of attachment for muscles, tendons and ligaments. With respect to each pair of adjacent vertebrae, the superior articular processes of the lower vertebra articulate by means of facets with the inferior articular processes of the upper vertebra (Figure 2.9b and Figure 2.10). These joints are called facet joints or apophysial joints. In most upright postures, the facet joints transmit some load. In general, the load transmitted by these joints decreases with flexion of the trunk (bending forward) and increases with extension of the trunk (bending backward).

The bodies of each pair of adjacent vertebrae, except the first two cervical vertebrae, are joined by a tough rubbery kidney-shaped disc of fibrocartilage, called an intervertebral disc, to form an intervertebral joint (Figure 2.10). Consequently, whereas the first two cervical vertebrae are joined by two facet joints, the other vertebrae are joined by one intervertebral joint and two facet joints. The type and range of movement between adjacent vertebrae is largely determined by the thickness of the intervertebral disc (which deforms in response to loading, rather like a pencil eraser) and the orientation of the facet joints (whose articular surfaces slide on each other). The different types of joints are described in Chapter 4.

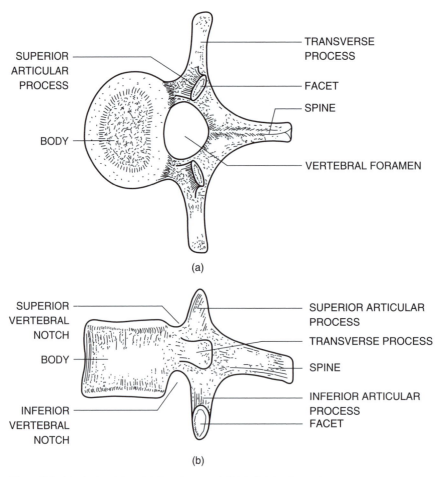

Figure 2.9 A typical vertebra. (a) Superior aspect. (b) Left lateral aspect.

On each side of the vertebral arch is a depression in the superior aspect of the pedicle, called the superior vertebral notch (Figure 2.9b). As the pedicle joins the posterior-superior aspect of the body, there is a much larger inferior vertebral notch beneath the pedicle. With respect to each pair of adjacent vertebrae, the inferior notch of the upper vertebra and the superior vertebral notch of the lower vertebra form a hole called the intervertebral foramen (Figure 2.10a). A spinal (peripheral) nerve occupies the intervertebral foramen (Figure 2.10b).

Distinguishing features of vertebrae

Whereas the vertebrae all have the same basic structure, there are differences between the different regions of the vertebral column in the size and shape of the bodies and in the size, shape and orientation of the processes and facet joints. The bodies and processes of the vertebrae gradually increase in size from the second cervical vertebra down to the sacrum; this increase reflects the gradual increase in weight that the vertebrae have to support (see Figure 2.7a).

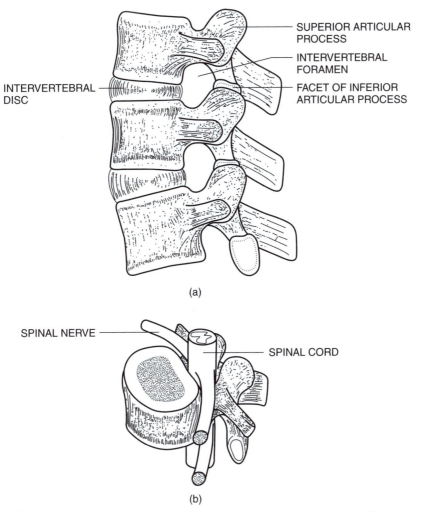

INTERVERTEBRAL
DISC

SUPERIOR ARTICULAR
PROCESS

INTERVERTEBRAL
FORAMEN

FACET OF INFERIOR
ARTICULAR PROCESS

(a)

SPINAL NERVE

SPINAL CORD

(b)

Figure 2.10 (a) Left lateral aspect of three articulated lumbar vertebrae. (b) Relationship of the spinal cord and spinal nerves to a lumbar vertebra.

The changes in the size, shape and orientation of the processes and facet joints are fairly gradual within each of the cervical, thoracic and lumbar regions but tend to be more marked at the junctions between the regions (Figure 2.7a). In the mature vertebral column the cervical, thoracic and lumbar vertebrae have characteristics that distinguish them from each other.

Cervical: All cervical vertebrae (C1 to C7) have a hole called a transverse foramen in each of their transverse processes (Figure 2.11a). Only cervical vertebrae have this characteristic. The facets of the superior and inferior articular processes of the cervical vertebrae articulate in oblique planes that slope downward laterally and posteriorly. The orientation of the facet joints, the short transverse processes, the relatively thick intervertebral discs and the relatively short spines of C3 to C6 all combine to give a fairly large range of movement in the cervical region as a whole compared with other regions of the column.

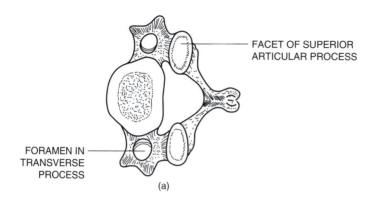

FACET OF SUPERIOR
ARTICULAR PROCESS

FORAMEN IN
TRANSVERSE
PROCESS

(a)

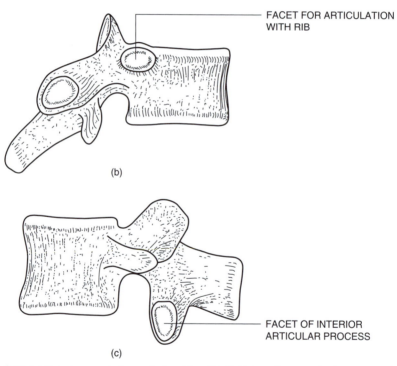

FACET FOR ARTICULATION
WITH RIB

(b)

FACET OF INTERIOR
ARTICULAR PROCESS

(c)

Figure 2.11 (a) Superior aspect of a cervical vertebra. (b) Right lateral aspect of a thoracic vertebra. (c) Left lateral aspect of a lumbar vertebra.

Thoracic: Thoracic vertebrae (T1 to T12) can be identified by the presence of facets on the lateral aspects of the bodies for articulation with the heads (posterior ends) of the ribs (Figure 2.11b). The spines of the thoracic vertebrae are fairly long and tend to overlap each other closely, especially in the middle of the region (see Figure 2.7a). The transverse processes are also fairly long and gradually decrease in length from T1 to T12. The superior and inferior articular facets articulate in a plane that slopes sharply downward posteriorly. The overlapping spines, relatively thin intervertebral discs and splinting effect of the ribs result in a smaller overall range of movement in the thoracic region than in the cervical region.

Lumbar: The lumbar vertebrae (L1 to L5) have fairly long transverse processes and large, flat, rectangular spines (Figure 2.11c). The main distinguishing feature of the lumbar verte-brae is the orientation of the facets on the superior and inferior articular processes. The facets on the superior articular processes face medially and posteriorly, and the facets on the inferior articular processes face laterally and anteriorly. The orientation of the facet joints severely limits rotation of the lumbar vertebrae about a vertical axis. However, the relatively thick intervertebral discs in the lumbar region ensure a much greater range of movement in other directions.

Sacrum: The sacral vertebrae (S1 to S5) become progressively smaller from S1 through to S5. The sacrum is formed by the fusion or partial fusion of the sacral vertebrae. When viewed from the front (or the back) the sacrum is more or less triangular with the apex pointing downward (Figure 2.12a). The anterior edge of the upper surface of the first sacral vertebra projects forward and is called the sacral promontory. The anterior aspect of the sacrum is concave, largely as a result of the orientation of S3, S4 and S5 (Figure 2.12b). In the anatomi-cal position, the large upper portion of the sacrum (S1 and S2) is tilted forward; this tilt tends to accentuate the lumbar curve (see Figure 2.7a).

On each superior-lateral aspect of the sacrum is a fairly large C- or L-shaped articular surface called the auricular surface (auricular = ear-shaped) (Figure 2.12b). The auricular sur-faces are formed by the lateral expansions of the fused transverse processes of S1, S2 and S3. The auricular surfaces of the sacrum articulate with the hip bones (innominate bones) to form the sacroiliac joints (Figure 2.1). The sacrum and the left and right hip bones form a complete bony ring called the pelvis or pelvic girdle. Consequently, the sacrum is an important part of the vertebral column and the pelvis.

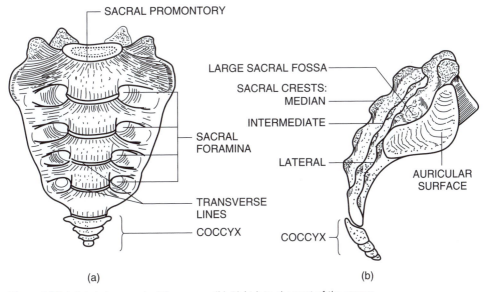

Figure 2.12 (a) Anterior aspect of the sacrum. (b) Right lateral aspect of the sacrum.

> Whereas the vertebrae all have the same basic structure, there are differences between the five regions of the vertebral column in the size and shape of the bodies, and in the size, shape and orientation of the processes and facet joints.

The rib cage

The rib cage, which consists of 12 pairs of ribs and the sternum, provides protection for the heart and lungs and facilitates breathing. The sternum is a fairly flat bone and the ribs are also fairly flat in cross section. As the ribs form the major part of the rib cage, they have a distinct curved shape. The heads (posterior ends) of the ribs articulate with the thoracic vertebrae. The anterior ends of the upper ten pairs of ribs are attached to the sternum by pieces of cartilage called costal cartilages (*costa* = rib). The upper seven pairs of ribs are attached to the sternum by separate costal cartilages and are sometimes referred to as true ribs. The costal cartilages of the eighth, ninth and tenth pairs of ribs fuse with each other before fusing with the costal cartilages of the seventh ribs (see Figure 2.13). Consequently, whereas the upper seven pairs of ribs have direct cartilaginous attachments to the sternum, the eighth, ninth and tenth pairs of ribs have an indirect cartilaginous attachment to the sternum. The lower two pairs of ribs do not attach onto the sternum; the anterior ends of these ribs are free, and these ribs are referred to as floating ribs. Because none of the lower five pairs of ribs has a direct

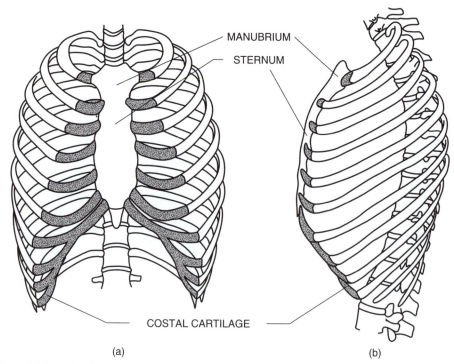

MANUBRIUM

STERNUM

COSTAL CARTILAGE

(a)   (b)

Figure 2.13 (a) Anterior aspect of the rib cage. (b) Left lateral aspect of the rib cage.

cartilaginous or other attachment to the sternum, these ribs are sometimes referred to as false ribs.

Movement of the ribs

The intercostal spaces (spaces between the ribs) are largely occupied by muscles (intercostal muscles) which, in association with other muscles of the thorax, move the ribs during breathing. During inspiration (breathing in), the ribs and sternum swing upward and outward; this decreases the pressure inside the thorax and simultaneously drives air into the lungs. During expiration (breathing out), the ribs and sternum are pulled back down by the elasticity of the surrounding soft tissues (costal cartilages, ligaments and muscles that are stretched during inspiration). The downward movement of the ribs and sternum increases the pressure inside the thorax and simultaneously drives air out of the lungs.

> The rib cage consists of the sternum and 12 pairs of ribs. It is a fairly flexible structure that provides protection for the heart and lungs and, in association with intercostal muscles, facilitates breathing.

THE APPENDICULAR SKELETON

The appendicular skeleton (126 bones) consists of the bones of the upper and lower limbs. In an adult, each upper limb consists of 32 bones and each lower limb consists of 31 bones.

The upper limb

There are five regions in each upper limb: the shoulder (scapula and clavicle), upper arm (humerus), lower arm (radius and ulna), wrist (8 carpals) and hand (5 metacarpals and 14 phalanges).

Shoulder

The shoulder region of each upper limb consists of a scapula (shoulder blade) and a clavicle (collarbone) (Figure 2.14). Together with the sternum, the scapulae and clavicles of both upper limbs form an incomplete ring of bone called the shoulder girdle (Figure 2.1). The arms are suspended from the shoulder girdle. The medial end of each clavicle articulates with the sternum to form a sternoclavicular joint, and the lateral end of each clavicle articulates with the acromion process of the corresponding scapula to form an acromioclavicular joint (Figure 2.1). The scapulae are not joined to the axial skeleton, but are held in position at the lateral-superior-posterior aspects of the rib cage by muscles. Consequently, each scapula has a considerable range of movement. Most movements of the shoulder region involve movements at the sternoclavicular and acromioclavicular joints.

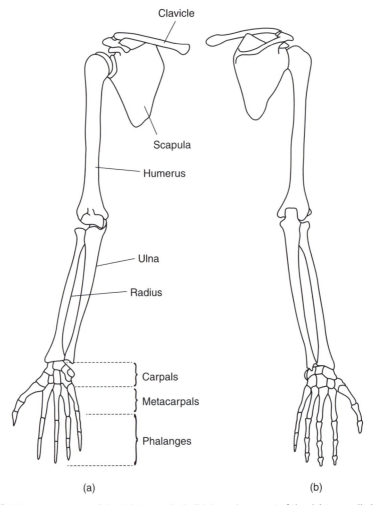

Clavicle

Scapula

Humerus

Ulna

Radius

Carpals

Metacarpals

Phalanges

(a)   (b)

Figure 2.14 (a) Anterior aspect of the right upper limb. (b) Posterior aspect of the right upper limb.

Upper arm

The humerus, the only bone in the upper arm, is a typical long bone consisting of a relatively long shaft between two fairly bulbous ends (Figure 2.15). The proximal end of the humerus is dominated by the head, which is an almost perfect hemisphere that articulates with the glenoid fossa of the corresponding scapula to form the shoulder joint. The distal end of the humerus has a cylindrical articular surface consisting of two condyles, the capitulum and trochlea, fused together side by side.

Lower arm

The lower arm consists of two long bones, the radius and the ulna. In the anatomical position, the radius is lateral to the ulna (Figure 2.16). The proximal end of the ulna is dominated

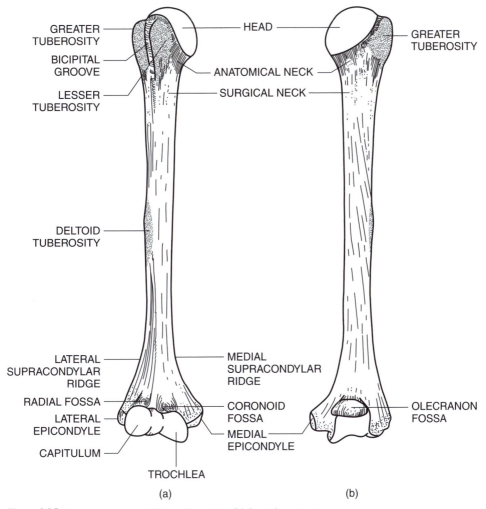

GREATER TUBEROSITY

BICIPITAL GROOVE

LESSER TUBEROSITY

DELTOID TUBEROSITY

LATERAL SUPRACONDYLAR RIDGE

RADIAL FOSSA

LATERAL EPICONDYLE

CAPITULUM

HEAD

ANATOMICAL NECK

SURGICAL NECK

MEDIAL SUPRACONDYLAR RIDGE

CORONOID FOSSA

MEDIAL EPICONDYLE

TROCHLEA

GREATER TUBEROSITY

OLECRANON FOSSA

(a)

(b)

Figure 2.15 The right humerus. (a) Anterior aspect. (b) Posterior aspect.

by a large pulley-shaped concave articular surface, the trochlea notch, which articulates with the trochlea of the humerus to form part of the elbow joint. The proximal end of the radius consists of a drum-shaped head separated from the main part of the shaft by a short cylindrical neck (Figure 2.16). The circular side of the head and the superior surface of the head form a continuous articular surface. The side articulates with the radial notch on the ulna, and the superior surface articulates with the capitulum on the humerus. The elbow joint consists of the joints between the trochlea and trochlea notch, and the capitulum and head of the radius.

The distal end of the ulna has a small drum-shaped head with a small projection on its posteromedial aspect called the styloid process of the ulna. The lateral part of the distal end of the radius forms a small projection called the styloid process of the radius. The inferior aspect of the distal end is dominated by a fairly large, more or less quadrangular, concave articular surface, which forms part of the wrist joint. Adjacent to and continuous with the medial edge

43

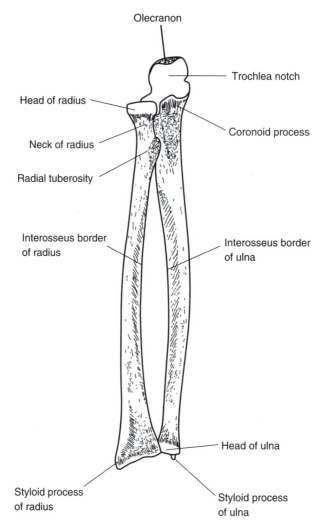

Olecranon

Trochlea notch

Head of radius

Coronoid process

Neck of radius

Radial tuberosity

Interosseus border
of radius

Interosseus border
of ulna

Head of ulna

Styloid process
of radius

Styloid process
of ulna

Figure 2.16 Anterior aspect of the right ulna and radius.

of this surface is the ulnar notch, a small articular surface. This notch articulates with the side of the head of the ulna.

Wrist and hand

The wrist consists of eight small irregular bones, called carpals, which articulate with each other to form the carpus (Figure 2.17). The carpals are arranged into a proximal and a distal row. The proximal row articulates with the distal ends of the radius and ulna to form the wrist joint. The series of joints between the proximal and distal rows of carpals is called the mid-carpal joint.

Each hand consists of 5 metacarpals and 14 phalanges (the bones of the digits) (Figure 2.17). In life, the metacarpals are joined together by soft tissues and form the palm of the hand on the

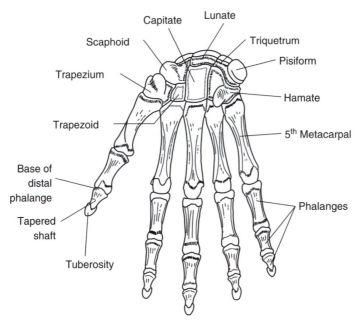

Figure 2.17 Anterior aspect of the right wrist and hand.

anterior aspect. The metacarpals are miniature long bones; each metacarpal consists of a base (the proximal end), a shaft and a head (the distal end). The bases of the metacarpals articulate with the distal row of carpals to form the carpometacarpal joints. The combined ranges of movement in the wrist, midcarpal and carpometacarpal joints facilitate a large range of movement for the hand as a whole. The heads of the metacarpals articulate with the bases of the proximal phalanges to form the metacarpophalangeal joints that link the thumb and fingers to the palm of the hand. Each of the four fingers consists of three phalanges (proximal, middle and distal), whereas the thumb has only two (proximal and distal).

> Each upper limb consists of 32 bones: shoulder (scapula and clavicle), upper arm (humerus), lower arm (radius and ulna), wrist (8 carpals) and hand (5 metacarpals and 14 phalanges)

The lower limb

There are five regions in each lower limb: the hip (innominate bone), pelvis (sacrum and right and left innominate bones), upper leg (femur and patella), lower leg (tibia and fibula) and foot (7 tarsals, 5 metatarsals and 14 phalanges).

Hip

Together with the sacrum, the right and left innominate bones form a complete ring of bone called the pelvis or pelvic girdle (Figure 2.18). Consequently, the innominate bones attach the lower limbs to the axial skeleton. Each innominate bone develops from three bones called the ilium, ischium and pubis, which fuse together at maturity. The region where the three bones fuse together is dominated by a large hemispherical concavity called the acetabulum, which articulates with the head of the femur to form the hip joint (Figure 2.19a).

The ilium comprises the upper two-fifths of the acetabulum and the large more or less flat portion of the innominate bone above the acetabulum (Figure 2.19a). The large flat upper part of the ilium is called the wing of the ilium. The superior border of the wing of the ilium forms a broad crest called the iliac crest that can be felt beneath the skin just above the hip joint. The iliac crest provides attachment for muscles comprising the wall of the abdomen. On the posterior-medial aspect of the wing of the ilium there is a large C-shaped or L-shaped auricular surface that articulates with the auricular surface on the corresponding side of the sacrum to form the corresponding sacroiliac joint (Figures 2.18 and 2.19). The large lateral and medial surfaces of the wing of the ilium provide attachment for muscles

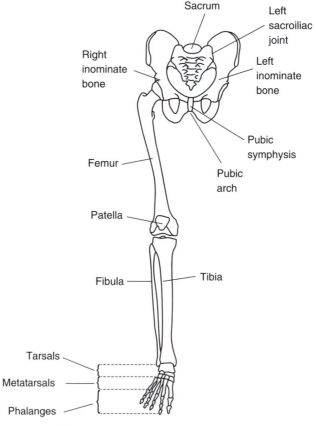

Figure 2.18 Anterior aspect of the pelvis and right lower limb.

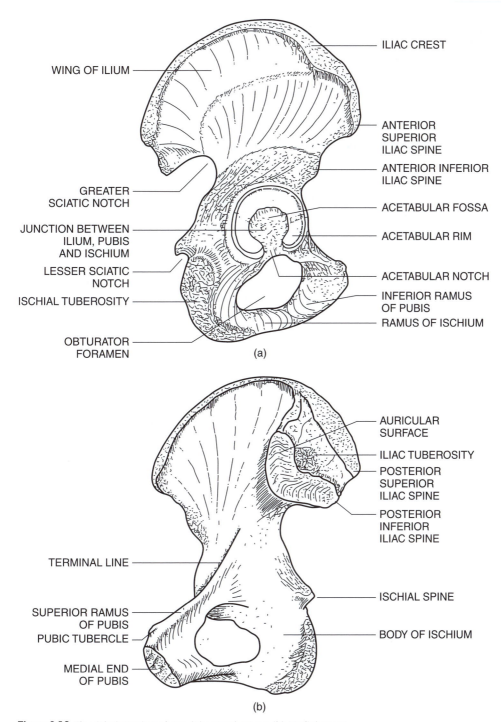

Figure 2.19 The right innominate bone. (a) Lateral aspect. (b) Medial aspect.

that move the hip joint. The medial surface of the wing also supports the contents of the abdomen.

The ischium, which forms the posterior-inferior portion of the innominate bone, consists of a body and a ramus. The body is a more or less vertical pillar that transmits the weight of the trunk, head and arms to the support surface when the individual is sitting. The superior part of the body forms the posterior-inferior two-fifths of the acetabulum. Below the acetabulum, the body of the ischium is characterised by a large ischial tuberosity on its posterior-inferior lateral aspect (Figure 2.19a). The ramus of the ischium is a broad, flat process that arises from the base of the body and projects medially, forward and upward to articulate with the pubis.

The pubis forms the anterior-inferior portion of the innominate bone. It consists of a body, a superior ramus and an inferior ramus. The body forms the anterior-inferior one-fifth of the acetabulum. The superior ramus extends medially and also slightly forward and downward from the body to join the medial end of the inferior ramus. The junction between the two rami of the pubis forms a fairly broad, flat region. The medial surface of this junction, the medial surface of the pubis, is elliptical in shape and lies in the median plane. The long axis of the ellipse is inclined at an angle of approximately 45° to the coronal plane. The medial surfaces of the right and left pubic bones articulate in the median plane to form the pubic symphysis joint (Figure 2.18). The inferior ramus of the pubis projects downward and backward laterally to join the anterior end of the ischium ramus (Figure 2.19). The inverted V-shaped notch formed by the inferior borders of the right and left inferior pubic rami is called the pubic arch (see Figure 2.18).

The pubis and ischium are both essentially V-shaped and joined at their free ends. Consequently, when fused together, the two bones create a large foramen. This is called the obturator foramen because of its close proximity to the obturator nerve.

The innominate bones link the lower limbs to the axial skeleton. Each innominate bone develops from three bones called the ilium, ischium and pubis, which fuse together at maturity.

Pelvis

Pelvis is a Latin word meaning basin (owing to the large wings of the ilia, which give the impression of an incomplete bowl when the pelvis is viewed from an anterior-superior aspect) (Figure 2.20). The upper part of the pelvis (the wings of the ilia and the upper two-thirds of the sacrum) provides a support base for the upper body. The lower part of the pelvis (ischium and pubis) transmits the weight of the upper body to the legs when standing and to the chair seat when sitting. The margin between the upper and lower parts of pelvis is delineated by a continuous ridge called the inlet or pelvic brim (Figure 2.20b,d).

Although the pelvis is similar in structure in men and women, there are four main differences in the shape of the pelvis between the sexes, due, it is assumed, to the woman's childbearing role (Figure 2.20):

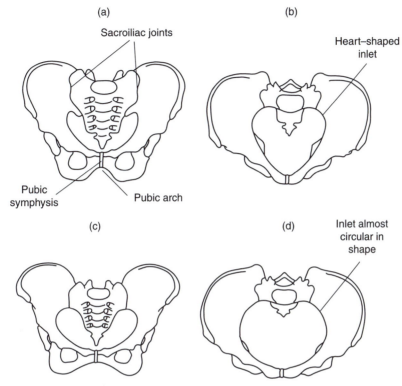

Figure 2.20 (a) Anterior aspect of the male pelvis. (b) Anterior-superior aspect of the male pelvis. (c) Anterior aspect of the female pelvis. (b) Anterior-superior aspect of the female pelvis.

1. The inlet of the male pelvis is heart-shaped, whereas that of the female pelvis is more circular.
2. The pubic bones are more in line with each other in the female pelvis than in the male. Consequently, the angle of the pubic arch is obtuse in the female pelvis and acute in the male.
3. The relative distance between the acetabulums is greater in the female pelvis than in the male. This results in a relatively greater girth around the hips in the female than in the male.
4. The anterior concavity of the sacrum is greater in the male pelvis than in the female, such that the lower half of the sacrum and the coccyx bend farther forward. This curvature reduces the front-to-back dimension of the lower pelvis. In the female pelvis, the sacrum is relatively straight, which tends to maintain a fairly constant front-to-back dimension in the lower pelvis.

Upper leg

The upper leg or thigh contains a long bone called the femur and a relatively small bone called the patella (kneecap), which articulates with the distal end of the femur. The femur is the longest and strongest bone in the skeleton. The proximal end of the femur consists of a nearly

49 ▪

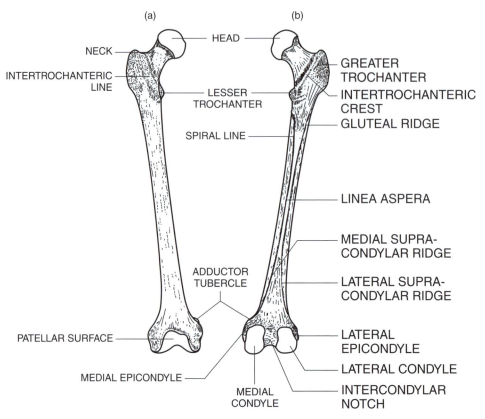

Figure 2.21 The right femur. (a) Anterior aspect. (b) Posterior aspect.

spherical head, which articulates with the acetabulum to form the hip joint (Figures 2.18 and 2.21). The head is joined obliquely to the shaft by a thick neck that runs laterally downward and backward from the head to the anterior-medial region of the proximal end of the shaft. A large process called the greater trochanter dominates the superior posterior-lateral region of the proximal end of the shaft. At the base of the neck on the posterior-medial aspect of the shaft is another fairly large process, called the lesser trochanter.

Like the humerus, the upper two-thirds of the shaft of the femur is cylindrical and the lower one-third gradually becomes broader (in the coronal plane) toward the distal end. In a paramedian plane, the anterior surface of the femur is slightly convex and the posterior surface is slightly concave (Figure 2.1b). The distal end of the femur consists of two large convex condyles, the lateral condyle and the medial condyle, fused together side by side anteriorly. The condyles are separated posteriorly by a large notch called the intercondylar notch (or intercondylar fossa). The upper part of the common anterior portion of the articular surface is called the patellar surface. The patellar surface is pulley-shaped (depressed in the middle in the parasagittal plane) and articulates with the posterior surface of the patella to form the patellofemoral joint. During extension and flexion of the knee joint, the patella slides up and down on the patellar surface and condyles of the femur.

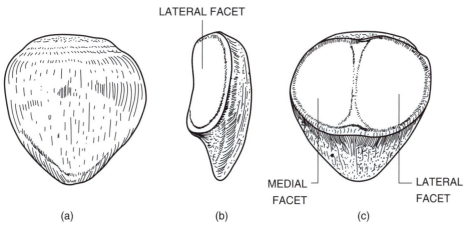

LATERAL FACET

MEDIAL FACET   LATERAL FACET

(a)   (b)   (c)

Figure 2.22 The right patella. (a) Anterior aspect. (b) Right lateral aspect. (c) Posterior aspect. Apart from its facets, the patella is embedded in the quadriceps tendon.

The patella is a sesamoid bone (so-called because it resembles a sesame seed), i.e. a bone that is partially embedded in a tendon (Figure 2.22). A sesamoid bone tends to increase the mechanical efficiency of the associated musculotendinous unit and prevent the tendon from rubbing on an adjacent bone. The whole of the anterior surface and the inferior quarter of the posterior surface of the patella are embedded in the quadriceps tendon. The upper three-quarters of the posterior surface articulates with the patellar surface of the femur when the knee joint is extended and with the condyles of the femur when the knee joint is flexed (Figure 2.23). The patella increases the mechanical efficiency of the quadriceps muscle group and prevents the quadriceps tendon from rubbing against the patellar surface of the femur.

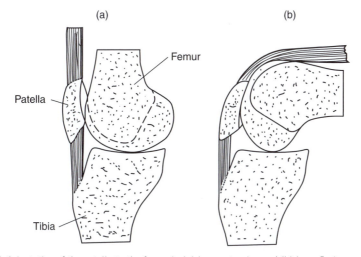

(a)   (b)

Femur

Patella

Tibia

Figure 2.23 Orientation of the patella to the femur in (a) knee extension and (b) knee flexion.

Lower leg

The lower leg or shank contains two long bones, the tibia and the fibula, aligned with their shafts more or less parallel to each other (Figure 2.24). The tibia is the larger of the two bones and is situated medial to the fibula. The proximal end of the tibia consists of two large condyles, the lateral and medial condyles, which are fused together side by side (Figure 2.24c).

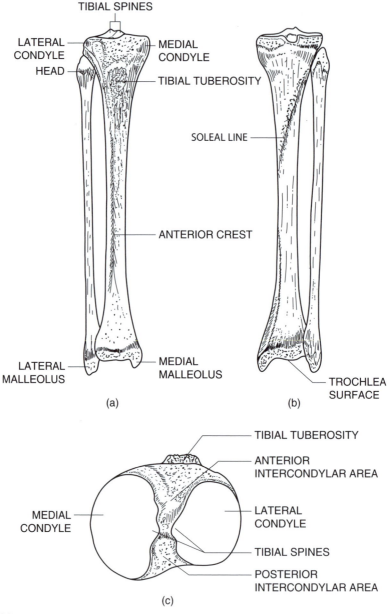

Figure 2.24 The right tibia and fibula. (a) Anterior aspect. (b) Posterior aspect. (c) Superior aspect of the tibia.

The tibial condyles articulate with the femoral condyles to form the tibiofemoral joint (knee joint). The articular surfaces of the tibial condyles are oval in outline and almost flat. The lateral surface is usually slightly convex and slightly smaller than the medial surface. The medial surface may be slightly convex. The surfaces occupy the same plane, more or less horizontally in the anatomical position. This orientation of the condylar surface gives rise to the term tibial table, sometimes used to describe the proximal end of the tibia.

The middle two-thirds of the shaft of the tibia is teardrop-shaped in cross section; the posterior aspect is rounded, whereas the anterior aspect consists of two fairly flat areas, anterior-lateral and anterior-medial, which converge anteriorly to form a distinct ridge, called the anterior crest. The anterior crest can easily be felt beneath the skin as a ridge running down the bone. The anterior-medial surface of the tibia, covered only by skin, is usually referred to as the shin. Above and below the anterior crest, the shaft broadens out toward the proximal and distal ends of the bone. Above the upper end of the anterior crest, on the anterior aspect of the shaft, is a fairly large process, called the tibial tuberosity.

On the medial side of the distal end of the tibia there is a downward projection called the medial malleolus. The lateral aspect of the medial malleolus articulates with the medial aspect of the talus to form the medial part of the ankle joint (Figure 2.24). The remainder of the distal end of the tibia is dominated by a large biconcave condylar surface, called the trochlea surface of the tibia. The trochlea surface articulates with the superior aspect of the talus to form the main part of the ankle joint. The trochlea surface of the tibia and the articular surface of the medial malleolus are continuous with each other. The tibia is almost completely responsible for transmitting loads from the upper leg to the foot, and vice versa.

The fibula is a thin, relatively weak bone that is only marginally involved in load transmission between the upper leg and foot. The main functions of the fibula are to provide lateral support to the ankle joint and to provide additional area for the attachment of muscles that move the ankle and foot. The proximal end of the fibula is called the head. The medial two-thirds of the superior aspect of the head articulates with the posterior-inferior lateral aspect of the lateral tibial condyle to form the proximal tibiofibular joint. The shaft of the fibula is characterised by four longitudinal ridges, which give rise to four faces of varying width and length along the shaft. The distal end of the fibula is called the lateral malleolus. The medial aspect of the lateral malleolus articulates with the lateral aspect of the talus to form the lateral part of the ankle joint. The medial part of the shaft of the fibula immediately above the articular surface of the lateral malleolus articulates with the lateral part of the distal end of the tibia to form the distal tibiofibular joint.

Foot

The foot consists of 7 tarsals, 5 metatarsals and 14 phalanges, often grouped into rear foot (talus and calcaneus), mid-foot (navicular, cuboid and cuneiforms) and forefoot (metatarsals and phalanges) (Briggs 2005) (Figure 2.25). When articulated, the tarsals form the tarsus. The tarsus corresponds to the carpus in the upper limb, but the tarsals are all much larger than the carpals. Whereas the carpus is not usually considered to be part of the hand, the tarsus forms the posterior half of the foot. The foot articulates with the lower leg at the ankle joint, i.e. the joint between the tibia, fibula and talus.

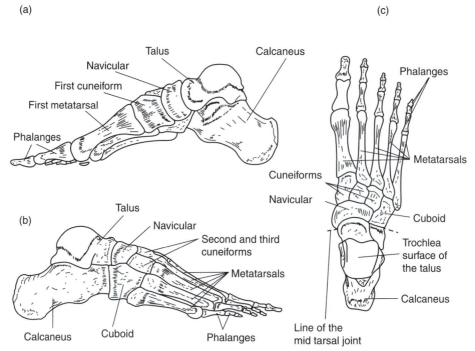

Figure 2.25 The right foot. (a) Medial aspect. (b) Lateral aspect. (c) Superior aspect.

The talus, the second largest tarsal, has a convex pulley-shaped articular surface on its superior aspect, called the trochlea surface of the talus (Figure 2.25c), which articulates with the trochlea surface of the tibia. The trochlea surface of the talus is continuous with articular surfaces on its lateral and medial aspects, which articulate with the lateral malleolus and medial malleolus, respectively.

The inferior aspect of the talus articulates with the anterior half of the superior aspect of the calcaneus by means of two or, in some cases, three articular facets, which together constitute the subtalar joint (talocalcaneal joint). The anterior aspect of the talus articulates with the posterior aspect of the navicular, on the medial aspect of the foot, to form the talonavicular joint.

The calcaneus, the largest tarsal, is often referred to as the heel bone. The anterior aspect of the calcaneus articulates with the posterior aspect of the cuboid, on the lateral aspect of the foot, to form the calcaneocuboid joint. The calcaneocuboid and talonavicular joints are continuous with each other and constitute the midtarsal joint, also referred to as the transverse tarsal joint (Figure 2.25c). The anterior aspect of the navicular articulates with the posterior aspects of the three cuneiforms (medial, middle, lateral), which lie side by side and articulate with each other. The posterior two-thirds of the lateral aspect of the lateral cuneiform articulates with the medial surface of the cuboid. The anterior aspects of the cuneiforms articulate with the bases of the first, second and third metatarsals. The anterior aspect of the cuboid articulates with the bases of the fourth and fifth metatarsals. The joints between the four anterior tarsals and the metatarsals are referred to as the tarsometatarsal joints. The lateral four metatarsals are similar in length, but tend to increase in girth from the second through to the fifth. In comparison, the first metatarsal is shorter but has a greater girth than the other four. The metatarsals are collectively referred to as the metatarsus. The heads of the metatarsals articulate with the proximal phalanges of the toes to form the metatarsophalangeal joints.

The distribution of phalanges in the foot is similar to that in the hand, two in the great toe (big toe) and three in each of the other toes. As in the hand, the phalanges of the toes become progressively shorter from proximal to distal. In comparison with the corresponding phalanges of the thumb, the phalanges of the great toe are slightly longer and have a much greater girth. However, the phalanges of the other four toes are much shorter and, in general, smaller in girth than the corresponding phalanges in the hand. The interphalangeal and meta-tarsophalangeal joints are similar in structure to their counterparts in the hand.

In addition to the tarsals, metatarsals and phalanges, a number of small accessory bones and sesamoid bones occur in fetal life (Standring 2008). There are normally about ten irregular-shaped accessory bones distributed around the tarsus and most of these bones fuse with one of the tarsal bones prior to skeletal maturity. There are normally about 12 sesamoid bones. Like the patella, each sesamoid bone in the foot is partially embedded in a tendon or ligament, with the free surface of the bone forming a synovial joint (sliding between the articular surfaces; see Chapter 4) with a bone over which the tendon or ligament slides during normal function.

REVIEW QUESTIONS

1. Describe the three main mechanical functions of the skeleton.

2. Describe the three main reference planes and define the spatial terminology associated with the planes.

3. List the bones of the axial skeleton.

4. Describe the primary and secondary curves of the vertebral column.

5. Describe the components of a typical vertebra.

6. Describe the difference between true ribs and false ribs.

7. List the bones of the upper limb.

8. Describe the shoulder girdle.

9. List the bones of the lower limb.

10. Describe the differences between the male pelvis and the female pelvis.

Chapter 3

Connective tissues

All of the cells of the body are joined by connective tissue into progressively larger units, i.e. tissues, organs and systems. The whole body consists of all of the systems joined together. Connective tissue maintains the integrity of the tissues, organs and systems by providing them with adequate strength and elasticity. Connective tissue also facilitates intercellular exchange of gases and nutrients. Connective tissue is continuous throughout the body, but its structure gradually changes from one part of a tissue, organ or system to another, depending on the function of the connective tissue at each location. The purpose of this chapter is to describe the structure and functions of connective tissues.

OBJECTIVES

After reading this chapter, you should be able to do the following:

1. Describe the structure and functions of ordinary connective tissues.
2. Describe the structure and functions of the three main types of cartilage.
3. Describe the growth and development of bone.
4. Describe the structure of mature bone.

FUNCTIONS OF CONNECTIVE TISSUES

In muscle tissue, nerve tissue and epithelial tissue, the cells predominate, i.e. the cells tend to be closely packed with little connective tissue between the cells. In contrast, connective tissues have relatively few cells distributed within a large amount of non-cellular material, called matrix, which is produced by the cells. The function of a connective tissue is determined by the properties of its matrix; these change from one part of a tissue, organ or system to another, depending upon the function of the connective tissue at each location. The matrix ranges from a viscous material (in areolar connective tissue) that provides a flexible join between cells and facilitates the intercellular exchange of gases and nutrients, to a very hard solid material (in bone) that provides strength. Connective tissues have two main functions: mechanical support and intercellular exchange.

Mechanical support

All connective tissues help maintain or transmit forces by providing variable amounts of strength and elasticity to facilitate a wide range of mechanical functions. These functions include the following:

- Binding together the cells of the body in the various tissues, organs and systems;
- Supporting and holding the various organs in place;
- Linking bones together at joints;
- Transmitting forces in joints;
- Providing smooth, tough joint surfaces in some joints and strong, flexible links between bones in other joints;
- Providing stability and shock absorption in joints;
- Transmitting muscle forces.

Intercellular exchange

In multicellular organisms, the cells rely on circulating body fluids, such as blood, to supply them with nutrients, oxygen and other substances and to carry away waste products, such as carbon dioxide. This involves the exchange of nutrients, gases and other substances between the vessels of the circulating body fluids and cells adjacent to the vessels, and between cells adjacent to each other. Intercellular exchange ensures that all cells can be supplied with nutrients, gases and other substances, and that they can excrete waste products, even if the cells do not receive a direct supply of the circulating body fluids.

> Connective tissues have two main functions: mechanical support and intercellular exchange.

Classification of connective tissues

Connective tissues are classified according to their level of specialisation into ordinary and special connective tissues (Standring 2008). Ordinary connective tissues are widely distributed throughout the body; at the tissue level, they provide mechanical support and intercellular exchange, and at the organ and system levels, they provide mechanical support. There are two special connective tissues, cartilage and bone. The function of cartilage is to transmit loads across joints efficiently and to allow movement between bones at certain joints. The functions of bone were described in Chapter 2.

ORDINARY CONNECTIVE TISSUES

The matrix of ordinary connective tissues consists of three components: elastin fibres, collagen fibres and ground substance. The main difference in structure of the various types of ordinary connective tissue is in the proportions of these basic components in the matrix.

Elastin and collagen fibres

Elastin fibres and collagen fibres are proteins. A protein molecule consists of a long chain of amino acids. In the unloaded state, the molecules in elastin are irregular in shape and arranged randomly in terms of orientation and attachment to one another (Alexander 1975) (Figure 3.1a). When elastin is subjected to tension, the elastin molecules straighten and are then stretched (Figure 3.2b). When the tension load is removed (assuming that the molecules have not been stretched to failure), the elastin molecules restore their original orientation and shape. Elastin is, therefore, elastic; hence its name.

An elastin fibril is formed by a number of elastin molecules and an elastin fibre consists of

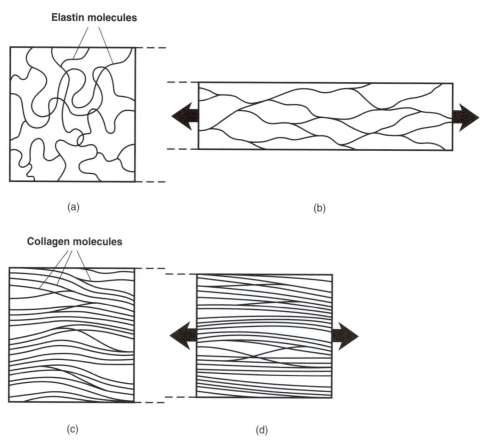

(a)   (b)

(c)   (d)

Figure 3.1 (a) Arrangement of molecules in elastin (unloaded). (b) Effect of stretching on elastin molecules. (c) Arrangement of molecules in collagen (unloaded). (d) Effect of stretching on collagen molecules.

a number of fibrils grouped together. An elastin fibre is similar in shape, strength and elasticity to a long, thin rubber band. Elastin fibres can be stretched by about 200% of their resting length before breaking (Nordin and Frankel 2001). They have a yellowish appearance and are often referred to as yellow elastic fibres or yellow fibres.

In contrast with elastin, collagen molecules are arranged in a more regular manner; they tend to run in the same overall direction and for the most part are aligned parallel to each other (Alexander 1975) (Figure 3.1c). Like elastin molecules, collagen molecules are attached to each other at various points. When subjected to tension in the direction of their main orientation, collagen molecules quickly straighten so that the amount of extension is limited (Figure 3.1d). Like elastin molecules, collagen molecules are elastic and, as such, return to their resting orientation when the tension load is removed. Each group of closely aligned parallel molecules constitutes an individual collagen fibril, and a collagen fibre consists of a number of fibrils grouped together. A collagen fibre is similar in shape, strength and elasticity to a shoelace; it is virtually inextensible and, in relation to elastin, it is extremely strong. Collagen fibres break after being stretched by approximately 10% of their rest length (Nordin and Frankel 2001). Collagen fibres are white and are often referred to as white collagen fibres or white fibres.

Ground substance

Ground substance forms the non-fibrous part of the matrix. It is a viscous gel, consisting mainly of large carbohydrate molecules (molecules consisting of carbon, hydrogen and oxygen) and carbohydrate–protein molecular complexes (molecules consisting of carbon, hydrogen, oxygen and nitrogen) suspended in a relatively large volume of water (Standring 2008). The actual volume of water is determined by the number and type of carbohydrate and carbohydrate–protein substances. Many of these substances are hydrophilic, i.e. they have an affinity for water and, as such, determine not only the volume of water in the ground substance, but also the viscosity of the ground substance. Viscosity refers to the resistance of a fluid to flowing (how quickly it changes shape in response to a load) and its stickiness (how strongly it adheres to adjacent structures). For example, oil is more viscous than water.

In contrast to elastin and collagen fibres, whose sole function is to provide mechanical support, ground substance is responsible not only for facilitating intercellular exchange, but also for providing some mechanical support. The glue-like viscosity of ground substance enables it to join cells together within the other main tissues (muscle, nerve and epithelia). Ground substance in ordinary connective tissues is sometimes referred to as tissue fluid or extracellular fluid. In addition, it is also referred to as amorphous ground substance (amorphous = without definite structure) as it appears, even under a microscope, as a featureless fluid.

> The matrix of ordinary connective tissues consists of elastin fibres, collagen fibres and ground substance. Elastin fibres provide elasticity and collagen fibres provide strength with a small amount of elasticity. Ground substance facilitates intercellular exchange and helps to join cells within the other main tissues.

59

Ordinary connective tissue cells

The number and type of cells found in ordinary connective tissues varies according to the type of connective tissue and the state of health of the individual (Standring 2008). When present, the various types of cells are found suspended in ground substance or, in some cases, attached to the collagen fibres. In general, there are six main types of cell in ordinary connective tissues:

> *Fibroblasts*: Fibroblasts, usually the most numerous cell type in a connective tissue, are responsible for producing the matrix.
>
> *Macrophages*: The macrophages are responsible for engulfing and digesting bacteria and other foreign bodies. They also dispose of dead cellular material that occurs as a result of injury, or as cells become old and die.
>
> *Plasma cells*: Plasma cells occur in large numbers in response to infection. They produce antibodies that inactivate and, with the macrophages, destroy harmful bacteria and other substances.
>
> *White blood cells*: The number and type of white blood cells increase in response to infection. They work with the plasma cells and macrophages to identify and destroy harmful bacteria and other substances.
>
> *Mast cells*: Mast cells, widespread throughout ordinary connective tissues, are responsible for producing heparin, which prevents the blood plasma from clotting inside blood vessels.
>
> *Fat cells*: Fat cells have a variety of functions and occur in large numbers in one particular type of ordinary connective tissue (adipose tissue).

The proportion of elastin fibres, collagen fibres and ground substance, and the number and type of cells within any particular ordinary connective tissue determine the function of the connective tissue. Collagen fibres predominate where great strength is required, whereas elastin fibres predominate where considerable elasticity is needed. Similarly, ground substance tends to predominate where intercellular exchange is of major importance. Under normal circumstances, a wide variety of cells are present within ordinary connective tissues. In response to infection, there is an increase in the number of cells responsible for identifying and destroying harmful bacteria.

Irregular ordinary connective tissues

Ordinary connective tissues are classified into irregular and regular tissues according to the arrangement of the fibrous content of the matrix. In irregular tissues, the fibres tend to run in all directions throughout the tissue with no set pattern. In contrast, the fibres in regular tissues tend to be orientated in the same overall direction. There are four types of irregular ordinary connective tissue (loose, adipose, irregular collagenous and irregular elastic) and two main types of regular ordinary connective tissue (regular collagenous and regular elastic). Figure 3.2 summarises the six main types of ordinary connective tissue in relation to dominant feature and fibre arrangement.

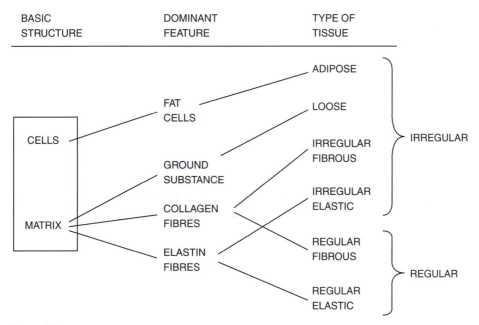

| BASIC STRUCTURE | DOMINANT FEATURE | TYPE OF TISSUE |

Figure 3.2 Ordinary connective tissues.

Loose connective tissue

Loose connective tissue is the most widely distributed of all the connective tissues. It is the connective tissue that joins the cells in the other main tissues (muscle, nerve and epithelia) and that joins tissues into organs. It consists of a loose irregular network of elastin fibres and collagen fibres, both of which branch freely, suspended within a relatively large amount of ground substance (Figure 3.3). The large amount of amorphous ground substance gives the impression of a lot of space between the fibres and cells of loose connective tissue. For this reason, loose connective tissue is also referred to as areolar tissue (areola = a small open area).

In addition to binding cells in tissues and tissues into organs, loose connective tissue provides a supporting framework for nerves, blood vessels and lymph vessels. The large amount of ground substance reflects the importance of loose connective tissue in the facilitation of intercellular exchange.

Adipose connective tissue

Adipose tissue has a loose network of elastin and collagen fibres, similar to loose connective tissue. However, in contrast with loose connective tissue, there is little ground substance and a large number of closely packed fat cells. Each fat cell consists of a thin cell membrane surrounding a relatively large globule of fat (Figure 3.4). Adipose tissue is widely distributed around the body, particularly in the following locations (McArdle *et al.* 2007):

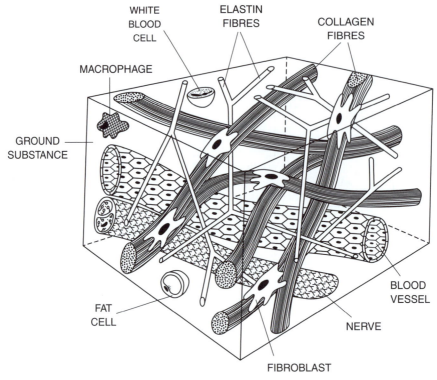

Figure 3.3 Loose connective tissue.

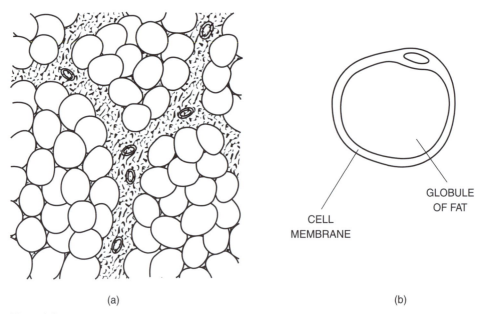

(a)   (b)

Figure 3.4 Adipose connective tissue. (a) Groups of fat cells held together by loose connective tissue. (b) Cross section of a single fat cell.

1. In bone marrow;
2. In association with the various layers of loose connective tissue within certain organs, especially skeletal muscles;
3. As padding around certain organs and joints;
4. As a continuous layer beneath the skin (the skin is sometimes referred to as cutaneous tissue and the layer of fat as the subcutaneous fat layer).

Adipose tissue is a poor conductor of heat and, consequently, the subcutaneous fat layer acts as an insulator, reducing the loss of body heat through the skin. Adipose tissue is moderately strong, owing to its collagen fibre content, and considerably elastic, owing to its elastin fibre content and the large number of elastic fat cells. Consequently, adipose tissue is well suited to provide mechanical support and protection (cushioning) in the form of padding around and between certain organs such as the heart, lungs, liver, spleen, kidneys and intestines. Adipose tissue also acts as padding in such joints as the knee and over certain bones, such as the calcaneus. In addition to its heat insulation and mechanical functions, adipose tissue is the body's main food store. Adipose tissue provides approximately twice as much energy per gram as any other tissue in the body (McArdle *et al.* 2007).

Irregular collagenous connective tissue

The matrix of irregular collagenous connective tissue is dominated by a dense, irregular network of bundles of collagen fibres with few elastin fibres and little ground substance (Figure 3.5). The collagen bundles and their irregular arrangement enable the tissue to resist

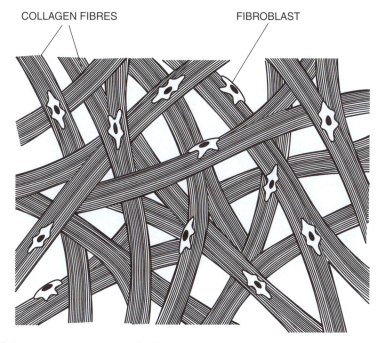

Figure 3.5 Irregular collagenous connective tissue.

tension in any direction. However, though it is strong, the tissue has a certain amount of elasticity, owing to the wavy orientation of the collagen bundles. When stretched in a particular direction, the collagen bundles tend to straighten in the direction of stretching. Irregular collagenous connective tissue is most frequently found as a tough cover around certain organs, where it provides mechanical support and protection. For example, it is found as:

■   A sheath around skeletal muscles (epimysium) and spinal nerves (epineurium);
■   A capsule or envelope around certain organs, such as the kidneys, liver and spleen, to hold the organs in place;
■   The perichondrium of cartilage (a fibrous tissue sheath around some cartilages, including the costal cartilages and embryonic long bones);
■   The periosteum of bones (discussed later in this chapter).

Irregular elastic connective tissue

The matrix of irregular elastic connective tissue is dominated by a dense, irregular network of branching interconnected elastin fibres, together with a few collagen fibres and a moderate amount of ground substance (Figure 3.6). In comparison with irregular collagenous connective tissue, irregular elastic connective tissue is not as strong, but it is much more elastic. It is found where moderate amounts of strength and elasticity are required in more than one direction as, for example, in the walls of arteries and the larger arterioles, the trachea (wind-

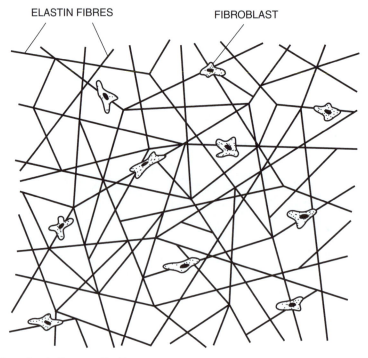

ELASTIN FIBRES   FIBROBLAST

Figure 3.6 Irregular elastic connective tissue.

pipe) and the bronchial tubes. There are few cells in irregular collagenous and irregular elastic connective tissues. The cells that are present are mainly fibroblasts.

Regular ordinary connective tissues

There are two main types of regular ordinary connective tissue: regular collagenous and regular elastic.

Regular collagenous connective tissue

Regular collagenous connective tissue consists almost entirely of bundles of collagen fibres arranged parallel to each other. Usually, there are few elastic fibres and little ground substance. The only cells present are fibroblasts arranged in columns between the collagen bundles (Figure 3.7). The collagen bundles are gathered together in the form of thick cords, bands or sheets of various widths. In the unloaded state, the collagen bundles have a slightly wavy orientation. When stretched, the bundles quickly straighten, and the tissue becomes taut. Regular collagenous connective tissue is extremely strong and virtually inextensible. It has three main forms:

1. Tendons and aponeuroses: mechanical links between skeletal muscle and bone;
2. Ligaments and joint capsules: mechanical links between bones at joints;
3. Retinacula: mechanical restraints on tendons that increase the mechanical efficiency of the musculotendinous units.

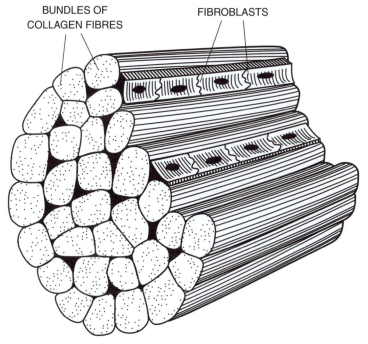

Figure 3.7 Regular collagenous connective tissue: part of a tendon.

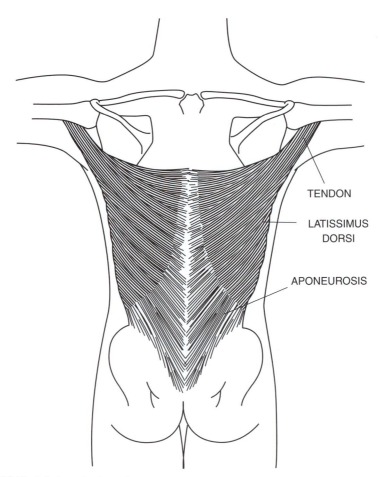

TENDON

LATISSIMUS DORSI

APONEUROSIS

Figure 3.8 The latissimus dorsi muscles.

Tendons and aponeuroses: Skeletal muscles are attached to the skeleton by regular collagenous connective tissue in the form of tendons and aponeuroses (Figure 3.8).

Ligaments and joint capsules: Skeletal muscles provide active (contractile) links between bones. Ligaments (Latin: *ligare* = to bind) and joint capsules provide passive (non-contractile) links between bones. In association with skeletal muscles, ligaments and joint capsules bring about normal movements in joints. Chapter 4 describes the different types of joints in the body. At this point it is sufficient to appreciate that each synovial (freely moveable) joint, i.e. each joint involving sliding and rolling between the joint surfaces of the ends of bones, as in the shoulder and hip, is enclosed within its own joint capsule (Figures 3.9 and 3.10).

The joint capsule encloses a space, usually quite small, called the joint cavity. A joint capsule is composed of two or more layers of regular collagenous connective tissue forming a sleeve around the joint, rather like a piece of rubber tubing joining two glass rods together. Whereas the collagen bundles in each layer are parallel to each other, the bundles in adjacent layers run in different directions. This arrangement enables the capsule to strongly resist

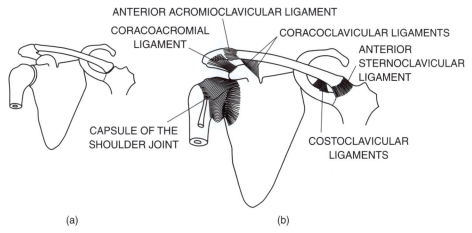

Figure 3.9 Ligaments of the shoulder girdle. (a) Right anterior aspect of the right shoulder girdle and right shoulder joint. (b) Shoulder joint capsule and ligaments supporting the shoulder girdle.

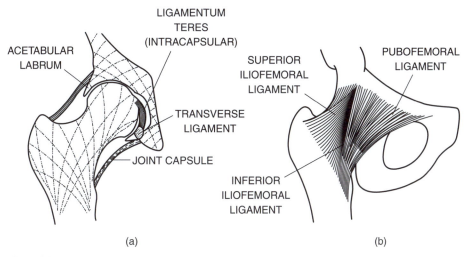

Figure 3.10 Ligaments of the hip joint. (a) Coronal section through the right hip joint showing the joint capsule and ligamentum teres. (b) Anterior aspect of the right hip joint showing the joint capsule and anterior capsular ligaments.

stretching in a number of different directions and, therefore, helps to maintain joint integrity (Figure 3.11).

In all synovial joints, the joint capsule is supported by a number of ligaments. These ligaments may be capsular or non-capsular. A capsular ligament is a distinct thickening in part of the joint capsule that provides additional strength in one direction. For example, the superior iliofemoral ligament, inferior iliofemoral ligament and pubofemoral ligament are capsular ligaments that strengthen the anterior aspect of the capsule of the hip joint (see Figure 3.10b). A non-capsular ligament is a distinct band separate from the joint capsule or only partially attached to it. Non-capsular ligaments may be extracapsular (outside the joint cavity) or intracapsular (inside the joint cavity). For example, the ligamentum teres of the hip joint is

67

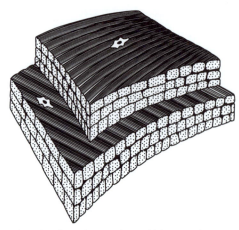

Figure 3.11 Three-dimensional section through a two-layered joint capsule.

intracapsular (Figure 3.10a), but the lateral ligament, medial ligament and cruciate ligaments of the knee joint are all extracapsular (Figure 3.12). Non-capsular ligaments usually consist of a single layer of tissue, but broad ligaments may consist of two or more layers, like a joint capsule.

In addition to the non-capsular ligaments associated with synovial joints, there are other ligaments similar in structure to non-capsular ligaments that help stabilise other parts of the skeleton; for example, the ligaments between the clavicle and scapula, and between the clavicle and first rib (Figure 3.9b).

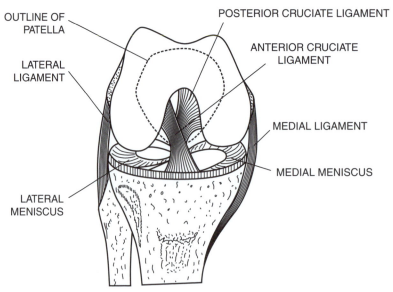

Figure 3.12 Extracapsular ligaments of the knee joint. Anterior aspect of the right knee, flexed at 90°, with patella removed to show the cruciate ligaments and femoral condyles slightly raised to show the menisci. The cruciate ligaments are located at the centre of the joint but lie outside the joint cavity.

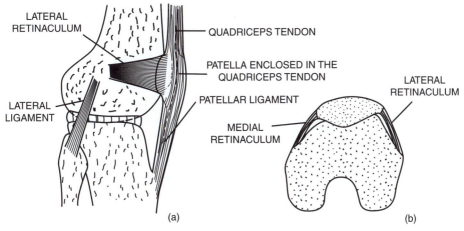

Figure 3.13 Retinacula of the patellofemoral joint. (a) Lateral aspect of the right knee joint. (b) Transverse section through the patellofemoral joint of the right knee joint.

Retinacula: A retinaculum (Latin: *retinere* = to retain) is a fairly broad single-layered sheet of regular collagenous connective tissue that restrains the tendons of some muscles so that the tendons operate close to the joints that they cross. There are two forms of retinacula.

The first form is like a guy rope that restricts the side-to-side movement of a tendon. For example, there are two retinacula, one on each side of the knee joint, that restrain the patella and, therefore, the quadriceps tendon (Figure 3.13). These retinacula help to maintain normal movement between the patella and the femur during flexion and extension of the knee.

The other form of retinaculum is like a pulley that prevents one or more tendons from springing away from a joint when the muscles contract. For example, the retinacula at the wrist and ankle hold down the tendons of the muscles that move these joints (Figure 3.14). The effect of this form of retinaculum is to considerably increase the mechanical effi-ciency of the associated muscles (see length–tension relationship of skeletal muscles in Chapter 5).

Regular elastic connective tissue

Regular elastic connective tissue consists largely of elastin fibres arranged parallel to each other. The proportion of collagen fibres and ground substance is usually fairly small. However, the proportion of collagen fibres and ground substance in regular elastic connective tissue is usually greater than the proportion of elastic fibres and ground substance in regular collagen-ous connective tissue (Akeson *et al.* 1985). Regular elastic connective tissue is found where moderate amounts of strength and elasticity are required, mainly in a single direction. Most ligaments consist of regular collagenous connective tissue, but a few consist of regular elastic connective tissue. Two of these so-called elastic ligaments (ligamentum nuchae, ligamentum flavum) help to stabilise the vertebral column and to allow a certain amount of movement between the vertebrae.

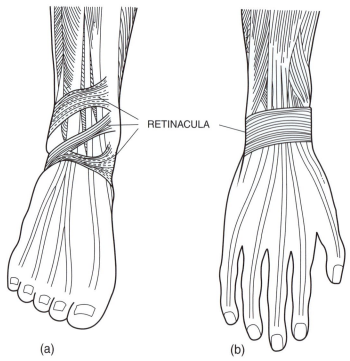

(a)   (b)

Figure 3.14 Retinacula at (a) ankle and (b) wrist.

Fibrous tissue, elastic tissue and fascia

Four of the six main types of ordinary connective tissue are dominated by collagen or elastin fibres: irregular collagenous, irregular elastic, regular collagenous and regular elastic. Whereas all of these tissues could be described as fibrous, the term fibrous tissue normally refers only to regular or irregular collagenous connective tissue. Elastic tissue normally refers only to regular or irregular elastic connective tissue.

The term fascia (Latin: *fascia* = band) refers to any type of ordinary connective tissue in the form of a sheet. In this sense, all aponeuroses are fascia. However, fascia most often refers to superficial fascia and deep fascia. Superficial fascia refers to the continuous layer of loose connective tissue that connects the skin to underlying muscle or bone. This layer of loose connective tissue is closely associated with the subcutaneous layer of fat referred to earlier. Deep fascia describes the sheets of irregular collagenous connective tissue that form sheaths around muscles and groups of muscles, separating them into functional units.

Ordinary connective tissues differ from each other in the proportions of elastin, collagen and ground substance, and in the arrangement of the fibrous content. There are four main types of irregular ordinary connective tissue: loose, adipose, irregular collagenous and irregular elastic and two main types of regular ordinary connective tissues: regular collagenous and regular elastic.

CARTILAGE

Like all connective tissues, cartilage is a composite material, i.e. a material that is stronger than any of the separate substances from which it is made (Alexander 1968). Fibreglass and the rubber used in the manufacture of tyres are examples of man-made composite materials. The matrix of cartilage is similar to that of fibrous and elastic ordinary connective tissues in that it consists mainly of collagen and elastin fibres embedded in ground substance. However, relative to ordinary connective tissues, the ground substance of cartilage is specialised to produce a material that is capable of resisting all forms of loading, not just tension (Caplan 1984). The matrix of cartilage consists of huge carbohydrate–protein molecular complexes called proteoglycans, which are highly hydrophilic; each proteoglycan complex is capable of attracting to itself a volume of water that is many times its own weight. Consequently, under normal circumstances, water is the chief constituent of cartilage. The proteoglycans and water produce a highly viscous gel, usually referred to as proteoglycan gel. In combination with collagen and elastin, the proteoglycan gel forms a tough rubbery material capable of strongly resisting all forms of loading.

The only cells found in cartilage are cartilage cells, called chondrocytes, which produce the cartilage matrix. The chondrocytes lie in fluid-filled spaces called lacunae, distributed throughout the matrix (Figure 3.15). The cells are arranged singly (parent cells) and in groups of two to five cells that each originate from a single parent cell. As the cells become mature they separate from their parent groups and start to produce new groups. Whereas collagen or elastin fibres dominate the matrix of all three main types of cartilage, the region around each lacuna is usually free of fibres. This distinct region, called the capsule of the lacuna, consists of proteoglycan gel that is denser than in other parts of the matrix.

Mature cartilage contains no blood vessels or nerves (Nordin and Frankel 2001). This reflects the mechanical functions of cartilage; blood vessels and nerves would be destroyed by the deformation of cartilage in response to loading. In the absence of a direct blood supply, the chondrocytes depend on intercellular exchange via blood vessels close to the

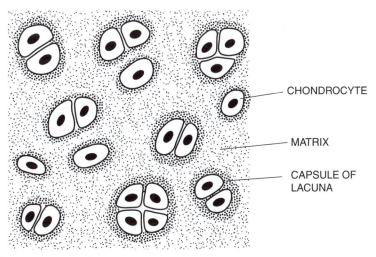

Figure 3.15 Typical structure of cartilage.

non-load-bearing surfaces of the cartilage for nutrition and excretion. For this reason, and the fact that cartilage is often under considerable load, repair of cartilage is slow and may not take place at all (Caplan 1984).

When cartilage is loaded (subjected to tension, compression, shear or any combination of these loads), water is gradually forced out of the cartilage and the cartilage deforms. The rate and extent of deformation depends on the size and duration of the load. When the load is removed, the proteoglycan structures gradually restore the original level of water saturation and, consequently, the original size and shape of the cartilage, by absorbing water into the cartilage. The ability of a material to deform gradually in response to a load and, following unloading, gradually to restore its original size and shape is referred to as viscoelasticity. In comparison, elasticity refers to a material's ability to deform immediately in response to a load and, following unloading, to immediately restore its original size and shape, like a rubber band. Cartilage tends to behave viscoelastically in response to prolonged loading and elastically in response to sudden impact loads.

The physical properties of cartilage, including viscoelasticity, elasticity and strength, depend on the proportions of collagen fibres, elastin fibres and proteoglycan gel in the matrix. In general, there are three main types of cartilage: hyaline cartilage, fibrocartilage and elastic cartilage.

Hyaline cartilage

Hyaline cartilage has a pearly bluish-white tinge; under a low-power microscope, the matrix appears amorphous and translucent (semitransparent), as in Figure 3.15. Under a high-power microscope, the matrix can be seen to consist of a dense network of very fine collagen fibrils and fibres embedded in proteoglycan gel (Standring 2008). Most of the skeleton is preformed in hyaline cartilage and, prior to maturity, the growth and development of many bones is largely determined by the hyaline cartilage content of the bones. The following structures consist of hyaline cartilage throughout life:

- Articular cartilage, which forms the smooth, tough, wear-resistant articular surfaces of bones in synovial joints;
- The costal cartilages that link the upper ten pairs of ribs to the sternum and provide the rib cage with flexibility and elasticity;
- Supporting rings within the elastic walls of the trachea (windpipe) and the larger bronchial tubes;
- Part of the supporting framework of the larynx (voice box);
- The external flexible part of the nose that forms the major part of the nostrils.

Fibrocartilage

In fibrocartilage, also referred to as white fibrocartilage, the matrix is dominated by a dense regular network of bundles of collagen fibres arranged parallel to each other in several layers. The bundles in adjacent layers run in different directions (like the layers in a joint capsule), to produce a strong material with moderate elasticity. Fibrocartilage is found in a number of locations and forms.

Articular discs: Complete or incomplete discs interposed between the articular surfaces of some synovial joints, including the knee joint, the sternoclavicular joint and the acromioclavicular joint (see Chapter 4). In these joints, the discs improve the congruence (area over which the joint reaction forces are distributed) and stability of the joints. In addition, the discs deform in response to loading and thereby provide shock absorption.

Symphysis joints: Complete discs that join the bones in symphysis joints (see Chapter 4). These joints include the pubic symphysis and the intervertebral joints. In these joints, deformation of the disc in response to loading allows movement between the articulated bones and provides shock absorption.

Labra in ball-and-socket joints: Extension to the concave articular surface in a ball-and-socket joint (e.g. shoulder and hip joints) in the form of a labrum (lip) around the border of the articular surface (see Chapter 4). A labrum deepens the socket, which increases the area of articulation and, therefore, the stability of the joint.

Lining of bony grooves: Lining of bony grooves and channels that are occupied by tendons. The grooves act as pulleys that normally increase the mechanical efficiency of the associated muscles.

Elastic cartilage

In elastic cartilage, also referred to as yellow elastic cartilage, the matrix is dominated by a dense network of elastin fibres. Elastic cartilage provides support with moderate elasticity. It is found mainly in the larynx, the external part of the ear (pinna), and the tube leading from the middle part of the ear to the throat (Eustachian or auditory tube).

> The physical properties of cartilage depend on the proportions of collagen fibres, elastin fibres and proteoglycan gel in the matrix. There are three main types of cartilage: hyaline cartilage, fibrocartilage and elastic cartilage.

BONE

The strongest and least flexible of all the connective tissues is bone. The matrix of bone consists of a dense, layered, regular network of collagen fibres embedded in a hard solid ground substance called bone salt. Bone salt consists of calcium phosphate and calcium carbonate with smaller amounts of magnesium, sodium and chlorine (Alexander 1975). In mature bone, bone salt makes up about 70% of the total weight of bone, with collagen making up the remaining 30%. Bone salt is denser than collagen, such that the bone salt and collagen both occupy about 50% of the total volume. The composite material made of bone salt and collagen produces a hard, tough, fairly stiff structure. Relative to cast iron, bone has the same tensile strength, is only one-third as heavy, and is much more elastic (Ascenzi and Bell 1971). The elasticity of bone, although slight relative to cartilage, is nevertheless important in enabling it to absorb sudden impacts without breaking.

Bone growth and development

Most of the embryonic skeleton, which appears around the third week of intrauterine life, is preformed in hyaline cartilage. Those parts of the embryonic skeleton that are not preformed in hyaline cartilage, which include the top of the skull, the clavicles and parts of the mandible, are preformed in a highly vascular fibrous membrane. By the eighth or ninth week of intrauterine life, the shapes of the embryonic bones are similar to their eventual adult shapes (Standring 2008). The developing bones constantly adapt their shapes and structures to withstand the forces (especially muscle forces and joint reaction forces) that act on them. After skeletal maturity (approximately 20–25 years of age) the bones experience negligible change in shape, but change in structure continues throughout life (Frost 2004).

Ossification

Ossification or osteogenesis (*osteo* = bone, *genesis* = creation) is the process that transforms the embryonic skeleton into bone. Ossification is a feature of normal growth and development and proceeds at different rates in different bones. In each bone, ossification is initiated at a particular location, referred to as the primary centre of ossification. In some bones, including the carpals and tarsals, ossification is completed from the primary centre of ossification, i.e. the volume of ossified bone around the primary centre of ossification gradually increases as the bone matures. In other bones, one or more secondary centres of ossification occur some time after the occurrence of the primary centre of ossification, i.e. ossification in these bones gradually progresses from two or more centres of ossification within the same bone. For example, in each metacarpal and metatarsal there is a primary centre of ossification and a secondary centre of ossification. In all of the large long bones there is a primary centre of ossification in the shaft and a secondary centre of ossification in each epiphysis. At birth, there are approximately 270 regions of the immature skeleton (associated with 270 primary and secondary centres of ossification) that are in a fairly advanced stage of ossification. The 270 regions normally result in 206 bones in the mature skeleton.

The ossification of hyaline cartilage is called intracartilaginous or endochondral ossification (*endo* = within, *chondral* = cartilage) and the ossification of fibrous membranes is called intramembranous ossification. Both forms of ossification are similar and produce the same type of bone tissue. The process of endochondral ossification is described with reference to a typical long bone.

Growth in girth

Each embryonic long bone is preformed in hyaline cartilage and covered in a fibrous perichondrium (*peri* = around, *chondrium* = cartilage), which contains blood vessels (Figure 3.16a). Between the fifth and twelfth weeks of intrauterine life, some fibroblasts in the perichondrium around the middle of the shaft of the cartilage model are transformed into osteoblasts.

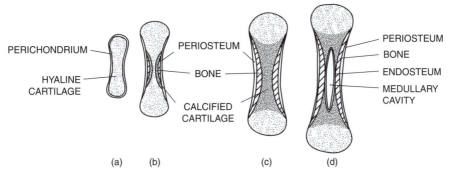

Figure 3.16 Early stages in the endochondral ossification of a long bone. (a) Embryonic long bone; hyaline cartilage enclosed within a fibrous perichondrium. (b) Establishment of a bony collar around the middle of the shaft. (c) Completion of a bony cylinder running the length of the shaft around the time of birth. (d) Formation of a medullary cavity.

Osteoblasts are one of three types of bone cell, the others being osteoclasts and osteocytes. Osteoblasts are responsible for the production of bone. The newly formed osteoblasts invade the hyaline cartilage immediately beneath the perichondrium and start to deposit calcium and other minerals in the matrix. Consequently, the hyaline cartilage is transformed into calcified cartilage. This process of mineralisation is called calcification; calcified cartilage represents an intermediate stage in the process of ossification of cartilage into bone. As calcification continues, a bony ring or collar is eventually formed around the middle of the shaft of the otherwise cartilage model (Figure 3.16b).

When the perichondrium starts to produce osteoblasts and, in turn, bone, it is called periosteum. The first site of bone formation, the middle of the shaft of the cartilage model, is called the primary centre of ossification. The process of ossification proceeds from the bony collar in two directions: across the shaft from the outside toward the centre, and toward the ends of the shaft. By the 36th week, around the time of birth, the bony collar has become a bony cylinder running the length of the shaft, but not progressing into the bulbous ends of the bone (Figure 3.16c). The bony cylinder is thickest at its middle and thinnest at its ends. By this time the remaining hyaline cartilage in the middle of the shaft has been transformed into calcified cartilage. Soon afterward, a second type of bone cells called osteoclasts invades this central portion of calcified cartilage. Whereas osteoblasts produce new bone, osteoclasts remove bone and calcified cartilage. The osteoclasts start to remove the calcified cartilage in the middle of the shaft thereby creating a space called the medullary cavity (Figure 3.16d). The medullary cavity gradually widens and extends toward both ends of the shaft. Simultaneously, the thickness of bone in the shaft gradually increases.

Eventually all of the calcified cartilage in the shaft is removed as a result of the combined effects of ossification across the shaft from the outside toward the centre and osteoclastic activity from the centre outward. By this time, the medullary cavity is occupied by yellow marrow consisting of loose connective tissue containing a large number of blood vessels, fat cells and immature white blood cells (Standring 2008). A layer of loose connective tissue containing many osteoblasts and a smaller number of osteoclasts lines the medullary cavity. This layer is called the endosteum.

Long bones are designed, above all, to resist bending. For a given amount of bone tissue, a hollow shaft is stronger in bending than a solid one, which would appear to be the main reason why the shafts of long bones are hollow (Alexander 1968). Growth in girth of the shaft of a long bone involves formation of new bone on the outside of the shaft by osteoblasts in the periosteum, and the removal of bone from the inside of the shaft by osteoclasts in the endosteum. The type of growth produced by the periosteum, which involves laying down new bone on the surface of older bone rather like the addition of rings in a tree, is called appositional growth. In mature bone, the periosteum consists of irregular collagenous connective tissue. In addition to appositional growth, the periosteum has three other main functions:

1. To provide a protective cover around the shaft of the bone;
2. To allow blood vessels to pass into the bone;
3. To provide attachment for muscles, tendons, ligaments and joint capsules.

Growth in length

Around the time of birth, a secondary centre of ossification occurs in the centre of each end of a long bone. These new centres of ossification are responsible for the ossification of the ends of the bones; ossification proceeds from the centre toward the periphery. After the secondary centres of ossification have been established, the only hyaline cartilage remaining from the original cartilage model is the cartilage that covers the bulbous ends of the bone and separates the ends of the bone from the shaft (Figure 3.17). These two regions of hyaline cartilage are continuous with each other and remain so until maturity.

Each end of a long bone is called an epiphysis and the shaft is called the diaphysis. Part of the cartilage covering each epiphysis forms an articular surface and, as such, is referred to as articular cartilage. The regions of cartilage that separate the epiphyses from the diaphysis are called epiphyseal plates (Figure 3.17). The epiphyseal plates are responsible for growth in length of the bone. During normal growth, they remain active until the bone has achieved its mature length.

An epiphyseal plate consists of four layers (Tortora and Anagnostakos 1984) (Figure 3.18). The layer adjacent to the epiphysis is called the reserve or germinal layer; this layer anchors the epiphyseal plate to the bone of the epiphysis. The second layer, called the proliferation layer, is responsible for chondrogenesis (production of new cartilage). The chondrocytes in this layer undergo fairly rapid cell division, and in turn, the cells produce new matrix that results in an increase in the amount of cartilage. Growth in length of the shaft of a bone is due to chondrogenesis in the proliferation layers of the epiphyseal plates. This type of growth, in which additional new tissue is produced from within the mass of existing tissue, is called interstitial growth.

The third layer of the epiphyseal plate is called the hypertrophic layer. In this layer, the chondrocytes are arranged in columns and gradually increase in size, with the larger and more mature cells furthest from the epiphysis. The fourth layer of the epiphyseal plate is called the calcified layer. In this layer, the hypertrophied chondrocytes and surrounding matrix are replaced by calcified cartilage. The calcified cartilage interdigitates with the underlying bone,

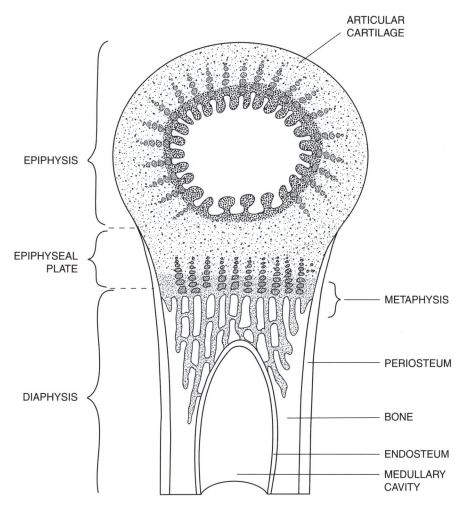

ARTICULAR
CARTILAGE

EPIPHYSIS

EPIPHYSEAL
PLATE

METAPHYSIS

DIAPHYSIS

PERIOSTEUM

BONE

ENDOSTEUM

MEDULLARY
CAVITY

Figure 3.17 Longitudinal section through the epiphysis and part of the diaphysis of a typical immature long bone.

forming a relatively strong bond (Figures 3.17 and 3.18) that is able to resist shear loading. As new cartilage is formed in the proliferation layer, the calcified cartilage in contact with the underlying bone is itself gradually transformed into bone. The net result of these processes is that the epiphyseal plates, which remain about the same thickness, gradually move farther from the middle of the shaft as the shaft increases in length.

The metaphysis is the region where the epiphysis joins the diaphysis; in a growing bone this corresponds to the calcified layer of the epiphyseal plate together with the interdigitating bone (Figure 3.17). The interface between the hypertrophic and calcified layers is sometimes referred to as the tidemark.

When a long bone has achieved its mature length, longitudinal growth in the epiphyseal plates ceases. Shortly afterward, the epiphyseal plates are replaced by bone so that the epiphyses are fused with the shaft. In most long bones, one end usually fuses with the shaft before

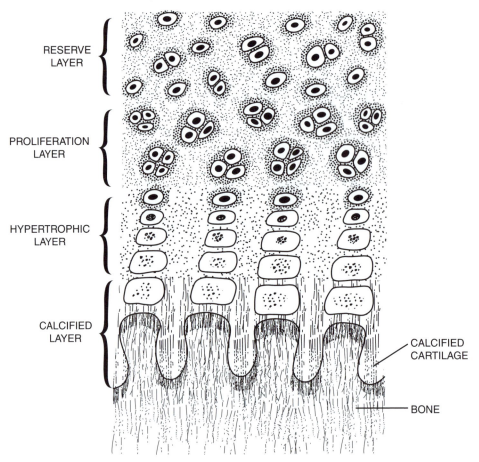

RESERVE LAYER

PROLIFERATION LAYER

HYPERTROPHIC LAYER

CALCIFIED LAYER

CALCIFIED CARTILAGE

BONE

Figure 3.18 A longitudinal section through an epiphyseal plate.

the other end. In the long bones of the arms and legs, fusion of both ends normally takes place between 14 and 20 years of age (Standring 2008). In some other bones, such as the innominate bones, fusion usually takes place between 20 and 25 years of age. Consequently, the epiphyseal plates of the various bones are vulnerable to injury for a relatively long period. Injury to an epiphyseal plate may, in severe cases, result in one of two types of bone deformity (Peterson 2001; Caine *et al.* 2006):

1. A complete cessation of growth and premature fusion, resulting in, for example, a limb length discrepancy;
2. An asymmetric cessation of growth across an epiphyseal plate, resulting in an angular deformity and joint incongruity.

The epiphyseal plates at each end of a long bone usually contribute different amounts to the length of the shaft. For example, the upper and lower epiphyseal plates of the humerus contribute approximately 80% and 20%, respectively, to the total length of the bone. In contrast,

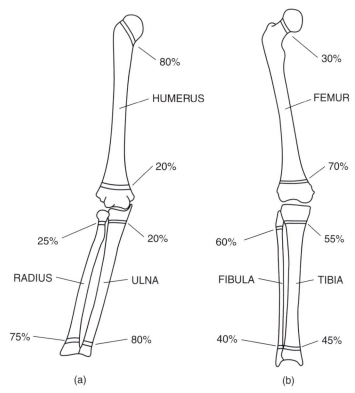

Figure 3.19 Contributions of the proximal and distal epiphyseal plates to growth in length of the long bones of (a) the upper limb and (b) the lower limb.

the upper and lower epiphyseal plates of the femur contribute approximately 30% and 70%, respectively, to the total length of the bone (Pappas 1983) (Figure 3.19).

The vulnerability of epiphyseal plates to injury is largely due to the plates being the weakest parts of the immature skeleton. For example, ligaments and joint capsules are two to five times stronger than epiphyseal plates (Larson and McMahan 1966). When a ligament supporting a particular joint is inserted into the epiphysis (rather than the diaphysis), a load applied to the joint that tends to stretch the ligament is, in a child, more likely to result in a fracture through the epiphyseal plate than in a tear in the ligament. In an adult, the same type of loading would tend to cause a ligament tear, since the epiphysis and diaphysis are fused (Pappas 1983) (Figure 3.20).

Growth of epiphyses

Just as the epiphyseal plates are responsible for growth in length of a bone, the articular cartilage is responsible for growth of the epiphyses (Figure 3.17). Like an epiphyseal plate, articular cartilage consists of four layers. The only real difference in structure between articular cartilage and an epiphyseal plate is in the arrangement of the fibres in the reserve layer. In an epiphyseal plate, the collagen fibres cross each other obliquely, forming a strong bond between the epiphyseal bone and the proliferation layer of the plate. In articular cartilage,

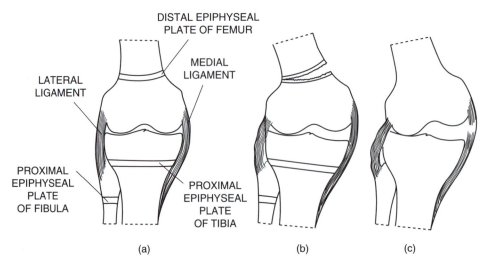

DISTAL EPIPHYSEAL
PLATE OF FEMUR

MEDIAL
LIGAMENT

LATERAL
LIGAMENT

PROXIMAL
EPIPHYSEAL
PLATE
OF FIBULA

PROXIMAL
EPIPHYSEAL
PLATE
OF TIBIA

(a)   (b)   (c)

Figure 3.20 Effect of degree of skeletal maturity on type of injury. (a) Anterior aspect of the right knee joint showing normal alignment of the femur, tibia and fibula. (b,c) Excessive abduction of the knee joint. In a child this is more likely to result in a fracture through the distal epiphyseal plate of the femur than tearing of the medial ligament. After maturity, it is likely to result in partial or complete tearing of the medial ligament.

the reserve layer is the outer layer. Whereas the majority of the layer is similar in structure to the reserve layer of an epiphyseal plate, the outer surface of articular cartilage is cell free and consists of densely packed collagen fibres and fibrils arranged parallel to the articular surface. This arrangement produces a tough wear-resistant surface.

The type of growth produced by articular cartilage is the same as that produced by an epiphyseal plate, i.e. interstitial growth. During the growth period, the rate of ossification of an epiphysis is greater than the rate of growth of the epiphysis. Consequently, the thickness of the articular cartilage becomes relatively thinner with age (Figure 3.21). At maturity, the thickness of articular cartilage is approximately 1–7 mm and this tends to decrease with age, owing to mechanical wear. Whereas bone growth is largely determined by genetic factors, the mechanical stress experienced by articular cartilage and epiphyseal plates, as a result of movement and the maintenance of an upright posture, also has a major effect on bone growth.

Growth of apophyses

Secondary centres of ossification occur not only in the epiphyses of long bones, but also in some of the rudimentary tuberosities of some bones, including the femur (greater trochanter and lesser trochanter), the innominate bones (ischial tuberosities, anterior-superior and anterior-inferior iliac spines), and the calcaneus (posterior calcaneal tuberosity) (Figures 3.22 and 3.23). The rudimentary tuberosities where these secondary centres of ossification occur (around 10 to 14 months after birth) are called apophyses. Each apophysis grows and ossifies in much the same way as an epiphysis. Apophyses provide areas of attachment for the tendons of powerful muscles, such as the quadriceps (tibial tuberosity), hamstrings (ischial tuberosity) and calf muscles (calcaneal tuberosity) (Figure 3.23). This form of attachment is different from that of most tendons, which attach directly onto the periosteum.

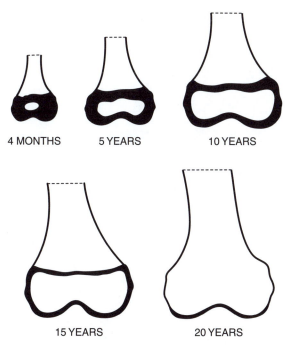

4 MONTHS   **5 YEARS**   **10 YEARS**

15 YEARS   **20 YEARS**

Figure 3.21 Successive stages in the ossification of the distal femoral epiphysis.

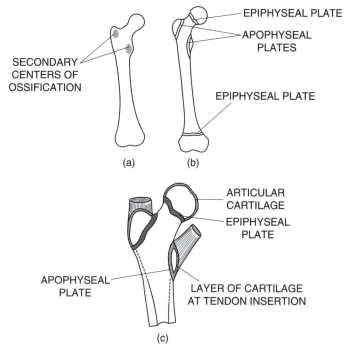

Figure 3.22 Apophyses of the femur: greater trochanter and lesser trochanter. (a) Occurrence of secondary centres of ossification. (b) Apophyseal and epiphyseal plates of the femur. (c) Growth areas of the head of the femur and the greater and lesser trochanters.

81

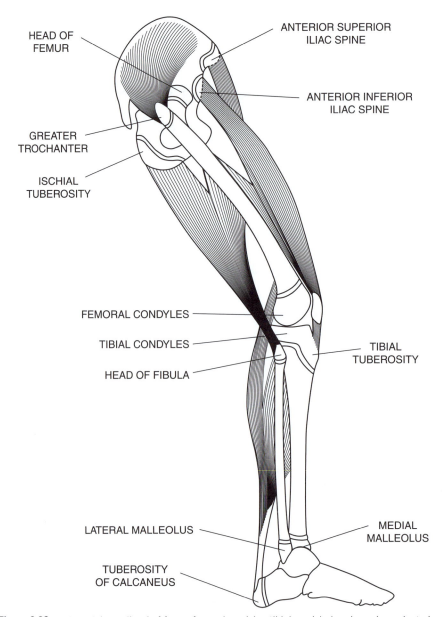

HEAD OF
FEMUR

ANTERIOR SUPERIOR
ILIAC SPINE

ANTERIOR INFERIOR
ILIAC SPINE

GREATER
TROCHANTER

ISCHIAL
TUBEROSITY

FEMORAL CONDYLES

TIBIAL CONDYLES

HEAD OF FIBULA

TIBIAL
TUBEROSITY

LATERAL MALLEOLUS

MEDIAL
MALLEOLUS

TUBEROSITY
OF CALCANEUS

Figure 3.23 Major epiphyses (head of femur, femoral condyles, tibial condyles) and apophyses (anterior-superior and anterior-inferior iliac spines, greater trochanter, ischial tuberosity, lateral malleolus, medial malleolus, tuberosity of the calcaneus) of the lower limb.

Prior to maturity, each apophysis is separated from the rest of the bone by an apophyseal plate, which is very similar in structure and function to an epiphyseal plate. Each apophyseal plate is responsible for growth of the bone adjacent to the non-apophyseal side of the plate. Growth of the apophysis itself is due to a layer of cartilage (mixture of hyaline cartilage and fibrocartilage) on the outside of the apophysis into which the fibres of the tendon insert (Figure 3.22c). At maturity, the apophyses fuse with the rest of the bone.

Epiphyses, especially those that form weight-bearing joints, are normally subjected to compression load and, as such, are often referred to as pressure epiphyses. In contrast, apophyses are normally subjected to tension load and are often referred to as traction epiphyses. Whereas apophyseal growth plates do not affect growth in bone length, they do affect the alignment and strength of the tendons attached to them. Consequently, injury to apophyseal plates may affect the mechanical characteristics of associated muscles, which, in turn, may affect normal joint function.

Studies of sport-related injuries in children show that the proportion of injuries involving growth plates (epiphyseal and apophyseal) is between 6% and 18% of the total number of injuries (Speer and Braun 1985; Krueger-Franke et al. 1992; Gross et al. 1994). About 5% of these growth-plate injuries result in some type of bone deformity (Larson 1973). On the basis of these figures, the number of growth-plate injuries resulting in bone deformity is in the region of three to nine per thousand. However, this estimate is likely to be conservative since many injuries that occur during free play and sports are not reported or are incorrectly diagnosed (Combs 1994).

Structure of mature bone

Different regions of a bone are subjected to different types and magnitudes of loading. For example, the epiphyses are mainly subjected to compression loads, whereas the shaft is mainly subjected to bending and torsion loads. Not surprisingly, the structure of a mature bone reflects the normal loading pattern on a bone.

Compact and cancellous bone

Mature bone consists of osteones, also referred to as Haversian systems (Figure 3.24). The only difference in the structure of bone in the different regions of a bone is in the extent to which the osteones are packed together; the closer the packing, the greater the density of the bone, the greater the strength of the bone and the lower the flexibility of the bone. In the hollow shaft of a long bone, the osteones are very closely packed. This high-density bone is called compact bone (Figure 3.25).

A single osteone is a column of bone that consists of three to nine concentric rings (or layers) of bone surrounding a central open channel (Figure 3.24). The concentric rings of bone are called lamellae and the central channel is called a Haversian canal. Each lamella consists of a single layer of closely packed collagen fibres arranged parallel to each other, embedded in bone salt. Whereas the collagen fibres in each lamella are parallel to each other, the orientation of fibres in adjacent lamellae is different. This arrangement, similar to the layers of collagen fibres in a joint capsule, enables the bone to strongly resist deformation in any direction.

Between the lamellae are a large number of osteocytes (Figure 3.24 and Figure 3.26a). Each osteocyte lies in a lacuna, a small space, and the lacunae are linked together by tiny channels called canaliculi (Figure 3.26b). The canaliculi run between the lamellae (circumferential canaliculi), across the lamellae from one side to the other (radial canaliculi), and in parallel with the osteones (longitudinal canaliculi). This three-dimensional network of canaliculi

83

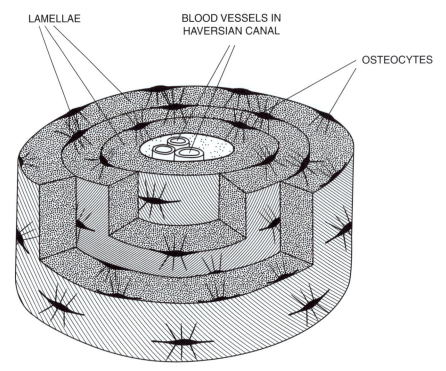

Figure 3.24 Structure of an osteone.

enables the osteocytes to connect with each other by means of projections from the cell bodies into the canaliculi. Consequently, all of the osteocytes in a bone are directly or indirectly connected to each other and to the osteoblasts and osteoclasts in the periosteum and endosteum. The main function of osteocytes is to monitor the strains in bone that arise from normal everyday activity and to use this information to control the growth, development and repair of bone by coordinating the activity of the osteoblasts and osteoclasts. Osteocytes also regulate the level of minerals, especially calcium and phosphorus, in the blood (Turner and Pavalko 1998; Bailey *et al.* 1986)

The Haversian canal at the centre of each osteone contains blood vessels and nerves supported by loose connective tissue (Figure 3.24). The canaliculi are linked to the Haversian canals, thereby facilitating intercellular exchange between blood vessels and osteocytes. In addition to being linked together by canaliculi, the Haversian canals of adjacent osteones are also linked together by channels called Volkmann canals, which are similar in size to Haversian canals (Figure 3.25a). Volkmann canals, like Haversian canals, contain blood vessels and nerves supported by loose connective tissue. In association with the Haversian canals, the Volkmann canals form a system of channels, which traverse the bone from the periosteum to the endosteum (Figure 3.25a). The system of Haversian and Volkmann canals enables blood vessels and nerves to pass along, around and across the bone.

The thickness of compact bone in the shaft decreases from the middle of the shaft toward the epiphyses as the osteones start to separate into groups, rather as the branches of a tree separate from the trunk (Figure 3.27). However, in contrast with the branches of a tree,

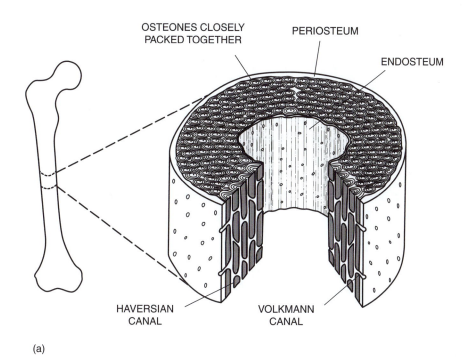

(a)

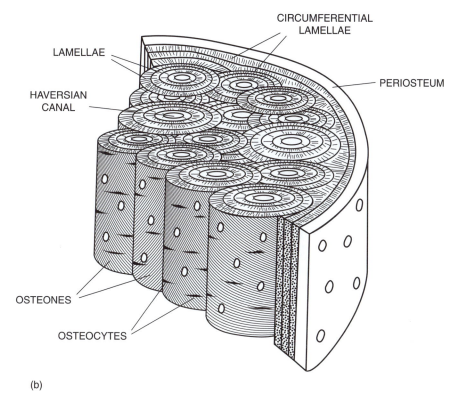

(b)

Figure 3.25 Structure of compact bone.

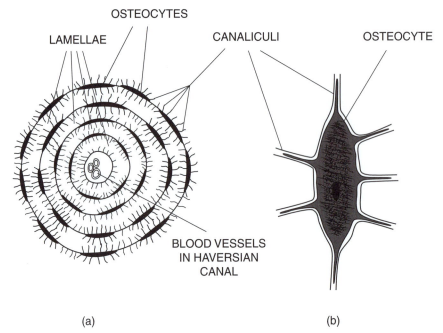

OSTEOCYTES

LAMELLAE

CANALICULI

OSTEOCYTE

BLOOD VESSELS
IN HAVERSIAN
CANAL

(a)

(b)

Figure 3.26 Osteocytes and canaliculi. (a) Cross section through an osteone, showing circumferential and radial canaliculi. (b) An osteocyte lying in a lacuna with projections of the cell body into the canaliculi.

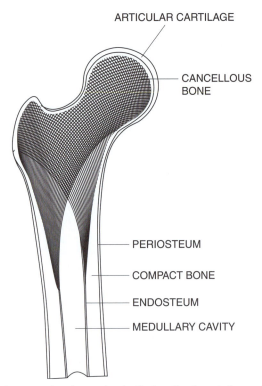

ARTICULAR CARTILAGE

CANCELLOUS
BONE

PERIOSTEUM

COMPACT BONE

ENDOSTEUM

MEDULLARY CAVITY

Figure 3.27 Structure of a mature long bone: a longitudinal section through the proximal third of the femur.

the groups of osteones, called trabeculae, form a distinct latticework pattern within each epiphysis (Figure 3.27). The latticework arrangement of the trabeculae is called trabecular bone, spongy bone or, most frequently, cancellous bone, owing to the large number of spaces between the trabeculae (*cancellous* = porous structure). The terminal branches of the trabeculae merge with a layer of calcified cartilage, called subchondral bone, adjacent to the articular cartilage.

The majority of the trabeculae cross each other at right angles; this arrangement maximises the strength of the trabecular bone and minimises the stress experienced by the epiphyses in all positions of the joint during habitual movements. The spaces between the trabeculae are filled with red marrow, i.e. loose connective tissue containing a large number of blood vessels, some white blood cells and fat cells, and a large number of cells called erythroblasts responsible for producing red blood cells. The spaces in cancellous bone are continuous with the medullary cavity and, therefore, the red marrow is continuous with the yellow marrow.

Cancellous bone is far less dense and, consequently, much more elastic than compact bone. The elasticity of cancellous bone is very important in ensuring congruity in joints during load transmission, thereby minimising stress within the epiphyses and on the articular cartilages (Frost 1999; Burr 2004).

Modelling and remodelling in bone

Growth, development and maintenance of bone are determined by the interaction of three subprocesses: skeletal genotype, modelling and remodelling. The skeletal genotype refers to the process of genetically programmed change in the external form (size and shape) and internal architecture of the bones. Modelling refers to the changes in the expression of the skeletal genotype that occur as a result of environmental factors, such as nutrition and, in particular, the mechanical strains imposed by normal habitual activity. Remodelling refers to the coordination of osteoblastic and osteoclastic activity responsible for the actual changes in external form and internal architecture of the bones, including repair of bones (Figure 3.28). As bone is continuously being absorbed from some places (by osteoclasts) and deposited in others (by osteoblasts), the process of remodelling is sometimes referred to as turnover. Prior to maturity, all bones are in a continual state of change in external form and internal architecture. After skeletal maturity is achieved (approximately 20 to 25 years of age), modelling of the external form decreases to negligible proportions, but modelling of the internal architecture continues throughout life (Frost 1979, 2004).

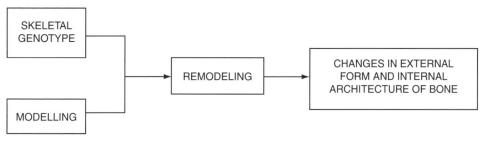

Figure 3.28 The relationship between skeletal genotype, modelling and remodelling in the growth, development and maintenance of bone.

Porosity, osteopenia and osteoporosis

Owing to the various channels and spaces within compact and cancellous bone, any particular region of a bone consists of certain amounts of bone tissue and non-bone tissue. The term porosity describes the proportion of non-bone tissue. At skeletal maturity, the porosity of compact and cancellous bone is approximately 2% and 50%, respectively; the density (amount of bone tissue per unit volume) of compact bone is approximately double that of cancellous bone (Radin 1984). The density of bone tissue depends on the degree of mineralisation. During ossification, the degree of mineralisation of bone tissue gradually increases and reaches a maximum level at skeletal maturity (Bailey *et al.* 1986). However, the amount of bone within the skeleton may continue to increase for five to ten years after skeletal maturity, especially in physically active individuals (Seeman 2008; Wang and Seeman 2008). Consequently, bone mass peaks in men and women between 25 and 30 years of age. In terms of turnover, this means that from skeletal maturity to the age at which peak bone mass occurs, more new bone is formed than old and damaged bone is absorbed.

Following peak bone mass, there is usually a stable period in which the amount of bone in the skeleton remains about the same, i.e. there is a balance between bone absorption and bone formation. This stable period is followed by a gradual decrease in bone mass for the rest of the life of the individual, i.e. the rate of bone absorption exceeds the rate of bone formation. Bone mass is the product of bone volume and bone density. The loss in bone mass that occurs with age following peak bone mass is the result of decreases in bone volume and bone density. Osteopenia refers to a level of bone density below the normal level for the age and sex of the individual (Frost 2004).

Bone mass starts to decrease earlier and at a greater rate in women than in men. In men, bone loss normally starts to occur between 45 and 50 years of age and proceeds at a rate of 0.4% to 0.75% per year (Bailey *et al.* 1986; Smith 1982). In women, bone loss has three phases. The first phase starts around 30 to 35 years of age and proceeds at a rate of 0.75% to 1% per year until the menopause. From menopause until about five years after menopause the rate of bone loss increases to between 2% and 3% per year. During the final phase, the rate of bone loss is approximately 1% per year. Thus, women may lose, on average, about 53% of their peak bone mass by the age of 80 years. In contrast, men may lose, on average, about 18% of their peak bone mass by the age of 80 years (Figure 3.29).

Even though body weight tends to decrease with age, the rate of bone loss is usually much greater than the rate at which body weight decreases. Consequently, the effect of bone loss is that the bones, especially weight-bearing bones, become progressively weaker relative to the weight of the rest of the body. In addition to a gradual decrease in strength, the bones also gradually lose their elasticity (owing to loss of collagen) and, as a result, become progressively more brittle. In some individuals, especially women, the loss of bone mass and elasticity may decrease to a level where some bones are no longer able to withstand the loads imposed by normal habitual activity. Consequently, these bones become very susceptible to fracture. This condition, the most common bone disorder in elderly people, is called osteoporosis (Frost 2004). Osteoporosis may cause severe disfigurement, especially of the trunk, owing to fractured or crushed vertebrae. Many deaths in the elderly are due to complications arising from bone fractures that occur as a result of osteoporosis (Cummings and Melton 2002).

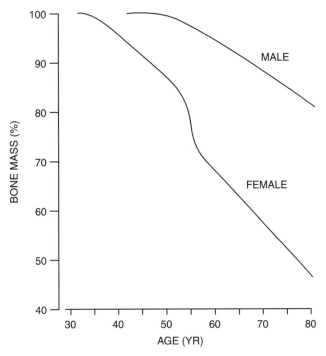

Figure 3.29 Effect of aging on bone mass.

Bone loss tends to occur earlier and to proceed at a faster rate in cancellous bone than in compact bone (Bailey *et al.* 1986). Consequently, regions of bones with a high proportion of cancellous bone, such as the bodies of the vertebrae, the head and neck of the femur, and the distal end of the radius, are particularly vulnerable to osteoporosis and, therefore, to fracture in elderly people. This vulnerability is reflected in studies indicating a rapid increase in the incidence of bone fractures with age, especially in women. For example, the results of one study showed that the incidence of fracture to the distal end of the radius was seven times higher in 54-year-old women than in 40-year-old women (Bauer 1960). In another study, the incidence of fracture of the neck of the femur was found to be 50 times higher in 70-year-old women than in 40-year-old women (Chalmers and Ho 1970). With regard to compact bone, bone loss occurs mainly on the endosteal surface so that bone width remains relatively unchanged into old age (Smith 1982; Seeman 2008).

Whereas the cause of osteoporosis is not yet clear, there is general agreement that four variables have a major influence on the onset and progression of osteoporosis: genetic factors, endocrine status, nutritional factors and physical activity (Bailey *et al.* 1986; Bergmann *et al.* 2011). The relative contribution of these variables has not yet been established, but the level of physical activity seems to have a major influence. In the absence of weight-bearing activity, no amount of endocrine or nutritional intervention will prevent rapid bone loss; there must be mechanical stress (Bailey *et al.* 1986; Frost 2004). Research suggests that regular moderate physical activity throughout life can help to prevent osteoporosis in three ways (Kohrt *et al.* 2004; Maddalozzo *et al.* 2007; Kemmler *et al.* 2007):

1. Peak bone mass is directly related to the level of physical activity prior to peak bone mass; the higher the peak bone mass, the lower the risk of osteoporosis.
2. An above-average level of physical activity after peak bone mass will delay the onset of bone loss.
3. An above-average level of physical activity after peak bone mass will reduce the rate of bone loss.

From about 30 years of age in women and about 45 years of age in men, bone mass and bone elasticity gradually decrease. Many people, especially women, develop osteoporosis, which may cause severe disfigurement and in some cases death due to complications arising from osteoporotic bone fractures. The cause of osteoporosis is not yet clear, but lack of mechanical stress appears to be a major influence. Regular physical activity throughout life appears to be the best way of preventing osteoporosis.

REVIEW QUESTIONS

1. Describe the two main functions of connective tissues.

2. Differentiate:

    (i)   Regular and irregular ordinary connective tissues;

    (ii) Intracapsular and extracapsular ligaments;

    (iii) Ligaments and retinacula;

    (iv) Fibrous tissue and elastic tissue.

3. Describe the different types of cell found in ordinary connective tissues.

4. Describe the two main functions of cartilage.

5. Differentiate elasticity and viscoelasticity.

6. Describe the three main mechanical functions of bone.

7. Differentiate:

    (i)   Primary and secondary centres of ossification;

    (ii) Appositional and interstitial growth;

    (iii) Epiphyseal and apophyseal plates;

    (iv) Osteoblasts, osteoclasts and osteocytes;

    (v)   Compact and cancellous bone;

    (vi) Osteopenia and osteoporosis.

Chapter 4

The articular system

The human body is capable of a broad range of movements facilitated by the combined effects of the open-chain arrangement of the bones, the number of joints linking the bones, the different types of joints and the range of movement in the joints. Most joints allow a certain amount of movement and all joints transmit forces. Joints differ in terms of the type and range of movement and the mechanism of force transmission; these differences are reflected in the structure of the joints. This chapter describes the structure and functions of the various types of joint.

OBJECTIVES

After reading this chapter you should be able to do the following:

1. Describe the structural classification of joints.
2. Describe the structure and specific functions of the different forms of fibrous and cartilaginous joints.
3. Describe the structure of a synovial joint.
4. Describe the stability–flexibility classification of joints.
5. Describe the different forms of synovial joint.
6. Describe the functions of joint capsules and ligaments.
7. Differentiate between flexibility, laxity, stability and congruence.

STRUCTURAL CLASSIFICATION OF JOINTS

A joint, also referred to as an articulation or an arthrosis, is defined as a region where two or more bones are connected. The adult skeleton normally has 206 bones linked by approximately 320 joints. The articular system refers to all of the joints of the body. Joints have two main functions: to facilitate relative motion between bones and to transmit forces from one bone to another.

In terms of structure, there are basically two types of joint:

1. Joints in which the articular (opposed) surfaces of the bones are united by either fibrous tissue or cartilage are called fibrous joints and cartilaginous joints, respectively (Figure 4.1a).

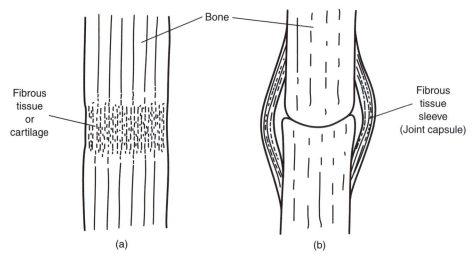

Bone

Fibrous tissue or cartilage

Fibrous tissue sleeve (Joint capsule)

(a)   (b)

Figure 4.1 Two basic types of joint structure. (a) Articular surfaces united by fibrous tissue or cartilage. (b) Articular surfaces not attached to each other but held in contact with each other by a fibrous tissue sleeve.

2. Joints in which the articular surfaces are not attached to each other but are held in contact with each other by a sleeve of fibrous tissue supported by ligaments (Figure 4.1b) are referred to as synovial joints, and the fibrous sleeve is the joint capsule (see Chapter 3).

Fibrous joints

Fibrous joints are often referred to as syndesmoses (*syn* = with, *desmo* = ligament). The degree of movement in a syndesmosis is largely determined by the amount of fibrous tissue between the articular surfaces. In general, the smaller the amount of fibrous tissue, the smaller the range of movement. There are two types of syndesmosis: membranous and sutural.

Membranous syndesmoses

In a membranous syndesmosis, the articular surfaces are united by a sheet of fibrous tissue called an interosseous membrane (*inter* = between, *osseous* = bone). The interosseous membrane functions rather like webbing; it forms a flexible but fairly inextensible link between the articular surfaces. The radius and ulna are connected by an interosseous membrane (Figure 4.2a). The majority of the fibres in the membrane run obliquely downward and medially from the medial border of the radius to the lateral border of the ulna. The remaining fibres run obliquely downward and laterally from the lateral border of the ulna to the medial border of the radius. The interosseous membrane between the radius and ulna has two main functions: to stabilise the bones in all positions of the lower arm, and to provide areas of attachment for muscles on the anterior and posterior aspects of the lower arm (Figure 4.2c). As in the lower arm, there is an interosseous membrane in the lower leg that connects the medial border of the shaft of the fibula and the lateral border of the shaft of the tibia (Figure 4.2b). The interosseous membrane between the fibula and tibia stabilises the bones in all positions

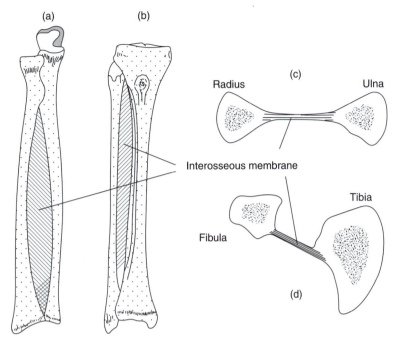

Figure 4.2 Anterior aspects and cross-sectional views of the membranous syndesmoses between (a,c) the right radius and ulna and (b,d) the right tibia and fibula.

of the ankle joint, and provides areas of attachment for muscles on the anterior and posterior aspects of the lower leg (Figure 4.2d).

Whereas the interosseous membranes in the lower arms and lower legs are permanent features, there is a particular group of syndesmoses, the sutures and fontanels of the skull (see Figure 2.6a,c), which originate as membranous syndesmoses and then change to sutural syndesmoses

Sutural syndesmoses

In a sutural syndesmosis the articular surfaces are united by a very thin layer of fibrous tissue. By late childhood, all of the sutures and fontanels of the skull are converted from membranous to sutural syndesmoses (see Figure 2.6). The thin layer of fibrous tissue, together with close interlocking of the articular surfaces, tends to severely restrict movement in these joints. With increasing age, the sutures usually undergo ossification and, as such, are converted to synostoses (*syn* = with, *osteo* = bone).

Cartilaginous joints

The degree of movement in cartilaginous joints is determined by the type and thickness of the cartilage. There are two kinds of cartilaginous joint: synchondroses and symphyses.

Synchondroses

In a synchondrosis (*syn* = with, *chondro* = cartilage), the articular surfaces are united by hyaline cartilage. There are two types of synchondrosis: temporary and permanent. The temporary synchondroses, sometimes referred to as physeal joints, include the following:

1. Joints between bones that eventually fuse together to form larger bones in the adult skeleton; for example, each innominate bone is formed by the fusion of the corresponding ilium, ischium and pubis;
2. Joints formed by epiphyseal plates;
3. Joints formed by apophyseal plates;
4. The joints between the first ribs and the manubrium.

All temporary synchondroses are converted to synostoses at maturity. A few synchondroses, the permanent synchondroses, remain moderately flexible throughout life. These joints include the joints between the anterior ends of the second to the tenth ribs and the sternum (see Figure 2.13).

Symphyses

In a symphysis (*sym* = with, *physis* = growth plate), the articular surfaces are united by a combination of hyaline cartilage and fibrocartilage. A layer of hyaline cartilage covers each articular surface, and a relatively thick piece of fibrocartilage is sandwiched between the layers of hyaline cartilage (Figure 4.3). The fibrocartilage is often referred to as a disc, even though it is usually kidney-shaped or oval. The joint is normally supported by a number of ligaments that cross the outside of the joint and attach onto the periphery of the fibrocartilage. The bone, hyaline cartilage and fibrocartilage in a symphysis joint are intimately connected; there is a gradual change from one region to another. In effect, the joint consists of a single piece of material whose flexibility varies across the joint.

Fibrocartilage readily deforms in response to bending and torsion loads. The degree of movement in a symphysis is largely determined by the thickness of the fibrocartilage; the

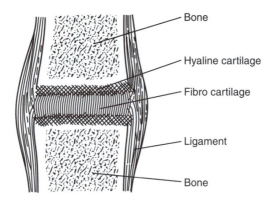

Figure 4.3 A typical symphysis.

thicker the fibrocartilage, the greater the flexibility. The joints between the bodies of the vertebrae (intervertebral joints) and the pubic symphysis are symphyses. Symphyses tend to remain moderately flexible throughout life.

Synovial joints

In the adult skeleton, approximately 80% of the joints are synovial. In general, synovial joints have greater range of movement than fibrous and cartilaginous joints. The body's capacity to adopt a broad range of postures is due largely to the range of movement in synovial joints. Virtually all of the joints in the upper and lower limbs are synovial.

In a synovial joint each articular surface is covered with a layer of articular (hyaline) cartilage. The surfaces are not attached to each other but, under normal circumstances, are held in contact with each other, in all positions of the joint, by a joint capsule and various ligaments (Figure 4.4). During movement of a synovial joint, the articular surfaces slide and roll on each other. The capsule encloses a joint cavity that, because of the close contact between the articular surfaces, is normally very small. In Figure 4.4, the joint cavity is shown much larger than normal to differentiate the features of the joint. The inner wall of the capsule and the non-articular bony surfaces inside the joint are covered with synovial membrane. Synovial membrane consists of areolar tissue (see Chapter 3) with specialised cells that secrete synovial fluid into the joint cavity. Synovial fluid is viscous and resembles raw egg white. It has two important functions:

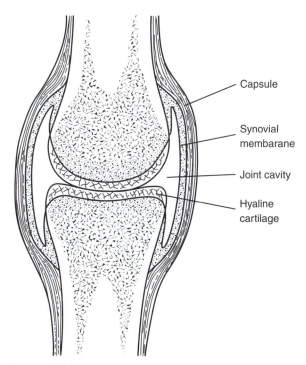

Capsule

Synovial membarane

Joint cavity

Hyaline cartilage

Figure 4.4 A typical synovial joint.

A mechanical function: The fluid lubricates the articular surfaces so that they slide over each other easily, thereby preventing excessive wear.

A physiological function: The fluid seeps into the articular cartilage and nourishes the cartilage cells.

In terms of structure, there are two basic types of joint:

- Joints in which the articular surfaces are united by either fibrous tissue (fibrous joints) or cartilage (cartilaginous joints);
- Joints in which the articular surfaces are not attached to each other, but are held in contact with each other by a joint capsule and ligaments (synovial joints).

Congruence, articular discs and menisci

The articular surfaces in most synovial joints are reciprocally shaped, which normally results in a large contact area (relative to the area of the articular surfaces) between the opposed articular surfaces in all positions of the joint (Frost 1999). For any particular joint position, the larger the contact area between the articular surfaces (the larger the area over which the joint reaction force is transmitted), the lower the compressive stress on the articular surfaces, and vice versa. Some synovial joints, such as the tibiofemoral joint, do not have reciprocally shaped articular surfaces so that, in the absence of other structures, the area of contact between the articular surfaces in any particular joint position would be relatively small and the compressive stress very high (see Figure 2.23). However, in such joints the effective area of contact between the articular surfaces is normally as large as in joints with reciprocally shaped articular surfaces, owing to the presence of fibrocartilaginous wedges between the unopposed parts of the articular surfaces that distribute the joint reaction force over a large area of the articular surfaces. The fibrocartilaginous wedges are not attached to the articular surfaces but are normally held in contact with the articular surfaces by attachment to the inner wall of the joint capsule or by attachment to bone adjacent to the articular surface (Figure 4.5).

In the acromioclavicular joint, and sometimes the ulnocarpal joint, there is a single fibrocartilage wedge in the form of a ring that tapers from the outside toward the centre (Figure 4.5a). In the tibiofemoral joint there are normally two C-shaped fibrocartilage wedges; each wedge is called a meniscus (for its crescent-moon shape; Figure 4.5b). In some joints, such as the sternoclavicular and ulnocarpal joints, there is usually a complete disc of fibrocartilage that effectively divides the joint into two joints (Figure 4.5c,d). A complete disc of fibrocartilage is referred to as an articular disc.

The congruence of a synovial joint refers to the area of contact between the articular surfaces; in any particular joint position, the greater the area of contact, the greater the congruence of the joint, and vice versa. Greater congruence will tend to improve joint function by:

(a)   (b)

(c)   (d)

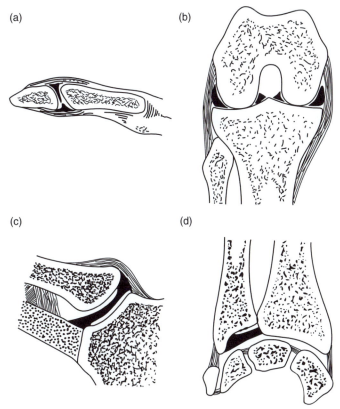

Figure 4.5 Articular discs and menisci. (a) Coronal section through the right acromioclavicular joint. (b) Coronal section through the right tibiofemoral joint with the joint flexed at approximately 90°. (c) Coronal section through the right sternoclavicular joint. (d) Coronal section through the left wrist joint.

- Reducing compressive stress on the opposed articular surfaces;
- Helping maintain effective distribution of synovial fluid over the articular surfaces and, in turn, normal joint movements (the normal combination of rolling and sliding between the opposed articular surfaces);
- Improving shock absorption.

One of the main functions of articular discs and menisci is to improve congruence in synovial joints. Damage to articular discs and menisci (usually as a result of tearing) is likely to adversely affect joint function and, in particular, result in progressive damage to the articular surfaces.

Whereas most joints fit exclusively into one of the main categories of joint (fibrous, cartilaginous, synovial), some joints have or develop characteristics of more than one category. Synovial joints with articular discs or menisci are examples of this variation and reflect the capacity of the skeletal system for structural adaptation, i.e. the capacity to modify structure to match changes in functional requirements (see Chapter 7).

JOINT MOVEMENTS

The type of movement that occurs in a joint, i.e. the direction and range of movement of an articular surface with respect to its opposed articular surface (and, therefore, the change in the orientation of the bones to each other), depends on the type of joint and the shape of the articular surfaces.

Degrees of freedom

Figure 4.6 shows the position of the reference axes (Figure 2.3) in relation to the shoulder joint. With respect to the reference axes, there are six possible directions, called degrees of freedom, in which the shoulder joint, or any other joint, might be able to move, depending upon its structure. The six directions consist of three linear directions (along the axes) and three angular directions (around the axes). A joint with six degrees of freedom could move in any direction by a combination of linear and angular movements. Some cartilaginous joints have six degrees of freedom, albeit with a small range of movement. In contrast, the larger synovial joints tend to have no linear degrees of freedom, but they usually have one to three angular degrees of freedom with a relatively large range of movement.

Most movements in everyday life, such as walking, bending and reaching, involve simultaneous or sequential movement in two or more joints. In such multijoint movements, the number of degrees of freedom in that part of the skeletal system responsible for the movement is the sum of the number of degrees of freedom of the individual joints involved.

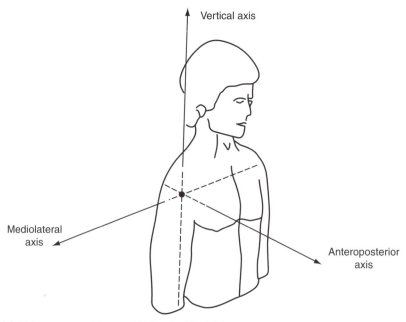

Figure 4.6 Reference axes with respect to the shoulder joint.

Consequently, there are an almost infinite number of combinations of joint movements that could be employed in all multijoint movements. Furthermore, temporary or permanent impairment in one joint can usually be compensated for by a change in the movement of other joints.

Angular movements

Angular movements in joints refer to rotations around the three reference axes. With the anatomical position as a reference position, special terms describe the various angular movements.

In most joints, the terms abduction and adduction refer to rotations around the anteroposterior axis. In the shoulder, wrist and hip joints, abduction and adduction refer to movement of the arm, hand and leg away from and toward the median plane, respectively (Figure 4.7a,b,c). In the hand and foot, abduction of the fingers and toes occurs when the fingers and toes are spread, and adduction occurs when the fingers and toes are returned to the reference position (Figure 4.7d).

In most joints, the terms flexion and extension refer to rotation around the mediolateral axis. In the shoulder, wrist and hip joints, flexion refers to movement of the arm, hand and leg forward, and extension refers to movement of the arm, hand and leg backward (Figure 4.8a,b,c). In the elbow, knee, and metacarpophalangeal and interphalangeal (hand and foot) joints, flexion occurs when the joints bend and extension occurs when the joints straighten (Figure 4.8d,e). In the trunk (the vertebral column as a whole), flexion refers to bending the trunk forward and extension refers to the reverse movement (Figure 4.9a,b). Lateral flexion of the trunk occurs when the trunk bends to the side about an anteroposterior axis (Figure4.9c).

Some bones, such as the humerus at the shoulder and the femur at the hip, can rotate axially, i.e. rotate about an axis along, parallel to, or close to parallel to the long axis of the

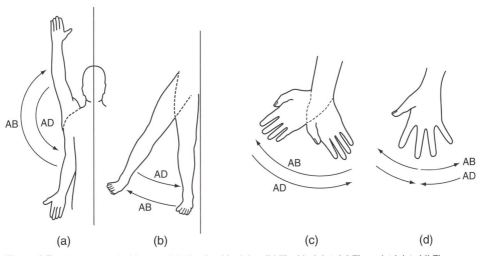

(a)   (b)   (c)   (d)

Figure 4.7 Abduction and adduction. (a) The shoulder joint. (b) The hip joint. (c) The wrist joint. (d) The fingers.

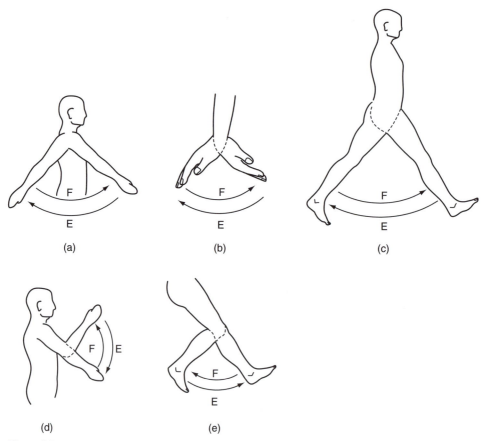

Figure 4.8 Flexion and extension. (a) The shoulder joint. (b) The wrist joint. (c) The hip joint. (d) The elbow joint. (e) The tibiofemoral joint.

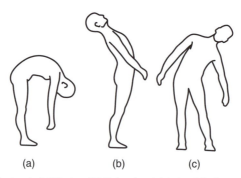

Figure 4.9 Movement of the trunk. (a) Flexion. (b) Extension. (c) Lateral flexion.

moving bone. For example, internal rotation (medial rotation) of the hip occurs when the anterior aspect of the femur is rotated toward (toes move toward the median plane) the median plane. Similarly, external rotation (lateral rotation) of the hip occurs when the anterior aspect of the femur is rotated away from (toes move away from the median plane) the median plane.

SYNOVIAL JOINT CLASSIFICATION

Synovial joints are classified according to the type of movement that occurs in the joints. There are two kinds of synovial joint:

1. Joints in which the main type of movement is linear. Sliding occurs in all synovial joints to a certain extent, but in these joints, called gliding or plane joints, the articular surfaces are normally fairly flat and slide on each other in one or more directions. Gliding joints include some intercarpal joints, some intertarsal joints and the facet joints of the vertebrae.
2. Joints in which the main type of movement is angular. Movement in these joints is normally a combination of rolling and sliding between the articular surfaces. There are three groups: uniaxial, biaxial and multiaxial.

Uniaxial

In uniaxial joints, movement normally takes place mainly about a single axis. There are two types of uniaxial joint, hinge joints and pivot joints. In a hinge joint, a convex, pulley-shaped (bicondylar) articular surface articulates with a reciprocally shaped concave surface. The elbow (humero-ulnar), interphalangeal and ankle joints are hinge joints (Figure 4.10). The

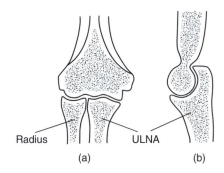

Radius   ULNA

(a)   (b)

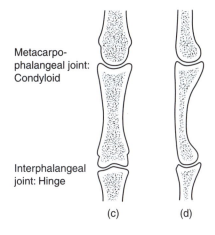

Metacarpo-
phalangeal joint:
Condyloid

Interphalangeal
joint: Hinge

(c)   (d)

Figure 4.10 Hinge and condyloid joints. (a) Coronal section through the right elbow joint in extension. (b) Sagittal section through the right humero-ulnar joint in extension. (c,d) Coronal and sagittal sections, respectively, through metacarpophalangeal and interphalangeal joints in extension.

101

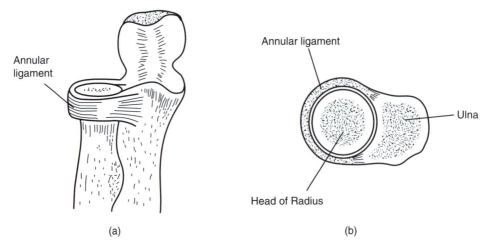

Annular
ligament

Annular ligament

Ulna

Head of Radius

(a)   (b)

Figure 4.11 A typical pivot joint. (a) Anterior aspect of the right proximal radio-ulnar joint. (b) Transverse section through the right proximal radio-ulnar joint.

notch of the pulley prevents (or severely limits) side-to-side movement. The tibiofemoral joint is usually regarded as a hinge joint, even though the articular surfaces of the femoral and tibial condyles are not very congruent. However, in the normal tibiofemoral joint, the congruence between the articular surfaces is considerably increased by the presence of menisci.

In a pivot joint, a cylindrical articular surface rotates about its long axis within a ring formed of bone and fibrous tissue. The proximal radio-ulnar joint is a pivot joint (Figure 4.11). The head of the radius is held against the radial notch by a ligament called the annular ligament (*annulus* = ring). During supination and pronation of the forearm (external and internal rotation of the forearm, as in using a screwdriver), the head of the radius rotates within the ring formed by the annular ligament and the radial notch.

Biaxial

In biaxial joints, movement mainly takes place about two axes at right angles to each other, usually the anteroposterior (abduction–adduction) and mediolateral (flexion–extension) axes. There are three types of biaxial joint: condyloid, ellipsoid and saddle. In a condyloid joint, a convex condylar surface articulates with a concave condylar surface. The metacarpophalangeal joints are condyloid joints. In an ellipsoid joint, such as the radiocarpal joint, an elliptical convex surface articulates with an elliptical concave surface. The articular surface on the distal end of the radius is elliptical, concave and shallow. This surface articulates with the proximal articular surfaces of the scaphoid and lunate, which together form a convex elliptical articular surface. Movements at the metacarpophalangeal joints and radiocarpal joints are normally combinations of flexion, extension, abduction and adduction. In a saddle (or sellar) joint, the articular surfaces are saddle-shaped. Each articular surface is convex in one direction and concave in a direction at right angles to the convex direction. Movement takes place mainly in two planes at right angles to each other. The carpometacarpal joint of the thumb and the calcaneocuboid joints are saddle joints.

Multiaxial

Some joints, such as the shoulder and hip, can rotate about all three reference axes. By combining rotations about the three reference axes, these joints can rotate about any axis in between the three. Consequently, these joints are referred to as multiaxial joints. In this type of joint, a hemispherical articular surface articulates with a cuplike concavity. Owing to the shapes of the articular surfaces, these joints are usually referred to as ball-and-socket joints.

> Synovial joints are classified according to the types of movement that they allow. Joints in which the main type of movement is linear are called gliding or plane joints. Joints in which the main type of movement is angular are classified into uniaxial (hinge and pivot), biaxial (condyloid, ellipsoid and saddle) and multiaxial (ball-and-socket) joints.

FLEXIBILITY, STABILITY AND LAXITY IN SYNOVIAL JOINTS

In previous sections of this chapter, the terms flexibility and stability have been used in a general sense. At this point it is necessary to define these terms more specifically in relation to synovial joints.

Flexibility

In a synovial joint, flexibility refers to the range of movement in those directions (degrees of freedom) considered normal for the joint. For example, the tibiofemoral joint is designed primarily to rotate about a mediolateral axis, i.e. for flexion and extension. Consequently, flexion and extension are considered normal movements at the tibiofemoral joint. However, rotations about an anteroposterior axis, abduction and adduction, are considered abnormal movements at the tibiofemoral joint. The flexibility of a joint is determined by four factors:

1. The shape of the articular surfaces;
2. Tension in the joint capsule and ligaments at the ends of the various ranges of motion;
3. Soft tissue bulk, mainly skeletal muscle, surrounding the bones forming the joint;
4. The extensibility of the skeletal muscles controlling the movement of the joint.

Shape of articular surfaces

In some joints, flexibility is limited by the impingement or interlocking of the non-articular surfaces of the bones at the end of certain ranges of motion. For example, elbow extension is restricted by the interlocking of the olecranon process of the ulna with the olecranon fossa of the humerus (Figure 4.12a). Similarly, elbow flexion is restricted by the interlocking of the coronoid process of the ulna with the coronoid fossa of the humerus (Figure 4.12b). Lateral and medial displacement of the radius and ulna relative to the humerus in the elbow joint is severely restricted by the interlocking of the articular surfaces (Figure 4.12c).

103

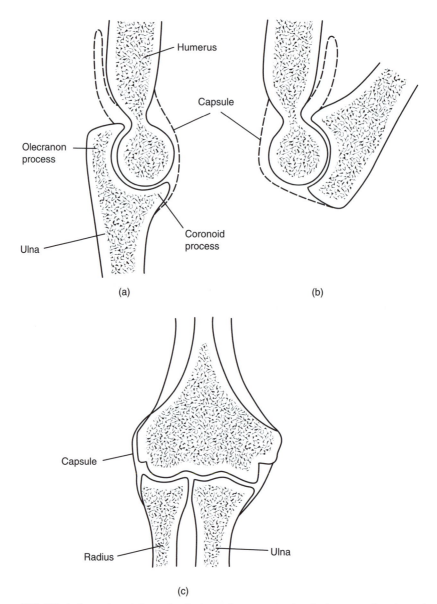

Figure 4.12 Effect of capsule and shape of articular surfaces on extension–flexion range of motion and abduction–adduction range of motion in the elbow joint. (a) Sagittal section through the elbow joint in extension. (b) Sagittal section through the elbow joint in flexion. (c) Coronal section through the elbow joint in extension.

Tension in joint capsule and ligaments

The function of ligaments is described in detail later in the chapter. At this point, it is sufficient to appreciate that in a normal joint, the joint capsule and some of the ligaments that support the joint become taut at the end of each range of movement, thereby restricting further movement (Figure 4.12).

Soft tissue bulk

Soft tissue bulk restricts flexibility in some joints. For example, elbow and knee flexion may be restricted in a heavily muscled individual by the impingement of the adjacent body segments.

Extensibility of muscles

The muscle extensibility is the maximum length that a musculotendinous unit can attain without injury. Muscle extensibility largely depends on the length range in which the muscle normally functions, i.e. the difference between its length when shortened and its length when extended. Generally speaking, the shorter the length range, the lower the extensibility. In the absence of regular flexibility training, games and sports involving highly repetitive and exclusive movement patterns are likely to result in reduced extensibility in some muscles. In most individuals, muscle extensibility is probably the main factor limiting joint flexibility (Nicholas and Marino 1987; Herbert 1988).

Stability and laxity

In a synovial joint, stability refers to the degree of congruence between the articular surfaces. During joint movement, different parts of the articular surfaces come into contact with each other. However, in all positions of a joint, the greater the congruence, the more stable the joint and the lower the risk of abnormal joint movements. The term laxity refers to the degree of instability in a joint, i.e. the range of movement in those directions considered abnormal for the joint. Joint congruence is determined by three factors:

1. The shape of the articular surfaces;
2. Suction between the articular surfaces;
3. Supporting structures: skeletal muscles, ligaments and the joint capsule.

Shape of articular surfaces

Most synovial joints have fairly congruent articular surfaces in all joint positions. In those joints where the articular surfaces are not very congruent, articular discs or menisci are usually present to improve congruence. Perfect congruence between articular surfaces would maximise joint stability and minimise joint laxity. However, perfect congruence would impair nutrition of the articular cartilage by restricting the flow of synovial fluid over the articular surfaces. Consequently, most joints are slightly incongruent and usually have a slight degree of laxity.

Suction between articular surfaces

In a normal joint, the articular surfaces are usually in close contact, with a thin film of synovial fluid between the surfaces. This film of fluid allows sliding between the surfaces but keeps the surfaces in contact with each other by suction. In a similar manner, it is often difficult to separate two sheets of glass held in contact with each other by a thin film of water, even though the two sheets will slide on each other.

Supporting structures

The supporting structures largely responsible for maintaining close contact between the articular surfaces in all positions of a joint are the skeletal muscles that control the movement of the joint and the ligaments of the joint.

Functions of joint capsule and ligaments

The joint capsule has two main functions:

1. To assist joint stabilisation by helping prevent (a) movement beyond normal ranges and (b) excessive laxity;
2. To provide a base for the synovial membrane.

At the end of each normal range of movement, part of the joint capsule will usually become taut to prevent movement beyond the normal range. For example, in full extension of the elbow, the anterior aspect of the capsule will be taut and the posterior aspect will be slack (Figure 4.12a). Similarly, in full flexion of the elbow, the posterior aspect of the capsule will be taut and the anterior will be slack (Figure 4.12b). With regard to abnormal ranges of movement, the regions of the joint capsule in the planes of abnormal ranges of movement are usually at their natural length, i.e. neither taut nor slack. However, these regions quickly become taut in response to abnormal movements, thereby helping to restrict the ranges of abnormal movements. For example, abduction and adduction are abnormal movements at the elbow, and the joint capsule normally helps to prevent these movements (Figure 4.12c).

In association with skeletal muscles, ligaments bring about normal movement in joints. In a normal joint, ligaments help to maintain maximum stability in all positions of the joint by guiding the movements of the joint. During normal movements, the tension in ligaments is low to moderate; ligaments only become taut to prevent or restrict abnormal movements. An abnormal movement may be defined as any movement that results in a decrease in normal congruence, i.e. any movement that results in complete distraction (separation) of the articular surfaces, referred to as luxation, or partial distraction, referred to as subluxation.

Subluxations are usually transient; normal congruence is usually restored as soon as the load causing the subluxation is removed. Subluxations often result in joint sprains, i.e. partial tearing of ligaments and the joint capsule, together with effusion (swelling) in the joint. Like subluxations, luxations are usually transient. A luxation that persists after the load causing it is removed is a dislocation (Figure 4.13). A dislocation usually requires manipulation by a physician or paramedic to restore the normal relationship between the articular surfaces (Grana *et al.* 1987). Dislocation usually results in considerable damage to ligaments and the joint capsule.

Considerable force is required to cause severe subluxations and luxations. Ligaments and joint capsules are likely to be subjected to very high forces in two particular situations:

106

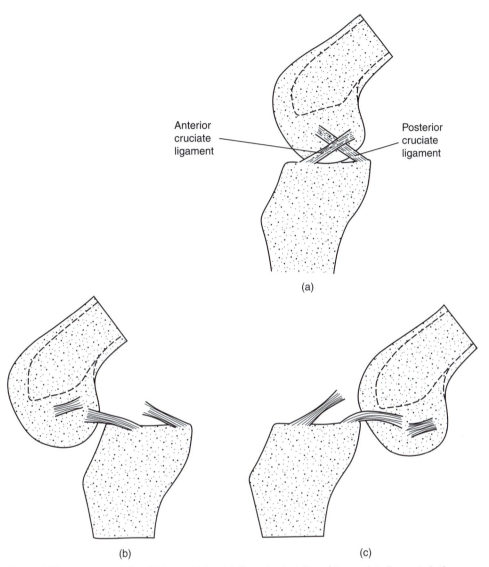

Anterior cruciate ligament

Posterior cruciate ligament

(a)

(b)

(c)

Figure 4.13 Dislocation of the tibiofemoral joint. (a) Normal orientation of the cruciate ligaments in the partially flexed tibiofemoral joint. (b) Anterior dislocation of the femur on the tibia, showing torn posterior cruciate ligament. (c) Posterior dislocation of the femur on the tibia, showing torn anterior cruciate ligament.

1. Unexpected situations in which the degree of muscular control of joint movement is less than adequate, for example, twisting an ankle by stepping on an uneven surface. In this situation, with the body moving forward over the foot, the ankle is likely to be rapidly and forcibly twisted.
2. High speed collisions, such as a tackle in football.

There are two kinds of abnormal movement in joints: hyperflexibility and excessive laxity. These will be described with reference to the tibiofemoral joint.

Hyperflexibility

Hyperflexibility may be defined as movement beyond the normal range of movement in a direction considered normal for the joint. Extension is a normal movement in the tibiofemoral joint. At full extension of the tibiofemoral joint, the four main ligaments that support the joint will become taut to prevent further movement. If the joint is forcibly extended beyond this position, i.e. hyperextended, the ligaments and joint capsule will be damaged (Figure 4.14). Hyperextension of the tibiofemoral joint is an example of hyperflexibility. In most individuals, full extension of the tibiofemoral joint normally corresponds to a position in which the leg is straight, i.e. the upper and lower legs are in line. Consequently, in most individuals, hyperextension of the tibiofemoral joint occurs when the joint is extended beyond the straight position. However, some individuals are able to voluntarily extend their tibiofemoral joints slightly beyond the straight position. In these cases, extension of the joints beyond the straight position would be considered normal for the individual, provided that normal congruence was maintained.

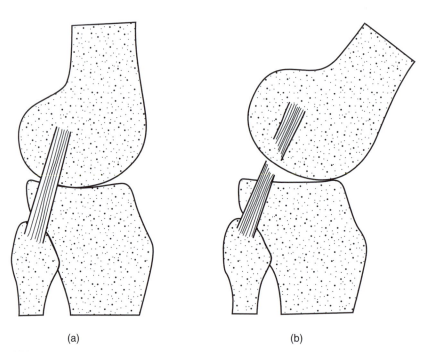

(a)   (b)

Figure 4.14 Hyperextension of the tibiofemoral joint. (a) Lateral aspect of the extended right tibiofemoral joint, showing the normal orientation of the lateral ligament. (b) Hyperextension of the tibiofemoral joint, showing torn lateral ligament.

Excessive laxity

Excessive laxity is defined as movement beyond the normal degree of laxity in directions considered abnormal for the joint. For example, abduction and adduction are abnormal movements in the tibiofemoral joint. In a normal tibiofemoral joint these movements are restricted to a minimal level by the medial and lateral ligaments, respectively (Figure 4.15). Abduction of the tibiofemoral joint beyond a minimal level will damage the medial ligament and joint

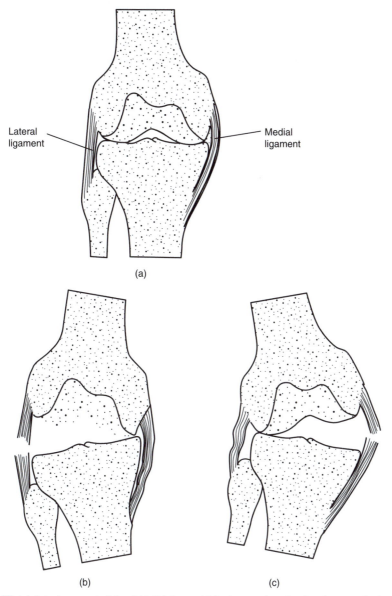

Figure 4.15 (a) Anterior aspect of the right tibiofemoral joint in extension, showing the normal orientation of the lateral and medial ligaments. (b) Adduction of the tibiofemoral joint, showing torn lateral ligament. (c) Abduction of the tibiofemoral joint showing torn medial ligament.

109

capsule. Similarly, adduction of the joint beyond a minimal level will damage the lateral ligament and joint capsule.

Movements of the femoral condyles backward and forward (along the anteroposterior axis) relative to the tibial condyles are abnormal movements. In a normal tibiofemoral joint, these movements are restricted to a minimal level by the anterior and posterior cruciate ligaments, respectively (Figure 4.13). Forward movement of the femoral condyles beyond a minimal level will damage the posterior cruciate ligament and the joint capsule. Similarly, backward movement of the femoral condyles beyond a minimal level will damage the anterior cruciate ligament and the joint capsule.

Any degree of hyperflexibility or excessive laxity in a joint tends to damage not only ligaments and joint capsules, but also the articular cartilage. The damage to articular cartilage is caused by localised overloading as a result the abnormal movements.

Movement between articular surfaces

Three types of movement occur between articular surfaces: spinning, sliding and rolling. In most joints, normal movement involves a combination of these three types of movement, either simultaneously or sequentially. Sliding, and to a lesser extent spinning, subjects the articular cartilage to compression and shear loading. Rolling subjects the articular cartilage to compression loading. These loads tend to cause mechanical wear of the articular cartilage in the form of damage to the surface of the cartilage and to the internal structure of the cartilage. Under normal circumstances, when the articular surfaces are congruent and properly lubricated, there is a balance between the amount of wear and the production of new cartilage. However, during subluxations, those parts of the articular cartilage that remain in contact are subjected to abnormally high loads. Over a period of time, the wear caused by the abnormal loads may outpace the production of new cartilage and result in permanent damage to the cartilage.

Flexibility training

In normal healthy individuals, ligaments and joint capsules, like musculotendinous units, adapt to the length range in which they normally function. Consequently, if a joint is not regularly moved through the full range of movement, the ligaments and joint capsule shorten, preventing full range of normal movement. In this context, the full range of normal movement is the range of movement between positions of the joint where subluxation of the articular surfaces occurs.

Flexibility training, in the form of a carefully prescribed programme of exercises designed to lengthen ligaments and joint capsules and to increase the extensibility of musculotendinous units, may restore full ranges of movement. As previously mentioned, lack of muscle extensibility, rather than shortened ligaments and joint capsules, is probably the main factor limiting flexibility in most individuals. During flexibility training, great care must be taken to ensure that ligaments and joint capsules are not stretched to the point where joints become hyperflexible. If this happens, the overstretched ligaments and joint capsules will not be able to function properly; the joints will be less stable in all joint positions, and abnormal movements will become more likely.

REVIEW QUESTIONS

1. Describe the two main functions of joints.

2. Describe the two main types of joint in terms of structure.

3. Differentiate a syndesmosis and a symphysis.

4. Describe the basic structure of a synovial joint.

5. With respect to synovial joints, differentiate the following:

   • Flexibility and laxity;

   • Stability and congruence;

   • Subluxation and dislocation.

6. Describe the function of ligaments in relation to synovial joints.

Chapter 5

The neuromuscular system

The muscular system is the interface between the nervous and skeletal systems. The muscles produce the forces that determine the movement of the joints, but the nervous system determines the intensity and timing of the muscle forces. The nervous system constantly monitors and interprets information from the various senses concerning body position and body movement, including information from muscles and joint supporting structures, and on the basis of this information sends instructions to the muscles to coordinate body movement. Those parts of the nervous and muscular systems responsible for bringing about coordinated body movement are referred to as the neuromuscular system. This chapter describes the structure and function of the neuromuscular system.

OBJECTIVES

After reading this chapter you should be able to do the following:

1. Differentiate the cerebrospinal nervous system, autonomic nervous system, central nervous system and peripheral nervous system.
2. Describe the events resulting in transmission of an impulse along a nerve fibre and from one nerve fibre to another.
3. Describe the general organisation of nerve tissue in the brain, spinal cord and spinal nerves.
4. Describe the structure of a skeletal muscle fibre and the organisation of fibres in pennate and non-pennate muscles.
5. Differentiate kinaesthetic sense and proprioception.
6. Describe the length–tension relationship in a sarcomere, muscle fibre and muscle–tendon unit.
7. Describe the force–velocity relationship and stretch–shorten cycle in skeletal muscle.

THE NERVOUS SYSTEM

The nervous system consists of approximately 13 000 million nerve cells, called neurons, and an equally large number of specialised connective tissue cells, called glial cells. Neurons are specialised to conduct electrochemical impulses rapidly throughout the body, to coordinate all the essential biological functions. The cells of the nervous system are organised into two functional divisions and two structural divisions (Standring 2008). The functional divisions are the cerebrospinal nervous system and the autonomic nervous system.

The cerebrospinal nervous system, also known as the somatic, craniospinal or voluntary nervous system, is under voluntary control except for reflex movements. A reflex movement provides protection by rapidly removing part of the body from a source of danger without conscious effort. The cerebrospinal nervous system includes those parts of the nervous system concerned with consciousness and mental activities, as well as control of skeletal muscle. The autonomic nervous system, also known as the visceral or involuntary nervous system, is not under voluntary control; it includes those parts of the nervous system that control the visceral muscles, the heart and the exocrine and endocrine glands.

The two structural divisions of the nervous system are the central nervous system and the peripheral nervous system. The central nervous system consists of the brain and spinal cord. The peripheral nervous system consists of 43 pairs of nerves (bundles of nerve fibres), which arise from the base of the brain and the spinal cord (Figure 5.1). The upper 12 pairs of nerves

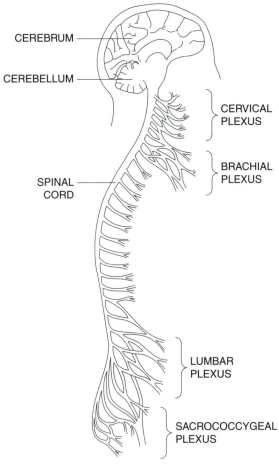

CEREBRUM

CEREBELLUM

CERVICAL PLEXUS

BRACHIAL PLEXUS

SPINAL CORD

LUMBAR PLEXUS

SACROCOCCYGEAL PLEXUS

Figure 5.1 The central nervous system consists of the brain (cerebrum and cerebellum) and spinal cord. The peripheral nervous system consists of the spinal nerves. Many of the spinal nerves link together to form plexuses. All of the spinal nerves and plexuses branch profusely throughout the regions of the body that they innervate.

113

arise from the base of the brain and are called cranial nerves. The other 31 pairs arise from the spinal cord and are called spinal nerves. The cranial and spinal nerves convey information between the central nervous system and the rest of the body.

Neurons

Neurons differ in size and shape, but they all have three common structural features: a cell body, processes of varying length that extend from the cell body and specialised sites for communicating with other neurons, with specialised receptors, such as pain receptors, and with specialised effectors, such as motor end plates in muscles. Neurons are classified by the direction in which they conduct impulses in relation to the brain. Sensory or afferent neurons conduct impulses toward the brain, and motor or efferent neurons conduct impulses away from the brain.

Nerve fibres

The processes that extend from the cell bodies of neurons are called nerve fibres. Nerve fibres vary in length from a few millimetres to more than one metre. There are two types of nerve fibre, dendrites and axons. Dendrites, or afferent fibres, conduct impulses toward the cell body. Axons, or efferent fibres, conduct impulses away from the cell body. In addition to the sensory and motor classification, neurons are classified on the basis of the number of processes arising from the cell body, that is, into pseudounipolar, bipolar and multipolar neurons.

In a pseudounipolar neuron, there appears to be one process arising from the cell body that quickly divides into an afferent fibre and an efferent fibre (Figure 5.2a). Sensory neurons

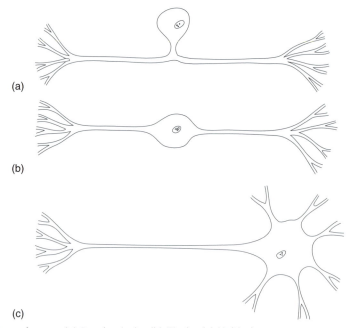

(a)

(b)

(c)

Figure 5.2 Types of neuron. (a) Pseudounipolar. (b) Bipolar. (c) Multipolar.

in the peripheral nervous system are pseudounipolar neurons. A bipolar neuron has two distinct processes, one afferent and one efferent (Figure 5.2b). Bipolar neurons are found in the sensory areas of the eye, ear and nose. Multipolar neurons have numerous relatively short dendrites with a single axon that may branch at various points (Figure 5.2c). Most of the neurons in the brain and spinal cord are multipolar neurons.

Myelinated and non-myelinated nerve fibres

Glial cells provide mechanical and metabolic support to neurons. In the central nervous system there are a variety of glial cells including astrocytes, which provide support for blood vessels, and oligodendrocytes, which provide support for nerve fibres. In the peripheral nervous system, there is only one type of glial cell, Schwann cells (Gamble 1988). All nerve fibres of the peripheral nervous system are enveloped by Schwann cells, which provide the same type of mechanical support as the oligodendrocytes provide for nerve fibres in the central nervous system. The Schwann cells around some fibres produce a fatty substance called myelin, which is deposited around the fibres as a multilayered myelin sheath. The sheath is in the form of a spiral, with up to 100 regularly spaced layers of myelin separated by folds of Schwann cell membrane. The outer fold of the Schwann cell membrane is referred to as the neurilemma (Figure 5.3).

The greater the number of layers of myelin in the sheath, the faster the speed of nerve transmission along the nerve fibre. Nerve fibres that have a myelin sheath are referred to as myelinated or medullated nerve fibres, and nerve fibres that do not are referred to as non-myelinated or non-medullated nerve fibres. Each myelinated nerve fibre is enclosed within a continuous chain of Schwann cells and each Schwann cell envelops approximately 1 mm of nerve fibre. At the junction between adjacent Schwann cells the myelin sheath is interrupted, such that the nerve fibre is only covered by the neurilemma; these regions are referred to as nodes of Ranvier (Figure 5.3a). The nodes of Ranvier facilitate intercellular exchange between the nerve fibres and the surrounding extracellular fluid, which is important for the nutrition of the nerve fibre and for the transmission of impulses along the nerve fibre. Myelinated nerve fibres in the central nervous system are different from those in the peripheral nervous system in that they are not surrounded by Schwann cells (there are no Schwann cells in the central nervous system) and have no neurilemma. It is thought that oligodendrocytes are responsible for the formation of the myelin sheath around these fibres at the embryonic stage (Standring 2008).

Non-myelinated nerve fibres of the peripheral nervous system are also enclosed within continuous chains of Schwann cells. However, in contrast with myelinated fibres, there are no nodes of Ranvier in non-myelinated fibres; as many as nine nerve fibres may be enveloped within the folds of the Schwann cells in the chain (Figure 5.3b).

Nerve fibre endings

The dendrites and axons of all neuron types have a large number of terminal branches or nerve endings devoid of Schwann cells and myelin sheath. There are three types of nerve ending:

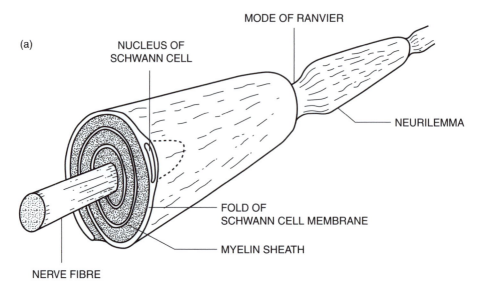

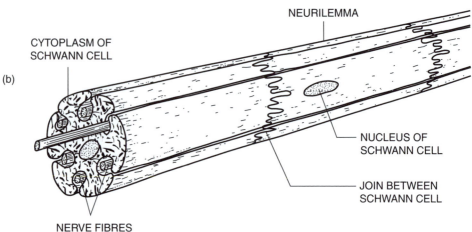

Figure 5.3 Nerve fibres. (a) Myelinated. (b) Non-myelinated.

Sensory: The nerve ending is in contact with a specialised receptor organ, such as a pain receptor;

Motor: The nerve ending is in contact with a specialised effector organ, such as a motor end plate in muscle;

Synapse: The nerve ending is in contact with another neuron.

Sensory and motor nerve endings are referred to as end organs. Neurons that only have synapses at their nerve endings are called association neurons or interneurons.

Nerve impulse transmission

The cytoplasm of a neuron and the extracellular fluid surrounding the neuron contain many different ions (electrically charged atoms). These include positively charged inorganic ions, such as sodium (Na^+) and potassium (K^+), negatively charged inorganic ions, such as chloride (Cl^-), and various organic anions (negatively charged amino acids and proteins (A^-)).

Like most membranes in the body, a nerve fibre membrane is semipermeable, i.e. it has a large number of tiny holes through which ions and small molecules (aggregations of ions) pass from one side of the membrane to the other. The movement of ions through the nerve fibre membrane depends on the permeability of the membrane (the number and size of the holes in the membrane) and the force tending to drive the ions through the membrane. The driving force has electrical, chemical and, in the case of Na^+ and K^+, mechanical components. The electrical component depends on the polarity of the ions; like charges repel each other and unlike charges attract each other. The chemical component depends on the concentration of ions in different regions; ions move from an area of high concentration to areas of lower concentration. The mechanical component results from specialised regions of the membrane collectively referred to as the Na^+-K^+ pump. The Na^+-K^+ pump transports Na^+ out of the cytoplasm and into the extracellular fluid and transports K^+ in the opposite direction.

Under resting conditions, when the nerve fibre is not transmitting an impulse, the net effect of the membrane permeability and the driving forces on the various ions is that the electrical charge on the outside of the fibre membrane is approximately 70 mV (millivolts) higher than on the inside; the potential difference across the membrane is approximately 70 mV, with the inside negative with respect to the outside (Figure 5.4a). This resting potential difference is referred to as the resting membrane potential (RMP) (Enoka, 2008).

The arrival of a stimulus at a nerve fibre in a state of rest alters the permeability of the fibre membrane to Na^+ and K^+ so that Na^+ flows into the cell and K^+ flows out of the cell. The flow of Na^+ into the cell is initially greater than the flow of K^+ out of the cell, so that the potential difference across the membrane decreases. If the decrease in potential difference, which depends on the strength of the stimulus, reaches a critical level, approximately 60 mV (with the inside of the membrane negative with respect to the outside), the membrane will be depolarised, i.e. the potential difference across the fibre membrane rapidly changes by approximately 100 mV from 70 mV, with the inside of the membrane negative with respect to the outside, to approximately 30 mV, with the inside of the membrane positive with respect to the outside (Figure 5.4a).

This change in potential difference constitutes an action potential, which results in a flow of electrical current, called a local current, between the depolarised region of the cell membrane and the adjacent unpolarised regions (both sides) (Figure 5.4b,c). The establishment of the local current results in progressive (rapid wave) depolarisation of the rest of the cell membrane so that the impulse is transmitted along the whole length of the fibre. After depolarisation, the membrane is rapidly repolarised, such that the action potential appears as a spike in a graph of the change in membrane potential with time (Figure 5.4a).

The duration of the action potential spike (depolarisation and repolarisation) is less than one millisecond (Gamble 1988). Repolarisation is due largely to a rapid decrease in the flow

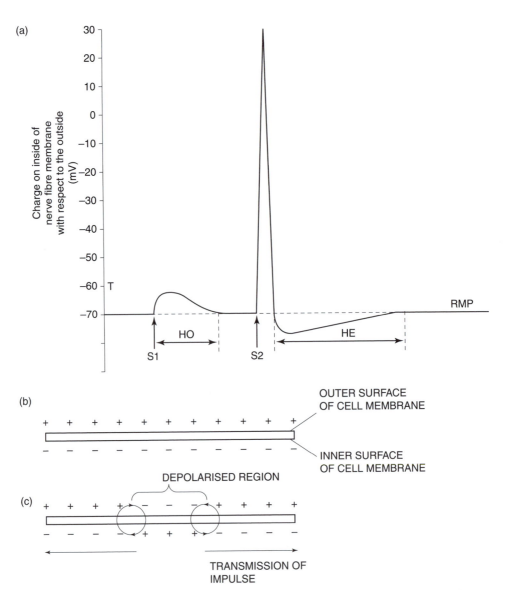

Figure 5.4 Resting membrane potential (RMP) and change in membrane potential. (a) Change in membrane potential in response to stimulation: T, level of hypopolarisation necessary to trigger depolarisation ($T \approx -60$ mV); S_1, a stimulus that results in hypopolarisation but not depolarisation; H_0, period of hypopolarisation following S_1; S_2, a stimulus that results in depolarisation; H_E, period of hyperpolarisation following repolarisation. (b) Electrical charge on nerve fibre membrane at RMP. The charge on the inside of the membrane is approximately −70 mV with respect to the outside. (c) Electrical charge on depolarised region of nerve fibre membrane; the charge on the inside of the membrane is approximately +30 mV with respect to the outside.

of Na^+ into the cell (due to reduced permeability of the membrane to Na^+ ions) and continued flow of K^+ out of the cell. Following repolarisation, there is usually a period (15–100 ms) of hyperpolarisation, in which the potential difference across the membrane is slightly greater than the RMP, as the RMP is gradually restored (Figure 5.4a). A stimulus not strong enough to cause depolarisation results in a period of hypopolarisation prior to restoration of the RMP, i.e. a period in which the potential difference across the membrane is slightly less than the RMP (Figure 5.4a).

Synapses

Each branch of an axon terminates in an end bulb (or end foot) that rests on the surface of a neighbouring neuron to form a synapse, a specialised region that facilitates one-way communication between the two neurons (Figure 5.5). Each neuron synapses with hundreds or thousands of other neurons (Standring 2008). The most common type of synapse is axodendritic (between an axon and a dendrite), but synapses may also be axosomatic (between an axon and a cell body) and axoaxonic (between two axons). A synapse consists of a presynaptic membrane (at the base of the end bulb), a postsynaptic membrane (at the corresponding region of the adjacent neuron), and an intervening synaptic cleft. The end bulb contains a number of synaptic vesicles full of neurotransmitters. Some of the vesicles contain excitatory transmitters and some contain inhibitory transmitters. The arrival of an action potential at a synapse results in the release of neurotransmitters into the synaptic cleft. If excitatory neurotransmitters are released, the postsynaptic membrane will be depolarised, resulting in an action potential and transmission of the impulse. If inhibitory transmitters are released, the postsynaptic membrane will be hyperpolarised, thereby preventing the development of an action potential so that the impulse will not be transmitted.

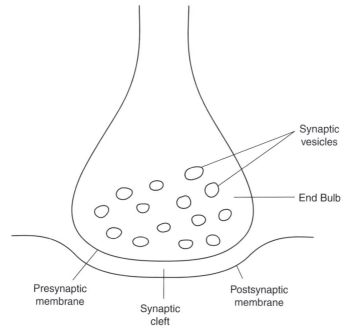

Figure 5.5 A synapse.

Table 5.1 Classification of peripheral nerve fibres (adapted from Gamble 1988).

Class	Speed (m/s)	Innervation
Afferent (sensory) fibres		
Ia	65–130	Muscle spindle intrafusal fibres
Ib	65–130	Golgi tendon organs
II	20–90	Muscle spindle intrafusal fibres, pressure receptors
III	12–45	Temperature and pain receptors
IV	0.2–2.0	Viscera, pain receptors
Efferent (motor) fibres		
Aα	65–130	Fast twitch extrafusal muscle fibres
Aβ	40–80	Slow twitch extrafusal muscle fibres, muscle spindle intrafusal fibres
Aγ	10–50	Muscle spindle intrafusal fibres
B	4–25	Presynaptic autonomics
C	0.2–2.0	Postsynaptic autonomics

Speed of nerve impulse transmission

The speed of transmission or conduction of impulses is directly proportional to the fibre diameter and the thickness of the myelin sheath; the larger the diameter and the thicker the myelin sheath, the faster the speed of conduction. Non-myelinated fibres do not have a myelin sheath and, thus, have much lower conduction speeds than myelinated fibres. Nerve fibres of the peripheral nervous system are classified on the basis of conduction speed and fibre diameter (Table 5.1). There are five main categories of afferent fibre: Ia, Ib, II, III and IV, and five main categories of efferent fibres: Aα, Aβ, Aγ, B and C. Skeletal muscle is innervated by the fastest afferent fibres (Ia and Ib) and the fastest efferent fibres (Aα, Aβ and Aγ).

Nerve tissue organisation in the brain

The brain is the largest and most complex aggregation of neurons in the nervous system. It consists of the cerebrum and the cerebellum (Figure 5.1). The cerebrum occupies most of the cranium and is bigger than the cerebellum. The region of the cerebrum close to and including its surface is called the cerebral cortex and consists of grey matter, i.e. the cell bodies of neurons and their processes, which are largely non-myelinated, together with their synapses and supporting glial cells. The cerebrum is heavily convoluted with fissures of varying depth. The largest fissure is the longitudinal central fissure that divides the cerebrum in the median plane into right and left cerebral hemispheres.

The cerebellum, which occupies the posterior inferior aspect of the cranium, is separated from the cerebrum by the transverse fissure. Like the cerebrum, the region of the cerebellum close to and including its surface consists of grey matter and is called the cerebellar cortex. The cerebellum is not convoluted but is traversed by numerous small furrows. The convolutions of the cerebrum and the furrows of the cerebellum significantly increase their surface areas and, thus, the volume of grey matter. The inner parts of the cerebrum and cerebellum consist of white matter, i.e. largely myelinated nerve fibres organised into groups that link the different parts of the cerebrum and cerebellum with each other and with the spinal cord.

> The brain is the largest and most complex aggregation of neurons in the nervous system. It consists of the cerebrum and the cerebellum. The cerebral cortex and cerebellar cortex consist of grey matter. The inner parts of the cerebrum and cerebellum consist of white matter.

Nerve tissue organisation in the spinal cord and spinal nerves

In transverse section, the spinal cord is roughly oval with an anterior median fissure and a posterior medial septum (Figure 5.6). The central area is dominated by a roughly H-shaped mass of grey matter, with the rest of the cord consisting of white matter in which the groups of fibres run parallel with the spinal cord. The posterior projections (or horns) of the grey matter are continuous with afferent fibres that enter the spinal cord via the left and right dorsal (posterior) roots of the corresponding left and right spinal nerves. The cell bodies of the afferent fibres are located in the dorsal root ganglia; a ganglion is an aggregation of cell bodies outside the spinal cord.

The anterior projections of the grey matter are continuous with efferent fibres that leave the spinal cord via the left and right ventral (anterior) roots of the corresponding spinal nerve. A spinal nerve is formed by the aggregation of the afferent and efferent fibres as they

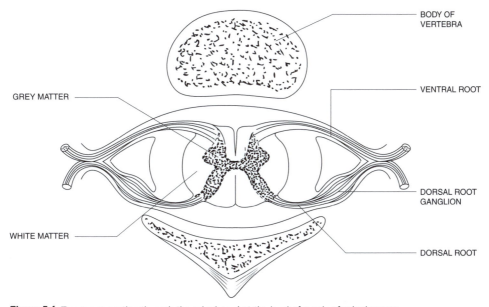

Figure 5.6 Transverse section through the spinal cord at the level of a pair of spinal nerves.

pass through the corresponding intervertebral foramen. Each spinal nerve divides into an anterior and posterior branch just outside the intervertebral foramen; the anterior branch is usually much larger than the posterior branch. In each branch, the individual nerve fibres are enveloped in a thin layer of connective tissue called the endoneurium, which supports a blood capillary network. The fibres are grouped together in bundles called fasciculi or funiculi and each fasciculus is sheathed within a layer of connective tissue called the perineurium. The fasciculi are grouped together and sheathed within another layer of connective tissue called the epineurium to form the complete spinal nerve (Figure 5.7). Each spinal nerve consists of a mixture of myelinated and non-myelinated nerve fibres.

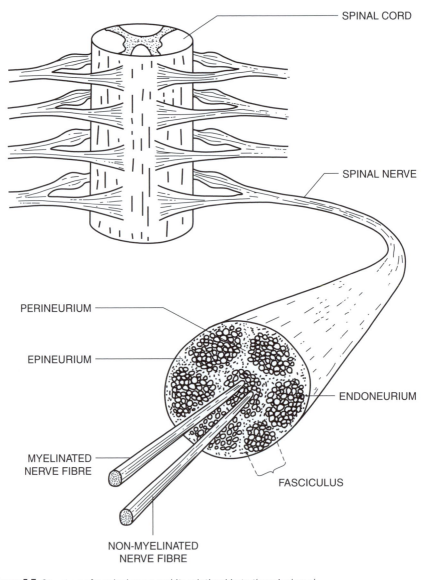

Figure 5.7 Structure of a spinal nerve and its relationship to the spinal cord.

In all regions of the spinal cord apart from most of the thoracic region, the spinal nerves link up with each other on each side of the spinal cord to form networks called plexuses (Figure 5.1). The upper four pairs of cervical nerves form the left and right cervical plexuses, which innervate the head and the upper part of the neck. The other cervical spinal nerves combine with the first pair of thoracic spinal nerves to form the left and right brachial plexuses, which innervate the upper limbs. The twelfth thoracic spinal nerves combine with the lumbar spinal nerves to form the lumbar plexuses, which innervate the lower trunk and pelvis. The sacral and coccygeal spinal nerves, with branches from the fourth and fifth lumbar spinal nerves, combine to form the left and right sacrococcygeal plexuses, which innervate the legs. The second to the eleventh thoracic spinal nerves, which innervate the trunk, do not form plexuses.

Voluntary and reflex movements

The brain interprets sensory information from the various receptors and, on the basis of this information, brings about appropriate responses via effectors to ensure normal bodily functioning. Whereas the autonomic nervous system operates largely at a subconscious level, the cerebrospinal nervous system normally operates at the level of consciousness, i.e. the individual consciously processes information, such as visual, auditory and kinaesthetic (sense of movement) information, and consciously brings about appropriate responses. For example, consider a child just about to touch a hot coffee pot resting on a stove.

1. As the child's hand moves close to the pot, the heat radiating from the pot may excite the heat receptors in the skin of her hand.
2. This information is transmitted by sensory neurons in the peripheral nervous system to the spinal cord, where the nerve endings of the axons of the sensory neurons synapse with many other neurons.
3. Some of these neurons relay the information to the brain centre responsible for heat sensation in the hand, and the child experiences the sensation of heat.
4. Having sensed the heat from the coffee pot, the child decides to move her hand away from the pot to avoid the danger.
5. Impulses are sent from the brain to motor neurons in the spinal cord that innervate the muscles of the arm.
6. The impulses are relayed to the muscles of the arm resulting in movement of the hand away from the coffee pot.

This sequence, illustrated in Figure 5.8, is typical of all voluntary movements. If the child had not sensed the danger and had actually touched the hot coffee pot, she would have jerked her hand away from the pot with lightning speed before she was even conscious of the heat. This extremely rapid involuntary reaction is called a reflex action and is one of a host of similar reflexes that result in instant reactions to protect the body from potentially harmful stimuli. In this particular case, the reflex action results in the child's hand being in contact with the coffee pot for only a fraction of the time it would have taken for the child to take her hand away from the pot voluntarily (and, therefore, consciously). Consequently, the child might

123

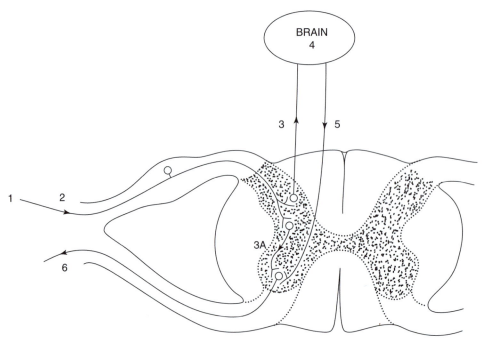

Figure 5.8 Pathway of impulses in voluntary and reflex movements (see text for description of stages).

sustain a relatively slight burn rather than a serious burn, which would have resulted from more prolonged contact with the coffee pot.

The increased speed of a reflex action compared with a voluntary action is due to a reduction in the distance over which the impulses travel from receptor to effector. In this particular case, the heat from the coffee pot is sensed by the heat receptors in the hand, which send impulses to the spinal cord. This is the same as in a voluntary action (Stages 1 and 2 in Figure 5.8). However, in a reflex action, the impulses are transmitted directly across the spinal cord to the motor neurons that innervate the muscles of the arm (Stage 3A in Figure 5.8). The impulses are relayed to the muscles of the arm and the reflex action is completed. Consequently, a reflex action is faster than a voluntary action because no time is spent in transmitting impulses up the spinal cord to the brain, making a decision, and transmitting impulses back down the spinal cord (Stages 3, 4 and 5 in Figure 5.8 are omitted). A reflex action is triggered when the intensity of the impulse output from the receptors is above a certain threshold, indicating extreme danger to the body. In this particular example, the hotter the coffee pot, the greater the intensity of output from the heat receptors and the greater the likelihood of a reflex action being triggered.

As the impulses are transmitted across the spinal cord (stage 3A in Figure 5.8), the impulses are simultaneously transmitted to the brain as in a voluntary action (stage 3 in Figure 5.8). However, stage 3 (transmission of impulses to the brain and sensation of heat) takes longer than stages 3A and 6, such that it is a fraction of a second after the child jerks her hand away from the coffee pot before she perceives any pain in her hand.

Nerve fibre injuries

Injuries to peripheral nerves usually occur as a result of compression or traction (stretching), or a combination of the two (Kleinrensink *et al.* 1994). Compression and traction may damage any or all of the main structures: connective tissue sheaths, Schwann cells, myelin sheaths (when present) and nerve fibres. Compression and traction damage the nerve structures directly, by crushing and tearing, respectively. Prolonged compression may also damage the nerve structures indirectly as a result of ischemia, i.e. a disruption of the local blood supply (due to compression of the local capillary network), which results in a deficiency of oxygen and nutrients to the affected tissues.

Injuries to peripheral nerves are classified according to the degree of structural and functional damage into neuropraxia, axonotmesis and neurotmesis (Seddon 1972). Neuropraxia is the slightest level of damage. It involves damage to Schwann cells and myelin sheaths but little or no damage to nerve fibres or the endoneurium. Neuropraxia is characterised by a disruption to impulse transmission, which is often associated with pain and tingling in the areas innervated by the affected nerves. Recovery of a nerve fibre from neuropraxia usually occurs within 10 to 14 days. In axonotmesis, the nerve fibre and Schwann cell covering or myelin sheath are severed, but the endoneurium remains intact. The severed part of the fibre degenerates. Recovery begins when fibre sprouts emerge from the severed end of the part of the fibre still attached to the cell body. One of the sprouts eventually dominates and gradually grows along the tube formed by the endoneurium. Growth occurs at a rate of approximately 2.5 cm per month, and function gradually returns to normal as the fibre and myelin sheath (when present) returns to normal. In neurotmesis, the nerve fibre, Schwann cell covering or myelin sheath, and endoneurium are all severed. The severed part of the fibre degenerates and without surgical repair it is unlikely that much recovery will occur. With surgical repair some recovery is likely in a manner that is similar to the way that a fibre recovers from axonotmesis, but functional outcome is often less than satisfactory.

> Compression and traction can damage nerves directly by crushing and tearing, respectively. Prolonged compression may damage the nerve structures indirectly as a result of ischemia.

SKELETAL MUSCLE

The composition and basic function of the muscular system are described in Chapter 1. This section describes the macrostructure of skeletal muscle.

Origins and insertions

Most of the muscles are attached to the skeletal system by tendons or aponeuroses. However, one or both attachments of some muscles attach directly onto bone without an

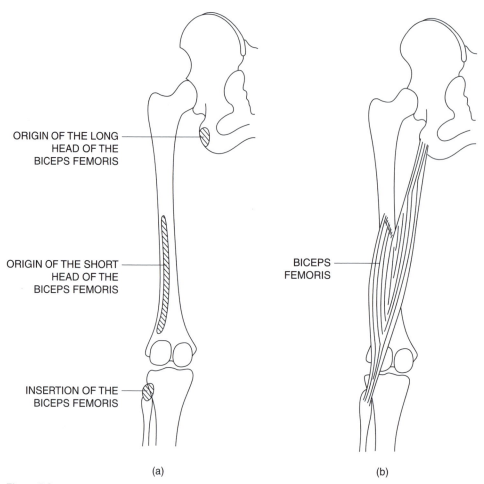

ORIGIN OF THE LONG
HEAD OF THE
BICEPS FEMORIS

ORIGIN OF THE SHORT
HEAD OF THE
BICEPS FEMORIS

INSERTION OF THE
BICEPS FEMORIS

BICEPS
FEMORIS

(a)

(b)

Figure 5.9 Attachments of the biceps femoris.

intervening tendon or aponeurosis. For example, the biceps femoris arises from two sites, a tendinous attachment to the ischial tuberosity, and directly from a long narrow area on the lateral aspect of the femur (Figure 5.9a). The muscle is attached by a single tendon to the head of the fibula and the adjoining posterior aspect of the lateral tibial condyle. Most of the muscles of the upper and lower limbs are arranged in line with the direction of the long bones. For descriptive purposes, the proximal and distal attachments of each of these muscles are referred to as the origins and insertions of the muscles, respectively. For example, the origin of the biceps femoris is on the ischial tuberosity (long head) and femur (short head) and the insertion is on the fibula and tibia (Figure 5.9b). The origins and insertions of the muscles of the trunk and the muscles that link the trunk to the limbs tend to be medial and lateral, respectively, but there are exceptions. The superficial muscles of the body are shown in Appendix I, together with descriptions of their origins and insertions.

Pennate and non-pennate muscles

A skeletal muscle is made up of skeletal muscle cells bound by various layers of connective tissue that support extensive networks of nerves and blood vessels. Muscle cells are long and thin and, as such, they are usually referred to as muscle fibres. The diameter of muscle fibres ranges between 0.01 mm and 0.15 mm (Lieber 1992; Andersen *et al.* 2000). All the fibres in an individual muscle are about the same length. In some muscles, the fibres are relatively short; for example, in the muscles that move the eyes, the fibres are 2–4 mm long. By contrast, the fibres in some other muscles are very long; for example, the fibres of the sartorius are approximately 30 cm long. The muscle fibre length in most muscles is between these two extreme values.

The fibres in all muscles are organised into bundles (as described later), and the fibres in each bundle run parallel with each other. However, the arrangement of the bundles of fibres with respect to the origin and insertion of the muscle is either pennate or non-pennate. In a pennate muscle, the fibres run obliquely with respect to the origin and insertion so that the line of pull of the fibres is oblique to the line of pull of the muscle (Figure 5.10). This arrangement gives pennate muscles a feather-like appearance and they are classified according to the number of groups of fibres into unipennate, bipennate and multipennate. In a unipennate muscle (Figure 5.10a), there is one group of fibres that inserts onto the sides of two tendons (or one bony attachment and one tendon). The flexors and extensors of the fingers are unipennate muscles. In a bipennate muscle, such as the gastrocnemius, there are two groups of fibres that insert onto the opposite sides of a central tendon (Figure 5.10b). A multipennate muscle such as the deltoid is, in effect, two or more bipennate muscles combined into a single muscle (Figure 5.10c).

In a non-pennate muscle the fibres run in line with the line of pull of the muscle. There are five main types: quadrilateral, strap, spiral, fusiform and fan-shaped (Figure 5.11). In a spiral muscle, the muscle curves around other muscles or bones. In a fusiform (or spindle-shaped) muscle, the

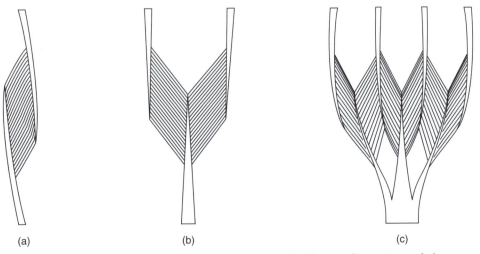

(a)   (b)   (c)

Figure 5.10 Pennate muscles. (a) Unipennate (e.g. finger flexors). (b) Bipennate (e.g. gastrocnemius). (c) Multipennate (e.g. deltoid).

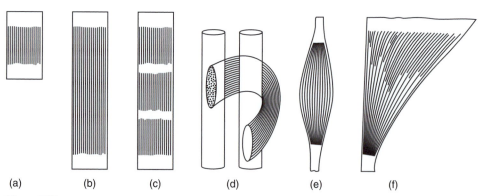

(a)   (b)   (c)   (d)   (e)   (f)

Figure 5.11 Non-pennate muscles. (a) Quadrilateral (e.g. pronator quadratus). (b) Strap (e.g. sartorius). (c) Strap with tendinous intersections (e.g. rectus abdominis). (d) Spiral (e.g. supinator). (e) Fusiform (e.g. biceps brachii). (f) Fan-shaped (e.g. pectoralis major).

fibres are gathered at each end to attach onto long, relatively narrow, tendons. In a fan-shaped muscle, the fibres converge from a broad origin to a relatively small insertion. The effect of pennate and non-pennate arrangements on muscle function is described later in this chapter.

Fusiform musculotendinous units

Figure 5.12 shows the structure of a fusiform musculotendinous unit. Each muscle fibre is enveloped in a layer of areolar tissue called the endomysium, which helps to bind the muscle fibres together and provides a supporting framework for blood capillaries and the terminal branches of nerve fibres. The muscle fibres are grouped together by irregular connective tissue (a mixture of collagenous and elastic) in bundles of up to 200 fibres; each bundle is called a fasciculus (or funiculus), and the connective tissue sheath is called the perimysium. The fasciculi are bound together to form the belly of the muscle by a layer of irregular collagenous connective tissue called the epimysium. The muscle fibres gradually taper at each end. The tapering of the fibres accompanies a gradual thickening in the epimysium and perimysium layers and a change in the composition of the epimysium and perimysium layers from irregular

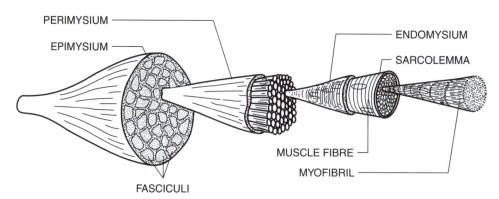

PERIMYSIUM
EPIMYSIUM
ENDOMYSIUM
SARCOLEMMA
MUSCLE FIBRE
MYOFIBRIL
FASCICULI

Figure 5.12 Structure of a fusiform muscle.

collagenous and irregular elastic connective tissue to regular collagenous connective tissue as the epimysium and perimysium layers merge to form a tendon or aponeurosis.

Each muscle receives one or more nerves (collections of sensory and motor nerve fibres), which usually enter the muscle together with the main blood vessels (arteries enter; veins leave) at a region of the muscle that does not move a great deal during normal movement; this region is referred to as the neurovascular hilus (Standring 2008). The blood vessels and nerves branch through the epimysium and perimysium layers down to the endomysium of the individual muscle fibres.

> A skeletal muscle is made up of skeletal muscle fibres bound together by connective tissue that supports extensive networks of nerves and blood vessels. The muscle fibres are organised into bundles that have a pennate or non-pennate arrangement.

Muscle fibres

A muscle fibre consists of hundreds or thousands of myofibrils embedded in sarcoplasm (muscle cytoplasm) and enclosed by a cell membrane called the sarcolemma (Figure 5.12 and Figure 5.13a,b). Each muscle fibre has a large number of nuclei that lie just beneath the sarcolemma. Each myofibril is approximately 0.001 mm wide; the myofibrils are arranged parallel to each other and run the whole length of the muscle fibre. The number of myofibrils in a muscle fibre and, consequently, the diameter of a muscle fibre, depends upon the type of fibre (described later) and state of training. In a muscle fibre with a diameter of 0.01 mm there will be approximately 100 myofibrils. In a muscle fibre with a diameter of 0.15 mm there will be approximately 25 500 myofibrils.

Each myofibril exhibits a characteristic pattern of alternate light and dark transverse bands owing to the way that the components of the myofibril reflect light (under an electron microscope). The light and dark bands are referred to as I (isotropic) and A (anisotropic) bands, respectively. Since the light and dark bands coincide in adjacent myofibrils, the muscle fibre has a striped or striated appearance; thus, skeletal muscle is often referred to as striated muscle (Figure 5.13a).

Each myofibril consists largely of four types of proteins (actin, troponin, myosin, titin) arranged in a highly ordered manner that gives rise to the light and dark bands. The four proteins form two distinct types of filament. One type of filament is thicker than the other. The thicker filaments occupy the A bands and are composed largely of myosin; these filaments are usually referred to as myosin filaments or A filaments (Figure 5.13c). The thinner filaments occupy the I bands and are composed largely of actin; these filaments are usually referred to as actin filaments or I filaments (Edman 1992). Each I band is divided by a transverse Z disc. The section of a myofibril between two successive Z discs is called a sarcomere, and is the basic structural unit of a muscle fibre. A myofibril consists of a chain of sarcomeres. The actin filaments project from each side of the Z discs and reach into the A bands of the corresponding sarcomeres, where they interdigitate with the myosin filaments (Figure 5.13c). The region between the ends of the two groups of actin filaments in the middle of a sarcomere is referred to as the H zone.

129

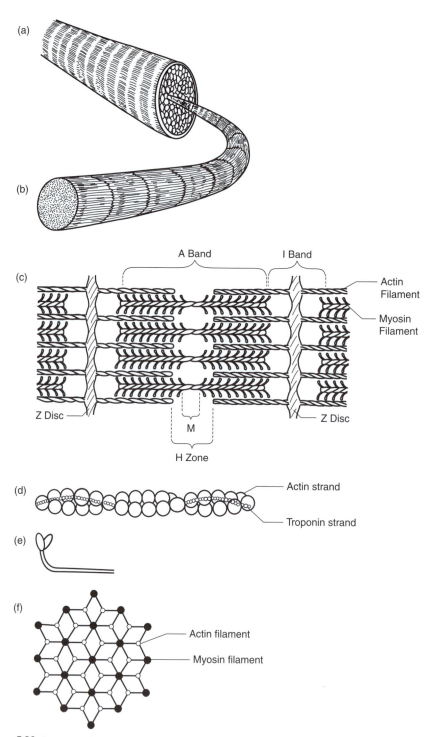

(a)

(b)

A Band   I Band

(c)

Actin Filament

Myosin Filament

Z Disc

Z Disc

M

H Zone

(d)

Actin strand

Troponin strand

(e)

(f)

Actin filament

Myosin filament

Figure 5.13 Structure of a muscle fibre. (a) Muscle fibre. (b) Myofibril. (c) Arrangement of actin and myosin filaments in a sarcomere. (d) Part of an actin filament. (e) Myosin molecule. (f) Hexagonal arrangement of actin and myosin filaments in a sarcomere.

Each actin filament consists of two strands of actin molecules and one strand of troponin molecules wound together longitudinally in a helical manner (Figure 5.13d) (Nishikawa *et al.* 2012). Each myosin filament is composed of three stands of myosin molecules and six strands of titin molecules wound together longitudinally in a helical manner. Each myosin molecule is a club-like structure consisting of two adjacent globular heads attached by a relatively short curved neck to a long shaft (Figure 5.13e). In a myosin filament, the myosin molecules are packed such that the shafts form the three strands of the filament with the heads projecting outward at regular intervals. The two halves of each myosin filament are mirror images of each other, i.e. the myosin molecules in one half of the filament are orientated in the opposite direction to the myosin molecules in the other half. This arrangement, significant in the functional interaction between the actin and myosin filaments (see next section on muscular contraction), is such that no myosin heads project from the central region of each filament; this central region is sometimes referred to as the inert zone, M band or M line (Figure 5.13c). In each half of a myosin filament, the myosin molecules are arranged in groups of six, such that a line joining the heads of the molecules in each group forms a spiral around the myosin filament. The corresponding head in each group faces the same actin filament. Each myosin filament is surrounded by six actin filaments in a regular hexagonal arrangement (Figure 5.13f). This arrangement is maintained by the six strands of titin in each myosin filament; the strands of titin, which are elastic, extend from the ends of the myosin filament across the I bands so that each of the six strands of titin joins one of the six actin filaments close to the corresponding Z disc (Figure 5.13c,f). The strands of titin in adjacent sarcomeres overlap in the Z discs, such that the titin strands are continuous along the entire length of every myofibril (Gregorio *et al.* 1999).

Muscular contraction

When a musculotendinous unit contracts it produces tension and tends to shorten, i.e. it tends to pull its origin and insertion closer together. However, while contracting, the muscle may shorten, lengthen or stay the same length depending on the external load on the muscle (the load tending to lengthen the muscle). If the tension produced by the muscle is greater than the external load, the muscle will shorten; this type of contraction is called a concentric contraction. In weight lifting, the lifting phase of a biceps curl exercise (elbow flexion) is an example of concentric contraction of the elbow flexor muscles. If the tension produced by the muscle is less than the external load, the muscle will lengthen; this type of contraction is called an eccentric contraction. The lowering phase of a biceps curl exercise (elbow extension) is an example of eccentric contraction of the elbow flexor muscles. Concentric and eccentric contractions are often referred to as isotonic contractions, i.e. contractions that involve a change in the length of the muscle. If the tension produced by the muscle is equal to the external load, as in holding the weight stationary in the middle of the flexion–extension range in a biceps curl exercise, the length of the muscle will not change; this type of contraction is called an isometric contraction.

During all types of muscular contraction, the actin and myosin filaments in the sarcomeres stay the same length, but in isotonic contractions the degree of interdigitation between the actin and myosin filaments changes as the length of the muscle fibres changes; the width of the

131

A bands stay the same, but the widths of the I bands and H zones vary. As the muscle fibres shorten, the region of interdigitation increases, and the widths of the I bands and H zones decrease. As the muscle fibres lengthen, the region of interdigitation decreases and the widths of the I bands and H zones increase. These observations led to the formulation of the sliding filament theory of muscular contraction (Huxley and Hanson 1954). The essential features of the theory, which is now generally accepted, are as follows:

1. When a muscle contracts, tension is generated in the muscle by the formation of cross bridges between the heads of the myosin molecules in the myosin filaments and specialised sites on the troponin strands of the actin filaments. Each cross bridge exerts a small amount of tension; the greater the number of cross bridges, the greater the tension.
2. In a concentric contraction, flexion of the necks of the myosin molecules while the heads are in contact with the actin filaments exerts a pulling force on the actin filaments, which causes the actin filaments to slide relative to the myosin filaments, so that the muscle shortens. After exerting their pulling action, the heads of the myosin molecules detach (or decouple) from the actin filaments and swing back to reattach (or recouple) onto the actin filaments farther along the actin filaments. The coupling and decoupling of different cross bridges occurs at different times so that sufficient tension can be maintained while the muscle shortens.
3. In an eccentric contraction, the cross bridges are stretched, which results in decoupling and recoupling at longer sarcomere lengths, as the muscle lengthens.

Isometric length–tension relationship in a sarcomere

The amount of tension generated in a sarcomere depends on the length of the sarcomere and the level of stimulation. Figure 5.14 shows the isometric length–tension relationship in a sarcomere (Gordon *et al.* 1966). The relationship between length and total tension was determined by maximally stimulating the sarcomere, but not allowing it to shorten, for a number of different sarcomere lengths, and recording the tension at each length. The relationship between length and passive tension was determined by stretching the sarcomere to a number of lengths without stimulation and recording the tension at each length. Passive tension is exerted by the titin strands; the greater the stretch, the greater the passive tension. The relationship between length and active tension (the tension due to cross bridges) was determined by comparing the relationship between length and total tension and that between length and passive tension.

With regard to active tension, when the sarcomere is extended to the point where there is no interdigitation between the actin and myosin filaments, no active tension is generated, since there are no myosin heads in a position to attach to form cross bridges. This situation is represented by the point L5 in Figure 5.14. As the sarcomere shortens and the degree of interdigitation gradually increases, there is a linear increase in the amount of active tension generated, up to the point L4, where the length–active tension relationship levels off. At L4, the maximum number of cross bridges has been formed, and active tension is a maximum. The region of the length–active tension relationship between L4 and L5 is referred to as the descending limb. At L4, the H zone corresponds to the inert zone of the myosin filaments (Figure 5.13c). As

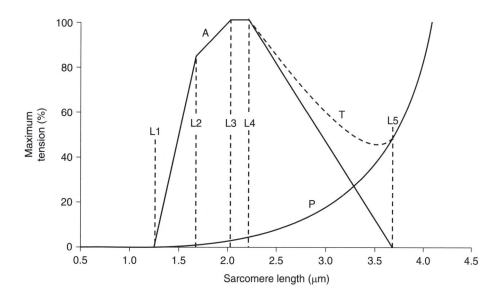

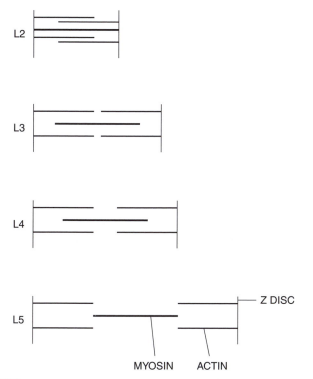

Figure 5.14 Isometric length–tension relationship in a sarcomere: A, active tension; P, passive tension; T, total tension.

the sarcomere shortens, between L4 and L3, the active tension stays the same, since no more cross bridges can be formed (the inert zones of the myosin filaments do not have myosin heads to attach cross bridges). The region of the length–active tension relationship between L3 and L4 is referred to as the plateau region. At L3, the ends of the actin filaments in each half of the sarcomere come together, i.e. the H zone is reduced to zero. As the sarcomere shortens, between L3 and L2, the actin filaments progressively overlap each other, resulting in a progressive drop in active tension because the overlapping actin filaments interfere with cross bridge formation in the region of overlap. The region of the length–active tension relationship, between L2 and L3, is referred to as the shallow ascending limb. At L2, the ends of the myosin filaments abut the Z discs. As the sarcomere shortens, between L2 and L1, there is a rapid and progressive drop in active tension due to progressive overlap of the actin filaments and progressive longitudinal compression of the myosin filaments, both of which reduce the number of myosin heads available to form cross bridges. At L1, no cross bridges can be formed and, consequently, no active tension is generated. The region of the length–active tension relationship between L1 and L2 is referred to as the steep ascending limb.

Isometric length–tension relationship in a musculotendinous unit

The length–tension relationship in a musculotendinous unit is similar to that in a sarcomere, with active (contractile) and passive (tension exerted by stretching of connective tissues) components. Figure 5.15 shows the isometric length–tension relationship in a musculotendinous unit. The contributions of the contractile and connective tissue components to the total tension at any particular length are shown in the separate curves. Some of the connective tissue components are parallel with the muscle fibres and some are arranged in series; this has given rise to the terms parallel elastic component and series elastic component (Huijing 1992). The parallel elastic component consists of sarcolemma, endomysia, perimysia and epimysium. The series elastic component consists of tendons, aponeuroses and titin.

In the absence of stimulation and any external load, the musculotendinous unit assumes a rest length at which the tension in the unit is zero, with no tension in the contractile component, and no tension (no stretch) in the connective tissue component. Figure 5.15 shows that the rest length is associated with that part of the isometric length–tension curve at which the tension in the contractile component is maximum. The tension tends to reduce to zero when the unit shortens to approximately 60% of its rest length (Figure 5.15). However, in practice, this is unlikely to occur, owing to the arrangement of the musculotendinous units on the skeleton. When a musculotendinous unit contracts in a very shortened state, and so generates a low force, it is said to be in a state of active insufficiency (Elftman 1966). This is more likely to occur with musculotendinous units that cross more than one joint. For example, the hamstrings extend the hip and flex the knee (Figure 1.5). However, the muscle fibres in the hamstrings are not long enough to fully extend the hip and flex the knee simultaneously. If you stand on one leg and attempt to fully extend the hip and fully flex the knee of the other leg at the same time, you will be unable to flex the knee much more than 90°; i.e. the hamstrings will be in a state of active insufficiency. In contrast, if you flex the hip and then flex the knee, you will be able to flex the knee approximately 140°. This is possible because the hamstrings operate closer to rest length and are therefore able to exert more force (Elftman 1966).

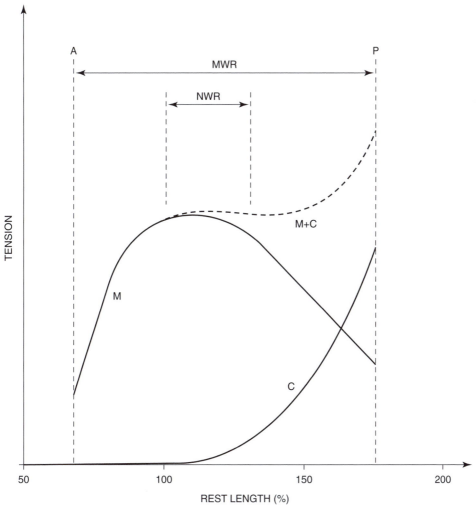

Figure 5.15 Isometric length–tension relationship in a musculotendinous unit: M, tension exerted by the contractile component; C, tension exerted by the connective tissue component; M+C, total tension; P, passive insufficiency; A, active insufficiency; MWR, maximum working range; NWR, normal working range.

Figure 5.15 shows that as a musculotendinous unit lengthens beyond its rest length, the isometric tension generated is fairly constant between 100% and 150% of the rest length and then increases to a maximum at approximately 175% of rest length. The change in isometric tension between rest length and maximum tension is associated with a gradual decrease in the amount of tension produced by the contractile component and a gradual increase in the amount of passive tension. Tension in the contractile component would be reduced to zero if the musculotendinous unit were lengthened to approximately 210% of rest length. However, the parallel elastic connective tissue components ensure that this situation does not arise by limiting the maximum length of the musculotendinous unit to approximately 175% of rest length. In this situation, the musculotendinous unit is said to be in a state of passive insufficiency (Elftman 1966).

135

When a musculotendinous unit lengthens, not all of the sarcomeres lengthen to the same extent. Theoretically, a situation could occur where some of the sarcomeres in a muscle fibre were fully extended, i.e. no interdigitation between the actin and myosin filaments, while other sarcomeres were not fully extended. If the muscle were stimulated to contract in this state, the fully stretched sarcomeres would not be able to contract, whereas the other sarcomeres would be able to contract. This would result in further stretching and, consequently, damage to the already fully stretched sarcomeres. This theoretical condition has been referred to as muscle instability, and may be prevented, at least in part, by passive insufficiency (Alexander 1989). Consequently, the maximum working length range of a musculotendinous unit is determined by the lengths at which active insufficiency and passive insufficiency occur, i.e. between approximately 60% and 175% of rest length. However, it is likely that the normal working range is between approximately 100% and 130% of rest length. This range incorporates the region of the length–tension curve where contractile tension is maximum and, as such, allows maximum flexibility in tension generation (Figure 5.15).

Motor units

The functional unit of skeletal muscle is the motor unit. A motor unit consists of a motor neuron with an Aα axon (sometimes referred to as an alpha motoneuron), together with all the terminal branches of the axon and the muscle fibres that they innervate (Gamble 1988) (Figure 5.16). The number of muscle fibres innervated by a single alpha motoneuron is referred to as the innervation ratio. The innervation ratio of different motor units varies con-

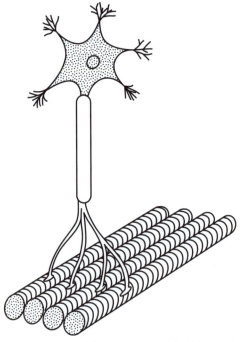

Figure 5.16 Composition of a motor unit: an alpha motoneuron with all the terminal branches of the axon and the muscle fibres that they innervate.

siderably, from approximately 1:4 in the muscles that move the eyes, to approximately 1:2000 in the large back extensor and leg extensor muscles. When an alpha motoneuron transmits an action potential, all of the fibres in the motor unit contract. Consequently, muscles associated with very fine motor control, such as the muscles that move the eyes, have motor units with low innervation ratios so that the amount of force produced can be finely controlled. Muscles associated with forceful movements are made up of motor units with relatively high innervation ratios. The fibres of a single motor unit are usually mixed with the fibres of other motor units, but are grouped within a relatively small area of the muscle.

> The number of muscle fibres in a motor unit is referred to as the innervation ratio. Muscles associated with fine motor control have motor units with low innervation ratios, whereas muscles associated with forceful movements are made up of motor units with relatively high innervation ratios.

A muscle fibre contracts when an action potential is generated in the sarcolemma at the junction with a motor end plate. The action potential is transmitted along and across the muscle fibre (by a system of tubules continuous with the sarcolemma), resulting in contraction. A single action potential produces a muscle twitch, i.e. a force that rapidly peaks and then equally rapidly dies away. If a series of action potentials is generated at a high enough frequency, the twitches fuse to produce tetanus, a sustained level of force.

Slow and fast twitch muscle fibres

Whereas the basic structure and function of all muscle fibres is the same, muscle fibres and, consequently, motor units vary in relation to the following:

1. The activation threshold, or the level of stimulus required to generate an action potential;
2. The contraction time, or the time from force onset to peak force;
3. Resistance to fatigue.

Muscle fibres are classified into slow twitch fibres and fast twitch fibres on the basis of their contraction times. Slow twitch fibres, also referred to as type I or red fibres, have contraction times of 100–120 ms. Fast twitch fibres, also referred to as type II fibres or white fibres, have contraction times of 40–45 ms (Gregor 1993; Gamble 1988). The metabolism of slow twitch fibres is essentially aerobic and, therefore, these fibres are resistant to fatigue. Fast twitch fibres are subdivided on the basis of their metabolic characteristics into type IIa (aerobic and fatigue resistant) and type IIb (anaerobic and fatigue sensitive; also referred to as IIx fibres). The muscle fibres in a particular motor unit have the same functional characteristics; thus, motor units can be classified into three categories:

■ Slow contracting, fatigue resistant (S);
■ Fast contracting, fatigue resistant (FR);
■ Fast contracting, fatigable (FF).

137

Table 5.2 Characteristics of slow and fast twitch motor units

	Slow twitch, fatigue resistant (S)	Fast twitch, fatigue resistant (FR)	Fast twitch, fatiguable (FF)
Activation threshold of muscle fibres	Low	Moderate	High
Contraction time of muscle fibres (ms)	100–120	40–45	40–45
Innervation ratio of motor unit	Low	Moderate	High
Types of muscle fibre	I	IIa	IIb
Type of axon	Aβ	Aα	Aα
Diameter of axon (μm)	7–14	12–20	12–20
Speed (m/s)	40–80	65–120	65–120
Duration and size of force	Prolonged low force	Prolonged relatively high force	Intermittent high force
Type of activity	Long-distance running and swimming	Kayaking and rowing	Sprinting, throwing, jumping and weight lifting

Individuals differ in the proportions of the different types of muscle fibres in their muscles. The average person has approximately 50% type I, 25% type IIa and 25% type IIb fibres in each calf muscle. By contrast, elite distance runners have a much higher proportion of type I fibres, and elite sprinters have a much higher proportion of type IIb fibres (Gamble 1988; Andersen *et al.* 2000).

Although the classification of muscle fibres into types I, IIa and IIb is widely used, the categories represent ranges of metabolic and functional characteristics rather than discrete categories (Sargeant 1994; Rome 2006). The metabolic and functional characteristics of muscle fibres appear to be influenced considerably by the type of innervation that the fibres receive. In experiments performed on animals, it has been shown that altering the type of innervation results, over time, in a change in the metabolic and functional characteristics of muscle fibres (Noth 1992; Rome 2006). Table 5.2 lists the characteristics of slow and fast twitch motor units.

MUSCLE ARCHITECTURE AND MUSCLE FUNCTION

All muscles are made up of muscle fibres. However, the length and the orientation of the fibres (pennate or non-pennate) have a considerable effect on the function of the muscles. The fundamental relationships between muscle architecture and muscle function are that excursion (the distance that the muscle can shorten) and velocity of shortening are proportional to fibre length, and force is proportional to the total physiological cross-sectional area of the muscle fibres (Lieber and Bodine-Fowler 1993).

All muscle fibres are composed of similar sarcomeres, and the number of sarcomeres determines the length of a muscle fibre. Each sarcomere in a muscle fibre is capable of shortening to the same extent as all the other sarcomeres in the muscle fibre. Consequently, the excursion of the muscle fibre is equal to the sum of the excursions of all the individual sarcomeres; the greater the number of sarcomeres, the longer the muscle fibre, and the greater the excursion. Excursion and velocity of shortening are directly related, since velocity of shortening is the rate of change of excursion, i.e. the rate of change in length of the muscle. The longer the muscle fibre (in terms of number of sarcomeres), the greater its excursion and velocity of shortening.

Theoretically, the ideal muscle (in terms of force and excursion capabilities) has a large cross-sectional area and very long fibres. However, such a muscle would be bulky and create considerable packing problems, owing to its girth and areas of attachment to the skeletal system. As there are no muscles with both of these characteristics, it is reasonable to assume that the architecture of the muscular system has evolved to provide the best compromise between structure and function. The muscles of the body represent a broad range of combinations of force and excursion capability (Lieber 1992), and it is, perhaps, not surprising that most movements of the body involve simultaneous activity in a number of muscles, with each muscle performing a particular role.

Roles of muscles

With regard to control of joint movements, muscles perform a number of different roles, including stabiliser, agonist, prime mover, assistant mover, antagonist, synergist and neutraliser. Each of the muscles that contributes to a particular movement may have more than one role and the relative importance of each role may change during the movement.

Joint stabilisation, the maintenance of joint congruence, is a major function of the muscular system. The extent to which a muscle contributes to joint stabilisation depends largely on the line of pull of the muscle in relation to the centre of the joint the muscle crosses. Generally, the closer the line of pull of the muscle to the centre of the joint, the greater the stabilising effect of the muscle.

An agonist is a muscle that moves a body segment in the intended direction. For example, the deltoid and supraspinatus are both agonists in abduction of the shoulder joint, with the deltoid as prime mover and the supraspinatus as the assistant mover (Figure 5.17a,b,c). An antagonist is a muscle that acts in the direction opposite to that of an agonist. For example, in abduction of the shoulder joint, the latissimus dorsi and pectoralis major are antagonists (Figure 5.17d,e).

A synergist assists the action of the prime mover. For example, in abduction of the shoulder, the trapezius and serratus anterior rotate and abduct the scapula so that complete abduction of the arm (180° with respect to the anatomical position) can be achieved (Figure 5.17f,g).

A neutraliser prevents unwanted action of a muscle. For example, the tendency would be for the flexors of the fingers to flex the wrist simultaneously as they flex the fingers (Figure 5.18). However, if the finger flexors performed both movements at the same time, the finger flexors would experience active insufficiency. Consequently, the wrist extensors neutralise the action by preventing wrist flexion. The length of the muscle fibres of the finger flexors is approximately 100 mm. To flex the wrist and hold a tight position, the finger flexors

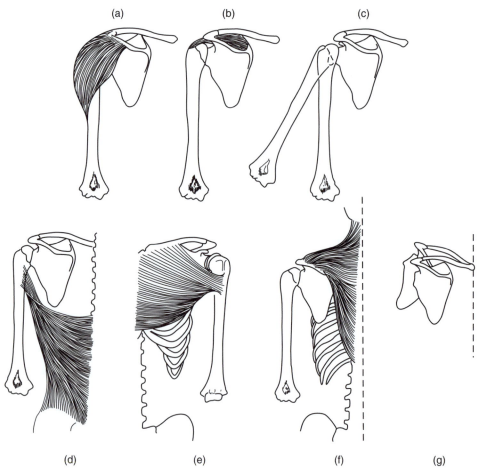

Figure 5.17 Roles of muscles in abduction of the arm. (a) Posterior aspect of the left shoulder showing the deltoid muscle (agonist and prime mover: shoulder abduction). (b) Posterior aspect of the left shoulder showing the supraspinatus muscle (agonist and assistant mover: shoulder abduction). (c) Action of the deltoid and supraspinatus (shoulder abduction). (d) Posterior aspect of the left shoulder and trunk showing the latissimus dorsi muscle (antagonist). (e) Anterior aspect of the left shoulder showing the pectoralis major muscle (antagonist). (f) Posterior aspect of the left shoulder showing the trapezius muscle (synergist: rotation of the clavicle and scapula). (g) Posterior aspect of the left shoulder showing the action of the trapezius muscle (rotation of the clavicle and scapula).

need to shorten by about 27 mm. To flex the fingers into a tight fist, the finger flexors need to shorten by about 37 mm. The finger flexors can perform both movements separately, since 27 mm to 37 mm is well within the normal working range of the muscles. However, the muscles cannot perform both movements simultaneously because, to do so, they would need to shorten by about 64 mm (27 mm plus 37 mm), which would produce active insufficiency (Alexander 1992). The finger flexors can only produce a tight fist when the wrist is held straight so that the tendency of the finger flexors to flex the wrist is neutralised. This is achieved by the wrist extensors (Figure 5.18).

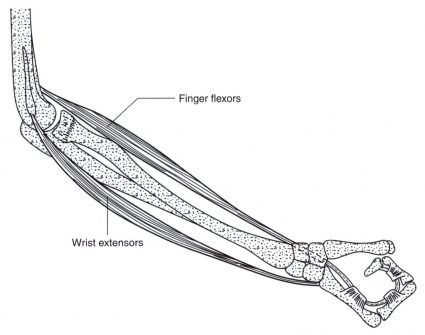

Finger flexors

Wrist extensors

Figure 5.18 The action of the wrist extensors in neutralising the tendency of the finger flexors to flex the wrist as they flex the fingers.

Muscle fibre arrangement and force and excursion

Figures 5.19a and c show two musculotendinous units with the same rest length and the same muscle mass (same volume of myofibrils). One muscle is a non-pennate parallel-fibred muscle (Figure 5.19a) and the other is a unipennate muscle (Figure 5.19b). The physiological cross-sectional area of each muscle is the cross-sectional area of all of the muscle fibres perpendicular to their line of pull. Assuming that the length of the muscle fibres in the pennate muscle is only half that of the fibres in the non-pennate muscle, it follows that the physiological cross-sectional area of the pennate muscle is double that of the non-pennate muscle (since the muscle mass is the same in both muscles). Consequently, the pennate muscle can exert double the force of the non-pennate muscle. However, as the fibres in the pennate muscle are oblique to the line of pull of the musculotendinous unit, not all of the force is in the line of pull of the musculotendinous unit. In a pennate muscle, the angle of the fibres with respect to the line of pull of the musculotendinous unit is usually 30° or less (Alexander 1968), such that 90% or more of the force exerted by the muscle is directed in the line of pull of the muscle. Consequently, pennate muscles are normally capable of exerting far more force in the line of pull of the musculotendinous unit than non-pennate muscles of the same muscle mass.

In contrast with their capacity to generate force, the excursion range of non-pennate musculotendinous units is usually much greater than that of pennate musculotendinous units of similar muscle mass. The increased excursion range of non-pennate muscles is the result of both an increased fibre length and a line of pull directly in line with the line of pull of the

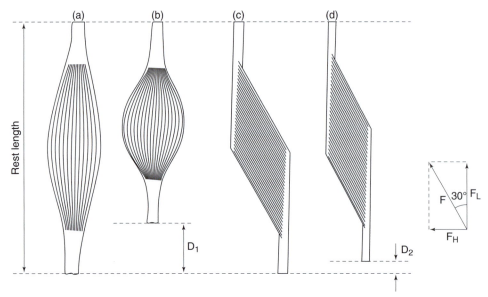

Figure 5.19 Effects of muscle structure on force and excursion. (a) Non-pennate muscle at rest length. (b) Non-pennate muscle of (a) with fibres shortened to 70% of rest length. (c) Pennate muscle at rest length. (d) Pennate muscle of (c) with fibres shortened to 70% of rest length. (e) Components of the muscle force F in the line of pull of the musculotendinous unit, F_L, and perpendicular to the line of pull, F_H. $D_1 = 20\%$ of rest length. $D_2 = 5\%$ of rest length.

musculotendinous unit. In Figures 5.19b and d, the muscles are shown with their fibres shortened to 70% of their rest length. The corresponding shortening of the musculotendinous units is 20% and 5%, respectively, in the non-pennate and pennate muscles.

> The fundamental relationships between muscle architecture and muscle function are that excursion and velocity of shortening are proportional to fibre length, and force is proportional to total cross-sectional area of the muscle fibres.

Biarticular muscles

Many of the skeletal muscles, especially those in the upper and lower limbs, span more than one joint (see Figure 5.18). These muscles are usually referred to as biarticular muscles because muscles that span more than two joints function in the same way as muscles that span two joints (Lieber 1992). Biarticular muscles are too short to fully flex or fully extend simultaneously all of the joints that they span. For example, the hamstrings are two-joint muscles that can extend the hip and flex the knee, but these actions (as described earlier in the chapter) cannot be performed maximally at the same time. Indeed, hip extension is normally associated with knee extension, and hip flexion is normally associated with knee flexion, as in walking and running. In this way, the length of the muscles stays within the normal working range of approximately 100% to 130% of rest length. The functional advantages of biarticular muscles are that tension is produced in one muscle rather than two (or more), which conserves energy, and that working within the 100% to 130% range allows maximal flexibility in tension generation (Burkholder and Lieber 2001; Lieber 1992).

KINAESTHETIC SENSE AND PROPRIOCEPTION

The central nervous system constantly receives sensory information from a wide variety of sources concerning the different aspects of physiological functioning. Awareness of body position and body movement is provided by a range of sensory organs, in particular, those concerned with the sensations of effort and heaviness, the timing of the movement of individual body parts, the position of the body in space, joint positions and joint movements.

The inputs from these sources contribute to what is referred to as kinaesthetic sense (or kinaesthesia) (Figure 5.20). Some aspects of kinaesthetic sensitivity, such as a sense of effort and heaviness, and a sense of timing of actions, are generated by sensory centres that monitor the motor commands sent to muscles. Other aspects of kinaesthetic sensitivity are generated largely by input from peripheral receptors that monitor the execution of motor commands, i.e. the actual movements. For example, inputs from the eyes and ears are responsible for generating a sense of the position of the body in space. The sense of the position and movement of a joint is generated by a group of receptors located in the skin and musculoskeletal tissues. These receptors are called proprioceptors, and the sensation they provide is called proprioception. Proprioceptors are mechanoreceptors; they are activated by physical distortion.

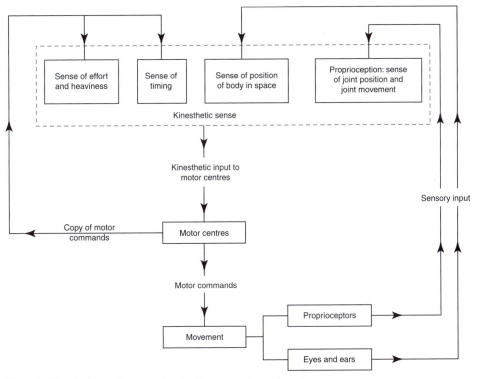

Figure 5.20 Relationship between kinaesthetic sense and proprioception.

Proprioceptors

The existence of proprioceptors in the skin, muscles, tendons, joint capsules and ligaments is well established, but the precise role of the different proprioceptors and the interrelationships between them is less clear (Grigg 1994). However, it appears that proprioceptors in joint capsules and ligaments are largely responsible for generating a sense of joint position and joint movement in the end ranges of joint movements, where joint capsules and ligaments may become taut. Between the end ranges it seems unlikely that the proprioceptors in joint capsules and ligaments provide much sensory information, since they are unlikely to be under sufficient tension to excite them.

Joint and ligament proprioceptors

There are two main types of proprioceptor in joint capsules, Ruffini end organs (or Ruffini corpuscles), which appear to be mainly responsive to tension, and Pacinian corpuscles, which appear to be responsive to compression. These are both widely distributed between the collagenous fibres of the joint capsule.

The proprioceptors in ligaments and skin are similar to those found in joint capsules. However, there are few proprioceptors in ligaments and skin compared with the number in joint capsules. In addition, since tension in ligaments and skin may be caused by movement in a number of different directions, it is unlikely that the proprioceptors can provide information on movement in specific directions. For these reasons, it is thought that the contribution of the proprioceptors in ligaments and skin to proprioception is relatively small (Grigg 1994). However, they may make a significant contribution to joint stabilisation in reflexive muscular activity.

Muscle and tendon proprioceptors

Whereas proprioceptors in joint capsules and, to a lesser extent, in ligaments appear to generate information on joint position and joint movement in the end ranges of joint movements, proprioceptors in muscles, called muscle spindles, and tendons, called Golgi tendon organs, seem to be responsible for generating this type of information for movement between end ranges. Golgi tendon organs and muscle spindles are responsive to tension.

Each muscle spindle consists of a number of tiny muscle fibres enclosed within a spindle-shaped connective tissue capsule (Figure 5.21). The muscle spindle fibres are referred to as intrafusal (inside the spindle) to distinguish them from the larger and more numerous extrafusal fibres that make up the vast majority of the muscle. Muscle spindles are embedded between extrafusal fibres. Intrafusal fibres are classified by the arrangement of their nuclei into nuclear bag fibres and nuclear chain fibres. In both types of fibre, the nuclei are located in the central region of the fibre, which is devoid of myofibrils. In nuclear bag fibres the nuclei cluster in a group, whereas in nuclear chain fibres the nuclei are arranged in a line parallel to the long axis of the fibre. The regions of the fibres on each side of the central region contain a large number of myofibrils and are referred to as the polar regions (Enoka 2008).

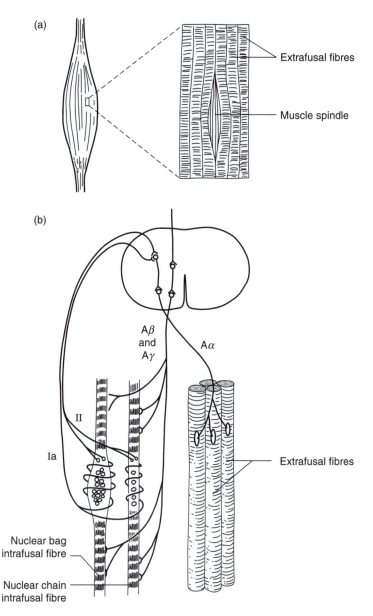

(a)

Extrafusal fibres

Muscle spindle

(b)

Aβ and Aγ

Aα

II

Ia

Extrafusal fibres

Nuclear bag intrafusal fibre

Nuclear chain intrafusal fibre

Figure 5.21 Structure of a muscle spindle. (a) Location of a muscle spindle. (b) Innervation of a muscle spindle.

Nuclear bag fibres and nuclear chain fibres are usually about 8 mm and 4 mm long, respectively; in a typical muscle spindle there are two bag fibres and four chain fibres (Roberts 1995). The central regions of both types of fibre are supplied with type Ia and type II sensory nerve endings. The endings of type Ia nerve fibres spiral around the intrafusal fibres and the endings of type II nerve fibres consist of a number of branches with end bulbs; the spirals and end bulbs adhere closely to the sarcolemma of each fibre.

145

The polar regions of the intrafusal fibres are supplied with motor nerve endings from Aα and Aγ motor nerve fibres. Stimulation of the intrafusal fibres via these nerves results in contraction of the polar regions, which stretches the central regions and excites the spiral and end bulb nerve endings. This results in sensory discharge via the type Ia and II sensory nerve fibres. The type Ia and II fibres synapse in the spinal cord directly with the Aα motor neurons that supply the extrafusal muscle fibres of the same muscle, resulting in contraction of the extrafusal fibres. The level of contraction of the extrafusal fibres depends on the level of activation, which, in turn, depends on the degree of tension in the intrafusal fibres. There is always a certain amount of tension in the intrafusal muscle fibres (activated by the sensory centres of the brain via the Aβ and Aγ fibres), which results in a certain amount of tension in the extrafusal muscle fibres. The resting level of tension in the intrafusal and extrafusal muscle fibres is called muscle tone; the level of muscle tone in the extrafusal fibres is determined by the level of muscle tone in the intrafusal fibres. Muscle tone can be regarded as the sensitivity of a muscle to a change in its length (Kandel *et al.* 2000).

Sensory output from muscle spindles occurs when the central regions of the intrafusal fibres are stretched. For the purpose of setting muscle tone, the central regions are stretched by contraction of the polar regions by the Aβ and Aγ motor nerve fibres (sometimes referred to as the fusimotor nerves). Sensory output from muscle spindles can also be generated by stretching the muscle as a whole, since this will stretch the muscle spindles and excite the spiral and end bulb nerve endings. Low-velocity stretching of active muscles, i.e. low-velocity eccentric muscle contraction, is an essential feature of normal movements; as a muscle group shortens, its antagonist partner lengthens. It is thought that the sensory information provided by muscle spindles and Golgi tendon organs as a result of stretching provides a sense of joint position and joint movement, especially during mid-range movements (Gandevia *et al.* 1992).

Whereas low-level stretching of a musculotendinous unit seems to be important in generating proprioceptive information concerning joint movement and joint position, rapid stretching results in reflex contraction of the musculotendinous unit (via the spindle afferent to muscle efferent loop) to prevent subluxation of the associated joints (Mynark and Koceja 2001). These stretch reflexes are important in protecting joints from injury. For example, recurrent inversion sprains of the ankle are associated with deficient stretch reflex of the evertors and dorsiflexors (Garn and Newton 1988). Excitation of muscle spindles appears to be mainly responsible for initiating reflex muscle contractions. However, there is evidence that proprioceptors in joint capsules and ligaments may also contribute to the initiation of such reflex contractions, especially at the ends of joint ranges of movement (Matthews 1988; Hall *et al.* 1994).

Role of proprioceptors

The precise roles of the various types of proprioceptors are not yet clear. However, there is general agreement that proprioceptive information aids coordination and balance and, in particular, maintains joint congruence (Grigg 1994; Wilkerson and Nitz 1994). It appears that injury to muscles, ligaments and capsules may damage proprioceptors, resulting in long-term proprioceptive deficits, which, in turn, contribute to the development of degenerative joint diseases, such as osteoarthritis (Freeman and Wyke 1967; Garn and Newton 1988; Hall *et al.* 1995). There is evidence that proprioceptive information from musculotendinous units can be enhanced by specific exercises that emphasise activation of muscle spindles and, thereby, improve muscle tone. Such enhancement may compensate for proprioceptive deficits in other structures, such as joint capsules and ligaments (Beard *et al.* 1994; Skinner *et al.* 1986; Steiner *et al.* 1986).

FORCE–VELOCITY RELATIONSHIP IN MUSCULOTENDINOUS UNITS

The everyday physical tasks that individuals perform are usually well within the strength capability of the musculotendinous units used. In such movements, the musculotendinous units generate just enough tension to overcome the external load acting on them so that they can move the external load. The external load may simply be the weight of a limb segment, such as the forearm in a movement involving elbow flexion. At other times, the external load consists of the weight of the limb segments together with any additional load that is being moved, such as something held in the hand.

When the amount of force produced by a muscle just matches the external load, the muscle contracts isometrically. The maximum load the muscle can sustain isometrically is called the isometric strength of the muscle. When the external load is less than isometric strength, the muscle is able to contract concentrically. The speed of shortening in a concentric contraction depends on how much force the muscle needs to produce to move the external load. The greater the external load, the greater the muscle force needs to be, and the greater the muscle force (as a proportion of isometric strength), the slower the speed of shortening. A muscle can shorten at maximum speed when the external load on the muscle is zero. When the external load on a muscle is greater than the isometric strength of the muscle, it is forced to lengthen, i.e. contract eccentrically.

In an eccentric contraction a muscle resists the stretching load. The attached cross bridges are themselves stretched, adding to the overall tension, such that the force produced by the muscle is greater than the isometric strength of the muscle. The force produced by a muscle during eccentric contraction depends on the speed of lengthening, which depends on the size of the external load. The greater the external load (in relation to the isometric strength of the muscle), the greater the speed of lengthening. The greater the speed of lengthening, the greater the effect of the stretch reflex, and, therefore, the greater the force produced by the muscle. When the external force exceeds the maximum strength of the muscle, the muscle, its tendons, or both will be injured. The relationship between muscle force and speed of shortening or lengthening is referred to as the force–velocity relationship (Figure 5.22). Figure 5.23 shows the effect of the force–velocity relationship on the length–tension relationship of a musculotendinous unit. The figure shows that at any particular length, the greater the speed of shortening, the lower the tension, and that the greater the speed of lengthening, the higher the tension.

> The amount of force generated by a musculotendinous unit depends on the length of the musculotendinous unit at the time of stimulation (length–tension relationship) and the speed with which it changes length in the ensuing contraction (force–velocity relationship).

147

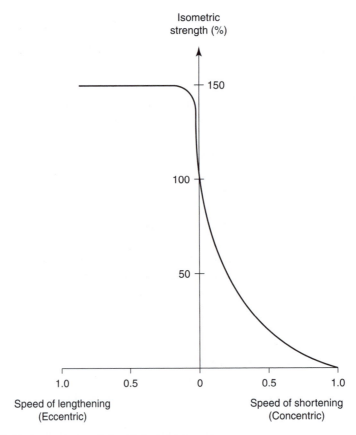

Figure 5.22 The force–velocity relationship in skeletal muscle.

Action and contraction in musculotendinous units

The contractile (muscle) and non-contractile (connective tissue) components of a musculotendinous unit function as a single unit. During contraction of the muscle component, the
length of the musculotendinous unit may increase, decrease or stay the same. An increase in
length could be due to an increase in both the muscle (eccentric contraction of the muscle)
and connective tissue components (elastic stretching), but it may also be due to an increase in
the connective tissue component while the muscle component stays the same length. In this
situation, the muscle *contracts* isometrically, but the musculotendinous unit *acts* eccentrically.
A musculotendinous unit acts eccentrically when it lengthens while its muscle component is
contracting. A decrease in the length of a musculotendinous unit in which the muscle component is contracting could be due to a decrease in both the muscle (concentric contraction of
the muscle) and connective tissue components (recoil following elastic stretch), but it may also
be due to a decrease in the connective tissue component while the muscle component stays
the same length. In this situation, the muscle *contracts* isometrically, but the musculotendinous
unit *acts* concentrically. A musculotendinous unit acts concentrically when it shortens while
its muscle component is contracting. The functional relationship between the contractile and

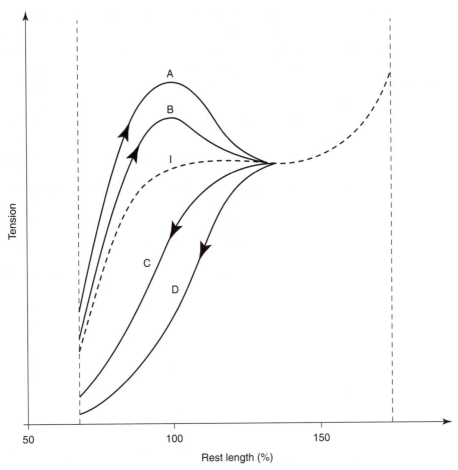

Figure 5.23 The effect of speed of shortening and speed of lengthening on the length–tension relationship in skeletal muscle. A and B show eccentric contractions: the speed of lengthening in A is greater than in B; C and D show concentric contractions: the speed of shortening in C is less than in D; I shows the isometric length–tension curve.

non-contractile components of a musculotendinous unit is clearly very complex (Ishikawa *et al.* 2005; Kawakami and Fukunaga 2006; Spanjaard *et al.* 2006). It is thought that one of the main functions of the muscle component is to continuously adjust the stiffness of the tendons in order to maximise energy conservation, i.e. minimise energy expenditure (Lindstedt *et al.* 2001; Roberts 2002).

Stretch–shorten cycle

When a concentric contraction occurs without prestretching, the initial phase of contraction takes up the slack in the series elastic connective tissue (SEC) components; it is only when the slack in the SEC components has been taken up, that is, when the SEC components have become taut, that the force produced by the muscle is transmitted to the skeleton. The need for the muscle to expend energy in taking up the slack in the SEC components before force

149

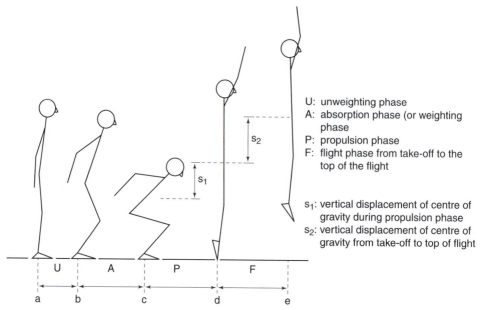

U: unweighting phase
A: absorption phase (or weighting phase)
P: propulsion phase
F: flight phase from take-off to the top of the flight

s_1: vertical displacement of centre of gravity during propulsion phase
s_2: vertical displacement of centre of gravity from take-off to top of flight

Figure 5.24 Sequence of movement in a countermovement vertical jump (a–e) and a squat jump from a stationary position (c–e). (a) Standing upright at rest. (b) Instant in countermovement when downward velocity of the body is at its maximum. (c) Instant at which the vertical velocity of the body is zero (maximum displacement downward). (d) Take-off. (e) Top of flight.

can be transmitted to the skeleton is not efficient. It is not surprising, therefore, that in most, if not all, preferred whole body movements, many of the musculotendinous units involved in controlling the various joints are initially stretched before they shorten. For example, jumping movements generally begin with a downward movement followed by upward movement (Figure 5.24). Similarly, in throwing actions, the arm is usually swung backward before being accelerated forward (see Figure 1.16).

In such actions, the initial movement in the opposite direction to that of the final movement is usually referred to as a countermovement. A countermovement involves two phases. In the first phase, the body (as in a vertical jump) or body segments (such as the arm in a throwing action) develop a speed of movement in the opposite direction to that of the final movement. Before the final movement can be initiated, the movement of the body or body segments in the opposite direction must be arrested. Consequently, in the second phase of a countermovement, the muscles contract to arrest the movement of the body or body segments; in doing so, they are forcibly stretched and, as such, act eccentrically. The eccentric phase is usually immediately followed by a concentric phase to produce the final movement. This pattern of eccentric action followed without a pause by concentric action is referred to as the stretch–shorten cycle (Komi 2003). Most whole body actions, including relatively slow walking, utilise the stretch–shorten cycle. However, the utilisation of the stretch–shorten cycle is more obvious in movements involving a distinct countermovement, as in jumping, throwing and striking. For example, in a golf swing, the backswing is arrested by eccentric action of the same muscles that then act concentrically to produce the downswing. The eccentric phase of the backswing is usually accentuated by starting to turn the trunk to face the flag before the backswing has been completed.

> For any given task, movements using the stretch–shorten cycle may be more effective (in terms of performance) and more efficient (in terms of utilisation of energy) than movements that rely on concentric contractions.

Storage and utilisation of elastic strain energy

A force does mechanical work when it moves its point of application in the direction of the force, that is, the work W done is the product of the magnitude of the force F applied and the distance d moved by the point of application of the force ($W = F \cdot d$). Consequently, when a muscle contracts isometrically, it expends energy (metabolic energy expenditure by the muscle cells to maintain the contraction), but it does no work, since the length of the musculotendinous unit does not change. When a muscle contracts concentrically it expends energy in creating tension and does work by pulling its skeletal attachments closer together. The amount of work done by a muscle in a concentric contraction is the product of the muscle force and the distance over which the musculotendinous unit shortens. When a muscle contracts eccentrically, it expends energy in creating tension, but in contrast to a concentric contraction, work is done on the musculotendinous unit; it is lengthened by the external load. The amount of work done on the musculotendinous unit by the external load is the product of the muscle force and the distance over which the musculotendinous unit is lengthened. When work is done on a musculotendinous unit, i.e. when energy is expended in stretching a musculotendinous unit, the energy is absorbed by the musculotendinous unit in the form of strain energy (like the energy stored in a drawn bow that is subsequently used to propel the arrow). The extent to which the strain energy can be used to move the body, rather than being dissipated as heat within the muscle, will depend on the speed of the changeover from eccentric to concentric activity within the stretch–shorten cycle.

For any given task, movements using the stretch–shorten cycle may be more effective (in terms of performance) and more efficient (in terms of energy expenditure) than movements relying on concentric contractions (Anderson and Pandy 1993; Komi 2003). For example, most people are able to jump higher using a countermovement jump (Figure 5.24a–e) than a squat jump (Figure 5.24c–e). In a countermovement jump, the person starts from a standing position and then performs a downward countermovement immediately followed by a maximum effort upward jump. The leg extensor musculotendinous units act eccentrically to arrest the countermovement and then act concentrically to drive the body upward into the jump. In a squat jump, the person performs a maximum effort jump from a stationary squat position. The leg extensor musculotendinous units act isometrically in the stationary squat position and act concentrically to drive the body upward into the jump. Assuming that the same level of squat is achieved in both the countermovement jump and the squat jump, the difference in performance, i.e. in height jumped, will be largely due to differences in the storage and utilisation of elastic strain energy in the connective tissues of the leg extensor

151

musculotendinous units and the amount of force produced by the muscle components of the leg extensor muscles.

In the countermovement of a countermovement jump, the connective tissue components (series elastic and parallel elastic) are forcibly stretched and, therefore, elastic strain energy builds up in them, like the energy stored in a stretched spring. The amount of elastic strain energy absorbed by the connective tissues ($= F \cdot d$) will be determined by the stretching force (F) and the amount of stretch (d = tension strain). However, the magnitude of the stretching force will largely determine the amount of stretch; the higher the force, the greater the stretch and the greater the amount of elastic strain energy absorbed. The magnitude of the stretching force will largely depend on the velocity of stretch, i.e. the rate at which stretching occurs. The higher the velocity of stretch, the greater the amount of elastic strain energy absorbed. However, a high velocity of stretch of the connective tissues can only be achieved if the force produced by the muscle components is high; a low-to-moderate force results in lengthening of the muscle components with little or no stretch on the connective tissues. With regard to amount of stretch, the muscle components can only produce a high force within the central region of the length–tension range; consequently, the amount of stretch should be low to moderate. In general, the amount of elastic strain energy absorbed in the connective tissues of the leg extensor musculotendinous units in the countermovement of a countermovement jump will be maximised by a low-to-moderate amount of stretch combined with a high velocity of stretch.

In the squat position of a squat jump, the leg extensor muscles will contract isometrically and their connective tissue components will be in a stretched position. Consequently, the connective tissues will have a certain amount of elastic strain energy (dependent on the amount of static stretch), but it is likely to be less than that stored during the countermovement of a countermovement jump (dependent upon the amount of dynamic stretch). In both the squat jump and the countermovement jump (and any other movement involving absorption of elastic strain energy by connective tissue components), the elastic strain energy can contribute to movement in the form of force (additional to that produced by the muscle components) exerted during the recoil of the connective tissue components from their stretched position.

It should be possible to absorb more elastic strain energy in the dynamic countermovement phase of a countermovement jump than in the static squat phase of a squat jump. However, the ability to utilise the additional strain energy depends on the delay between the eccentric and concentric phases of the movement. Some of the additional strain energy is inevitably converted to heat and, therefore, is not available to contribute to movement. The amount of elastic strain energy converted to heat depends on the speed of the changeover from eccentric to concentric action. Generally, the faster the changeover, the smaller the proportion of strain energy converted to heat, and, consequently, the greater the proportion available to contribute to movement (Gregor 1993; Komi, 2003).

The amount of elastic strain energy absorbed in the connective tissues of musculotendinous units in a countermovement will be maximised by a low-to-moderate amount of stretch combined with a high velocity of stretch.

Sometimes the elastic strain energy that is converted to heat is referred to as lost energy. However, this is misleading, since energy can never be completely lost; it can only be converted from one form of energy to another. For example, the muscles convert energy in the form of chemical substances (such as adenosine triphosphate) into mechanical energy in the form of movement (kinetic energy), which itself may be converted into another form of mechanical energy (strain energy). With regard to elastic strain energy in musculotendinous units, the proportion of this energy converted to heat is only lost in the sense that it is not available to contribute to movement.

The concentric phase of the squat jump is preceded by isometric contraction of the leg extensor muscles, whereas the concentric phase of the countermovement jump is preceded by eccentric action. Elicitation of the stretch reflex during the eccentric phase of the countermovement jump is likely to enhance performance over the squat jump in two ways:

1. The high force during the eccentric phase (greater than isometric force) is likely to increase the possibility of a high velocity of stretching of the connective tissues and, consequently, increase the amount of elastic strain energy absorbed in the connective tissues, compared with the squat jump.
2. The force generated during the concentric phase of the countermovement jump is likely to be greater than that generated in the concentric phase of the squat jump.

Stretch load and jump performance in drop jumping

A person's ability to make use of the stretch–shorten cycle in jumping activities depends on her ability to tolerate stretch loading, i.e. the force exerted in the musculotendinous units undergoing eccentric action. As stretch load and velocity of stretch increases, performance increases up to a particular optimum velocity of stretch, and then decreases with further increases in velocity of stretch. For example, it has been shown that in drop jumping, i.e. when subjects are asked to drop onto the floor from various heights and then immediately perform a maximum vertical jump, performance (jump height) increases as drop height increases, up to approximately 50 cm to 60 cm, and then decreases as drop height increases further (Komi and Bosco 1978). As drop height increases, the stretch load (reflected in the magnitude of the ground reaction force) during the eccentric phase of ground contact tends to increase. However, for each individual there is a drop height D that corresponds to a maximum tolerable stretch load (a maximum stretch load at which maximal effort in the drop jump can be maintained). This drop height may be associated with maximal performance due to the beneficial effects of the stretch–shorten cycle. At drop heights greater than D, the individual is unable to tolerate the stretch load associated with maximal effort and may reduce the stretch load by increasing the amount of hip, knee and ankle flexion during the eccentric phase of landing. This increases the magnitude of stretch of the leg extensors. The increased magnitude of stretch reduces the velocity of stretch of the leg extensors and thus reduces the potential benefits of increased muscle force and elastic strain energy, resulting in decreased performance. Not surprisingly, jump training based on drop jumping has been shown to increase performance and the size of the stretch load that can be tolerated (Komi 2003).

153

Utilising the stretch–shorten cycle in movements without a countermovement

In movements such as the countermovement jump, it is only possible to use the stretch–shorten cycle by incorporating a countermovement. In some whole-body movements, it may be possible to use the stretch–shorten cycle to accelerate the relevant body parts in the intended direction during the eccentric phase as well as during the concentric phase. In such actions there is no countermovement, but there is a premovement that results in eccentric action of the relevant musculotendinous units. For example, in the final stage of throwing a javelin, the javelin is pulled by the throwing arm from a position behind the trunk to a release point in front of the trunk (Figure 5.25). If, at the start of this pulling action, the (right-handed) thrower can thrust his right shoulder forward fast enough (Figure 5.25c–d), the inertia of the arm and javelin results in eccentric action of the shoulder flexors and abductors and elbow flexors, which are (in association with muscles in the legs and trunk) responsible for the pulling action. The arm and javelin are accelerated forward though the shoulder and elbow muscles act eccentrically. The eccentric phase of the elbow flexors is relatively short, and the elbow flexes and then extends prior to release of the javelin. In contrast, the eccentric phase of the shoulder flexors and abductors may last for most of the pulling action with only a short concentric phase just prior to release (see Figure 5.25e,f). Ideally, the thrower should thrust his right shoulder forward for as long as possible during the pulling action, as this will maximise the force exerted on the javelin by prolonging the eccentric (high-force) phases of

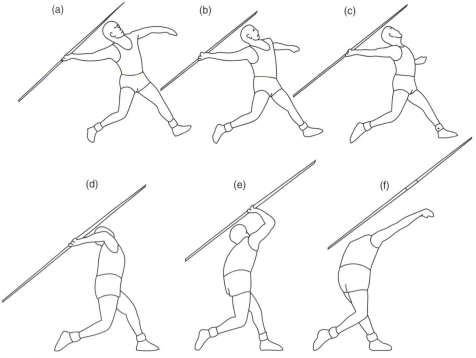

Figure 5.25 The delivery phase in throwing a javelin.

the shoulder and elbow muscles and increasing the force exerted in the concentric phases of the muscles by decreasing their speed of shortening.

REVIEW QUESTIONS

1. Differentiate between the cerebrospinal nervous system and the central nervous system.

2. Differentiate between resting potential and action potential.

3. Describe the general organisation of nerve tissue in the spinal cord and spinal nerves.

4. Describe the sequence of events within the nervous system in a typical voluntary movement.

5. Describe the various categories of pennate and non-pennate muscles.

6. Describe the sliding filament theory of muscular contraction.

7. Differentiate between kinaesthetic sense and proprioception.

8. Differentiate between active and passive insufficiency in skeletal muscle.

9. Describe the fundamental relationships between muscle architecture and muscle function.

Chapter 6

Mechanical characteristics of musculoskeletal components

All materials deform in response to loading in a manner that reflects their mechanical characteristics, including, for example, their stiffness and their strength. The components of the musculoskeletal system (musculotendinous units, ligaments, cartilage and bone) have different mechanical characteristics, but they combine to serve two main mechanical functions: as brakes to dissipate energy in impacts, and as springs to minimise energy expenditure by recycling stored energy. This chapter describes the mechanical characteristics of the musculoskeletal components and the response of the musculoskeletal components to loading.

OBJECTIVES

After reading this chapter you should be able to do the following:

1. Differentiate between a load–deformation curve and a stress–strain curve.
2. Describe the general stress–strain behaviour of compact bone and ligaments.
3. Differentiate work, strain energy, gravitational potential energy and kinetic energy.
4. Describe the difference in function of musculotendinous units in landing and rebound activities.
5. Describe the mechanism of shock absorption in synovial joints.

STRESS–STRAIN RELATIONSHIPS IN SOLIDS

All materials deform to a certain extent in response to loading; the greater the load, the greater the deformation. A material's load–deformation relationship reflects its mechanical characteristics. To compare the mechanical characteristics of different materials, it is usual to express load and deformation in terms of stress (load per unit cross-sectional area) and strain (deformation as a proportion of the dimensions of the material when unloaded), respectively. Stress is denoted by the lower case Greek letter sigma (σ), and strain is denoted by the lower case Greek letter epsilon (ε). Figure 6.1 shows a generalised stress–strain curve.

In response to tension loading, a material tends to lengthen in the direction of the tension load. Consequently, tension strain refers to an increase in length of the material as a proportion of the length of the material when it is not loaded. Similarly, in response to compression

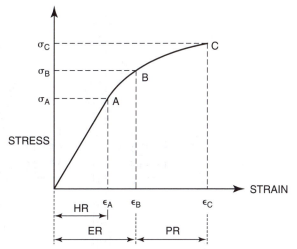

Figure 6.1 Generalised stress–strain curve. ER, elastic range; PR, plastic range; HR, Hookean range; A, proportional limit; B, yield point (elastic limit); C, failure point (complete rupture).

loading, a material tends to shorten in the direction of the compression load; compression strain refers to a decrease in length of the material as a proportion of the length of the material when it is not loaded. Note that stress is measured in units of force per unit cross-sectional area, such as N/cm^2, but that strain has no units, since it is the ratio of two lengths.

All materials deform in response to loading. The load–deformation relationship of a material reflects its mechanical characteristics. To compare the mechanical characteristics of different materials, load is expressed in terms of stress and deformation in terms of strain.

Most materials are elastic to a certain extent; that is, they deform in response to loading and then restore their original dimensions when the load is removed. In Figure 6.1, the point B represents the yield point or elastic limit, i.e. the point at which the material starts to tear or fracture. The strain range between zero strain and the strain at B (ε_B) is the elastic range; that is, provided that the strain on the material is within the elastic range, the material will not be damaged and will remain perfectly elastic. However, if the strain on the material exceeds the elastic range, the material will be deformed plastically; that is, in the case of an inanimate object, it will be permanently damaged to a degree corresponding to the amount of strain. As such it will lose some of its elasticity and will not return to its original dimensions when the load is removed. If the amount of strain is allowed to increase progressively beyond the yield point, the material will eventually fail completely; this is the failure point and is represented by the point C in Figure 6.1. The strain range between ε_B and ε_C is the plastic range. The stress at C (σ_C) is the ultimate stress or strength of the material.

157

Units of force

The *Système International d'Unités*, usually referred to as the SI system or the metric system, is the most widely used system of units in commerce and scientific communication. In the SI system, the unit of force is the newton (N). In accordance with Newton's second law of motion ($F = m \cdot a$, where a is the acceleration experienced by a mass m when acted upon by a force F), a newton is defined as the force acting on a mass of 1 kg (kilogram) that accelerates it at 1 m/s^2 (metre per second per second), i.e.

$$1\,N = 1\,kg \times 1\,m/s^2 \text{ (i.e.} 1\,N = 1\,kg \cdot m/s^2\text{)}.$$

The weight W of an object is the product of its mass m and the acceleration due to gravity g, i.e.

$$W = m \cdot g, \text{ where } g = 9.81\,m/s^2.$$

Consequently, the weight of a mass of 1 kg, referred to as 1 kgf (kilogram force) is 9.81 N, i.e.

$$1\,kgf = 1\,kg \times 9.81\,m/s^2 = 9.81\,N.$$

The kgf is referred to as a gravitational unit of force. Most weighing machines in everyday use, such as kitchen scales and bathroom scales, are graduated in kgf or lbf (pounds force). Thus the weight of a man of mass 70 kg can be expressed as 70 kgf or 686.7 N, i.e.

$$70\,kgf = 70\,kg \times 9.81\,m/s^2 = 686.7\,N.$$

In calculations using SI units, the unit of force is the newton, and all forces, including weights, must be expressed in newtons.

Stiffness and compliance

In most materials, all or part of the stress–strain curve within the elastic range is linear, i.e. the increase in strain is directly proportional to the increase in stress. Any material that behaves in this way is said to obey Hooke's Law (after Robert Hooke, 1635–1703). Consequently, the linear region of the stress–strain curve is referred to as the Hookean region. The upper limit of the Hookean region is the proportional limit. In some materials the proportional limit and the yield point coincide, but in most materials the proportional limit occurs before the yield point. The gradient of the stress–strain curve in the Hookean region reflects the stiffness of the material, that is, the resistance of the material to deformation. The greater the stress required to produce a given amount of strain, the stiffer the material.

The gradient of the stress–strain curve in the Hookean region is referred to as the Young modulus of elasticity (or the elastic modulus) for the material. The Young modulus (after Thomas Young, 1773–1829) indicates the amount of stress needed to produce 100% strain. Most materials fail long before 100% strain, but the Young modulus provides a standard measure of stiffness for comparing different materials. The Young modulus is denoted by E. With reference to Figure 6.1, if $\sigma_A = 6000 \text{ N/cm}^2$ and $\varepsilon_A = 0.015$ (1.5% strain), then

$$E = \frac{\sigma_A}{\varepsilon_A}$$

$$= \frac{6{,}000 \text{N/cm}^2}{0.015} = 400\,000 \text{ N/cm}^2 = 400 \text{ kN},$$

where 1 kN = 1 kilonewton = 1000 N.

The larger the Young modulus, the stiffer the material. Slight changes in the composition of a material may affect its stiffness (and other mechanical characteristics). For example, different kinds of steel have different levels of stiffness. Similarly, the stiffness of musculoskeletal components depends considerably on the age, nutrition and physical activity level of the person. Furthermore, the mechanical characteristics of similar musculoskeletal components vary with location in the body. For example, the stiffness of compact bone in the femur is different from that in the tibia of the same individual (Burstein and Wright 1994). Owing to the variation in the magnitude of the mechanical properties of different types of the same material there are no standard reference data. Table 6.1 shows some data reported in the literature concerning the stiffness of certain materials in tension.

Figure 6.2 shows generalised stress–strain curves for bone and ligament. It is clear that bone is stiffer and stronger than ligament. However, bone tends to fail suddenly, whereas ligament exhibits progressive, albeit rapid, failure following the proportional limit. Furthermore, in contrast to bone, ligament has a characteristic 'toe' region in which a relatively small increase in stress results in a relatively large increase in strain during the first 1% of strain. The toe region reflects the straightening out of the collagen fibres, which, under resting

Table 6.1 Young modulus for some materials under tension (kN/cm^2).

Material		Mean	Range
Normal compact bone (6th decade)[1]	Femur	1700	
	Tibia	2000	
Normal compact bone[2]	Femur	1569	1269–1943
Osteoporotic compact bone[2]	Femur	1155	397–1834
Patellar ligament[1]		40	
Elastin[3]		0.06	
Tool steel[4]		19 000	
Stainless steel[4]		17 000	
Glass[4]		7000	
Oak[3]		1000	
Lightly vulcanised rubber[3]		0.14	

[1] (Burstein and Wright 1994)
[2] (Dickenson et al. 1981)
[3] (Alexander 1968)
[4] (Frost 1967)

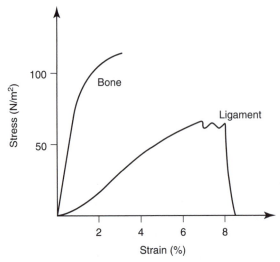

Figure 6.2 Generalised stress–strain curves for bone and ligament in tension.

conditions, have a wavy arrangement. Tendons and cartilage respond to loading in a similar manner to ligament.

In real-life situations, many materials, like bone, are loaded simultaneously in tension, compression and shear. The Young modulus can be calculated for each type of loading. When the Young modulus of a particular material is the same in all three forms of loading, the material is said to exhibit strain isotropy. When the Young modulus is different for the three forms of loading, the material is said to exhibit strain anisotropy. Most materials with a physical grain, like wood, bone, tendon, ligament and cartilage, exhibit strain anisotropy (Frost 1967). For example, bone is stiffer in compression than in tension, and stiffer in tension than in shear.

Compliance is the reciprocal of stiffness; that is, increasing the stiffness of a material decreases its compliance, and vice versa. The greater the strain produced by a given amount of stress, the more compliant the material. The yield point of the load–deformation (or stress–strain) curve of a material is usually signified by a marked increase in compliance (decrease in stiffness).

Toughness, fragility and brittleness

For any given piece of material, the area under the load–deformation curve represents the strain energy absorbed by the material. The toughness of a material is defined as the amount of strain energy that the material absorbs prior to failure; the greater the amount of energy absorbed, the tougher the material. For the purpose of comparing the toughness of different materials, the toughness modulus is defined as the strain energy absorbed per unit volume of the material prior to failure. The toughness modulus of a material is represented by the area under the stress–strain curve of the material.

Figure 6.3 shows typical stress–strain curves for normal compact bone and osteoporotic compact bone. The area under the osteoporotic curve is much smaller than that under the normal curve, which shows that normal bone is much tougher than osteoporotic bone. Fragility refers to a low level of toughness, i.e. a fragile material absorbs relatively little strain

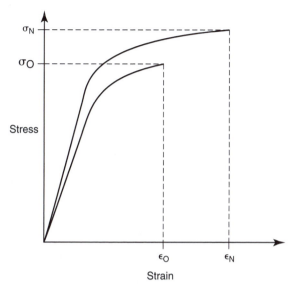

Figure 6.3 The effects of osteoporosis on the stress–strain characteristics of compact bone: N, normal bone; O, osteoporotic bone.

energy prior to failure. It follows that osteoporotic bone is more fragile than normal bone. Figure 6.3 shows that the greater toughness of normal bone is due to greater strength (ultimate stress) and greater strain to failure compared with osteoporotic bone. A brittle material fails after relatively little strain; the lower the strain to failure, the more brittle the material. It follows that osteoporotic bone is more brittle than normal bone.

ENERGY

There are a number of different forms of energy, including heat, light, sound, electricity, chemical energy and various forms of mechanical energy. The total amount of energy in the universe is constant; it cannot be created or destroyed, it can only be transformed from one form to another. All interactions in nature are the result of transformation of energy from one form to another. Living organisms digest food to release nutrients that are contained in the food. Some of the nutrients, in particular, carbohydrates and fats, are used to produce chemical energy, i.e. substances which, when required, break down into their constituent components and simultaneously release energy to maintain all of the processes that sustain life. In human beings, the majority of the energy obtained from nutrients is used to produce muscular contractions.

Work, strain energy and kinetic energy

As described in Chapter 5, a force does work when it moves its point of application in the direction of the force and the amount of work done is defined as the product of the force and the distance moved by the point of application of the force. For example, in drawing a bow, the archer does work on the bow by pulling on the arrow, which, in turn, pulls on the bowstring (Figure 6.4a). Figure 6.4b shows the corresponding load–deformation curve of the

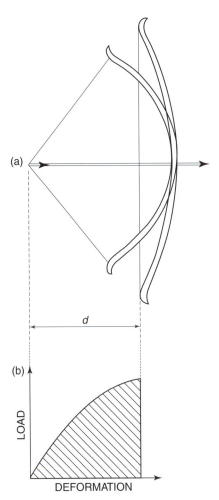

Figure 6.4 Storage of strain energy in a bow. (a) Deformation of a bow through a distance d.(b) Load–deformation curve of the force exerted on the bow and the corresponding deformation of the bow. The work done on the bow, i.e. the strain energy stored in the bow, is represented by the shaded area under the load–deformation curve.

force exerted on the bow. As the bow is drawn, the work done on the bow, represented by the area under the load–deformation curve, is stored in the bow, which deforms like a spring. The work done on the bow is stored in the bow as strain energy, i.e. energy that can be used to do work on the arrow (propel the arrow forward via the bowstring) when the bowstring is released. Strain energy is a form of mechanical energy, i.e. energy that can do work. The amount of work done by the archer on the bow, i.e. the amount of strain energy stored in the bow, is $F \cdot d$, where F is the average force exerted on the bowstring and d is the distance that the bow is drawn back. When the arrow is released, the bow recoils and the strain energy stored in the bow is transformed into work on the arrow via the bowstring. The arrow separates from the bowstring with kinetic energy equivalent to the strain energy stored in the drawn bow. Kinetic energy, another form of mechanical energy, is the energy possessed by a body due to its speed of movement. An object of mass m and speed of movement v has kinetic energy equal to $m \cdot v^2 / 2$. Consequently, in the bow and arrow example, $F \cdot d = m \cdot v^2 / 2$, where F is the average force exerted on the arrow by the bowstring, d is the distance over which F is applied, m is the mass of the arrow, and v is the release speed of the arrow.

Many materials store strain energy in response to loading, for example, a stretched elastic band, a trampoline, a springboard in diving, a beat board in vaulting, a pole in pole vaulting or a musculotendinous unit in an eccentric action. Strain energy is a form of potential energy, i.e. stored energy, that, given appropriate conditions, may be used to do work.

In the SI system, the unit of work is the joule (J) (after James Prescott Joule, 1818–1889). One joule is the amount of work done by a force of 1 N when it moves its point of application a distance of 1 m in the direction of the force, i.e. $1 J = 1 N \cdot m$ (newton metre).

Human movement is brought about by coordinated actions of the skeletal muscles. The muscles do work in moving the body segments. In doing work, the muscles transform chemical energy stored in the muscles into kinetic energy of the moving body segments. The stored energy in the muscles is potential energy in the form of complex chemical substances (chiefly adenosine triphosphate and creatine phosphate). When a muscle contracts isometrically (no change in length) it expends energy but does no work. When a muscle contracts concentrically (shortens) it expends energy in doing positive work, i.e. it pulls its skeletal attachments closer together. When a muscle contracts eccentrically (lengthens) it expends energy, but in contrast to a concentric contraction, work is done on the muscle, i.e. it is forcibly stretched; this type of work by muscles is called negative work. As a musculotendinous unit lengthens in an eccentric action, the elastic components of the musculotendinous unit absorb energy in the form of strain energy. For example, when landing from a jump or vault in gymnastics, the kinetic energy of the body is transformed into strain energy in the support surface and strain energy in the musculotendinous units that control the hip, knee and ankle joints by eccentric action of these units. When the purpose of the landing is to bring the body to rest, the strain energy in the musculotendinous units is rapidly dissipated as heat in the musculotendinous units and subsequently in the rest of the body and the surrounding air. However, if the landing is immediately followed by a rebound, some of the strain energy in the musculotendinous units may be recycled in the subsequent movement in the form of work (additional to that produced by concentric contraction of the muscles) resulting from recoil of the elastic components of the musculotendinous units. As described in Chapter 5, the use of this strain energy depends largely on the speed of changeover from eccentric to concentric muscle action. Generally, the faster the changeover, the smaller the proportion of strain energy dissipated as heat and, consequently, the greater the proportion available to contribute to the subsequent movement.

Gravitational potential energy

If an object is held above ground level and then released, it will fall to the ground due to the force of its own weight. The work done on the object by the force of its own weight W when it falls a distance h is given by $W \cdot h$. Consequently, when an object of weight W is held a distance h above the ground, it possesses gravitational potential energy equivalent to $W \cdot h$, which can be transformed into kinetic energy if it is allowed to fall. Gravitational potential energy is usually expressed as $m \cdot g \cdot h$ (where $W = m \cdot g$; m is the mass of the object and g is the acceleration due to gravity).

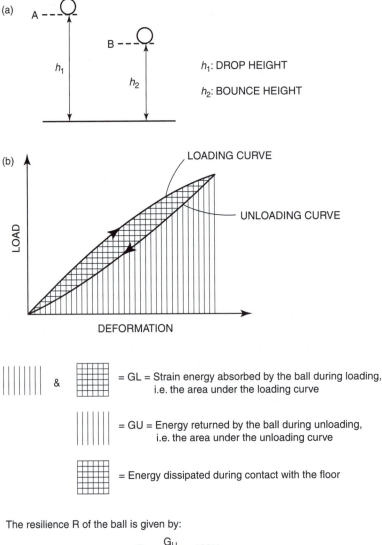

(a)

A - - -

B - - -

h_1

h_2

h_1: DROP HEIGHT

h_2: BOUNCE HEIGHT

(b)

LOADING CURVE

UNLOADING CURVE

LOAD

DEFORMATION

||||||| & ▦ = GL = Strain energy absorbed by the ball during loading, i.e. the area under the loading curve

||||||| = GU = Energy returned by the ball during unloading, i.e. the area under the unloading curve

▦ = Energy dissipated during contact with the floor

The resilience R of the ball is given by:

$$R = \frac{G_U}{G_L} \times 100\%$$

If G_L = 180 J and G_U = 153 J, then:

$$R = \frac{153\ J}{180\ J} \times 100\%$$

$$R = 85\%$$

Figure 6.5 Load–deformation characteristics of a bouncing rubber ball.

Figure 6.5a shows a rubber ball held at rest at a height h_1 above the floor where the floor is the reference level ($h = 0$) for the measurement of gravitational potential energy. While it is held at rest, the ball has no kinetic energy, but its gravitational potential energy will be equal to $m \cdot g \cdot h_1$. If the ball is allowed to fall, its gravitational potential energy will be transformed into kinetic energy, i.e. its gravitational potential energy will decrease and its kinetic energy will increase. When the ball hits the floor, its gravitational potential energy will be zero and its kinetic energy will be equal to $m \cdot v^2/2$ where v is the velocity of the ball at impact, i.e.

$$m \cdot g \cdot h_1 = m \cdot v^2/2$$

$$v = \sqrt{2g \cdot h_1},$$

If $h_1 = 1\text{m}$ then $v = \sqrt{2 \times 9.81\text{m/s}^2 \times 1\text{m}} = 4.43\,\text{m/s}^2$.

Hysteresis, resilience and damping

In the preceding example, the ball strikes the floor with kinetic energy equivalent to the gravitational potential energy it possessed at release. During contact with the floor the ball will undergo a loading phase in which it is compressed and the kinetic energy of the ball is transformed into strain energy in the compressed ball. Following the loading phase, the ball undergoes an unloading phase, in which it recoils and the strain energy is released as kinetic energy in the form of the upward bounce of the ball. However, the ball will not bounce as high as the point from which it was dropped. This situation is shown in Figure 6.5a, where h_1 is the drop height and h_2 is the bounce height. As the ball is at rest at A and B, some of the energy of the ball was dissipated during contact with the floor in the form of, for example, heat and sound. The amount of energy dissipated is reflected in the load–deformation curves of the ball during loading and unloading (Figure 6.5b).

The amount of strain energy absorbed by the ball during loading, the area under the loading curve, is greater than the amount of energy returned during unloading, the area under the unloading curve. The loop described by the loading and unloading curves is a hysteresis loop (from the Greek word *husteros*, meaning later or delayed). The area of the hysteresis loop represents the energy dissipated. The extent of hysteresis in a material is reflected in the resilience of the material, which is defined as the amount of energy returned during unloading as a percentage of the amount of energy absorbed during loading. All materials exhibit hysteresis to a certain extent; there are no 100% resilient materials.

Figure 6.6a shows the load–deformation characteristics of highly resilient material such as ligament and tendon, and Figure 6.6b shows the load–deformation characteristics of low-resilience material, such as some forms of vinyl acetate foam. Damping refers to a low level of resilience; a damping material returns very little energy during unloading compared with the amount of energy that it absorbs during loading. For protection during transportation, fragile goods are usually packed in materials with good damping properties. Similarly, in walking and running, shock-absorbing soles and insoles in shoes are used to protect the body from high-impact loads at heel-strike. In human movement, shock absorption refers to the dissipation of the work done on the body as a result of a collision with the environment in a way that prevents high-impact loads. Shock absorption systems are low-resilience energy absorption systems.

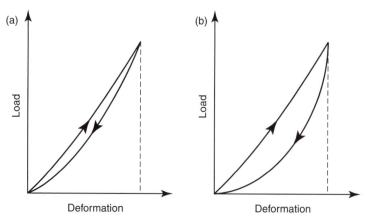

(a)

Load

Deformation

(b)

Load

Deformation

Figure 6.6 Load–deformation characteristics of materials. (a) High resilience and low damping. (b) Low resilience and high damping.

> The human body converts chemical energy into three forms of mechanical energy: kinetic energy, gravitational potential energy and strain energy.

Resilience of the lower limbs in running

The amount of strain energy absorbed by the different components of a system during deformation depends on the toughness and volume of the components. The tougher the component and the greater its volume, the more strain energy it is likely to absorb. Of the various musculoskeletal components and related structures, such as the heel pad (the approximately 2 cm thick layer of subcutaneous fat over the inferior aspect of the calcaneus), muscle has the least capacity for absorbing strain energy and tendon has the highest capacity (approximately 65 times that of muscle), while the capacity of bone (approximately 55 times that of muscle) is between that of muscle and tendon (Evans 1971). Whereas the energy-absorbing capacity of muscle is very much lower than that of tendon, the musculotendinous unit has the highest energy-absorbing capacity of all musculoskeletal and associated tissues (Evans 1971). During the mid-stance phase in running (Figure 6.7a,b), the system of support surface, shoe (including sock and insole), and musculoskeletal system (including associated structures, such as heel pad and skin) deforms in response to the force of the impact following the heel strike. The leg is forcibly flexed and the arch of the foot is forcibly flattened, such that strain energy is stored in the bones (bending of long bones and compression of short bones), joints (compression of epiphyses), musculotendinous units (eccentric actions of leg extensor and foot arch support musculotendinous units) and ligaments supporting the arch of the foot. Figure 6.7 shows a model of the movement of the lower leg and foot from flat foot (Figure 6.7a,c) to peak force (Figure 6.7b,d) during the mid-stance phase, which illustrates the strain on the calf muscles and arch support mechanisms.

The gravitational and kinetic energy of an athlete running at a middle-distance pace (7–8 m/s) is estimated to decrease by about 100 J during the absorption phase and then

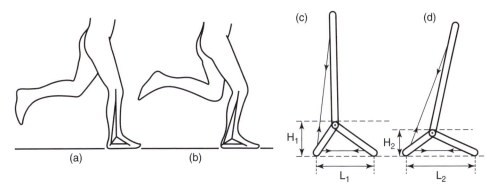

Figure 6.7 Storage of strain energy in the calf muscles and arch support mechanisms during mid-stance in running.

Table 6.2 Energy storage and resilience in system components during the ground contact phase in middle-distance running.

Material	Energy absorbed (J)	Resilience (%)	Energy returned (J)
1. Calf muscles	35	93*	32.5
2. Arch support mechanism	17	78	13.2
3. Heel pad	3	20	0.6
4. Shoe	5	60	3.0
5. Track	7	90	6.3
6. Other[†]	33	64**	21.1
Total	100		76.7

* Resilience of Achilles tendon
** Average of 1, 2 and 3
[†] Energy stored in other parts of the body

increase by about 100 J during the propulsion phase (Ker *et al.* 1987). The same researchers also estimate that during the absorption phase energies of approximately 35 J, 17 J and 5 J are stored in the calf musculotendinous units, arch support mechanisms and shoe, respectively. The heel pad is estimated to store approximately 3 J (Cavanagh *et al.* 1984) and a specially designed indoor running track can store in the region of 7 J (McMahon and Greene 1978). These findings are summarised in the second column of Table 6.2, while the resilience of the materials (reported in the same sources) is shown in the third column of the table. The fourth column shows the theoretical potential for the release of strain energy in the form of useful mechanical work during the propulsion phase (from heel-off to toe-off). Whereas the estimate for the release of useful strain energy is probably higher than that which occurs in real situations, the figures do indicate the considerable energy-saving potential of the system.

Clearly, the energy-absorbing capacity and resilience of musculotendinous units is likely to be a major determinant of the quality of a person's performance in games and sports. However, musculotendinous units can only function efficiently when the muscles are not fatigued. A fatigued muscle is limited in its ability to apply tension to its tendons, which, in turn, limits the ability of the tendons to absorb strain energy. Consequently, muscle fatigue

167

reduces the energy-absorbing capacity of a musculotendinous unit; the greater the degree of muscle fatigue, the greater the reduction in energy-absorbing capacity. In any movement involving the absorption of gravitational potential energy and kinetic energy, such as in the absorption phase of running (from heel strike to mid-stance), or landing from a jump, the extent to which a particular musculotendinous unit has to lengthen to make its contribution to energy absorption is determined by the force the muscle can produce. The greater the muscle force, the shorter the distance the musculotendinous unit must lengthen to absorb a given amount of energy. Fatigue reduces the amount of contractile force a muscle can produce; a fatigued muscle has to lengthen farther than a non-fatigued muscle to absorb a given amount of energy.

It has been shown that a muscle yields at the same degree of strain irrespective of its level of fatigue. Consequently, a fatigued muscle is more likely to be stretched beyond its yield point than a non-fatigued muscle (Mair *et al.* 1996). Furthermore, when the level of effort remains fairly constant, as when running at a constant speed, the gradual reduction in energy-absorbing capacity of musculotendinous units due to fatigue inevitably results in increased strain on associated structures, especially bones and joints, because the amount of energy absorbed in each absorption phase of the activity is likely to remain fairly constant. Consequently, the greater the degree of muscular fatigue, the greater the risk of injury to all components of the musculoskeletal system (Grimston and Zernicke 1993).

The musculotendinous unit has the highest energy-absorbing capacity of all the musculoskeletal tissues, but the capacity to absorb energy decreases with increasing fatigue. The gradual reduction in energy-absorbing capacity of musculotendinous units due to fatigue results in increased strain on associated structures, especially bones and joints.

VISCOSITY AND VISCOELASTICITY

As described previously, stiffness is a measure of the resistance of a solid material to deformation by a load. The viscosity of a liquid or semi-liquid substance is a measure of the resistance of the substance to shear deformation in response to a shear load. Figure 6.8 shows a flat, square piece of wood separated from a larger flat surface by a layer of liquid or semi-liquid substance. If the area of the piece of wood is A and a horizontal force F is applied to the piece of wood, then the shear stress on the substance is given by F/A. The movement of the wood is resisted by the viscosity of the substance; the greater the viscosity, the greater the resistance. The viscosity V of the substance is defined as:

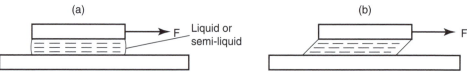

Figure 6.8 Response of a liquid or semi-liquid to shear stress. (a) At the start of application of force F. (b) Some time after the start of application of force F.

$$V = \frac{\text{shear stress}}{\text{shear strain rate}}.$$

Consequently, for a given level of shear stress, the lower the shear strain rate, the higher the viscosity of the substance and vice versa (Alexander 1968).

In contrast with an elastic material, which deforms immediately in response to loading and restores its original size and shape immediately in response to unloading, a viscoelastic material deforms gradually in response to loading and gradually restores its original size and shape when unloaded. Most biological materials, including all the musculoskeletal components, behave elastically or viscoelastically depending on the rate at which they are loaded; they tend to behave elastically in response to high rates of loading and viscoelastically in response to low-to-moderate rates of loading.

Mechanical model of viscoelasticity

In mechanical models of viscoelastic materials, the elastic elements are usually represented by springs and the viscous elements by Newton's model of a hydraulic piston (a 'dashpot') (Taylor *et al.* 1990; Figure 6.9). Figure 6.9c shows a mechanical model of a viscoelastic material based on a piston and three springs; one of the springs is in series with the piston and the other two springs are in parallel with the piston. In response to tension loading, the model gradually lengthens in the direction of T at a rate that depends on the stiffness of the springs and the viscosity of the piston. When the load is removed, the model gradually restores its

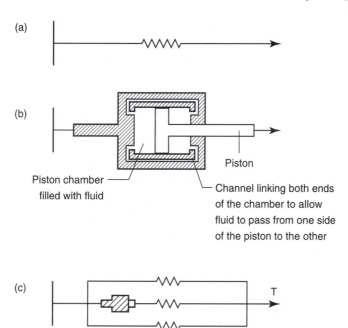

Figure 6.9 A mechanical model of viscoelastic behaviour. (a) A spring represents elastic behaviour. (b) A piston represents viscoelastic behaviour. (c) Model of a viscoelastic material that incorporates a piston and three springs, one spring in series with the piston and the other two in parallel with the piston.

169

original length at a rate depending on the force exerted by the springs and the viscosity of the piston.

Properties of viscoelastic materials

The response of a viscoelastic material to loading is always time dependent. However, the actual response depends on the type of load. When a viscoelastic material is subjected to a constant load (lower than yield stress), the material deforms asymptotically with time, i.e. it gradually deforms at a progressively decreasing rate until a point at which further deformation ceases. This property of viscoelastic materials is called creep. If the load is then removed, the material gradually restores its original dimensions. For example, if a viscoelastic material is subjected to a constant tension load (lower than the yield stress), the material gradually lengthens until a point is reached where lengthening ceases (Figure 6.10a). If the load is then removed, the material gradually restores its original dimensions.

If a viscoelastic material is deformed (within its elastic range) and then held in the deformed position, the stress experienced by the material decreases asymptotically with time until a point at which no further decrease in stress occurs. This property of viscoelastic materials is called stress relaxation. If the load is then removed, the material gradually restores its original dimensions. For example, if a viscoelastic material is stretched within its elastic range and then held at a constant length, the tension stress experienced by the material decreases with time until a point where no further decrease in tension stress occurs (Figure 6.10b). If the load is then removed, the material gradually restores its original dimensions.

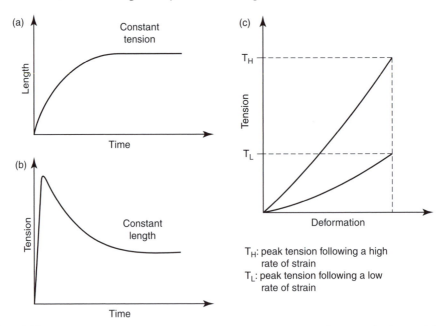

Figure 6.10 Properties of viscoelastic materials. (a) Creep: length–time curve for a viscoelastic material subjected to a constant tension load. (b) Stress relaxation: tension–time curve for a viscoelastic material stretched and then held at a constant length. (c) Strain rate dependency: effect of strain rate on stiffness, peak tension and energy absorption in a viscoelastic material (at the same degree of deformation).

In addition to creep and stress relaxation, viscoelastic materials also exhibit strain rate dependency, i.e. the mechanical characteristics of a viscoelastic material depend on the rate of strain. The higher the rate of strain, the smaller the degree to which creep and stress relaxation can occur during deformation, which, in turn, increases the stiffness, strength (ultimate stress) and toughness of the material (Garrett *et al.* 1987; Taylor *et al.* 1990) (Figure 6.10c). In general, the higher the strain rate, the greater the stiffness, strength and toughness of the material. The increased toughness of a viscoelastic material in response to an increased strain rate enables it to absorb more energy. With regard to the musculoskeletal system, the increased toughness of the components, especially musculotendinous units and bone, in response to increased strain rates may enable the body to dissipate large amounts of energy as heat. However, if the large amounts of stored energy associated with high strain rates are dissipated in the form of failure, then the damage to the musculoskeletal system may be considerable. For example, when a bone fails in response to a low rate of strain, the amount of energy dissipated is relatively low and the bone may fracture in the form of a clean break with relatively little damage to the surrounding soft tissues. However, if the bone fails in response to a high rate of strain, a large amount of energy is dissipated and the bone may shatter into many small pieces, resulting in considerable damage to the bone and surrounding soft tissues. Bones may be subjected to very high rates of strain, for example, in high-speed collisions.

SHOCK ABSORPTION IN JOINTS

During foot strike in walking and running, and in similar foot-ground impacts, such as landing from a jump in gymnastics, some or all of the kinetic energy of the body is transformed into strain energy in all of the materials that are deformed during the impact with the floor; these include the support surface, the musculoskeletal system and, in the case of walking and running, shoes and socks. In these impacts, the joints of the lower limbs and vertebral column are compressed and absorb some energy, i.e. they contribute to shock absorption. Whereas the intervertebral joints and pubic symphysis joint (all symphysis joints) are specifically designed to function as shock absorbers, the hip, knee and ankle joints (all synovial joints) are not. Figure 6.11 shows a section through a typical synovial joint. In response to loading,

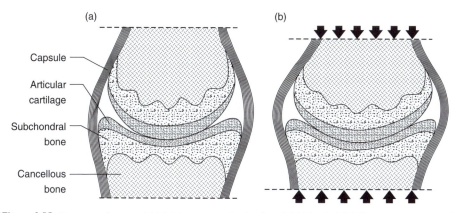

(a)   (b)

Capsule
Articular cartilage
Subchondral bone
Cancellous bone

Figure 6.11 Response of a synovial joint to compression loading. (a) Unloaded. (b) Response to compression loading.

both epiphyses deform to a certain extent. Cancellous bone is stiffer than subchondral bone, which is stiffer than articular cartilage. Consequently, articular cartilage and subchondral bone absorb shock better than an equivalent amount of cancellous bone. However, in a typical synovial joint, the volume of cancellous bone is greater than the volume of articular cartilage and subchondral bone, such that in healthy synovial joints the cancellous bone may be the major contributor to shock absorption (Radin and Paul 1971; Hoshino and Wallace 1987).

High-impact loads increase the likelihood of microfractures to trabeculae in cancellous bone. Healing of fractured trabeculae increases the stiffness of the cancellous bone and, consequently, decreases its shock-absorbing capacity (Radin and Paul 1971; Simon et al. 1972; Radin et al. 1973). Repeated microfracture and healing of cancellous bone progressively increases its stiffness and progressively decreases its shock-absorbing capacity. As the stiffness of cancellous bone increases, the subchondral bone and articular cartilage are subjected to increased strain (in both rate and amount), thereby increasing the likelihood of microtrauma, i.e. crushing or tearing of the matrix in subchondral bone and articular cartilage. Such microtrauma decreases the shock-absorbing capacity of the subchondral bone and articular cartilage. Not surprisingly, it has been shown that the shock-absorbing capacity of healthy joints is greater than that of degenerated joints (Voloshin and Wosk 1982). Progressive damage to articular cartilage can culminate in osteoarthritis (Figure 6.12).

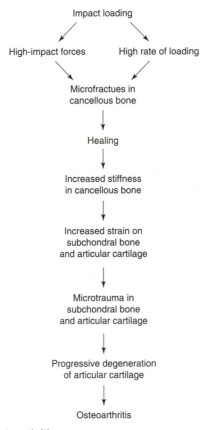

Figure 6.12 Development of osteoarthritis.

> Repeated microfracture and healing of cancellous bone results in a progressive increase in stiffness, which, in turn, increases the strain on subchondral bone and articular cartilage.

Heel strike during walking is the most common source of impact loading on the human body, and repeated exposure to high levels of shock resulting from walking heel strike appears to be a major cause of joint degeneration (Radin *et al.* 1973; Wosk and Voloshin 1985). Viscoelastic inserts in shoes have been shown to reduce the amplitude of heel-strike-induced shock waves and may compensate to a certain extent for the decreased shock-absorbing capacity of degenerated joints (Voloshin and Wosk 1981; Johnson 1988). Voloshin and Wosk (1981) showed that prolonged use (for 18 months) of viscoelastic heel inserts can significantly reduce clinical symptoms, especially pain, in adults suffering from chronic degenerative joint conditions such as osteoarthritis and intervertebral disc damage.

REVIEW QUESTIONS

1. Describe the stress–strain characteristics of bone and ligament.

2. Differentiate between toughness, fragility and brittleness.

3. Differentiate between hysteresis, resilience and damping.

4. Describe the effects of strain rate dependence on the mechanical characteristics of viscoelastic materials.

5. Describe the difference in function of musculotendinous units in landing (to rest) and rebound activities.

6. Describe the effects of muscle fatigue on the stress experienced by other musculoskeletal components.

Chapter 7

Structural adaptation

In response to the loads imposed on the musculoskeletal system as a result of normal everyday physical activity (ranging from activities of daily living to manual labour and training for sport), the musculoskeletal components (muscles, tendons, ligaments, cartilage and bone) experience strain. A certain level of strain is necessary to ensure normal growth and development, but excessive strain results in abnormal growth and development and injury. Under normal circumstances the musculoskeletal components continuously adapt their external form (size and shape) and internal architecture in response to the time-averaged strain. This chapter describes the effects of changes in time-averaged loading on the external form and internal architecture of the musculoskeletal components.

OBJECTIVES

After reading this chapter, you should be able to do the following:

1. Describe the relationship between genetic and environmental influences on growth and development.
2. Differentiate biopositive and bionegative effects of loading on musculoskeletal components.
3. Differentiate chronic injury and acute injury.
4. Describe structural adaptation in bone, regular fibrous tissues and skeletal muscle.

ADAPTATION

Two types of factor influence growth and development of the human body: genetic and environmental factors. The genes determine the pattern of growth and development in a set of 'genetic instructions' called the genotype. However, the body is constantly subjected to a variety of environmental influences, including nutritional state, changes in body temperature and the physical stress imposed by movement of the body. These environmental influences affect the genotype by modifying the timing, rate, extent and type of growth and development that occur, such that the body normally becomes adapted to function effectively in relation to the environmental conditions (Malina *et al.* 2004; Wackerhage and Rennie 2006; Seynnes *et al.* 2008). Adaptation to environmental conditions is continuous throughout life.

174

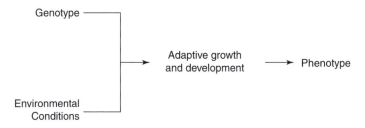

Figure 7.1 Model of adaptation.

The combination of size, shape and structure of the body that results from the effect of environmental conditions on the genotype is called the phenotype. The phenotype reflects both the general effects of the genotype and the specific effects of the environmental influences. We can actually see and measure the phenotype. Identical twins have identical genotypes and tend to look similar to each other throughout life. However, they obviously have different phenotypes because they are not subjected to exactly the same environmental influences. This is usually more apparent during adulthood, when differences in lifestyle, especially in terms of nutrition and physical exercise, can result in marked differences in phenotype. Figure 7.1 illustrates the concept of adaptation.

Biopositive and bionegative effects of loading

The effects of loading on the musculoskeletal system tend to be either bionegative or biopositive (Nigg *et al.* 1981). Bionegative effects result from insufficient loading and excessive loading (Figure 7.2). Prior to maturity, insufficient loading can result in abnormal growth and development of the musculoskeletal system. In adults, insufficient loading can

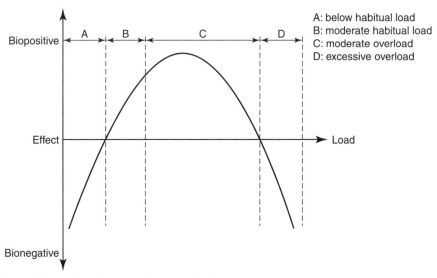

Figure 7.2 Relationship between load and effect on the musculoskeletal system.

175

result in decreased functional capacity of musculoskeletal components. Like insufficient loading, excessive loading may also result in abnormal growth and development of the musculoskeletal system prior to maturity. In addition, excessive loading may result in injury to musculoskeletal components at any age. Biopositive effects, including normal growth and development of the musculoskeletal system prior to maturity and increased functional capacity of musculoskeletal components due to physical training, result from moderate loading.

Effects of insufficient loading

A certain amount of loading is essential to promote normal growth and development of the musculoskeletal system (Zernicke and Loitz 1992; Lieber 2002). This is clearly demonstrated in children with diseases of the nervous system, such as polio, which prevent normal muscular activity and, therefore, normal patterns of loading. The muscles of such children are usually poorly developed and the bones are usually abnormal in shape and much smaller than in a normal child (Jurimae and Jurimae 2001; Malina *et al.* 2004). To grow and develop normally, the musculoskeletal system needs the mechanical stimulation provided by a normal pattern of motor-skill development, i.e. the postures, movements and levels of physical activity associated with an active childhood.

After maturity, the maintenance of the musculoskeletal system still depends on the mechanical stimulation provided by regular exercise. Lack of use results in atrophy, i.e. a decrease in mass of musculoskeletal components and, consequently, decreased functional capacity. With regard to muscle, loss of strength is rapid in totally inactive muscles. For example, studies of bed rest and unilateral limb suspension have shown that a strength loss is evident after only one day of inactivity and that loss in strength proceeds at the rate of 1% to 1.5% per day (Muller 1970). Immobilisation of a limb in a plaster cast results in a loss of strength of about 22% in the first seven days (Muller 1970; Booth 1987). Similarly, lack of weight bearing due to bed rest (Donaldson *et al.* 1970), immobilisation in a plaster cast (Anderson and Nilsson 1979), denervation of muscle (Brighton *et al.* 1985) and space flight (LeBlanc *et al.* 2007) have been found to decrease bone mass substantially and, therefore, to decrease the strength and toughness of bone.

To grow and develop normally, the musculoskeletal system needs the mechanical stimulation provided by a normal pattern of motor-skill development. After maturity, the maintenance of normal musculoskeletal function depends on the mechanical stimulation provided by regular physical activity.

Effects of moderate loading

Moderate loading generally has a biopositive effect on growth, development and maintenance of the musculoskeletal system. The moderate range can be subdivided into a moderate habitual range, i.e. loading associated with normal daily activity (Figure 7.2), and a moderate overload range, i.e. loading associated with physical training. The moderate habitual range promotes normal growth and development of the musculoskeletal system prior to maturity and maintains a healthy level of musculoskeletal function consistent with normal daily activity after maturity. Loading within the moderate overload range has a biopositive effect on the musculoskeletal system, resulting in hypertrophy, i.e. an increase in mass, of musculoskeletal components and, consequently, increased functional capacity in terms of strength and toughness of musculotendinous units, ligaments, cartilage and bone (Zernicke and Loitz 1992; Lieber 2002). These changes occur in response to moderate overloading at all ages, but they are far more noticeable in adults than in children.

Effects of excessive loading

The upper part of the moderate overload range is associated with a progressive decrease in biopositive effect, and the excessive overload range is associated with a progressive increase in bionegative effect (Figure 7.2). Excessive overload, in the form of continuous or highly repetitive non-impact loading, may result in severe angular deformities in joints or reduced bone lengths prior to maturity and degenerative joint disease in adults (Frost 1990; Forwood 2001; Duyar 2008). Excessive overload in the form of impact loading may result in injury, i.e. structural damage to one or more components of the musculoskeletal system, resulting in decreased functional capacity.

The basic relationship between load and effect on the musculoskeletal system, shown in Figure 7.2, is similar for everyone. However, the actual amount (magnitude and frequency) of loading corresponding to insufficient loading, moderate habitual loading, moderate overloading and excessive overloading for a particular individual depends on stage of maturity and level of physical conditioning. In other words, a particular amount of loading that corresponds to moderate overload for one person may correspond to insufficient loading or excessive loading for someone else.

Bionegative effects result from insufficient and excessive loading. Biopositive effects result from moderate loading.

Physical training and injury

An athlete's performance largely depends on her physical fitness and motor ability. The need for a certain level of physical fitness, i.e. cardiorespiratory endurance, local muscular endurance, strength and flexibility, reflects the physiological demands of the sport. Similarly, the need for a certain level of motor ability, i.e. the ability to perform specific skills, reflects the technical demands of the sport. A high level of motor ability (skill) requires a high level of neuromuscular coordination in the form of a combination of speed, agility, balance and power.

Clearly, the physiological and technical demands of different sports vary considerably. For example, performance in long-distance running events requires cardiorespiratory endurance, whereas performance in springboard diving requires more technical ability. A training

177

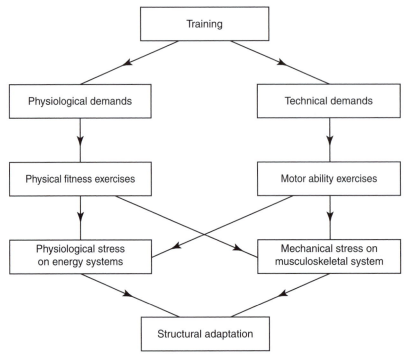

Figure 7.3 The training process.

programme, i.e. a set of exercises designed to improve an athlete's performance in a sport, should reflect the balance between the physiological and technical demands of the sport. However, whether a particular training exercise is designed to improve physical fitness or technique, the effect on the musculoskeletal system is basically the same; the musculoskeletal system experiences overload (Figure 7.3). The effect of training depends on the level of overload.

A fairly high level of physical effort is necessary to generate a large enough physiological stimulus to improve cardiorespiratory endurance in an already well trained endurance athlete. The intensity of such effort almost certainly subjects the musculoskeletal system to loads at the upper end of the moderate overload range and probably to loads in the lower end of the excessive overload range. This level of loading inevitably results in minor damage (microtrauma) to the musculoskeletal tissues, especially muscle and connective tissue. Given adequate rest, these tissues not only heal, but also adapt their structures over time to more readily withstand loads imposed on them during training. However, when rest periods are inadequate, the rate at which microtrauma occurs outpaces the processes of repair and structural adaptation such that microtrauma gradually accumulates and eventually results in a chronic injury; i.e. an injury that develops over a period of time (cumulative microtrauma) and is characterised by a gradual increase in pain and functional impairment (Watkins and Peabody 1996).

The main cause of chronic injuries appears to be overtraining, i.e. a training and competition schedule involving training sessions that are too long or rest periods between training sessions that are too short (Jones *et al.* 1994). Proper progression in the amount of exercise and, therefore, the level of loading on the musculoskeletal system is essential to avoid injury. The amount of exercise should increase gradually, so that the musculoskeletal and cardiorespiratory systems have sufficient time to adapt to the increase in the intensity of the training exercises. Although it is possible to significantly increase cardiorespiratory fitness relatively quickly, similar changes in the musculoskeletal system take much longer, especially if the individual has been sedentary for a number of years (Micheli 1982; Hootman *et al.* 2001).

Jumper's knee is a common chronic injury in sports such as volleyball and basketball, which involve high-frequency jumping and landing. The condition is characterised by pain at one or more of three sites: the insertion of the quadriceps tendon to the upper pole of the patella and the insertion of the patellar ligament to the lower pole of the patella or the tibial tuberosity (Ferretti *et al.* 1990). Ferretti and colleagues (1990) describe three stages of jumper's knee. Stage 1 is characterised by pain after a practice or after a game. Stage 2 is characterised by pain at the beginning of activity that disappears after warm-up and reappears after completion of activity. Stage 3 is characterised by fairly persistent pain that is usually severe enough to prevent participation in games and sports. Continuing to train or play at this stage may result in complete failure of the patellar ligament (Ferretti *et al.* 1990). Complete failure of the ligament is usually referred to as an acute injury, i.e. an injury that occurs suddenly (sudden macrotrauma) and is severe enough in terms of pain or functional disablement to prevent further participation, at least temporarily (Watkins and Peabody 1996). Acute injuries range in severity from minor (e.g. a minor muscle tear) to severe (e.g. a complete ligament rupture or complete bone fracture). It has been shown that many acute injuries, especially severe muscle, tendon and ligament injuries, are the sudden end result of progressive degeneration of the structure concerned (Ferretti *et al.* 1990). Continuing to train or play when suffering from a minor injury significantly increases the risk of a severe acute injury.

Response and adaptation of musculoskeletal components to loading

The response of a musculoskeletal component to loading refers to the immediate changes in stress and strain experienced by the component. Provided the load (or change in load) is not prolonged, the stress and strain experienced by the component in response to loading are unlikely to result in any structural change in the external form (size and shape) or internal architecture of the component, even if the load is within the moderate overload range. For example, it is unlikely that the changes in stress and strain experienced by the elbow extensor musculotendinous units during the performance of a single press-up exercise will result in a change in the external form or internal architecture of the elbow extensor musculotendinous units. However, if the press-up exercise is performed more frequently, for example, as part of a fitness training programme, and the load on the elbow extensor musculotendinous units is within the moderate overload range in each repetition, the elbow extensor musculotendinous units may experience structural changes that enable them to more readily withstand the time-averaged increase in load. Structural change in external form or internal architecture of musculoskeletal components that occurs as a result of changes in the time-averaged loads exerted on them is referred to as structural adaptation (Carter *et al.* 1991).

179

Optimum strain environment

The period of growth and development prior to maturity is associated with a gradual increase in the range and complexity of movement patterns and an almost continuous increase in body weight. Consequently, the total load on the musculoskeletal system increases during this period. To a certain extent, this increase in loading is balanced by an increase in the size of the musculoskeletal system. However, the period of growth and development is also associated with considerable changes in the relative size and shape of the various body segments (Figure 7.4). For example, up to about 2 years of age, the length of the lower limbs is about the same length as the upper limbs. Thereafter, the lower limbs increase in length and weight more rapidly than the upper limbs. The change in the complexity of movement patterns, change in relative size of body segments and gradual increase in body weight combine to produce an almost continuous change in the pattern of loading on the musculoskeletal system.

The musculoskeletal system adapts to these changes and continues to adapt to such changes throughout life. It is well established that all components of the musculoskeletal system adapt (or try to adapt) their external form or internal architecture to the time-averaged loads exerted on them, to maintain an optimal strain environment (Taber 1995; Frost 2003; Doschak and Zernicke 2005). The genetically determined optimal strain environment of each component appears to be maintained by a negative-feedback system that is similar in operation to a thermostat; a change in time-averaged load that produces a level of strain outside the strain limits of the optimal strain environment results in a change in the external form or internal architecture of the component so that the optimal strain environment is restored. For example, in a long bone, an increase in the time-averaged load above the upper limit of the optimal strain environment range will result in one or more of the following structural adaptations to restore the optimal strain environment: an increase in the cross-sectional area of compact bone, a change in the shape of the shaft and a realignment of the trabeculae in one or both epiphyses. Similarly, a decrease in the time-averaged load below the lower limit of the

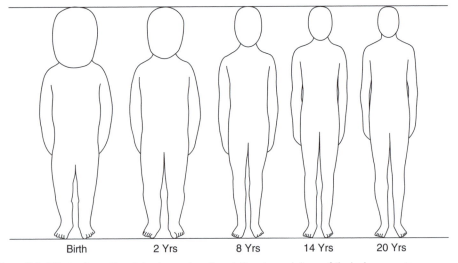

| Birth | 2 Yrs | 8 Yrs | 14 Yrs | 20 Yrs |

Figure 7.4 Effects of growth and development on the relative size and shape of the body segments.

optimal strain environment range will result, for example, in a decrease in the cross-sectional area of compact bone such that the optimal strain environment is restored. Prolonged absence of load or minimal load, for example, because of paralysis (Eser et al. 2004), prolonged immobilisation following injury (Sievänen 2010), or spaceflight (LeBlanc *et al.* 2007) will result in fairly rapid adaptation in the form of reduced mass. However, the loss of mass eventually ceases at a level referred to as the genetic baseline, i.e. the genetically determined mass that results from growth and development in the absence of loading (Rubin 1984; Frost 2003).

STRUCTURAL ADAPTATION IN BONE

The last 40 years have produced much of the present knowledge concerning the adaptation of musculoskeletal components to changes in time-averaged load (Frost 1988a, 1988b, 1990, 2003). However, the fundamental concepts concerning the adaptation of bone were established more than 100 years ago (Gross and Bain 1993). In 1892, Julius Wolff (1836–1902) summarised the contemporary views of bone adaptation to changes in time-averaged load in what came to be known as Wolff's law (Wolff 1988). Wolff's law, shown to be more or less correct, hypothesised that:

- Bone adapts its external form and internal architecture to the time-averaged load exerted on it.
- Adaptation in bone provides optimal strength with minimal bone mass.
- Adaptation in bone occurs in an ordered and predictable manner.

Stereotypical loading and optimal bone mass

As described in Chapter 3, the adaptation of bone to environmental influences, in particular to time-averaged load, is referred to as modelling. In normal growth and development, modelling has been estimated to account for 20% to 50% of the dimensions of mature bones (Frost 1988b; Schoenau and Frost 2003). Some of the load experienced by bone is attributable to the weight of body segments. However, this source of loading is small relative to the loads exerted by muscles, owing to the generally low mechanical advantages of the muscles (Burr 1997; Schiessl *et al.* 1998). Across the full range of human movement, the mechanical advantages of the muscles range from about 1:2 to 1:10, i.e. muscle forces are usually 2 to 10 times greater than the associated external forces. Consequently, it is reasonable to assume that modelling in a particular bone reflects the time-averaged loads exerted by the muscles controlling the movement of the bone, and thus modelling strengthens the bone to withstand the habitual load exerted by the muscles. Because bones, especially long bones, are stronger in axial compression than in any other form of loading (Frost 2003), the habitual form of loading exerted by muscles on long bones is mainly axial compression, i.e. compression along the long axis of the bones. There is general agreement that the muscles controlling the movement of each long bone act synergistically stereotypically, i.e. they exert an axial compression load on the bone in all body movements even though the magnitude of the load can vary (Rubin 1984; Frost 2003). Stereotypical loading produces a restricted strain environment in which the type of strain experienced by a bone is similar whenever it is loaded, even though the amount of strain can vary. A bone requires less bone mass in a restricted strain environment than it would in a broad strain environment. It is generally agreed that all bones function in restricted strain environments and that modelling optimises a bone's strength (provides maximum strength with minimal bone mass) for its particular restricted strain environment (Gross and Bain 1993; Frost 2003).

> In normal growth and development, modelling accounts for an estimated 20% to 50% of the dimensions of mature bones.

Bone modelling throughout life

From birth to maturity, bone has the capacity to model external form and internal architecture. However, the capacity to model external form gradually decreases and virtually ceases at maturity. The capacity to model internal architecture also decreases with age but is retained to some extent throughout life. Bone generally adapts to changes in time-averaged loads in the same way as other musculoskeletal components, i.e. by increasing or decreasing bone mass to maintain an optimum strain environment. In bone, the optimum strain environment is characterised by minimal flexure (or bending) strain and an even distribution of stress (usually compression stress) across articular areas. Minimal flexure strain is maintained by modelling in accordance with the phenomenon of flexure-drift. An even distribution of stress across articular areas is maintained by modelling in accordance with the phenomenon of chondral modelling (see later in this chapter) (Frost 1979).

> The capacity of bone to model external form gradually decreases from birth and virtually ceases at maturity. The capacity to model internal architecture also decreases with age but is retained to some extent throughout life.

Flexure-drift phenomenon

At birth, long bone shafts and the interarticular regions of many other bones, such as the vertebrae, are straight. However, prior to skeletal maturity, the bone shafts adopt a narrow-waisted shape, such that the diameter of the shaft is smaller at the middle than at the ends. The change from a straight to a narrow-waisted shape reflects the shaft's modelling to minimise flexure strain. This is illustrated in Figure 7.5 with respect to the development of a vertebra.

Figure 7.5a shows a frontal cross section through the body of a vertebra of a young child. In an unloaded state, as in Figure 7.5a, the sides of the body of the vertebra are basically straight. Figure 7.5b shows the vertebra subjected to a vertical compression load. The compression load reduces the vertical height of the vertebra (from h_1 to h_2), and the increased pressure on the cancellous bone and surrounding marrow bends the side walls of the vertebra outward. The greater the compression load, the greater the pressure exerted by the cancellous bone and marrow on the side walls. As the side walls bend in response to the pressure exerted by the cancellous bone and marrow, the compression load adds to the bending load exerted on

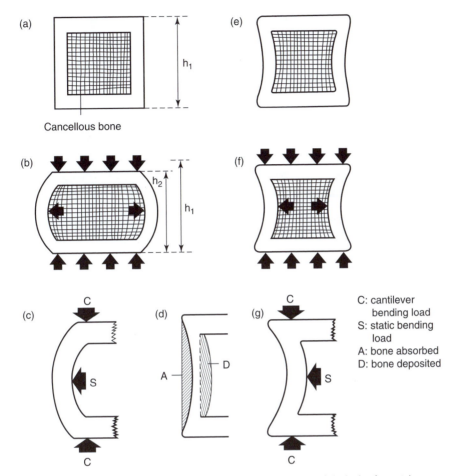

Figure 7.5 The flexure-drift phenomenon in relation to the development of the body of a vertebra.

the side walls. The type of load exerted on the side walls by the compression load (which occurs after the side walls have started to bend) is referred to as a cantilever (indirect) bending load. The type of bending load exerted on the side walls by the pressure of the cancellous bone and marrow is referred to as a static (direct) bending load (Figure 7.5c).

When a bone (or part of a bone) is subjected to flexure strain above the upper limit of the optimum strain environment, flexure drift occurs, i.e. bone is absorbed (removed) from the convex-tending surface of the bone and new bone is deposited on the concave-tending surface of the bone. The flexure-drift phenomenon is sometimes referred to as the flexure-drift law (Frost 1979). In the bodies of vertebrae, the flexure-drift phenomenon results in bone absorption from the periosteal surfaces of the side walls and deposition of new bone on the endosteal surfaces, such that each vertebra adopts a narrow-waisted shape (Figure 7.5d,e). When this shape is subjected to a vertical compression load, the side walls experience a cantilever bending load that bends them farther inward and a static bending load exerted by the cancellous bone and marrow that bends them outward. Thus, the cantilever and static bending loads oppose each other, which minimises the amount of flexure strain on the side walls

183

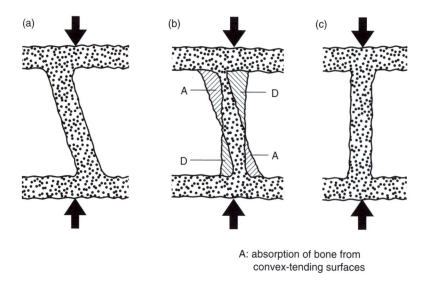

A: absorption of bone from convex-tending surfaces

D: Deposition of new bone on concave-tending surfaces

Figure 7.6 Adaptation of trabeculae to a change in time-averaged loading. The normal loading on trabeculae is axial loading. (a) Change in load on the bone, resulting in non-axial load on the trabecula. (b) Adaptation of the trabecula to restore axial loading. (c) Axial load on the trabecula restored.

(Figure 7.5f,g). Consequently, whereas the thickness of the compact bone in the side walls of the vertebrae reflects the time-averaged compression load exerted on them, the shape of the walls reflects the time-averaged bending load exerted on them.

Trabeculae in cancellous bone adapt to axial loads (loads in line with the trabeculae) and bending loads in the same way as compact bone. The thickness of trabeculae reflects the magnitude of the time-averaged compression or tension loads experienced by the trabeculae, and the orientation of the trabeculae reflects the normal line of action of the compression or tension loads. A change in time-averaged loading on trabeculae can change the thickness or orientation of the trabeculae, as shown in Figure 7.6.

In accordance with the flexure-drift phenomenon, the shafts of long bones and the inter-articular regions of many other bones, such as the vertebrae, develop narrow-waisted shapes, minimising the flexure strain on the bones. Trabeculae in cancellous bone also model in accordance with the flexure-drift phenomenon.

Chondral modelling phenomenon

All bones that develop from hyaline cartilage via endochondral ossification (Chapter 3) experience chondral modelling, i.e. the effect of loading on the rate and amount of new bone formed by hyaline cartilage. Chondral modelling applies to the following regions of bones:

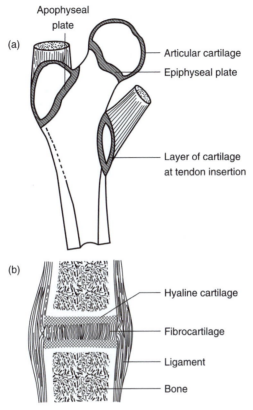

Figure 7.7 Regions of bone at which chondral modelling occurs. (a) Coronal section through the proximal end of the femur. (b) Coronal section through a typical intervertebral joint; only the hyaline cartilage region experiences chondral modelling.

Articular cartilage: Growth of epiphyses (Figure 7.7a);

Epiphyseal plates: Growth of metaphyses (Figure 7.7a);

Layers of hyaline cartilage at the insertion of tendons and ligaments: Growth of apophyses, non-apophyseal insertions of tendons, insertions of ligaments (Figure 7.7a);

Apophyseal plates: Growth of shaft adjacent to apophyseal plate (Figure 7.7a);

Layers of hyaline cartilage at the bone–cartilage interfaces in symphysis joints: Growth of bony end plates (Figure 7.7b);

Hyaline cartilage surrounding sesamoid bones: Growth of sesamoid bones.

The effect of change of load on rate of growth in these regions is shown in the chondral growth–force relationship (Frost 1979) (Figure 7.8). The relationship has the following main features:

Genetic baseline rate of growth: A certain amount of growth occurs in response to zero load.

Ascending tension limb: Increasing tension tends to increase rate of growth.

Ascending compression limb: Increasing compression tends to increase rate of growth.

Descending compression limb: Excessive compression tends to decrease the rate of growth and can result in the cessation of growth.

185

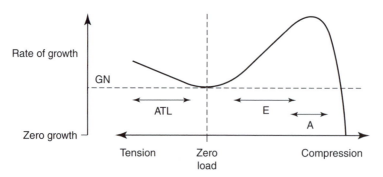

Figure 7.8 The chondral growth–force relationship: GN, genetic baseline rate of growth; ATL, normal range of loading on apophyseal plates, tendon insertions and ligament insertions; E, normal range of loading on epiphyseal plates; A, normal range of loading on articular cartilage.

Growth of epiphyses and metaphyses in bones forming synovial joints

In a long bone, the size and shape of the epiphyses and metaphyses and the orientation of the epiphyses of a bone to its shaft are determined by chondral modelling in articular cartilage and epiphyseal plates. Epiphyseal plates normally load to the left of the peak of the compression component of the chondral growth–force relationship, whereas articular cartilage normally loads around the peak (Figure 7.8). Consequently, the rate of growth of epiphyses is greater than that of metaphyses when congruence between the articular surfaces is a maximum.

However, incongruence tends to have a more marked effect on the rate of growth of the epiphyses than on the associated metaphyses. Incongruence decreases the rate of growth of the epiphyses below that of the associated metaphyses such that the orientation of the epiphyses to the shaft is largely determined by metaphyseal growth. Metaphyseal growth not only determines the orientation of the epiphyses of a bone to its shaft but also affects the alignment of bones at joints.

Changes in the alignment of the long bones of the legs are particularly noticeable from birth to about 6.5 years of age (Salenius and Vankka 1975) (Figure 7.9). At birth, most children have genu varum (bow-leggedness) with an angle between the femur and tibia of about 15° (Figure 7.9a). Between birth and about 2 years of age, the genu varum gradually decreases to zero; the femur and tibia become directly in line (Figure 7.9b). During the third year, genu valgum (knock knees) develops. This reaches a maximum of about 12° of valgus between the femur and tibia at about 3 years of age (Figure 7.9c). During the next 3.5 years, the genu valgum gradually decreases, reaching about 5° of valgus at about 6.5 years of age (Figure 7.9d). The changes in the degree of genu varum and genu valgum from birth to approximately 6.5 years of age reflect the considerable changes in body weight, relative size of body segments and complexity of movement patterns occurring during this period (Wearing et al. 2006).

When a synovial joint is maximally congruent, the loading on articular cartilage and epiphyseal plates tends to be evenly distributed. Incongruence results in an unequal distribution of load across the articular cartilage and epiphyseal plates. If prolonged, such unequal loading results in modelling to restore maximal congruence. However, the actual changes that occur depend on the extent of the changes in the patterns of loading on the articular cartilage and

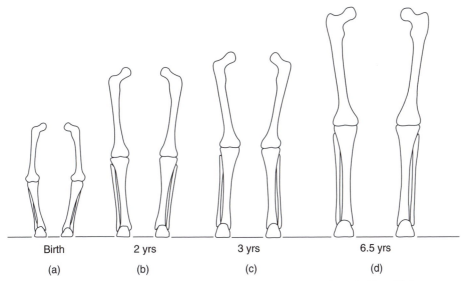

Figure 7.9 Changes in the alignment between the femur and the tibia during the period from birth to 6.5 years.

epiphyseal plates. If the changes in loading remain within the normal range, as indicated by the chondral growth–force relationship, then maximal congruence is usually restored, perhaps with some degree of abnormal alignment of the bones. However, changes in loading that are outside the normal range are likely to aggravate the condition, resulting in progressively worsening misalignment.

Modelling of metaphyses

A functionally normal joint is a congruent joint that transmits loads across the articulating surfaces in a normal manner. An anatomical misalignment at the knee, or any other joint, will be functionally normal if the misalignment stabilises (does not get progressively worse). In these cases, the anatomical misalignments represent normal modelling in response to abnormal patterns of loading imposed on the skeleton by the combined effects of muscle forces and body weight. The skeletal adaptations ensure normal transmission of loads across the joints. The anatomical misalignments must be normal functionally, or the joints will become painful. Figure 7.10 illustrates the effect of a hip abductor–adductor muscle imbalance on modelling of the metaphyses of the distal femoral epiphysis and the proximal tibial epiphysis. A hip abductor–adductor muscle imbalance can result, for example, from a decrease in physical activity in association with an increase in age or body weight (Johnson et al. 2004) or repetitive actions in sport combined with inadequate abductor–adductor strength training (Tyler et al. 2001; Heinert et al. 2008).

Figure 7.10a illustrates normal balance between the abductor and adductor muscles at the hip such that the resultant horizontal force at the knee is zero, that is, there is no tendency to pull the femoral epiphysis medially (which would increase genu valgum) or laterally (which would decrease genu valgum). This situation is associated with normal alignment between the

187

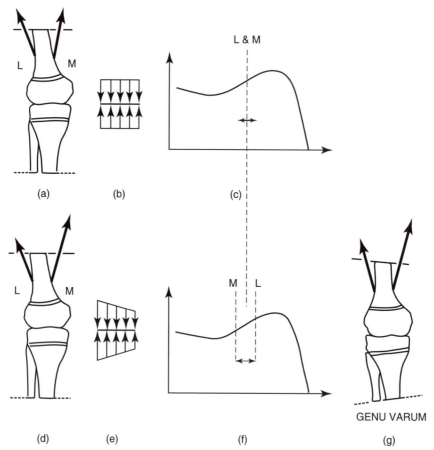

Figure 7.10 Chondral growth–force relationship: effect of a hip abductor–adductor muscle imbalance on modelling of the metaphyses of the distal femoral epiphysis and the proximal tibial epiphysis: L, lateral; M, medial. (a) Normal balance between abductor and adductor muscles at the hip such that the resultant horizontal force at the knee is zero. (b) Even distribution of load across the epiphyseal plates. (c) Loading (even distribution) on the epiphyseal plates in relation to the chondral growth–force curve. (d) The same knee with an abductor–adductor imbalance such that there is a net medially directed horizontal force at the knee tending to increase the degree of genu valgum. (e) Uneven distribution of load on the epiphyseal plates associated with the muscle imbalance. (f) The range of uneven load (within the normal range) on the epiphyseal plates in relation to the chondral growth–force curve. (g) Restoration of functional alignment at the expense of an abnormal anatomical alignment.

femur and tibia and an even distribution of load across the epiphyseal plates (Figure 7.10b). Figure 7.10c shows the loading (even distribution) on the epiphyseal plates in relation to the chondral growth–force curve. Figure 7.10d shows the same knee with an abductor–adductor imbalance such that there is a net, medially directed, horizontal force at the knee tending to increase the degree of genu valgum. Figure 7.10e shows the unequal pattern of loading on the epiphyseal plates associated with the muscle imbalance. Figure 7.10f shows the range of loading on the epiphyseal plates in relation to the chondral growth–force curve.

Because the unequal range of loading is within the normal range, the rate of growth of the lateral aspects of the metaphyses is increased and the rate of growth of the medial aspects of

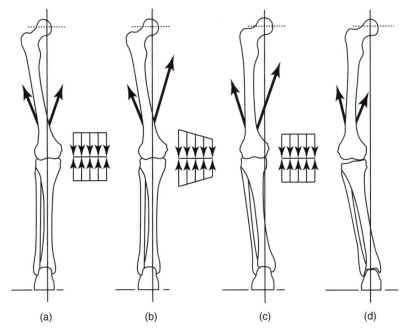

Figure 7.11 Effect of a hip abductor–adductor muscle imbalance prior to and after skeletal maturity on the orientation of the femur to the tibia in the coronal plane. (a) Normal muscle balance, normal anatomical alignment and functional alignment. (b) Abnormal muscle balance resulting in abnormal functional alignment. (c) Restoration of normal functional alignment at the expense of the development of slight genu varum by modelling of the metaphyses. (d) Change in muscle balance after maturity, resulting in worsening anatomical and functional alignments.

the metaphyses is decreased such that normal congruence is restored (with net zero horizontal force at the knee) at the expense of an abnormal alignment between the femur and tibia, that is, a much reduced genu valgum or even slight genu varum relative to most people (Figure 7.10g).

Whether or not a particular joint is anatomically misaligned during childhood, the only time it can become painful (excluding injuries and pathological conditions not attributable to loading) is during adulthood, when the bones are no longer capable of modelling in response to abnormal loading. In most adults, abnormal patterns of loading are the result of an increasingly sedentary lifestyle in which body weight gradually increases and muscle strength gradually decreases. Figure 7.11 shows the likely effect of a hip abductor–adductor muscle imbalance prior to and after skeletal maturity on the orientation of the femur to the tibia in the coronal plane. Figure 7.11a shows normal muscle balance (between the abductors and adductors on the femur), normal anatomical alignment (normal angle between the femur and tibia) and normal functional alignment (even distribution of load across the epiphyseal plates of the distal femoral epiphysis and the proximal tibial epiphysis). Figure 7.11b shows the same knee following the development of a hip abductor–adductor muscle imbalance that results in an uneven distribution of load across the epiphyseal plates. In response to the uneven distribution of load across the epiphyseal plates, modelling of the metaphyses occurs so that functional alignment is restored at the expense of the development of slight genu varum (Figure 7.11c).

189

Following skeletal maturity, a further change in the abductor–adductor muscle balance is likely to result in anatomical and functional misalignments that cannot be compensated by modelling (Figure 7.11d).

Some of the world's best athletes have marked genu varum or genu valgum, but they train and perform without injury (Micheli 1982). Similarly, some of the world's best ballet dancers have severely pronated feet, but they practice and perform without injury (Micheli 1982). In these cases, it must be assumed that the abnormalities are functionally normal and arose during childhood. Anatomical misalignments that develop after maturity are the result of a combination of muscle weakness, ligament laxity and progressive bone collapse (Frost 1979).

> Anatomically misaligned but functionally normal joints represent normal modelling in response to abnormal patterns of loading imposed on the skeleton by the combined effects of muscle forces and body weight.

Modelling of articular surfaces

Because articular surfaces in synovial joints are not physically attached to each other, even minor incongruences result in large changes in the load experienced by different parts of the articular surfaces. This is especially the case in joints with pulley-shaped articular surfaces, such as the ankle joint (Figure 7.12). Under normal circumstances, the subtalar joint contributes to inversion and eversion of the foot (Figure 7.12a,b). However, if movement at the joint is absent or limited, inversion and eversion of the foot twists the talus in the tibiofibular mortise, resulting in excessive loading on those parts of the articular surfaces of the ankle joint that remain in contact (Figure 7.12c). The excessive loading on the impinging

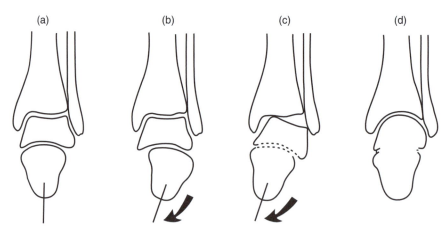

Figure 7.12 Effect of modelling of the articular surfaces of the ankle joint. (a) Normal orientation of the tibia, fibula, talus and calcaneus in the coronal plane. (b) Normal movement of the calcaneus in inversion of the foot. (c) Effect of restricted movement of the subtalar joint during inversion of the foot; the talus is twisted in the tibiofibular mortise resulting in excessive loading on those parts of the articular surfaces of the ankle joint that remain in contact. (d) Modelling of the articular surfaces of the ankle joint in response to the abnormal loading.

areas reduces or halts growth in these areas, while growth of the unloaded areas proceeds at the genetic baseline rate (Figure 7.8). Consequently, the shapes of the articular surfaces of the ankle joint adapt to the abnormal loading conditions by forming a rounded surface in the frontal plane rather than a trochlear-shaped surface, and the ankle joint as a whole resembles a ball-and-socket joint rather than a hinge joint (Figure 7.12d) (Frost 1979).

Modelling of vertebral bodies

The load experienced by the articular regions of vertebral bodies in intervertebral joints in upright postures tends to be evenly distributed compression (Figure 7.13a,b). Bending the vertebral column in any direction produces a pattern of loading on the discs and the hyaline cartilage interfaces between the end plates of the vertebrae and the fibrocartilage of the discs, ranging from relatively high compression on the concave-tending side of the column

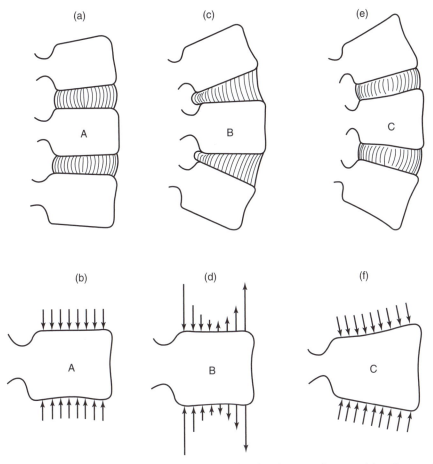

Figure 7.13 Effect of modelling of vertebrae. (a,b) Evenly distributed compression on vertebrae in normal upright posture. (c,d) Bending of the vertebral column, resulting in high compression on the concave-tending side of the column and high tension on the convex-tending side of the column. (e,f) Wedging of vertebrae caused by modelling in response to prolonged unidirectional bending stress.

to relatively high tension on the convex-tending side of the column (Figure 7.13c,d). This loading pattern in response to bending the column is normal. However, if part of the column is subjected to higher-than-normal, unidirectional, bending stress during the period of growth and development, the vertebral bodies in the affected region can become wedge-shaped to restore a more normal pattern of loading (Figure 7.13e,f). Wedging of vertebrae occurs in the thoracic and lumbar regions in the median and frontal planes.

Effects of age on modelling capacity

The modelling capacity of bone decreases with age. Whereas the ability to adapt internal architecture to changes in patterns of loading is somewhat retained throughout life, the ability to adapt size and shape decreases more rapidly and is negligible in the adult (Frost 1979; Lanyon 1981). Consequently, during childhood a change in the normal pattern of loading on bones usually results in adaptive bone growth to restore normal loading. However, in an adult, adaptive bone growth cannot accommodate a change in the normal pattern of loading that results, for example, from an increase in body weight or a change in the muscle strength balance about a joint. Unless corrected by specific forms of treatment, such as physiotherapy or orthotics, the abnormal pattern of loading increases the likelihood of degenerative joint disease. An orthosis is a musculoskeletal support, i.e. an external appliance, such as leg calipers, a foot arch support or a heel raise designed to improve musculoskeletal function by helping to maintain normal transmission of loads in joints (Redford 1987). Orthotics is the theory and practice of development, manufacture and use of orthoses (Redford 1987).

The following examples illustrate the rate at which the modelling capacity of bone decreases with age and the possible effects of a lack of modelling capacity in the adult.

Tibial torsion: Tibial torsion is an abnormality of the tibia in which the lower end of the tibia is excessively rotated internally or externally with respect to the upper end about the long axis of the shaft. Internal and external tibial torsion are characterised by abnormal toeing in and toeing out, respectively (Figure 7.14). The normal degree of rotation of the lower end of the tibia with respect to the upper end is 15° to 20° of external rotation (the foot is turned out 15° to 20° with respect to the knee; Figure 7.14b). Tibial torsion can be corrected easily in an infant by applying a constant torsion load to the tibia by means of special splints (Frost 1979). The torsion load is applied in the direction opposite to that of the abnormality. The bone adapts to the torsion stress by modelling to relieve the torsion stress. This process gradually reduces the tibial torsion, provided the torsion load and stress are maintained. However, the effect of this type of treatment decreases fairly rapidly with age. For example, 30° to 40° of correction of an internal tibial torsion can be produced in ten weeks of treatment when applied to a 5-month-old child. The same amount and duration of treatment has a negligible effect in a 5-year-old child (Frost 1979).

Bone fracture: Following an injury to a bone involving two or more fractures, the chances of the broken pieces knitting together in exactly the same orientation to each other as existed prior to the injury are remote. Consequently, after healing, the line of action of the muscles crossing the joints formed by the two ends of the bone is altered. This can result in abnormal

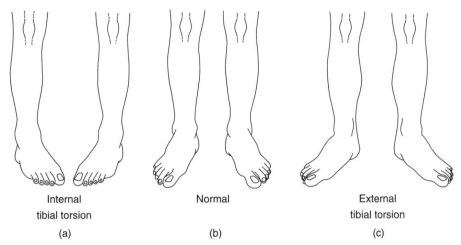

Internal	Normal	External
tibial torsion		tibial torsion
(a)	(b)	(c)

Figure 7.14 Tibial torsion. (a) Internal tibial torsion: excessive internal rotation of the distal end of the tibia with respect to the proximal end. (b) Normal degree of rotation of the distal end of the tibia with respect to the proximal end: 15° to 20° of external rotation. (c) External tibial torsion: excessive external rotation of the distal end of the tibia with respect to the proximal end.

loading on the articulating surfaces of the joints. In a child, the articulating surfaces usually restore normal loading by modelling. In an adult, the abnormal loading increases the likelihood of degenerative joint disease, especially in weight-bearing joints (Radin 1986).

Anatomically misaligned but functionally normal joints that develop in childhood can become painful during adulthood when the bones are no longer capable of modelling in response to abnormal loading. In most adults, abnormal patterns of loading result from an increasingly sedentary lifestyle, in which body weight gradually increases and muscle strength gradually decreases.

STRUCTURAL ADAPTATION IN REGULAR FIBROUS TISSUES

Regular fibrous tissues, and particularly ligaments and tendons, are designed to provide strength in tension. The effect of changes in time-averaged tension load on regular fibrous tissues depends on the change in magnitude and type of load. When subjected to continuous tension at a level exceeding the optimum strain environment, regular fibrous tissues experience creep (Chapter 6). When subjected to intermittent tension at a level exceeding the optimum strain environment, regular fibrous tissues hypertrophy to restore the optimal strain environment (Elliot 1965; Magnusson *et al.* 2008). For example, increasing the strength of a muscle increases the time-averaged tension load exerted on the associated tendons, which experience an increase in strain. The tendons adapt to the increased strain by increasing their cross-sectional areas to a level that restores the optimal strain environment. The capacity of regular fibrous tissues to adapt to increases in time-averaged tension load is called the stretch–hypertrophy rule (Frost 1979).

Just as an increase in time-averaged intermittent tension on regular fibrous tissue results in hypertrophy, a decrease in time-averaged tension results in atrophy to restore the optimal strain environment. Atrophy in regular fibrous tissue involves a decrease in cross-sectional area and shortening (Akeson et al. 1977; Frost 1990). Immobilisation, which can occur because of paralysis or injury, results in considerable atrophy in ligaments. Noyes (1977) studied the effects of immobilisation and subsequent rehabilitation on the strength of the anterior cruciate ligament in rhesus monkeys. The results of the study showed that immo- bilisation in a whole body cast for eight weeks produced an average decrease of 39% in the strength of the anterior cruciate ligament, and after five months and 12 months of rehabili- tation the average strength of the anterior cruciate ligament was still only 79% and 91%, respectively, of the preimmobilisation level. In human beings, rehabilitation of ligaments following immobilisation and injury is a lengthy process (Frost 1990; Sharma and Maffulli 2006).

Under normal circumstances, the load experienced by ligaments is markedly reduced by ligament-muscle stretch reflex mechanisms; stretching a ligament tends to result in reflex contraction of associated muscles, which relieves the load on the ligaments (Cohen and Cohen 1956; Kondradsen et al. 1993; Roberts et al. 2007). For example, hyperextension of the knee results in a reflex contraction of the hamstrings, which is triggered, at least in part, by stretch reflex loops between the knee ligaments (cruciate and collateral) and the hamstrings. Injury to ligaments can impair the stretch reflex mechanism by delaying the elicitation of muscular contraction. This can occur directly in the form of damage to nerves or indirectly in the form of laxity in the ligaments such that greater movement is necessary in the joint to stretch the ligaments sufficiently to elicit the stretch reflex. The greater the delay in the elicitation of the stretch reflex, the greater the likelihood of ligaments being excessively overloaded or associ- ated joints being dislocated. Injury to ligaments can also impair their blood supply, which can reduce the rate of hypertrophy.

It is perhaps not surprising that many ligament reconstructions based on grafts from other parts of the body fail because it takes time to develop an adequate blood supply, which is essential for hypertrophy, and stretch reflex loops, which protect the ligaments from overload (Frost 1973).

Under normal circumstances, the load experienced by ligaments is markedly reduced by ligament-muscle stretch reflex mechanisms. Injury to ligaments can impair the function- ing of the stretch reflex mechanisms by delaying the elicitation of muscular contraction, which increases the likelihood of excessively overloading ligaments or dislocating associ- ated joints.

Structural adaptation at ligament and tendon insertions

All ligaments and tendons insert onto bone via a hyaline cartilage interface, and thus the bone adapts to the tensile load exerted via the tendons and ligaments in accordance with the chon- dral modelling phenomenon (Figure 7.15). Just before entering the layer of hyaline cartilage,

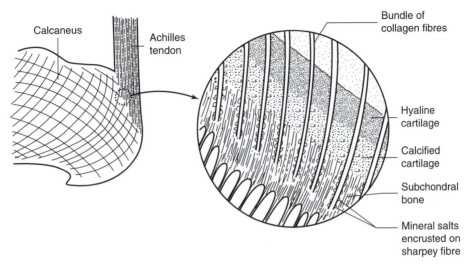

Figure 7.15 Sharpey fibres.

the ligament or tendon separates into bundles of collagen fibres. Each bundle of fibres passes through and is embedded within all three layers of the region of insertion: hyaline cartilage, calcified cartilage and subchondral bone. In the layer of subchondral bone, the collagen fibre bundles become encrusted with mineral salts. At this stage, each bundle is referred to as a Sharpey fibre (Frost 1973; Hamrick 1999).

The ultimate shear stress between a Sharpey fibre and the surrounding subchondral bone determines the fibre's resistance to being pulled out of the insertion. The deeper the penetration of the fibre, the greater the area of fibre presented to the surrounding bone and therefore the lower the shear stress on the fibre. The lower the shear stress on the fibre, the greater the amount of tension required to pull out the fibre. It is therefore not surprising that each ligament and tendon insertion consists of a very large number of Sharpey fibres; the larger the number of fibres, the lower the shear stress on each fibre. Furthermore, the fibres are distributed over a relatively large area (much larger than that generally indicated on bony specimens and models) and merge with adjacent fibrous tissues. This is referred to as fibre fan-out (Frost 1973; Myers 2001). The larger the area of insertion, the lower the tensile stress on the region of insertion.

The combination of fibre fan-out and Sharpey fibres produces strong attachments that, in the case of apophyses, are stronger than the apophyseal plate. Avulsion fractures occur along the apophyseal plate, i.e. the tendon stays intact with the apophysis and the apophysis is displaced along with the tendon. This can reasonably be compared to pulling up a plant that has an extensive root system; usually a lot of soil is still attached to the roots. In this sense, a tendon or ligament can be described as having a very extensive root system. The insertions of ligaments and tendons adapt to changes in time-averaged tension loads by varying the degree of fibre fan-out and the number of Sharpey fibres. Increases in time-averaged loading increase the area of fibre fan-out and the number of fibres, and decreases in loading reduce the area of fan-out and number of fibres.

STRUCTURAL ADAPTATION IN MUSCLE

As in other musculoskeletal components, skeletal muscles adapt to a time-averaged increase in intermittent load that exceeds the optimal strain environment of the muscles by increasing in strength and to a time-averaged decrease in load that falls below the optimal strain environment by decreasing in strength.

Strength changes

Unlike the non-contractile components of the musculoskeletal system, connective tissue and bone, which passively transmit loads applied to them, a skeletal muscle only functions (i.e. produces tension) when it is stimulated to contract. Furthermore, the amount of tension that a muscle produces depends upon the degree of activation; the greater the activation, the greater the tension. Consequently, changes in strength are the result of neuromuscular adaptations, i.e. changes in structure and function of both the neural and muscle components of the neuromuscular system (Häkkinen 1994).

Change in structure is mainly reflected in an increase in the cross-sectional area of muscle fibres. The latter is due to an increase in the number of actin and myosin filaments, which increases the potential number of cross bridges and, therefore, the capacity for tension generation (Reeves *et al.* 2006; Narici and Maganaris 2006). Change in function is mainly reflected in increased capacity for synchronous recruitment of motor units and increased rate of discharge of motor units (Moritani 1993; Enoka 1997; Aagaard *et al.* 2002).

The number of motor units recruited and, by inference, the level of stimulation of a muscle, corresponds to the net sum of all the action potentials of all the motor units in a muscle at a particular point in time (Kamen and Caldwell 1996). It is not possible to measure the sum of all the action potentials directly, but the sum can be estimated from an electromyogram (EMG), i.e. a recording of the electrical activity in the muscle by means of electrodes located on the skin (surface electrodes) overlying the target muscles or electrodes inserted into the target muscles (intramuscular electrodes).

In previously untrained people who start a prolonged strength training programme, the first few weeks of training result in a significant increase in strength without any significant muscle hypertrophy. This initial increase in strength, reflected in an increase in an integrated EMG (IEMG: the area under the EMG), is attributed to neural adaptation (Moritani 1993). After this initial phase, further increases in strength are associated with a progressive increase in the contribution of muscle hypertrophy.

The pattern of strength gain in response to strength training in women is similar to that in men, i.e. an initial phase dominated by neural adaptation followed by a longer period in which hypertrophy progressively dominates. However, in women the initial neural adaptation phase is shorter than in men and ultimate strength gains in women tend to be lower than in men. This is largely due, it would appear, to hormonal differences, especially lower levels of testosterone in women than in men.

In women and men, decreases in strength subsequent to a period of detraining (time-averaged loading below the optimal strain environment) follow a similar two-phase pattern, i.e. a rapid and significant decrease in strength (associated with a decreased IEMG) without any significant atrophy (decrease in muscle mass) followed by more a gradual decrease in strength that is associated with significant atrophy. As with strength gain, the initial period of strength loss is attributed to neural adaptation (Moritani 1993).

Strength in normal, healthy, untrained women and men normally reaches its peak between the ages of 20 and 30, remains fairly constant or declines slightly between the ages of 30 and 40 and then progressively declines, with increase in age associated with a marked increase in the rate of decline. For most people, strength declines by 30% to 50% between the ages of 30 and 80 years (Häkkinen 1994; Akima *et al.* 2001). Loss of strength decreases the ability of individuals to undertake activities of daily living and, in particular, decreases speed of movement and speed of reaction to postural perturbations, which significantly increases the risk of falling (Grabiner and Enoka 1995). Loss of postural stability and the ability to walk without assistance are the main causes of elderly people being permanently admitted to nursing homes (Schultz *et al.* 1992).

As shown in Figure 7.16, the age-related decline in strength tends to be associated with three interrelated changes: change in hormone balance, progressive degeneration in the structure and function of the neuromuscular system, and a decrease in physical activity.

Some of the deterioration in the structure and function of the neuromuscular system that occurs with age is a natural consequence of aging (Tanaka and Seals 2008). However, the effect of aging *per se*, relative to environmental factors, is not yet clear. In normal healthy people, the neuromuscular system retains the capacity to adapt positively to strength training and motor ability training throughout life (Reeves *et al.* 2006; Narici and Maganaris 2006; Baker *et al.* 2007; Capodaglio *et al.*, 2007). In the absence of intervention, age-related decline in the structure and function of the neuromuscular system is associated with a decrease in muscle mass, a decrease in the ability to control the amount of force produced, especially in manipulative tasks, and a decrease in coordination (Figure 7.16). In old age, the decrease in muscle mass is often associated with severe impairments in muscle function (strength, endurance and balance) and an inability to respond positively to well-designed programmes for conditioning and rehabilitation; this condition is referred to as sarcopenia (Cruz-Jentoft *et al.* 2010).

Muscle extensibility changes

The muscle fibre length determines a muscle's extensibility, and the number of sarcomeres in each myofibril determines the length of each muscle fibre. Changes in the length of muscle fibres and, therefore, in the extensibility of muscles occur as a result of changes in the time-averaged range of movement of the muscles (Goldspink 1992; Herzog 2000). Muscles adapt to changes in time-averaged range of movement by increasing or decreasing the number of sarcomeres in each myofibril in order to maintain optimal function of muscle fibres in terms of length–tension characteristics. For example, immobilising the ankles of cats in full dorsiflexion, i.e. with the soleus muscles in a stretched position, increased the number of sarcomeres in the fibres of the soleus muscle by about 20% in four weeks. The same researchers found that immobilising the ankles of cats in full plantar flexion, i.e. with the soleus muscles in a shortened position, decreased the number of sarcomeres in the fibres of the soleus muscle by about 40% in four weeks (Williams and Goldspink 1973, 1978).

197

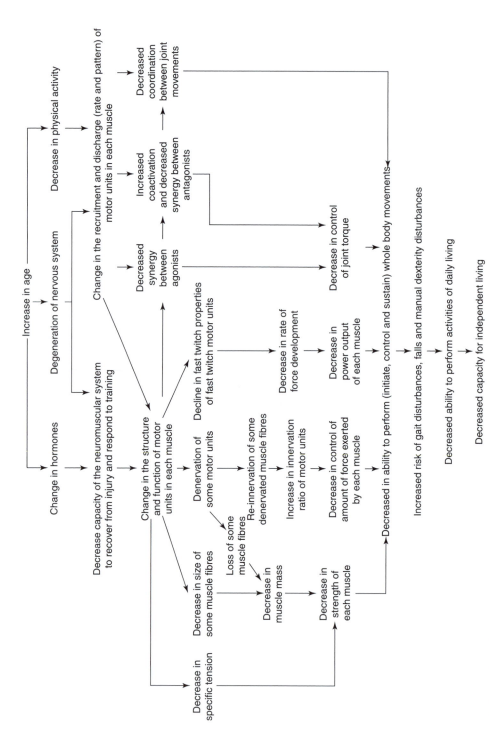

Figure 7.16 Effect of aging and decrease in physical activity on voluntary control of movement.

To maximise performance (by increasing the potential for strength of musculotendinous units) and reduce the risk of muscle and tendon injuries (by increased muscle extensibility), flexibility training should be undertaken to ensure that muscles are long enough to facilitate full ranges of whole body movement. Lengthening a muscle through appropriate flexibility training will increase the length of its myofibrils which, in turn, will increase its potential for strength development and reduce the risk of overstretching the muscle.

> Muscles adapt to changes in time-averaged range of movement by increasing or decreasing the length of muscle fibres to maintain optimal function in terms of length–tension characteristics.

REVIEW QUESTIONS

1. Differentiate between biopositive and bionegative effects of loading on musculoskeletal components.

2. Differentiate between moderate habitual load and moderate overload.

3. Differentiate between acute and chronic injury.

4. Differentiate between response to loading and adaptation to loading.

5. Describe the chondral growth–force relationship.

6. Differentiate between anatomical and functional alignment in normal joints.

7. Describe the effects of age on the modelling capacity of bone.

8. Describe structural adaptation in regular fibrous tissues.

9. Describe structural adaptation in skeletal muscle.

Part II

Biomechanics of movement

By coordination of the various muscle groups, the forces generated by our muscles are transmitted by our bones and joints to enable us to apply forces to the external environment, usually by our hands and feet, so that we can adopt upright postures, transport the body and manipulate objects, often simultaneously. The forces generated and transmitted by the musculoskeletal system are referred to as internal forces. Body weight and the forces that we apply to the external environment are referred to as external forces. Internal forces change the position of the body segments relative to each other, but it is the resultant of the external forces that determines the movement of the body as a whole. Biomechanics of movement is the branch of biomechanics concerned with the effect of external forces on the movement of the body. The key to understanding biomechanics of movement is a thorough knowledge of force, Newton's laws of motion, work and energy. Part II, Biomechanics of movement, develops knowledge and understanding of these fundamental concepts through consideration of the biomechanics of a wide range of human movements.

Chapter 8 – Introduction to biomechanics of movement – reviews the fundamental concepts of force, mechanics and biomechanics, and describes the different forms of motion (linear and angular) and units of measurement that underlie the study of biomechanics. Chapter 9 – Linear motion – develops the fundamental concepts that underlie the study of linear motion, in particular, generation and absorption of linear momentum. The concepts are developed through an in-depth application to a wide range of movements including standing, walking, running, jumping, landing, falling, throwing and catching. Chapter 10 – Angular motion – develops the fundamental concepts that underlie the study of angular motion, in particular, generation and transfer of angular momentum. The concepts are developed through an in-depth application to a wide range of movements, including strength training exercises, hammer throwing, long jumping, somersaulting, diving and twisting. Chapter 11 – Work, energy and power – develops the fundamental concepts of work, energy and power. The concepts are developed through an in-depth application to a wide range of movements, including kicking, hitting, cycling, swinging and pole vaulting. Chapter 12 – Fluid mechanics – develops the fundamental concepts of buoyancy, water resistance and air resistance. The concepts are developed through an in-depth application to a wide range of movements, including floating, ball flight, swimming, skiing and skydiving.

Chapter 8

Introduction to biomechanics of movement

The capacity of the body to move and carry out all of the activities that constitute daily living depends upon the capacity of the musculoskeletal system to generate and transmit forces. The forces generated and transmitted by the musculoskeletal system are referred to as internal forces. Body weight and the forces that we apply to the external environment are referred to as external forces. Internal forces change the position of the body segments relative to each other, but it is the resultant of the external forces that determines the movement of the body as a whole. The purpose of this chapter is to review the concepts of force, mechanics and biomechanics, describe the two fundamental forms of motion, and describe the units of measurement used in the study of biomechanics.

OBJECTIVES

After reading this chapter, you should be able to do the following:

1. Describe the two ways that forces tend to affect bodies.
2. Describe the four subdisciplines of mechanics.
3. Describe the two fundamental forms of motion.
4. Convert units of measurement between the international system (SI) and the British imperial system.

FORCE

All bodies, animate and inanimate, are continuously acted upon by forces. A force can be defined as that which alters or tends to alter a body's state of rest or type of movement. The forces that act on a body arise from interaction of the body with its environment. There are two types of interaction, contact interaction, which produces contact forces, and attraction interaction, which produces attraction forces.

Contact interaction refers to physical contact between the body and its environment. In contact interactions, the forces exerted by the environment on a body are referred to as contact forces. The environment consists largely of three main types of physical phenomenon: solids, liquids and gases. In sport and exercise, the main sources of contact forces are implements (e.g. balls and rackets), the ground (e.g. walking, running and jumping), water (e.g. swimming and diving), air (e.g. skydiving, ski jumping and downhill skiing) and the forces exerted by opponents, usually in the form of pushes and pulls.

Attraction interaction refers to naturally occurring forces of attraction between certain bodies that tend to make the bodies move toward each other and to maintain contact with each other after contact is made. For example, the electromagnetic attraction force maintains the configuration of atoms in molecules and the configuration of molecules in solids, liquids and gases. Similarly, a magnetised piece of iron attracts other pieces of iron to it by the attraction force of magnetism. The human body is constantly subjected to a very considerable force of attraction, i.e. body weight, the force due to the gravitational pull of the earth. It is body weight that keeps us in contact with the ground and that brings us back to the ground should we leave it, for example, following a jump into the air.

All bodies, animate and inanimate, are continuously acted upon by forces, which arise from interaction of the body with its environment. The environment exerts two kinds of force, contact forces and attraction forces.

MECHANICS

Forces tend to affect bodies in two ways:

- Forces tend to deform bodies, i.e. change the shape of the bodies by, for example, stretching (pulling force), squashing (pushing force) and twisting (torsion force).
- Forces determine the movement of bodies, i.e. the forces acting on a body determine whether it moves or remains at rest and determine its speed and direction of movement if it does move.

Mechanics is the study of the forces that act on bodies and the effects of the forces on the size, shape, structure and movement of the bodies (Watkins 2008). The actual effect that a force or combination of forces has on a body, i.e. the amount of deformation and change of movement that occurs, depends upon the size of the force in relation to the mass of the body and the mechanical properties of the body. The mass of a body is the amount of matter (physical substance) that comprises the body. The mass of a body is the product of its volume and its density. The volume of a body is the amount of space that the mass occupies and its density is the concentration of matter (atoms and molecules) in the mass, i.e. the amount of mass per unit volume. The greater the concentration of mass, the larger the density. For example, the density of iron is greater than that of wood and the density of wood is greater than that of polystyrene. Similarly, with regard to the structure of the human body, bone is more dense than muscle and muscle is more dense than fat.

The mass of a body is measure of its inertia, i.e. its resistance to start moving if it is at rest and its resistance to change its speed or direction if it is already moving. The larger the mass, the greater the inertia and, consequently, the larger the force that will be needed to move the mass or change the way it is moving. For example, the inertia of a stationary soccer ball (a small mass) is small in comparison to that of a heavy barbell (a large mass), i.e. much more force will be required to move the barbell than to move the ball.

Whereas the effect of a force on the movement of a body is largely determined by its mass, the amount of deformation that occurs is largely determined by its mechanical properties, in particular, its stiffness (the resistance of the body to deformation) and strength (the amount of force required to break the body). For a given amount of force, the higher the stiffness and the greater the strength of a body, the smaller the deformation that will occur.

> Mechanics is the study of the forces that act on bodies and the effects of the forces on the size, shape, structure and movement of the bodies.

Subdisciplines of mechanics

The different types and effects of forces are reflected in four overlapping subdisciplines of mechanics: mechanics of materials, fluid mechanics, statics and dynamics. Mechanics of materials is the study of the mechanical properties of materials including, for example, the stiffness and resilience of materials used to make running tracks and other playing surfaces and the strength of bone, muscle and connective tissues. Fluid mechanics is the study of the movement of liquids and gases, such as blood flow in the cardiovascular system, and the effect of liquids and gases on the movement of solids, such as the movement of the human body through water and air.

Statics is the study of bodies under the action of balanced forces, i.e. the study of the forces acting on bodies that are at rest or moving with constant speed in a particular direction. In these situations, the resultant force (the net effect of all the forces) acting on the body is zero. Figure 8.1 shows a book resting on a table. Since the book is at rest, there are only two forces acting on the book (discounting the force exerted by the surrounding air which is negligible), the weight of the book W acting downward and the upward reaction force R exerted by the table. The magnitudes of W and R are the same, but they act in opposite directions and, therefore, cancel out, such that the resultant force acting on the book is zero.

Figure 8.2 shows a skydiver falling to earth. After jumping out of the aeroplane, she is accelerated downward (her downward speed increases) by the force of her weight W. However, as her downward speed increases, so does the upthrust of air on the underside of her body, i.e. the air resistance R. After falling for a few seconds, R will be equal in magnitude, but opposite in direction to W. Consequently, the resultant force acting on the skydiver will

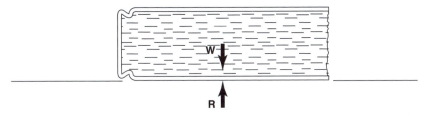

Figure 8.1 Forces acting on a book resting on a table: W, weight of book; R, force exerted on book by table.

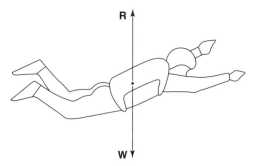

Figure 8.2 Forces acting on a skydiver: *W*, weight of skydiver, clothing and parachute; *R*, air resistance.

be zero and provided that she does not alter the orientation or shape of her body, she will continue to fall with constant speed until she opens her parachute.

Dynamics is the study of bodies under the action of unbalanced forces, i.e. bodies moving with non-constant speed. In this situation, the resultant force acting on the body will be greater than zero, i.e. the body will be accelerating (speed increasing) or decelerating (speed decreasing) in the direction of the resultant force. For example, Figure 8.3a shows a sprinter in the set position, i.e. when the body is at rest. In this situation, the resultant force acting on the sprinter will be zero. However, following the starting signal, the sprinter accelerates away from the blocks under the action of the resultant force acting on his body, i.e. the resultant of his body weight and the forces acting on his feet (Figure 8.3b). The determination of the resultant force is described in detail in Chapter 9.

Kinematics is the branch of dynamics that describes the movement of bodies in relation to space and time (Greek *kinema*, movement). A kinematic analysis describes the movement of a body in terms of distance (change in position), speed (rate of change of position) and acceleration (variability in the rate of change of position). Kinetics (Greek *kinein*, to move) is the branch of dynamics that describes the forces acting on bodies, i.e. the cause of the observed kinematics.

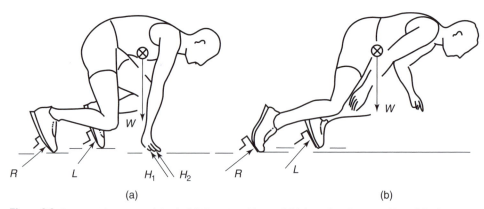

(a)   (b)

Figure 8.3 Forces acting on a sprinter in (a) the set position and (b) just after the start: H_1 and H_2, forces acting on the hands; *W*, weight of the sprinter; *L*, force exerted on the left foot; *R*, force exerted on the right foot.

206

Biomechanics

Biomechanics is the study of the forces that act on and within living organisms and the effect of the forces on the size, shape, structure and movement of the organisms. Biomechanics of sport and exercise is the study of the internal forces (muscle forces and the forces in bones and joints that result from transmission of the muscle forces through the skeleton), the external forces (e.g. the ground reaction force) that result from the internal forces, the effects of the internal forces on the size, shape and structure of the musculoskeletal components (structural adaptation) and the effects of the external forces on the movement of the body (biomechanics of movement) in sport and exercise.

FORMS OF MOTION

There are two fundamental forms of motion, linear motion and angular motion. Linear motion, also referred to as translation, occurs when all parts of a body move the same distance in the same direction in the same time. In all types of self-propelled human movement, such as walking, running and swimming, the orientation of the body segments to each other continually changes and, therefore, pure linear motion seldom occurs in human movement. The human body may experience pure linear motion for brief periods in activities such as skating (Figure 8.4) and ski jumping (Figure 8.5). When the linear movement is in a straight line, the motion is called rectilinear motion (Figures 8.4 and 8.5a). When the linear movement follows a curved path, the motion is referred to as curvilinear motion (Figure 8.5b).

Angular motion, also referred to as rotation, occurs when a body or part of a body, such as an arm or a leg, moves in a circle or part of a circle about a particular line in space, referred to as the axis of rotation, such that all parts of the body move through the same angle in the same direction in the same time. The axis of rotation may be stationary or it may experience linear motion (Figure 8.6). Figure 8.7 shows a gymnast rotating about a horizontal bar. Provided that the orientation of the body segments with respect to each other does not change, the gymnast as a whole and each of the body segments will experience angular motion about the bar. Most

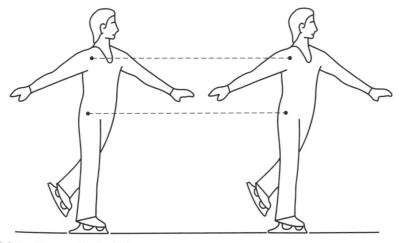

Figure 8.4 Rectilinear motion in skating.

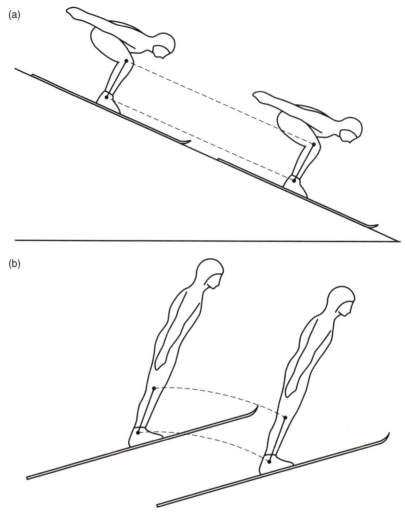

(a)

(b)

Figure 8.5 Linear motion: a ski jumper is likely to experience: (a) rectilinear motion on the runway; (b) curvilinear motion during flight.

whole body human movements are combinations of linear and angular motion. For example, in walking, the movement of the head and trunk is fairly linear, but the movements of the arms and legs involve simultaneous linear and angular motion as the body as a whole moves forward (Figure 8.8). Similarly, in cycling, the movement of the trunk, head and arms is fairly linear, but the movements of the legs involve simultaneous linear and angular motion (Figure 8.9). The movement of a multisegmented body, like the human body, which involves simultaneous linear and angular motion of the segments, is usually referred to as general motion.

There are two fundamental forms of motion, linear motion and angular motion. Most whole body human movements are combinations of linear and angular motion.

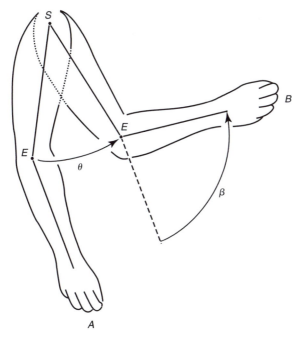

Figure 8.6 Angular motion: as the arm swings from position A to position B, the upper arm rotates through an angle θ about the transverse (side-to-side) axis S through the shoulder joint and the lower arm and hand rotate through an angle β about the transverse axis E through the elbow joint.

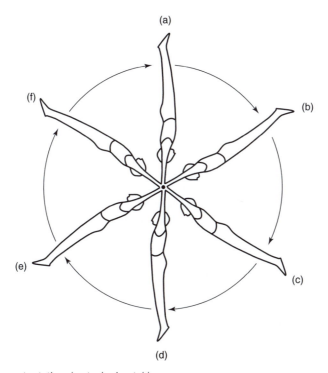

Figure 8.7 A gymnast rotating about a horizontal bar.

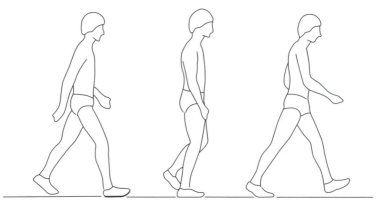

Figure 8.8 General motion: in walking, the movement of the head and trunk is fairly linear, but the movements of the arms and legs involve simultaneous linear and angular motion.

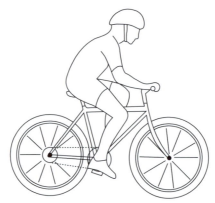

Figure 8.9 General motion: in cycling, the movement of the trunk, head and arms is fairly linear, but the movements of the legs involve simultaneous linear and angular motion.

UNITS OF MEASUREMENT

Commerce and scientific communication are dependent on the correct use and interpretation of units of measurement. With the advent of the industrial revolution in the eighteenth century and the progressive increase in international trade that resulted from it, the need for uniformity in measurement became increasingly evident. At that time, one of the most widely used systems of units was the British imperial system, but lack of clarity and consistency with regard to definitions and symbols for many variables resulted in resistance to the use of this system internationally (Rowlett 2004). The metric system of measurements originated in France around 1790. The name of the system is derived from the base unit for length, i.e. the metre, which was defined as one 10-millionth of the distance from the equator to the North Pole. In contrast to the British imperial system, each unit in the metric system has a unique definition and a unique symbol. Largely for this reason, the metric system progressively gained ground internationally. The metric system was officially adopted in the Netherlands and Luxembourg in 1820 and in France in 1837. In 1875, many of the industrialised countries signed the Treaty of the Metre which established the International Bureau of Weights and Measures (BIPM for *Bureau International des Poids et Mesures*) and a single system of units, the international system of units, to include all physical and chemical, metric and non-metric units. The system is usually referred to as the SI system after its French-language name *Système International d'Unités*. The SI system is now the most widely used system of units, especially in science and international commerce. The system is maintained and updated by the BIPM as new units are proposed and accepted. The system now consists of a large number of units, but all of the units are derived from a set of base units. The base units for mechanical variables in the SI system are the metre (length), the kilogram (mass) and the second (time). These three units give rise to a subsection of the SI system called the metre-kilogram-second (m-kg-s) system. The corresponding subsection of the British imperial system is the foot-pound-second (ft-lb-s) system. These two subsystems are shown in Table 8.1. With the exception of a few examples, the m-k-s system is used throughout this book.

Table 8.1 Mechanical units and (symbols) of measurement.

Quantity	British imperial system	SI system
Distance	foot (ft)	metre (m)
Time	second (s)	second (s)
Speed	feet per second (ft/s)	metres per second (m/s)
Acceleration	feet per second per second (ft/s^2)	metres per second per second (m/s^2)
Mass	pound (lb)	kilogram (kg)
Linear momentum	pounds feet per second (lb·ft/s)	kilogram metres per second (kg·m/s)
Force	poundal (pdl) 1 pdl = 1 lb × 1 ft/s^2	newton (N) 1 N = 1 kg × 1 m/s^2
Weight*	pound force (lbf) 1 lbf = 1lb × 32.2 ft/s^2 = 32.2 pdl	kilogram force (kgf) 1 kgf = 1 kg × 9.81 m/s^2 = 9.81 N
Pressure	pounds force per square inch (lbf/in^2)	pascal (Pa) 1 Pa = 1 N/m^2
Angular distance	radian (rad)	radian (rad)
Angular speed	radians per second (rad/s)	radians per second (rad/s)
Angular acceleration	radians per second per second (rad/s^2)	radians per second per second (rad/s^2)
Moment of inertia	pound foot squared (lb·ft^2)	kilogram metres squared (kg·m^2)
Angular momentum	pound foot squared per second (lb·ft^2/s)	kilogram metres squared per second (kg·m^2/s)
Turning moment	poundal foot (pdl·ft)	newton metre (N·m)
Energy and work	foot poundal (ft·pdl)	joule (J) (J = N·m)
Power	horsepower (hp) 1 hp = 550 ft·lb/s**	watt (W) (W = J/s)

* pound force (lbf) and pound weight (lbwt) are different names for the same unit, i.e. the weight of a mass of 1 lb; kilogram force (kgf), kilopond (kp) and kilogram weight (kgwt) are different names for the same unit, i.e. the weight of a mass of 1 kg.

** The horsepower symbol is usually written as ft·lb/s, but the 'lb' is actually 'lbf' (pound force). Consequently, the correct symbol for horsepower is ft·lbf/s (foot pounds force per second). Fortunately, the horsepower is rarely used in biomechanics.

> The international system of units (SI system) includes all physical and chemical, metric and non-metric units. It is the most widely used system of units, especially in science and international commerce.

Unit symbols in the SI system

Units in the SI system are represented by symbols, which are derived according to mathematical rules, rather than abbreviations that follow grammatical rules (Rowlett 2004). The mathematical rules include:

- A symbol is not followed by a full-stop (period) except at the end of a sentence.
- The letter 's' is not added to a symbol to indicate more than one. For example, 2 kilograms is reported as 2 kg, not 2 kgs.
- Superscripts are used to indicate 'squared' or 'cubed'. For example, 4 square metres is written as 4 m^2, not 4 sq m.
- A raised dot (also referred to as a middle dot, centred dot and half-high dot), a decimal point or a space is used to indicate multiplication of one SI unit by another. For example, the symbol for a newton metre is N·m, N.m or N m, but not Nm. The raised dot format is used in this book.
- A forward slash or raised dot with a negative power is used to indicate division of one unit by another. For example, the symbol for metres per second is m/s or m·s^{-1}. However, only one slash or raised dot is permitted. For example, the symbol for metres per second per second is m/s^2 or m·s^{-2}, not m/s/s. The slash format is used in this book.
- A space is placed between the number and the associated symbol. For example, 2.4 kg and 3.25 s are correct, but 2.4 kg and 3.25 s are incorrect. In addition, the signs for percentage and degrees Celsius, which are widely used in scientific literature although they are not part of the SI system, should be spaced, as in 7.6 % and 5.5 °C. However, angle symbols (degrees °, minutes ′ and seconds ″) should be closed up; an angle is correctly reported as 53° 32′ 23″.
- In numbers with five or more digits either side of the decimal point, groups of three digits are separated by a space instead of a comma (which is used as a decimal point in some countries) as, for example, 10 000 m or 0.123 46 kg.

Conversion of units

Whereas most countries use the SI system, units from the British imperial system are still widely used in the UK and the USA. These units include, for example, inches (in), feet (ft), yards (yd) and miles (as in miles per hour, mph) for distance, and pounds (lb) and tons for mass. Table 8.2 shows some frequently used equivalences between SI and British imperial system units.

To convert units, it is necessary to replace the units to be converted by their numerical

Table 8.2 Equivalences between SI and British imperial system units.

Mass	1 lb	0.4536 kg	
	1 kg	2.2046 lb	
	1 ton	2240 lb	
	1 ton	1016.05 kg	
Length	1 in	25.4 mm	(mm = millimetre: 1 m = 1000 mm)
	1 in	2.54 cm	(cm = centimetre: 1 m = 100 cm)
	1 in	0.0254 m	
	1 ft	0.3048 m	
	1 yd	0.9144 m	
	1 mile	1609.34 m	
	1 mile	1.609 34 km	(km = kilometre: 1 km = 1000 m)
	1 cm	0.3937 in	
	1 cm	0.0328 ft	
	1 m	39.37 in	
	1 m	3.2808 ft	
	1 m	1.0936 yd	
	1 m	6.2137×10^{-4} miles = 0.000 621 37 miles	
	1 km	0.621 37 miles	
Angular distance	360°	2π rad	
	1°	0.017 45 rad	
	1 rad	57.296°	
Time	1 s	0.0167 min	
	1 s	2.7778×10^{-4} h (hours) = 0.000 277 78 h	
	1 min	60 s	
	1 h	60 min	
	1 h	3600 s	
Force	1 kgf	9.81 N	
	1 N	0.1019 kgf	
	1 kgf	2.2046 lbf	
	1 lbf	0.4536 kgf	
	1 lbf	4.4498 N	
	1 N	0.2247 lbf	
	1 tonf (ton force)	2240 lbf	
	1 tonf	1016 kgf	
	1 tonf	9964 N	
Speed	1 m/s	3.2808 ft/s	
	1 m/s	2.2369 mph (miles per hour)	

Table 8.2 (continued)

	1 m/s	3.6 km/h	
	1 km/h	0.277 78 m/s	
	1 ft/s	0.3048 m/s	
	1 ft/s	0.6818 mph	
	1 mph	0.4470 m/s	
	1 mph	1.609 34 km/h	
	1 km/h	0.6214 mph	
Area	1 m²	10.7639 ft²	
	1 m²	1550 in²	
	1 m²	1.1960 yd²	
	1 yd²	0.8361 m²	
	1 ft²	0.0929 m²	
	1 in²	$0.000\ 645\ 16\ m^2 = 6.4516 \times 10^{-4}\ m^2$	
	Surface area of a sphere	$4\pi \cdot r^2$	r, radius of the sphere
Volume	1 yd³ (cubic yard)	0.764 555 m³ (cubic metre)	
	1 ft³ (cubic foot)	0.028 316 m³	
	1 in³ (cubic inch)	16.387 cm³	
	1 m³	35.3144 ft³	
	1 m³	1.307 95 yd³	
	1 cm³	0.061 023 7 in³	
	1 l (litre)	$10^3\ cm^3 = 1000$ ml (millilitres)	
	1 m³	$10^6\ cm^3 = 10^3$ l	
	1 l	$10^{-3}\ m^3$	
	Volume of a sphere	$4\pi \cdot r^3/3$	r, radius of the sphere
	Volume of an ellipsoid	$4\pi \cdot a \cdot b^2/3$	a, length radius; b, width radius
Pressure	1 Pa (pascal)	1 N/m²	
	1 Pa	$0.000\ 144\ 988$ lbf/in² $= 1.449\ 88 \times 10^{-4}$ lbf/in²	
	1 lbf/in²	6897.15 Pa	
	1 atm (atmosphere)	101 325 Pa	
	1 atm	14.69 lbf/in²	
Density	Water (at sea level)	1000 kg/m³	
	Air (at sea level)	1.25 kg/m³	
Viscosity	1 P (poise)	$1\ g/(cm \cdot s) = 1\ g \cdot cm^{-1} \cdot s^{-1}$	
	1 Pa·s (pascal second)	$1\ kg/(m \cdot s) = 1\ kg \cdot m^{-1} \cdot s^{-1} = 10$ P	
	Water (at 20°C)	0.1002 P $= 0.010\ 02$ Pl	
	Air (at 20°C)	0.0018 P $= 0.000\ 18$ Pl	

equivalent in the units required. For example, the maximum speed of elite male sprinters in a 100 m race is approximately 12 m/s. This is equivalent to a speed of 26.84 mph:

As 1 m/s = 2.2369 mph (Table 8.2),

then 12 m/s = 12 × 2.2369 mph = 26.84 mph.

Similarly, the standard road vehicle speed limit in built-up areas in the UK is 30 mph. This is equivalent to a speed of 48.28 km/h:

As 1 mph = 1.609 34 km/h,

then 30 mph = 30 × 1.609 34 km/h = 48.28 km/h.

REVIEW QUESTIONS

1. Define the following terms: force, contact force, attraction force, resultant force, mechanics, biomechanics, mass, inertia, volume, density, stiffness, strength, kinematics and kinetics.

2. Describe the two ways in which forces tend to affect bodies.

3. Describe the four main subdisciplines of mechanics.

4. Describe the two fundamental forms of motion.

5. List the base units for length, mass and time in the international system of units.

6. Convert:

    *   150 m/s to mph;

    *   10 mph to km/h;

    *   25 km/h to m/s.

Chapter 9

Linear motion

The human body, like any other body, will only begin to move or, if is already moving, change its speed or direction, when the resultant force acting on it (the resultant of all the external forces acting on it) becomes greater than zero. Furthermore, the amount of change in speed or direction that occurs will depend upon the magnitude and direction of the resultant force, i.e. there is a direct relationship between change of resultant force and change in movement. Isaac Newton (1642–1727) described this relationship in what have come to be known as Newton's laws of motion. In addition to the three laws of motion, Newton's law of gravitation describes the naturally occurring force of attraction that is always present between any two bodies. A body falls to the ground because of the gravitational attraction between the body and the earth and the planets are maintained in their orbits round the sun by the gravitational attraction between the planets and the sun. The purpose of this chapter is to introduce the fundamental mechanical concepts underlying the study of linear motion, in particular, Newton's laws of motion and gravitation.

OBJECTIVES

After reading this chapter, you should be able to do the following:

1. Differentiate linear kinematics and linear kinetics.
2. Differentiate scalar and vector quantities.
3. Determine resultant force using the vector chain method and the method of trigonometry.
4. Differentiate active and passive loading.
5. Differentiate mass and weight.
6. Describe the linear impulse–linear momentum relationship in relation to jumping and landing.
7. Use the equations of uniformly accelerated motion in relation to the motion of projectiles.

SPACE AND THE NEWTONIAN FRAME OF REFERENCE

In mechanics, the position and change in position of a body in space are defined in relation to a Newtonian frame of reference (after Isaac Newton). In a Newtonian frame of reference, the three dimensions of space (forward and backward, side to side, up and down) are represented by three orthogonal axes (three lines at right angles to each other) that intersect at a point

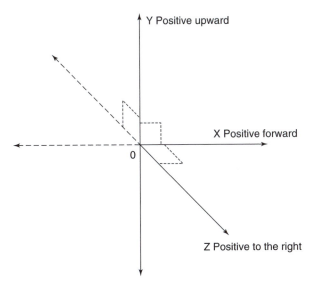

Figure 9.1 The right-handed axis system: 0 = origin.

called the origin (Figure 9.1). The three axes are usually referred to as X (forward–backward), Y (vertical) and Z (side-to-side) axes. Each axis has a positive and a negative sense with respect to the origin. Forward is positive and backward is negative on the X axis, upward is positive and downward is negative on the Y axis. Positive Z may be to the left or to the right, giving rise to the so-called left-handed and right-handed axis systems, respectively. In the right-handed axis system, as shown in Figure 9.1, positive Z is to the right. If the thumb and first two fingers of the right hand are held at right angles to each other with the index finger pointing forward (positive X) and the second finger pointing upward (positive Y), then the thumb will point to the right (positive Z); hence the name right-handed axis system. The right-handed axis system is the most widely used system. The right-handed axis system will be used in this book.

In a Newtonian frame of reference, the position of a point is defined by the coordinates of the point with respect to the three axes, i.e. the lengths x, y and z along the X, Y and Z axes that correspond to the point. The coordinates of a point are listed in the order x, y and z. For example, the coordinates of the points A, B and C in Figure 9.2 are (0, 0, 2), (0, 3, 2) and (4, 3, 2) respectively. The three axes give rise to three orthogonal planes, XY, YZ and XZ (Figure 9.3). Analysis of human movement may be concerned with movement along an axis (such as the movement of the body as a whole along the X axis in a 100 m sprint), in a plane (such as the movement of the head in the XY plane in a 100 m sprint) or in three-dimensional space.

> In a Newtonian frame of reference, the three dimensions of space are represented by three orthogonal axes that intersect at a point called the origin.

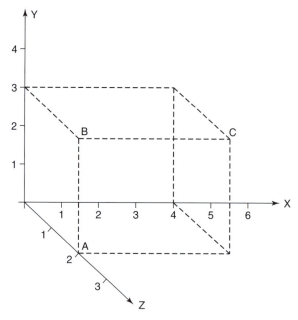

Figure 9.2 Coordinates of points in the right-handed axis system: A (0, 0, 2), B (0, 3, 2), C (4, 3, 2).

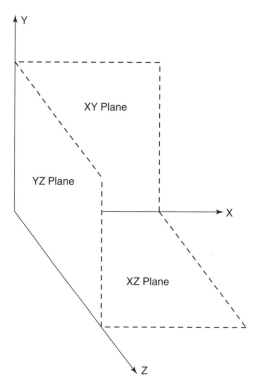

Figure 9.3 Reference planes in the right-handed axis system.

ANATOMICAL FRAME OF REFERENCE

To describe the spatial orientation of a particular part of the body in relation to another, it is necessary to use standard terminology with reference to a standard body posture. The generally accepted convention, referred to as the anatomical, relative or cardinal frame of reference, utilises the right-handed Newtonian frame of reference axis system in relation to a standard body posture called the anatomical position. In the anatomical position, the body is upright with the arms by the sides and the palms of the hands facing forward. The anatomical frame of reference (Figure 9.4) describes three principal planes (median, coronal and transverse) and three principal axes (anteroposterior, vertical and mediolateral).

The median plane is a vertical plane that divides the body down the middle into more-or-less symmetrical left and right portions. The median plane is also frequently referred to as the sagittal plane; the terms sagittal, paramedian and parasagittal (*para* = beside or beyond)

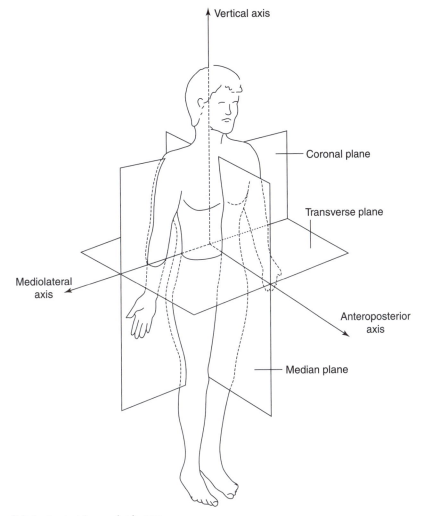

Figure 9.4 Anatomical frame of reference.

are also sometimes used to refer to any plane parallel to the median plane. In this book, the term sagittal is used to refer to any plane parallel to the median plane. The mediolateral axis is perpendicular to the median plane. The terms lateral and medial are used to describe the position of structures with respect to the mediolateral axis. Lateral means farther away from the median plane and medial means closer to the median plane. For example, in the anatomical position, the fingers of each hand are medial to the thumbs (and the thumbs are lateral to the fingers). Lateral and medial are also used to describe the direction of forces acting on the body in a mediolateral direction. For example, a laterally directed force acting on the right foot tends to move the body to the right, and a medially directed force acting on the right foot tends to move the body to the left.

The coronal plane (or frontal plane) is a vertical plane perpendicular to the median plane that divides the body into anterior and posterior portions. The anteroposterior axis is perpendicular to the coronal plane. The terms anterior (in front of) and posterior (behind) are used to describe the position of structures with respect to the anteroposterior axis. For example, in the anatomical position, the toes of each foot are anterior to the heels (and the heels are posterior to the toes). The terms ventral and dorsal are synonymous with anterior and posterior, respectively.

The transverse plane is a horizontal plane, perpendicular to both the median and coronal planes, which divides the body into upper and lower portions. The vertical axis is perpendicular to the transverse plane. The terms superior (above) and inferior (below) are used to describe the position of structures with respect to the vertical axis. For example, in the anatomical position, the head is superior to the shoulders (and the shoulders are inferior to the head).

Some spatial terms apply to some segments but not to others. For example, the terms proximal and distal are normally only used in reference to the limb segments (upper arm, forearm, hand, thigh, shank and foot). Superior parts or features of the segments (with respect to the anatomical position) are referred to as proximal, whereas inferior parts or features are referred to as distal. For example, the proximal end of the right upper arm articulates with the trunk to form the right shoulder joint. Similarly, the distal end of the right upper arm articulates with the proximal end of the right forearm to form the right elbow joint.

> The anatomical frame of reference describes three principal planes (median, coronal and transverse) and three principal axes (anteroposterior, vertical and mediolateral).

DISTANCE AND SPEED

The length of the line between two points in three-dimensional space is referred to as the distance between the points. Similarly, the length of the path followed by a body as it moves from one position to another in three-dimensional space is referred to as the distance travelled by the body. Speed is defined as rate of change of position, i.e. the distance travelled in moving from one position to another divided by the length of time taken to change position. For example, if a cross-country runner completes a race distance of 10.7 km (6.65 miles) in 37 min 2.5 s, his average speed during the run is given by:

$$\text{average speed} = \frac{\text{distance}}{\text{time}}$$

37 min 2.5 s = 2222.5 s = 0.6174 h

i.e. average speed $= \dfrac{10.7 \text{ km}}{0.6174 \text{ h}} = 17.33 \text{ km/h } (10.77 \text{ mph}).$

When the speed of an object is constant over a certain period of time, the object is said to move with uniform speed. When the speed of an object varies over a certain period of time, the object is said to move with non-uniform speed.

Analysis of the speed of human movement is important in all sports where time is the determinant of performance, such as track athletics and swimming. Knowledge of the average speed and the variation in speed of an athlete during a race can be helpful in the training of the athlete. For example, an endurance athlete aiming to run 5000 m in 13 min would need to achieve an average speed of 6.41 m/s, i.e.

$$\text{average speed} = \frac{5000 \text{ m}}{780 \text{ s}} = 6.41 \text{ m/s}.$$

However, average lap time would probably be more useful to the athlete and coach. Since there are 12.5 laps (1 lap = 400 m) in a 5000 m race, an average speed of 6.41 m/s corresponds to an average lap time of 62.4 s/lap, i.e.

$$\text{average lap time} = \frac{780 \text{ s}}{12.5 \text{ laps}} = 62.4 \text{ s/lap}.$$

> Analysis of the speed of human movement is important in all sports where time is the determinant of performance, such as track athletics and swimming.

Average speed in a marathon race

Table 9.1 shows the 5 km split times and average speeds in the 5 km splits of the winner of the 2005 women's London marathon, Paula Radcliffe (UK). Her average speed over the whole race was 5.11 m/s (11.43 mph), i.e.

distance = 26 miles 385 yd = 42.195 km,

time = 2 h 17 min 42 s = 8262 s,

$$\text{average speed} = \frac{42\ 195 \text{ m}}{8262 \text{ s}} = 5.11 \text{ m/s}.$$

The distance–time data (Columns 1 and 2 of Table 9.1) are plotted in the distance–time graph in Figure 9.5. The graph is close to linear, indicating little variation in speed throughout the

221

Table 9.1 Race time, time after each 5 km, 5 km split times and average speed in the 5 km splits of the winner (Paula Radcliffe, UK) of the 2005 women's London marathon.

Distance (km)	Time(min: s)	5 km split time (min: s)*	Average speed in each 5 km split (m/s)*
5	15:47	15:47	5.28
10	32:17	16:30	5.05
15	48:34	16:17	5.12
20	65:55	16:21	5.10
25	81:03	16:08	5.17
30	97:27	16:24	5.08
35	114:07	16:40	5.00
40	130:26	16:19	5.11
42.195	137:42	7:16	5.03

*The time for the final 2.195 km of the race was 7 min 16 s, resulting in an average speed of 5.03 m/s.

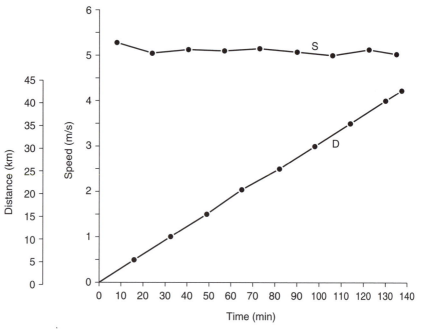

Figure 9.5 Distance–time graph (D) and average speed–time graph (S) of the winner of the 2005 women's London marathon: see data in Table 9.1.

race. This is reflected in the 5 km split times, which range between 15 min 47 s and 16 min 40 s and the corresponding average speed in the 5 km splits, which ranges between 5.00 m/s and 5.28 m/s. The average speed over the final 2.195 km of the race was 5.03 m/s. The average speed–time data are plotted in the average speed–time graph in Figure 9.5. Since the speed data are average speeds, each data point is plotted at the midpoint of the corresponding time interval.

Effect of running wide in middle-distance track events

A runner's energy reserves are fixed at the start of a race and, consequently, to maximise perform-ance, correct pace judgement is essential. Ideally, the runner would be completely exhausted, i.e. have used all his/her available energy reserves as s/he crosses the finish line. The runner's fixed energy reserves will determine the maximum average speed that s/he can maintain during the race. The runner's maximum average speed will also depend upon the distance covered, i.e. the longer the distance, the lower the average speed that can be maintained. Whereas the race distance is ostensibly fixed, the distance covered by the runner is not, i.e. it is likely, if only due to overtaking, that a runner will run farther than the race distance. For example, if a runner completes one lap of a 400 m track on the inside of the second lane, s/he will run 7.04 m farther than if s/he had run on the inside of the first lane (Jones and Whipp 2002).

In the finals of the men's 800 m and 5000 m races at the Sydney 2000 Olympic Games, the pre-race favourite in each race was beaten into second place. Jones and Whipp (2002) investi-gated the possible effect of actual distance covered on the performances of the first and second placed runners in each race. Using slow-motion video playback, the actual distances covered by the runners were calculated. The results are shown in Tables 9.2 and 9.3.

The 800 m race was won by Schumann (Germany) in 1 min 45.08 s. Schumann ran close

Table 9.2 Distance covered, race time, average speed and time to cover race distance at average speed of the gold and silver medal winners in the men's 800 m race at the Sydney 2000 Olympic Games.

	Schumann (Germany)	Kipketer (Denmark)	Schumann relative to Kipketer
Position in race	1	2	
Distance run (m)	802	813	−11
Race time (min: s)	1:45.08	1:45.14	−0.06
Average speed (m/s)	7.63	7.73	−0.10
Time to cover 800 m at average speed (min:s)	1:44.84	1.43.49	+1.35

Table 9.3 Distance covered, race time, average speed and time to cover race distance at average speed of the gold and silver medal winners in the men's 5000 m at the Sydney 2000 Olympic Games.

	Wolde (Ethiopia)	Saïdi-Sief (Algeria)	Wolde relative to Saïdi-Sief
Position in race	1	2	
Distance run (m)	5022	5028	−6
Race time (min: s)	13:35.49	13:36.20	−0.71
Average speed (m/s)	6.158	6.160	−0.002
Time to cover 5000 m at average speed (min: s)	13:31.95	13:31.69	+0.26

to the kerb throughout the race and covered a total distance of 802 m at an average speed of 7.63 m/s. Kipketer (Denmark) finished in second place in a time of 1 min 45.14 s. In contrast with Schumann, Kipketer ran in lanes 2 and 3 throughout the race and covered a total distance of 813 m at an average speed of 7.73 m/s. Schumann won the race even though his average speed during the race was 0.1 m/s slower than Kipketer, but he ran 11 m less than Kipketer. Based on their average velocities, Schumann and Kipketer should have been able to cover the actual race distance of 800 m in times of 1 min 44.84 s and 1 min 43.49 s, respectively. This suggests that Kipketer may have been able to win the race if his race tactics had been more closely related to his energy reserves.

The situation in the 5000 m race was similar to that in the 800 m race. The race was won by Wolde (Ethiopia) in 13 min 35.49 s at an average speed of 6.158 m/s. Saïdi-Sief (Algeria) finished in second place in 13 min 36.2 s at an average speed of 6.160 m/s. Whereas Wolde ran close to the kerb whenever possible, Saïdi-Sief tended to run on the outside shoulder of the leader. Wolde won the race even though his average speed during the race was 0.002 m/s slower than Saïdi-Sief, but he ran 6 m less than Saïdi-Sief.

Based on their average velocities, Wolde and Saïdi-Sief should have been able to cover the actual race distance of 5000 m in times of 13 min 31.95 s and 13 min 31.69 s, respectively. This suggests that Saïdi-Sief may have been able to win the race if his race tactics had been more closely related to his energy reserves. Jones and Whipp (2002) concluded that performance in middle-distance running events is dependent not only on energy reserves, but also on race tactics in terms of total distance covered.

LINEAR KINEMATIC ANALYSIS OF A 100 M SPRINT

Whereas an analysis of performance based on average speed is likely to be useful to athlete and coach in middle-distance and long-distance running events, average speed is of limited value in the short sprints of 100 m and 200 m. In these events, the aim of the sprinter is to achieve maximum speed as soon as possible and then maintain it to the end of the race. Consequently, analysis of the variation in speed during the race rather than average speed is likely to provide the most useful performance indicators. These include:

- Time taken to achieve maximum speed;
- Maximum speed;
- Length of time that maximum speed is maintained;
- Difference between maximum speed and speed at the finish.

To produce a speed–time graph, it is first of all necessary to obtain distance–time data. The most frequently used method of recording sprint performance for the purpose of obtaining distance–time data is video.

Video recordings for movement analysis

A video recording consists of a series of discrete images of the subject, each separated by a fixed time interval. The time interval between images is determined by the frame rate setting of the camera, i.e. the number of images (frames) recorded per second. In the SI system of units, frequency (the rate at which a periodic event or cycle of events occurs) is measured in hertz (Hz), i.e. the number of times that the event occurs per second (1 Hz = 1/s). The minimum frame rate available on most standard digital video cameras is 25 Hz. The human eye cannot detect discrete changes in the environment that occur more frequently than approximately 15 Hz. Consequently, to the human eye, a video playing at 25 Hz appears to be continuous rather than a series of discrete images. Whereas the frame rate of a digital video camera may be 25 Hz, the way that the images are stored by the camera allows the user to view discrete images at twice the frame rate, i.e. 50 Hz. Many analyses of human movement are based on measurements taken from sequences of discrete images in video recordings.

The type of analysis that can be carried out will depend upon the frame rate (which will determine the number of discrete images of the action under consideration) and the exposure (which will determine the sharpness and brightness of the images). The required frame rate of a recording will be determined by the duration of the action under consideration. For example, whereas 25 Hz is adequate for most types of human locomotion, such as walking and running (Winter 1990), a much higher frame rate is normally needed to record high-speed or short-duration events, such as impacts, adequately. For example, the contact time between club-head and ball during a golf drive is approximately 0.0005 s, i.e. half a millisecond (0.5 ms) or one two-thousandth of a second (Daish 1972). A frame rate in the region of 10 000 Hz would provide only five images of this type of impact:

$$\begin{aligned} \text{number of images} &= \text{frame rate} \times \text{contact time} \\ &= 10\ 000\ \text{Hz (images/s)} \times 0.0005\ \text{s} \\ &= 5\ \text{images.} \end{aligned}$$

The contact time between a tennis racket and ball during impact is approximately 0.005 s i.e. 5 ms or one two-hundredth of a second (Daish, 1972). A frame rate of 2000 Hz would provide approximately ten images of this type of impact:

$$\begin{aligned} \text{number of images} &= \text{frame rate count} \times \text{contact time} \\ &= 2000\ \text{Hz (images/s)} \times 0.005\ \text{s} \\ &= 10\ \text{images.} \end{aligned}$$

Exposure determines the sharpness (of contours and particular reference points) and brightness of the images. Sharpness is determined by the shutter speed setting of the camera, i.e. the length of time that the image sensor of the camera is exposed to the image. The faster the shutter speed, the sharper the image. A shutter speed of 0.002 s (one five-hundredth of a second) is usually adequate to capture sharp images in fast human movement. However, the faster the shutter speed, the shorter the duration of the exposure. This has to be balanced with the aperture setting of the camera (referred to as the f-stop), which determines the amount of light entering the camera during the exposure to ensure that the images are not too light or too dark.

Many analyses of human movement are based on measurements taken from sequences of discrete images in video recordings. The type of analysis that can be carried out will depend upon the frame rate and the exposure.

Distance–time and speed–time data from video analysis

Video was used to record the performance of a 19-year-old male junior international sprinter as he sprinted 100 m with maximum effort on a straight level track (frame rate = 25 Hz; shutter speed = 0.002 s; aperture = f8). Figure 9.6 shows the layout of the camera and track. The camera was placed close to the centre of the in-field area, in line with the 50 m mark on the track.

Prior to videotaping the sprint, the inside lane, i.e. the lane nearest to the camera, was marked at 10 m intervals from the start line. The sprinter was then asked to stand at the 10 m mark while a white wooden pole was placed in the in-field area approximately 1 m away from the track on a line between the camera lens and the sprinter. This procedure was repeated at each of the other nine 10 m marks, the last one being the finish line. The sprinter was then videotaped as he ran 100 m flat out under normal race start conditions. By viewing the video frame by frame (50 Hz) from the start of the run, the time taken by the sprinter to run the first 10 m, the first 20 m, the first 30 m, etc. up to 100 m was estimated by counting the frames and multiplying the number of frames by the frame rate, i.e. 0.02 s (1/50th of a second). The results are presented in the second column of Table 9.4. Column 3 of Table 9.4 shows the time for each successive 10 m of the sprint. Based on these data, the average speed of the sprinter in each successive 10 m is shown in Column 4 of Table 9.4. For example,

$$\text{average speed over the first 10 m} = \frac{10\,\text{m}}{1.92\,\text{s}} = 5.21\,\text{m/s}.$$

Elite performance in the 100 m sprint is characterised by a rapid increase in speed just after the start followed by a more gradual increase in speed up to maximum speed, which is then

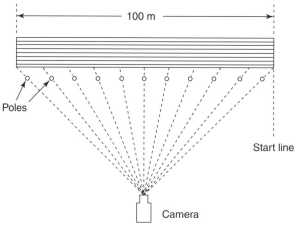

Figure 9.6 Layout of video camera, track and sighting poles for recording a 100 m sprint, to obtain distance–time data.

Table 9.4 Cumulative distance, cumulative time, time for each successive 10 m and average speed during each successive 10 m in a 100 m sprint by a male junior international athlete.

Distance (m)	Cumulative time (s)	Time for 10 m (s)	Average speed for 10 m (m/s)
10	1.92	1.92	5.21
20	3.10	1.18	8.47
30	4.16	1.06	9.43
40	5.06	0.90	11.11
50	6.08	1.02	9.80
60	7.00	0.92	10.87
70	8.02	1.02	9.80
80	9.04	1.02	9.80
90	10.02	0.98	10.20
100	11.12	1.10	9.09

maintained till the end of the race (Wagner 1998; Murase *et al.* 1976). The average speed–time data in Column 4 of Table 9.4 do not indicate a smooth change in speed; indeed the data indicate marked fluctuations in speed during the last 60 m, involving two phases of increasing speed alternating with three phases of decreasing speed. This almost certainly reflects errors in the distance–time data from which the average speed–time data was obtained. Timing errors could be related to the variation in body position of the sprinter at each 10 m marker and the restriction of the frame rate which both create difficulties in trying to locate the same point on the body, such as the pelvic region, at each marker post. More accurate distance–time data can be obtained from a 'line of best fit' distance–time graph. The line of best fit is a line drawn through the distance–time data that more accurately reflects the normal changes in speed during a 100 m sprint, i.e. a progressive smooth change in speed (absence of marked fluctuations in speed) involving an increase in speed up to maximum speed followed by maintenance of maximum speed or slight decrease in speed toward the end of the race. Figure 9.7 shows the distance–time data (Columns 1 and 2 of Table 9.4) and the corresponding line of best fit distance–time graph. Some of the distance–time data points lie on the line of best fit graph, but others do not. Very small errors in the distance–time data will result in much larger errors in speed–time data derived from them.

To obtain more accurate distance–time data from the line of best fit distance–time graph, parallel lines, perpendicular to the distance axis, are drawn to intersect the distance axis at intervals of one second (Figure 9.8). The points of intersection with the distance axis indicate the cumulative distance after successive intervals of one second (Column 2 of Table 9.5). The distance covered in each one-second interval (Column 3 of Table 9.5) and, therefore, the average speed in each one-second interval (Column 4 of Table 9.5) can then be calculated. Unlike the average speed–time data obtained directly from the original distance–time data (Column 4 of Table 9.4), the average speed–time data obtained from the line of best fit distance–time graph (Column 4 of Table 9.5) indicate that the speed of the sprinter increased fairly smoothly to a maximum value and then gradually decreased. This is typical of maximal effort sprinting over 100 m.

The average speed–time data obtained from the line of best fit distance–time graph (Column 4 of Table 9.5) are plotted in Figure 9.9, together with the line of best fit average

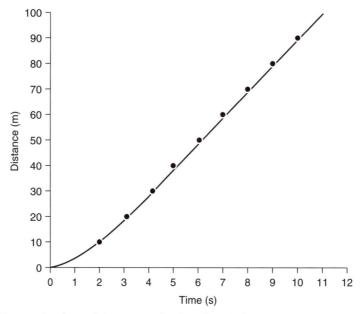

Figure 9.7 Distance–time data and the corresponding line of best fit distance–time graph.

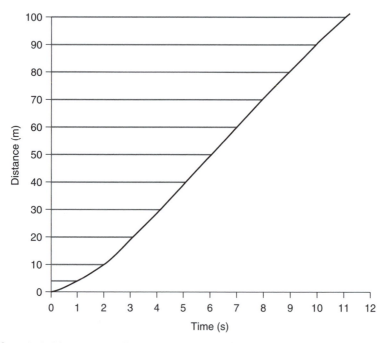

Figure 9.8 Method of determination of distance–time data from the line of best fit distance–time graph.

Table 9.5 Cumulative time, cumulative distance, distance covered in each one-second interval and average speed in each one-second interval in a 100 m sprint by a male junior international athlete.

Time (s)	Cumulative distance (s)	Distance travelled in each second (m)	Average speed in each second (m/s)
1	3.8	3.8	3.8
2	10.3	6.5	6.5
3	18.9	8.6	8.6
4	28.7	9.8	9.8
5	39.0	10.3	10.3
6	49.5	10.5	10.5
7	60.0	10.5	10.5
8	70.4	10.4	10.4
9	80.6	10.2	10.2
10	90.3	9.7	9.7
11	99.2	8.9	8.9

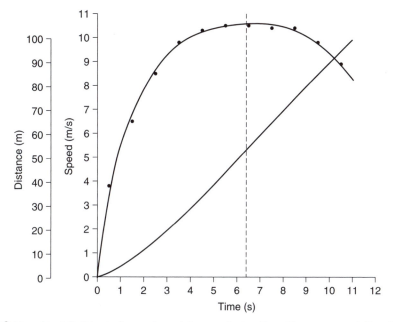

Figure 9.9 Line of best fit distance–time and speed–time graphs, together with average speed–time data points obtained from the line of best fit distance–time graph.

speed–time graph. Since the average speed–time data represent average speeds, each data point is plotted at the mid-point of the corresponding time interval. The line of best fit distance–time graph is also shown in Figure 9.9. Note the shallow S shape of the distance–time graph (look along the graph at eye level). The dotted vertical line distinguishes the two main phases of the run. The first phase is characterised by a progressive increase in the slope of the distance–time graph, corresponding to a progressive increase in speed to maximum speed of

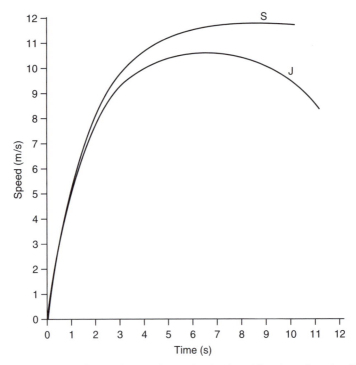

Figure 9.10 Speed–time graphs for a male junior international sprinter (J) and a male senior elite sprinter (S) in the 100 m sprint.

about 10.5 m/s (0 s to 6.4 s, 0 m to 53 m). The second phase is characterised by a progressive decrease in the slope of the distance–time graph, corresponding to a steady decrease in speed to a finishing speed of approximately 8.2 m/s (6.4 s to 11.12 s, 53 m to 100 m). The average speed–time data in Column 4 of Table 9.5 indicate a brief period of constant maximum speed (5.5 s to 6.5 s), but this is not evident in the line of best fit average speed–time graph.

To show that the distance–time and speed–time graphs in Figure 9.9 were truly representative of the sprinter's performance, it would be necessary to repeat the process on a number of trials, not just the one described here. However, assuming that the graphs in Figure 9.9 were representative, it would be useful to compare the speed–time graph with that of a senior elite sprinter in order to highlight areas for improvement. Figure 9.10 shows the junior international sprinter's speed–time graph (as in Figure 9.9) in relation to that of Carl Lewis (USA) in the final of the 100 m at the 1987 World Athletics Championships in Rome (Wagner 1998). Lewis finished second in a time of 9.93 s. Table 9.6 shows a comparison of the performances of the two sprinters. Whereas Lewis took longer to achieve maximum speed (7.5 s, 6.4 s), he was far superior to the junior athlete in relation to maximum speed (11.7 m/s, 10.5 m/s), length of time that maximum speed was maintained (2.4 s, 0 s) and finishing speed (11.7 m/s, 8.2 m/s).

Acceleration

Acceleration is defined as rate of change of speed, i.e. change in speed divided by the length of time in which the change in speed occurred:

Table 9.6 Comparison of performance of a male junior international (time = 11.12 s) with that of a senior elite sprinter (Carl Lewis, USA, final of the 1987 World Athletics Championships in Rome; time = 9.93 s) in the 100 m sprint.

	Junior international	Senior elite
Time taken to achieve maximum speed (s)	6.4	7.5
Maximum speed (m/s)	10.5	11.7
Length of time that maximum speed was maintained (s)	0	2.4
Finishing speed (m/s)	8.2	11.7
Difference between maximum speed and speed at the finish (m/s)	−2.3	0

$$a = \frac{v - u}{t_2 - t_1},$$

where a = acceleration, u = speed at time t_1 and v = speed at some later time t_2.

When the speed of a body increases during a particular period of time, the acceleration is positive. When the speed of a body decreases during a particular period of time, the acceleration is negative. Negative acceleration is usually referred to as deceleration.

The speed–time graph of the junior international sprinter shown in Figure 9.10 shows that his speed increased from zero at the start to a maximum speed of about 10.5 m/s in about 6.0 s. Consequently, his acceleration during this period is given by:

$$a = \frac{v - u}{t_2 - t_1} = \frac{10.5 \text{ m/s} - 0 \text{ m/s}}{6.0 \text{ s} - 0 \text{ s}} = 1.75 \text{ m/s}^2 \text{ (metres per second per second)},$$

i.e. his speed increased by an average of 1.75 m/s for each second between the start and 6.0 s into the run. Figure 9.10 also shows that his speed decreased from a maximum speed of 10.5 m/s at about 6.5 s to about 8.2 m/s at the end of the run, which was completed in 11.12 s,

$$\text{i.e. } a = \frac{v - u}{t_2 - t_1} = \frac{8.2 \text{ m/s} - 10.5 \text{ m/s}}{11.12 \text{ s} - 6.5 \text{ s}} = \frac{-2.3 \text{ m/s}}{4.62 \text{ s}} = -0.50 \text{ m/s}^2.$$

The negative sign indicates that the sprinter was decelerating during the period under consideration, i.e. his speed decreased at an average of 0.50 m/s for each second during the period 6.5 s to the end of the run.

Using the same method used to obtain distance–time data from the line of best fit distance–time graph, the speed of the junior international sprinter after each second of the run was obtained from the line of best fit speed–time graph in Figure 9.9. These data are shown in Column 2 of Table 9.7. Column 3 of Table 9.7 shows the change in speed during each second of the run; the corresponding average acceleration of the sprinter in each one-second interval is shown in Column 4 of Table 9.7. The average acceleration–time data (plotted at the mid-points of the corresponding time intervals) and line of best fit acceleration–time graph are shown in Figure 9.11, together with the corresponding distance–time and speed–time

231

Table 9.7 Cumulative time, cumulative speed, change in speed in each one-second interval and average acceleration in each one-second interval in a 100 m sprint by a male junior international athlete.

Time (s)	Cumulative speed (m/s)	Change in speed in each second (m/s)	Average acceleration in each second (m/s^2)
1	5.35	5.35	5.35
2	7.80	2.45	2.45
3	9.25	1.45	1.45
4	10.00	0.75	0.75
5	10.38	0.38	0.38
6	10.50	0.12	0.12
7	10.50	0	0
8	10.30	−0.20	−0.20
9	9.90	−0.40	−0.40
10	9.30	−0.60	−0.60
11	8.25	−1.05	−1.05

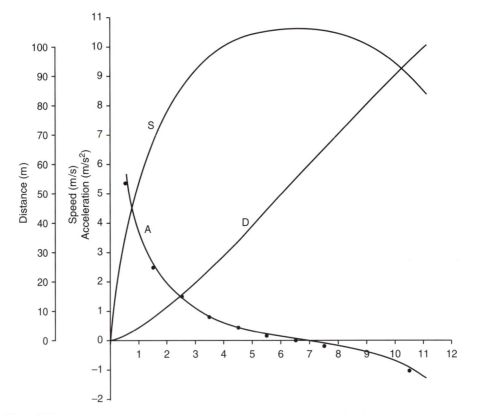

Figure 9.11 Distance–time (D), speed–time (S) and acceleration–time (A) graphs of a male junior international sprinter in the 100 m sprint.

graphs. The acceleration–time graph shows that the sprinter's acceleration was positive for about 6.4 s, i.e. his speed increased progressively during this period up to a maximum speed of about 10.5 m/s. During the remainder of the sprint, the sprinter's acceleration was negative, resulting in a steady decrease in speed. Whereas it was not possible to estimate the acceleration of the sprinter just after the start, data reported by Baumann (1976) indicate that 0.2 s after the start, acceleration would be approximately 13 m/s² for this standard of sprinter (100 m time of 10.9 s to 11.4 s). This is consistent with the acceleration–time data given in Figure 9.11.

In Practical Worksheet 1, students collect distance–time data over a 15 m sprint and analyse the data to present the corresponding distance–time, speed–time and acceleration–time graphs.

VECTOR AND SCALAR QUANTITIES

All quantities in the physical and life sciences can be categorised as either scalar or vector quantities. Quantities that can be completely specified by their magnitude (size) are called scalar quantities. These include volume, area, time, temperature, mass, distance and speed. Quantities that require specification in both magnitude and direction are called vector quantities. These include displacement (distance in a given direction), velocity (speed in a given direction), acceleration and force. A vector quantity can be represented by a straight line with an arrow head. The length of the line, with respect to an appropriate scale, corresponds to the magnitude of the quantity and the orientation of the line and arrow head, with respect to an appropriate reference axis (usually horizontal or vertical) that indicates the direction.

> All quantities in the physical and life sciences can be categorised as either scalar or vector quantities. Quantities that can be completely specified by their magnitude (size) are called scalar quantities. Quantities that require specification in both magnitude and direction are called vector quantities.

Displacement vectors

If a man runs 3 miles from a point A to a point B and then walks 2 miles from point B to a point C, it is clear that he has travelled a total distance of 5 miles. However, it is not possible to determine the position of C with respect to A, since no information is given concerning the directions in which he ran and walked. However, if we are given the directions as well as the distances, we are then dealing with vector quantities, i.e. displacements, and can, therefore, determine the position of C in relation to A. For example, if we are told that the man ran 3 miles due north from A to B and then walked 2 miles due east from B to C, the position of C in relation to A can be determined by considering the displacement vectors *AB* and *BC*. The bold italic typeface indicates a vector. The displacements *AB* and *BC* are shown in Figure 9.12a. The position of C in relation to A is specified by the vector *AC*, which is the vector sum of *AB* and *BC*, i.e. *AC* = *AB* + *BC*. The distance between A and C can be

233

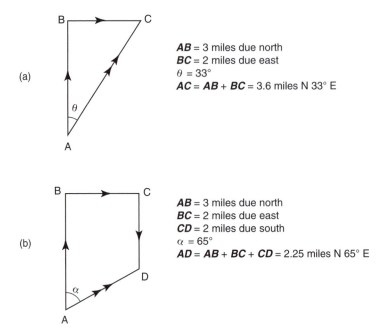

(a)

AB = 3 miles due north
BC = 2 miles due east
θ = 33°
$AC = AB + BC$ = 3.6 miles N 33° E

(b)

AB = 3 miles due north
BC = 2 miles due east
CD = 2 miles due south
α = 65°
$AD = AB + BC + CD$ = 2.25 miles N 65° E

Figure 9.12 Resultants of displacement vectors.

determined by measuring the line AC and converting this to miles using the distance scale. The direction of C in relation to A is specified by the angle θ. AC is referred to as the resultant vector of AB and BC, and AB and BC are referred to as component vectors. AC (3.6 miles N 33° E) is the resultant displacement of the man from the point A. Vector addition is clearly not the same as arithmetic (scalar) addition.

If the man walked 2 miles due south from C to a point D, the position of D in relation to A would be specified by the vector AD (Figure 9.12b). In this case, the resultant vector AD is the resultant of the three vectors AB, BC and CD. This example illustrates that irrespective of the number of component displacement vectors used to describe the movement of a body, the net result of all the component vectors can be specified by a single resultant displacement vector. This general principle applies to all vector quantities.

The method used in Figure 9.12 to determine the resultant of the component vectors is called the vector chain method, i.e. the component vectors are linked together in a chain (in any order) and the resultant vector runs from the starting point of the first component vector to the end point of the last component vector.

Velocity vectors

In addition to the vector chain method of determining the resultant of a number of component vectors, there is another method, the parallelogram of vectors, that is useful when there are only two component vectors, but somewhat laborious when there are three or more component vectors. In this method two component vectors extend from the same point to form adjacent sides of a parallelogram. The resultant of the two component vectors is given

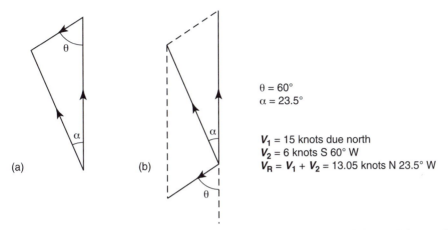

$\theta = 60°$
$\alpha = 23.5°$

$V_1 = 15$ knots due north
$V_2 = 6$ knots S 60° W
$V_R = V_1 + V_2 = 13.05$ knots N 23.5° W

(a)   (b)

Figure 9.13 Resultant velocity of a ship without a keel. (a) Vector chain method. (b) Parallelogram of vectors method.

by the diagonal of the completed parallelogram. For example, if a ship without a keel starts to sail due north in a wind blowing S 60° W, the resultant velocity of the ship is specified by the resultant of the velocity V_1 of the ship resulting from the drive of the engines and the velocity V_2 of the ship resulting from the wind. The vector chain and parallelogram of vectors methods of determining the resultant velocity of the ship are shown in Figure 9.13. If $V_1 = 15$ knots due north and $V_2 = 6$ knots S 60° W, the resultant velocity of the ship $V_R = 13.05$ knots N 23.5° W.

When using the parallelogram of vectors method to determine the resultant of three or more component vectors, the first step is to find the resultant R_1 of any two component vectors. The resultant of R_1 and another component vector is then found and the process repeated until the resultant of all the component vectors is found.

In this example of the ship without a keel, the component velocities were constant. However, component velocities are frequently variable, resulting in variable resultant velocities. Consider a rugby player attempting a penalty kick at goal. If there is no crosswind, the kicker has only to kick the ball in the direction of the middle of the posts (Figure 9.14a). However, if there is a crosswind, the movement of the ball will be determined by the velocity K imparted by the kick and the velocity W imparted by the wind. If the kicker does not

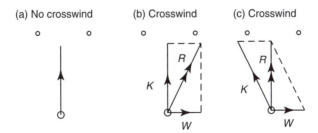

(a) No crosswind   (b) Crosswind   (c) Crosswind

Figure 9.14 Effect of a crosswind on the direction of a rugby ball following a place kick: K, velocity due to the kick; W, velocity due to the wind; R, resultant of K and W.

235

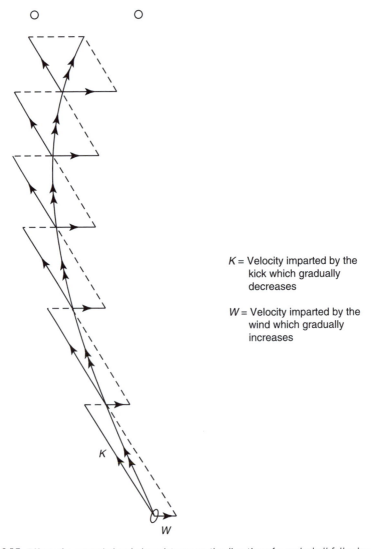

K = Velocity imparted by the
kick which gradually
decreases

W = Velocity imparted by the
wind which gradually
increases

Figure 9.15 Effect of a crosswind and air resistance on the direction of a rugby ball following a place kick.

take account of the wind, the ball will not travel in the direction of the middle of the posts (Figure 9.14b). A good kicker will take account of the wind, such that the combined effect of the kick and the wind will direct the ball between the posts (Figure 9.14c). Even then, the ball does not travel in a straight line, but along a curve, as shown in Figure 9.15. Assuming that the wind continues to blow throughout the period of ball flight, the speed of the ball imparted by the wind will gradually increase during the flight. However, the speed of the ball imparted by the kick will gradually decrease during the flight due to air resistance. Consequently, the direction of the ball will continually change (Figure 9.15). In this example, it is assumed that the kick does not impart spin to the ball. The mechanics of a spinning ball are considered in Chapter 12.

CENTRE OF GRAVITY

The human body consists of a number of segments linked by joints. Each segment contributes to the body's total weight (Figure 9.16a). Movement of the body segments relative to each other alters the weight distribution of the body. However, in any particular body posture, the body behaves (in terms of the effect of body weight on the movement of the body) as if the total weight of the body is concentrated at a single point, called the centre of gravity (also referred to as the centre of mass) (Figure 9.16b). Body weight acts vertically downward from the centre of gravity along a line called the line of action of body weight. The concept of centre of gravity applies to all bodies, animate and inanimate.

> The centre of gravity of an object is the point at which the whole weight of the object can be considered to act.

The position of an object's centre of gravity depends on the distribution of the weight of the object. For a regular-shaped object (of uniform density), such as a cube, oblong or sphere, the centre of gravity is located at the object's geometric centre (Figure 9.17).

For an irregular-shaped object, the centre of gravity may be inside or outside the object. For example, consider a triangular card with sides 15 cm, 20 cm and 25 cm in length, and vertices A, B and C. Figure 9.18a shows the card suspended from a freely moveable pin joint

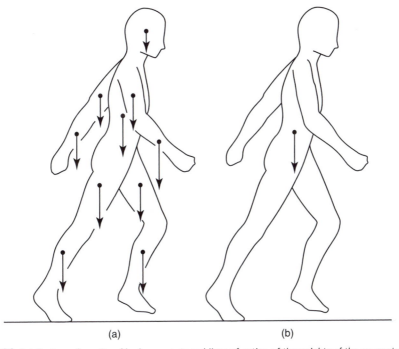

(a)　　　　　　　　　　(b)

Figure 9.16 (a) Centres of gravity of body segments and lines of action of the weights of the segments. (b) Centre of gravity of the whole body and line of action of body weight.

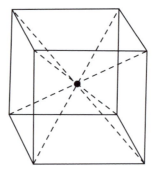

Figure 9.17 The centre of gravity of a regular-shaped object, such as a cube, is located at the geometric centre of the object.

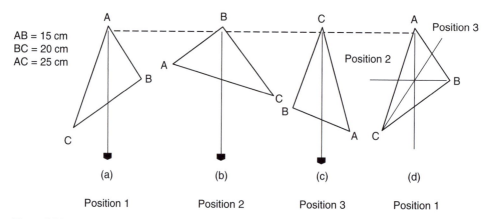

AB = 15 cm
BC = 20 cm
AC = 25 cm

(a)   (b)   (c)   (d)

Position 1   Position 2   Position 3   Position 1

Figure 9.18 Suspension method for locating the centre of gravity of an irregular-shaped object: a triangular shaped piece of card.

close to vertex A. The line of action of the weight of the card coincides with the vertical line through the point of suspension. By suspending a plumbline in front of the card from the same pin joint, the line of action of the weight of the card can be determined. Figures 9.18b and c show this process repeated from points of suspension close to vertices B and C, respectively. In Figure 9.18d, the lines of action of the weight of the card in positions 2 and 3 are shown superimposed on the line of action in position 1. The lines of action of the weight of the card in the three positions intersect at a single point, the centre of gravity of the card. In this example, the card's centre of gravity lies inside the body of the card.

Figure 9.19 shows the same process carried out with an L-shaped card with width 4 cm and arms of length 15 cm and 20 cm. In this case, the centre of gravity of the card is found to lie outside the body of the card (Figure 9.19d).

The human body is an irregular shape. When standing upright, the centre of gravity of an adult is located inside the body close to the level of the navel (56.4 $\pm$ 2.8% of stature for women and 57.1 $\pm$ 2.3% of stature for men) and midway between the front and back of the body (Figure 9.20a) (Watkins 2000). Moving the arms forward to a horizontal position will move the centre of gravity slightly forward and upward (Figure 9.20b). Moving the

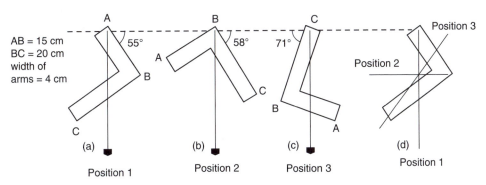

AB = 15 cm
BC = 20 cm
width of
arms = 4 cm

Figure 9.19 Suspension method for locating the centre of gravity of an irregular-shaped object: an L-shaped piece of card.

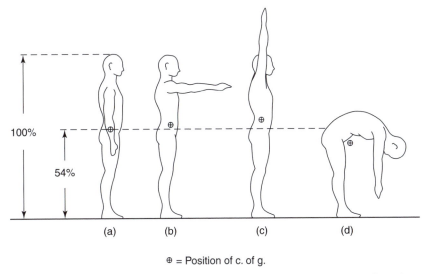

⊕ = Position of c. of g.

Figure 9.20 Movement of the location of the centre of gravity of the human body, resulting from changes in the mass distribution of the body.

arms from this position to overhead (Figure 9.20c) will move the centre of gravity slightly backward and upward. Since the combined weight of both arms comprises about 11% of body weight, any movement of the arms results in a fairly slight change in the position of the centre of gravity. However, movement of the trunk, which comprises approximately 50% of body weight, will result in a relatively large change in the position of the centre of gravity. For example, full flexion of the trunk will result in the centre of gravity being located outside the body (Figure 9.20d). This position is similar to the position adopted by a pole vaulter when clearing the bar (Figure 9.21a). The body's centre of gravity may also be located outside the body during postures involving full extension of the trunk, as in clearing the bar using the Fosbury flop technique in high jumping (Figure 9.21b). Movements involving continuous change in the orientation of body segments to each other, such as walking and running, result in a continuous change in the position of the body's centre of gravity.

239

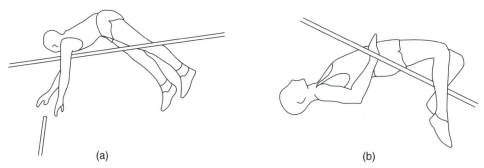

Figure 9.21 During bar clearance in (a) pole vault and (b) high jump, the centre of gravity of the body may lie outside the body.

STABILITY

Figure 9.22 shows a regular cube-shaped block of wood resting on a horizontal surface. The centre of gravity of the block of wood is located at its geometric centre and the line of action of the weight of the wood intersects the base of support ABCD on which it is resting. If the block of wood is tilted over on any of the edges of the base of support, AB, BC, CD or AD, it will return to its original position provided that, at release, the line of action of its weight intersects the plane of the original base of support ABCD. This situation is shown in Figure 9.22c with respect to the edge BC. However, if, at release, the line of action of its weight does not intersect the original base of support, the block of wood will fall onto one of its other faces, as shown in Figures 9.22d and e. With respect to a particular base of support, an object is stable

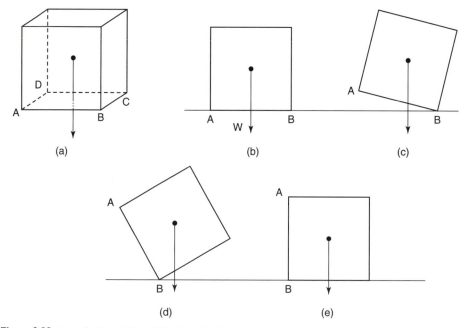

Figure 9.22 Line of action of the weight of a cube in relation to its base of support.

when the line of action of its weight intersects the plane of the base of support and unstable when it does not. Consequently, the block of wood in Figure 9.22 is stable with respect to the base of support ABCD in the positions shown in Figure 9.22b and c, and unstable with respect to the base of support ABCD in the position shown in Figure 9.22d.

> With respect to a particular base of support, an object is stable when the line of action of its weight intersects the plane of the base of support and unstable when it does not.

The stability of an object with respect to its base of support depends on the size of the base of support and the height of the object's centre of gravity above the base of support. Figure 9.23 shows two blocks of wood, 10 cm and 20 cm long, respectively, with the same square cross section of 4 cm × 4 cm. When the two pieces of wood rest on any of their larger faces, the heights of their centres of gravity above the base of support are the same, i.e. 2 cm. With respect to the X axis (CD in the longer block of wood and RS in the shorter block of wood) the stability of the longer block of wood is greater than that of the shorter block of wood, since the longer one would need to be tilted through a larger angle (79°) than the shorter one (68°) before it became unstable (Figure 9.23c,d). However, with respect to the Y axis (AD in the longer block of wood and PS in the shorter block of wood) the stability of the two blocks is the same; each block would need to be tilted through an angle of 45° before it became unstable (Figure 9.23e).

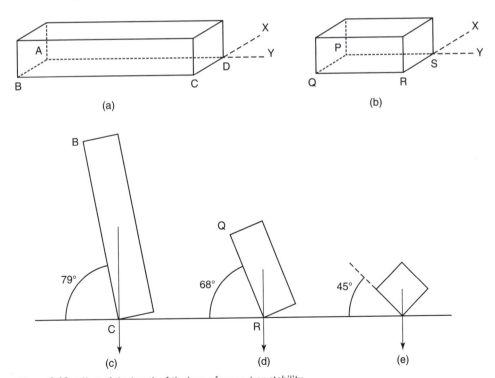

(a)   (b)

(c)   (d)   (e)

Figure 9.23 Effect of the length of the base of support on stability.

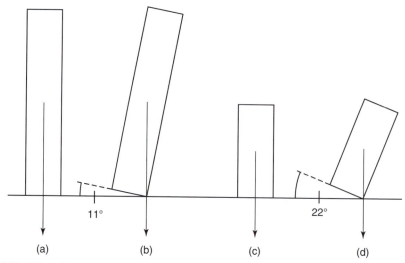

11° 22°

(a) (b) (c) (d)

Figure 9.24 Effect of the height of the centre of gravity above the base of support on stability.

Clearly, for a given height of centre of gravity, the broader the base of support with respect to a particular axis of tilt, the greater the object's stability. In Figure 9.24a the longer block of wood is shown standing on one of its ends, and in Figure 9.24c the shorter block is shown standing on one of its ends. In this situation, the dimensions of the base of support of each block are the same, but the centre of gravity of the taller block is 10 cm above its base and that of the shorter block is 5 cm above its base. When both blocks are tilted on one edge, the taller block becomes unstable after being tilted through a much smaller angle (11°) than the shorter block (22°). Consequently, in this situation, the taller block is less stable than the shorter block.

It follows from these examples that for any particular object the lower the ratio of the height of the centre of gravity to the length of the base of support (with respect to each possible tilt axis), the greater the stability of the object. This principle is used, for example, in the design of vehicles, to minimise their risk of overturning during normal use.

With regard to human movement, the terms stability and balance are often used synonymously. Maintaining stability of the human body is a fairly complex, albeit largely unconscious, process (Roberts 1995). In upright standing, the line of action of body weight intersects the base of support formed by the area beneath and between the feet (Figure 9.25a,b). The size of the base of support can be increased by moving the feet farther apart. For example, moving one foot in front of the other increases anteroposterior stability, and moving one foot laterally increases side-to-side stability (Figure 9.25c,d). Combining these movements with a degree of flexion of the hips, knees and ankles, as in certain movements in wrestling and boxing, reduces the height of the centre of gravity and, thereby, further increases stability.

Movement of the body from one base of support to another, such as in moving from standing to sitting, illustrates the unconscious way in which the balance systems of the body automatically redistribute body weight to maintain stability. Figure 9.26 shows a person moving from a standing position to sit on a chair. The person moves his feet close to the front of the chair and then lowers his body by flexing his knees and bending his trunk forward while maintaining the same base of support, i.e. the area beneath and between his feet (Figure 9.26a,b).

242

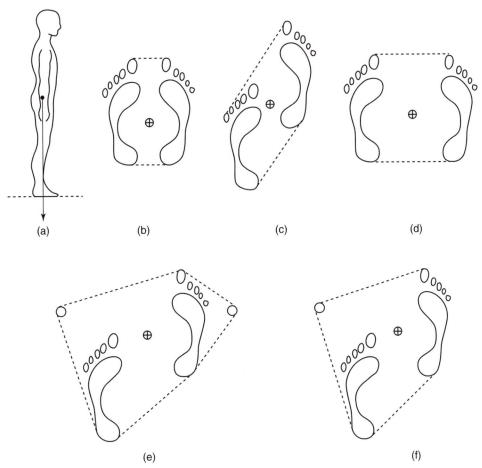

Figure 9.25 Line of action of body weight in relation to the base of support. (a,b) Standing upright. (c) Standing upright with the right foot in front of the left foot. (d) Standing upright with feet apart, side by side. (e) Standing with the aid of crutches or two walking sticks. (f) Standing with the aid of a walking stick in the left hand. The symbol ⊕ denotes the point of intersection of the line of body weight with the base of support.

He may or may not take hold of the sides of the chair as his thighs approach the seat of the chair. If he does take hold of the chair, his base of support immediately increases to include the area bounded by the legs of the chair as well as that beneath and between his feet, but the line of action of his body weight will still be over the area between his feet (Figure 9.26c). When his thighs come close to the seat of the chair he begins to transfer his weight from over his feet to over the seat by gently rocking the trunk backward (Figure 9.26d). These movements are reversed when moving from a sitting to a standing position.

Figure 9.27 shows a person stepping onto a chair. He initiates the movement by putting one foot on the chair. To step up with the other foot, he must move his centre of gravity forward so that the line of action of his weight passes within a new base of support provided by the foot of the leading leg. He can then extend the leading leg and stand up on the chair. Therefore, in walking up a flight of stairs, the centre of gravity is continually shifted forward over the leading foot.

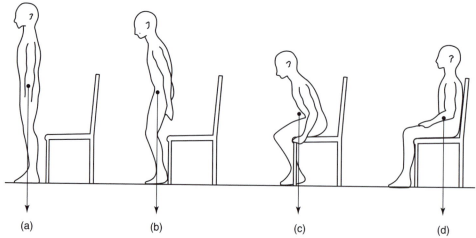

Figure 9.26 Line of action of body weight in relation to the base of support when moving from standing to sitting.

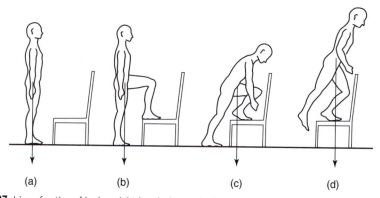

Figure 9.27 Line of action of body weight in relation to the base of support when stepping onto a chair.

When bending forward from an upright position, a person's buttocks move backward in relation to his feet so that the line of action of his weight remains over his base of support (Figure 9.28a,b). This can easily be demonstrated by asking someone to bend forward while standing with his back and heels against a wall. Since his buttocks are prevented from moving backward, the line of action of his weight soon passes in front of his base of support and he will fall forward unless he takes a step forward (Figure 9.28c,d).

In general, the lower the centre of gravity and the larger the area of the base of support, the greater stability is likely to be. For example, by moving from a standing to a sitting position, the body's centre of gravity is lowered and the area of the base of support is increased (Figure 9.29a–c). The recumbent position is one of the most stable positions of the human body since the area of the base of support is large and the centre of gravity is at its lowest (Figure 9.29d). Spreading the arms and legs on the floor would further increase stability. As the area of the base of support increases, the degree of muscular effort needed to maintain stability tends to decrease. For example, it is usually easier,

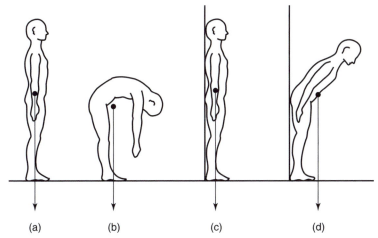

Figure 9.28 Line of action of body weight in relation to the base of support. (a) Standing. (b) Bending forward. (c) Standing against a wall. (d) Bending forward from a standing position against a wall.

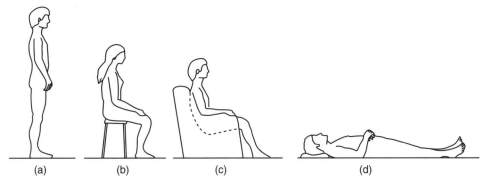

Figure 9.29 (a) Standing. (b,c) Sitting. (d) Lying down.

in terms of muscular effort, to maintain stability when standing on both feet than when standing on one foot. Similarly, it is usually less tiring to sit than to stand, and less tiring to lie down than to sit. A person recovering from a leg injury may use crutches or a walking stick in order to relieve the load on the injured limb. The use of crutches also increases the area of the base of support and makes it easier for the user to maintain stability (Figure 9.25e,f).

Adequate stabilty is vital for good performance in all sports. For example, in boxing, to apply a rapid powerful forward jab (Figure 9.30), the boxer needs to ensure that he has adequate stability so that he can apply a large force without losing his balance as a result of the equal and opposite force exerted on his fist. This is achieved by putting one foot in front of the other, which considerably increases his stabilty in the direction of the punch. Similarly, a baseball or softball player will tend to place one foot well in front of the other when hitting the ball so that he can hit the ball hard without losing his balance (Figure 9.31).

245

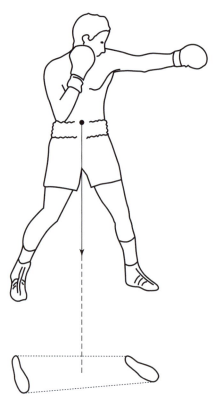

Figure 9.30 Line of action of the weight of a boxer in relation to his base of support when making a punch.

In certain situations in sport, good performance may depend on unstable rather than stable postures. For example, in the set position of a sprint start, the sprinter tends to move his centre of gravity as far forward as possible without overbalancing in order to obtain the best position from which to drive his body forward when the gun goes (Figure 9.32). In this position, the line of action of his body weight passes close to the anterior limit of his base of support.

As the area of the base of support decreases, the degree of tolerance in the movement of the line of action of body weight also decreases if stability is to be maintained. When the base of support becomes a knife edge or something similar, such as a tightrope or very narrow beam, the amount of tolerance in the movement of the centre of gravity is zero in any direction other than along the line of support. Consequently, when an object is in a balanced position on a knife-edge support, the centre of gravity of the object is located in the vertical plane through the line of support. By balancing an object in a number of different positions and noting the orientation of the vertical support plane to the object in each position, it may be possible to determine the position of the centre of gravity of the object, which will be located at the point of intersection of the support planes. This method could be used with the triangular piece of card in Figure 9.18.

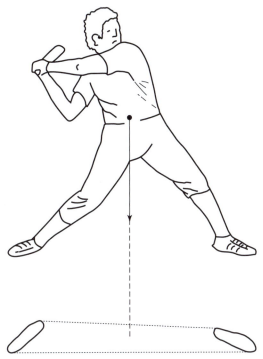

Figure 9.31 Line of action of the weight of a baseball player in relation to his base of support when hitting the ball.

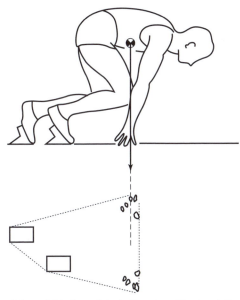

Figure 9.32 Line of action of the weight of a sprinter in the set position in relation to his base of support.

FRICTION

When one object moves or tends to move across the surface of another, there will be a force parallel to the surfaces in contact, which will oppose the movement or tendency to move. This force is called friction. Consider a block of wood resting on a level table (Figure 9.33). The only forces acting on the block are the weight of the block **W** and the force **R** exerted by the table on the block. Since the block is at rest, **R** is equal and opposite to **W** (Figure 9.33a). If an attempt is made to push the block along the surface of the table by applying a horizontal force **P**, the frictional force **F** between the contacting surfaces will begin to operate and oppose the tendency of the block to move (Figure 9.33b). As **P** increases, so does **F**, until the block begins to move, i.e. **F** has a maximum value. This value is directly proportional to the degree of roughness of the two surfaces in contact and the force **R**. The three variables are related as follows:

$$\mathbf{F} = \mu\mathbf{R} \tag{9.1}$$

where μ (Greek letter mu) is a measure of the roughness of the two surfaces in contact and is called the coefficient of friction between the two surfaces. The force **R** is referred to as the normal reaction force and is perpendicular to the plane of contact between the two surfaces.

The magnitude of μ depends on the types of surface in contact and whether the surfaces are sliding on each other. Surfaces are never perfectly smooth, and the minor irregularities of the contacting surfaces interdigitate and resist sliding between the surfaces (Figure 9.34a). To initiate sliding, the minor irregularities have to be dragged over each other. In doing so, the

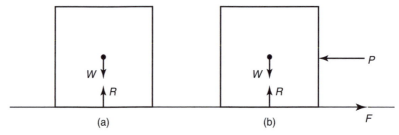

(a)   (b)   *F*

Figure 9.33 (a) Forces acting on a block of wood resting on a level table. (b) Forces acting on a block of wood resting on a level table, but tending to slide horizontally. *W*, weight of the block; *R*, normal reaction force; *P*, horizontal force applied to the side of the block; *F*, friction.

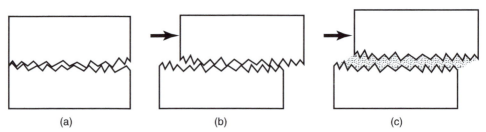

(a)   (b)   (c)

Figure 9.34 (a) Interdigitation of surface irregularities. (b) Slight separation of surfaces as a result of sliding. (c) Complete separation of surfaces as a result of lubrication.

surfaces tend to separate slightly which reduces the resistance to sliding, providing that the sliding is maintained (Figure 9.34b). Consequently, for any two surfaces in contact, μ (and therefore **F**) will be slightly less when the surfaces are sliding on each other than when the surfaces are not sliding on each other but tending to slide. Therefore, for any two surfaces, there is a coefficient of limiting (static) friction and a coefficient of sliding (dynamic) friction.

When no sliding occurs, the normal reaction force is distributed over those parts of the adjacent surfaces that are in contact; this will include the irregularities and some of the surfaces between the irregularities (Figure 9.34a). However, during sliding, the normal reaction force is exerted almost entirely by the irregularities (Figure 9.34b). Consequently, during sliding, the pressure exerted by the irregularities of one surface on the other surface is likely to be considerably increased and result in wear of the surface (similar to the effect of sandpaper on wood). The introduction of a fluid between the surfaces tends to separate not only the surfaces, but also the surface irregularities, resulting in a considerable reduction in friction and wear. This is the principle of lubrication (Figure 9.34c).

In the absence of lubrication, μ is about 0.25–0.50 for wood on wood, 0.15–0.60 for metal on metal, 0.20–0.60 for wood on metal and 0.4–0.9 for wood on rubber (Serway and Jewett 2004). The difference between limiting and sliding friction between different pairs of materials can be easily demonstrated with a spring balance and a block of wood. For example, place a block of wood weighing about 1 kgf on a level wooden table. Apply a horizontal force to the block very gradually with a spring balance and note the maximum force recorded just before the block begins to move. The coefficient of limiting friction μ_L between the block and the table can then be estimated by using Equation 9.1, i.e. $\mu_L = F_1/R$ where F_1 is the maximum force recorded on the spring balance just before the block begins to move and **R** is the weight of the block. Repeat the experiment and observe the force F_2 required to maintain sliding. The coefficient of sliding friction μ_S between the block and the table can then be estimated from $\mu_S = F_2/R$. Results similar to those shown in the first row of Table 9.8 will be obtained.

Different combinations of materials have different coefficients of friction and this can be demonstrated by varying the support surface in the experiment. The second, third and fourth rows of Table 9.8 show the results obtained for μ_L and μ_S for the same block of wood and three other materials.

Equation 9.1 shows that the amount of friction, limiting and sliding, between two surfaces is independent of the area of contact when the normal reaction force stays the same. The

Table 9.8 Coefficient of limiting friction (μ_L) and sliding friction (μ_S) for a number of materials with wood.

Support surface	Limiting friction		Sliding friction	
	F (kgf)	μ_L	F (kgf)	μ_S
Polished wooden table	0.55	0.50	0.23	0.21
Formica	0.33	0.30	0.18	0.16
Resin floor tile	0.80	0.70	0.38	0.34
Plain rubber mat	0.90	0.80	0.45	0.41

Normal reaction force = 1.1 kgf; F = horizontal force.

compression stress on the surfaces will vary with the area of contact, but the amount of friction will not change if the normal reaction force remains constant.

The development of adequate friction between the human body and the environment is essential for most actions of daily living, in particular, body transport (friction between the feet and the floor) and manipulation of objects (friction between the fingers and objects). The importance of the need for adequate friction in these types of actions is, perhaps, more obvious in sport, where the quality of performance is likely to depend largely upon the ability of the players to create adequate friction between feet and playing surface and between hands and racket or other implement. In such cases, adequate friction is maintained by using materials that have appropriate coefficients of friction with the playing surface and with the hands. For example, in volleyball, basketball, squash and badminton, the soles of shoes are normally made of materials that will provide adequate friction with the playing surface. It follows that for most indoor sports, the playing surfaces should not be highly polished, since this will reduce the coefficient of friction and increase the possibility of slipping. However, too much friction is likely to impair performance and result in injury, especially in sports that require rapid changes in speed or direction. Ideally, the sole of the shoe should turn as the player turns, but excessive friction may prevent the shoe turning and result in a twisting injury to the ankle or knee. This is also a potential problem in sports played on grass pitches, where the players use studded boots. In these situations, the horizontal forces produced between boots and playing surface are largely shear forces on the studs rather than friction. However, if the studs are too long and sink fully into the pitch, the sole of the boot may not turn as the player turns, and this will increase the risk of injury.

There are many non-sporting situations in which it is important to ensure adequate friction in order to reduce the risk of injury. For example, an injured or aged person may rely heavily on walking sticks or crutches for support. It is very important that the sticks or crutches do no slip on the floor. Rubber has a high coefficient of friction with most materials and, consequently, rubber tips are usually fitted to the ends of the walking sticks and crutches to reduce the risk of slipping.

In some activities, skilful performance depends upon reducing friction between shoes and floor. For example, in ballroom dancing, good technique is largely dependent on the ability to slide and turn the feet on the floor with as little resistance as possible. Consequently, not only is the floor highly polished, but so are the soles of the dancer's shoes. Similarly, elite skiers wax the underside of their skis in order to reduce the amount of friction between the skis and the snow.

Whereas the development of adequate friction between the human body and the environment is essential for daily living, friction between the different body tissues inside the body must be reduced as much as possible in order to minimise the risk of injury or wear. The human body is composed of a number of different tissues that lie adjacent to each other. Even the slightest movement involves a certain amount of sliding of the various tissues on each other. Unless the adjacent surfaces are adequately lubricated, frictional forces will operate when sliding occurs. Whenever friction develops, a certain amount of heat is generated. Too much heat will injure or wear body tissues. In machines, parts that slide on each other are usually highly polished and friction is reduced even more by lubricating the sliding surfaces with oil or grease. Similar mechanisms exist within the human body. All the synovial joints of

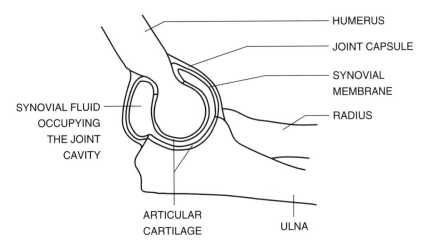

Figure 9.35 Vertical section through elbow joint.

the body are lined by synovial membrane, which produces synovial fluid (Figure 9.35). This is a transparent viscous fluid, resembling the white of an egg, that lubricates and nourishes the articular surfaces (articular cartilage) of the joints. The articular surfaces are normally extremely smooth so that in association with the synovial fluid $\mu_L \approx 0.01$ and $\mu_S \approx 0.003$ (Serway and Jewett 2004). Consequently, the amount of friction developed in healthy synovial joints during normal movements is usually extremely small. Joint injury, disease and degeneration due to aging may reduce the quality of lubrication in synovial joints, resulting in excessive wear and, eventually, painful joints.

Adequate lubrication in synovial joints is particularly important in the major weight-bearing joints of the body, i.e. the hips, knees and ankles. The articular surfaces of these joints are under considerable pressure, even when the person is just standing upright, and any kind of propulsive movement of the legs will increase the pressure even more. The greater the pressure, the greater the friction between the articular surfaces. Therefore, it is extremely important that any kind of injury to these joints is treated promptly in order to restore normal lubrication as soon as possible. Wearing of articular surfaces is similar to the wearing of brake pads in the wheels of a motor vehicle. When braking occurs, an enormous amount of friction and, therefore, heat is generated between brake pad and wheel. Consequently, the brake pads eventually wear out and have to be replaced. In a healthy synovial joint, any wear is usually repaired by normal metabolic processes. However, progressive joint degeneration will occur when the rate of wear outpaces the rate of repair.

As well as in synovial joints, synovial membranes are located in other parts of the body where different tissues slide over each other. For example, most of the tendons of muscles that cross the wrists and ankles pass over, through or around bones and ligaments. To reduce friction between the tendons and adjacent structures, the tendons are enclosed within synovial sheaths (Figure 9.36). A synovial sheath consists of a closed flattened sac composed of synovial membrane, which contains a capillary film of synovial fluid. The synovial sheath forms a protective sleeve around the tendon. Unaccustomed overuse of the associated muscles is likely to result in tenosynovitis, i.e. a condition characterised by inflammation of the synovial sheaths.

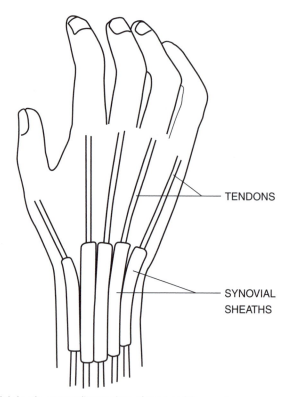

Figure 9.36 Synovial sheaths surrounding tendons of wrist and finger extensors.

Squash and badminton players are particularly prone to this type of injury to the flexor and extensor tendons of the wrist.

A synovial bursa is a closed sac composed of synovial membrane containing synovial fluid that is interposed between different tissues that slide on each other. Bursae are located most frequently between the deeper layers of the skin and underlying bone (subcutaneous bursa), between tendons and bone (subtendinous bursa) and between individual muscles (submuscular bursa). For example, there is a large subcutaneous bursa between the skin and the patella (the prepatellar bursa) (Figure 9.37). Unaccustomed pressure on a bursa is likely to result in bursitis, i.e. a condition characterised by inflammation of the bursa.

A blister on the skin is a form of bursa that occurs in response to unaccustomed friction. A blister is a short-term safety mechanism that protects the deep layers of the skin from sustained or excessive friction resulting from relatively infrequent experiences, such as stiff shoes rubbing against the feet or the handle of a screwdriver rubbing against the hand. The body responds to this friction by producing a layer of fluid between the superficial and deep layers of the skin, thereby protecting the deep layers from further damage. The body will adapt to a sustained increase in friction on a particular part of the skin by thickening the superficial layer of the skin. For example, in comparison with other parts of the body, the skin on the heel and ball of each foot is subjected to fairly sustained pressure or frictional force. Not surprisingly, the skin on the heel and ball of each foot is usually

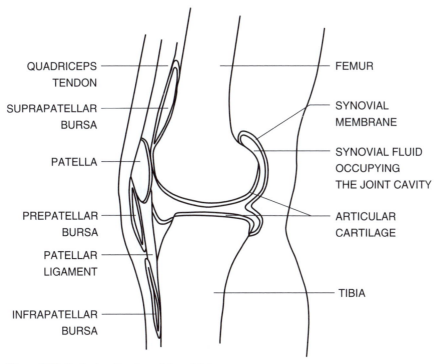

QUADRICEPS TENDON

SUPRAPATELLAR BURSA

PATELLA

PREPATELLAR BURSA

PATELLAR LIGAMENT

INFRAPATELLAR BURSA

FEMUR

SYNOVIAL MEMBRANE

SYNOVIAL FLUID OCCUPYING THE JOINT CAVITY

ARTICULAR CARTILAGE

TIBIA

Figure 9.37 Vertical section through knee joint.

much thicker than in other places, except, perhaps, for the palmar surfaces of the hands of manual workers.

> Whereas the development of adequate friction between the human body and the environment is essential for daily living, friction between the different body tissues inside the body must be reduced as much as possible, to minimise the risk of injury or wear.

FORCE VECTORS AND RESULTANT FORCE

When standing upright, three forces act on the human body, body weight **W**, the ground reaction force **L** on the left foot and the ground reaction force **R** on the right foot (Figure 9.38). The point of application of W in Figure 9.38 and subsequent figures is the centre of gravity of the body. In Figure 9.38, the resultant ground reaction force (resultant of L and R) is equal in magnitude but opposite in direction to W, i.e. the resultant force acting on the body is zero. In Figure 9.39a the force F_1 is the resultant ground reaction force (resultant of the ground reaction forces acting on the left and right feet). An additional load on the body, such as the object in Figure 9.39b, simply increases the total downward load on the body and results in a corresponding increase in the magnitude of the ground reaction force.

253

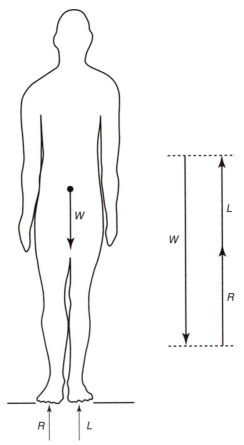

Figure 9.38 Forces acting on the human body when standing upright and corresponding vector chain: *W*, body weight; *L*, force on left foot; *R*, force on right foot.

Figure 9.40 shows the forces acting on a man sitting on a chair. In this case, there are three upward forces counteracting body weight, the force exerted by the chair and the ground reaction forces on the feet. In the examples in Figures 9.38 to 9.40, all of the forces are vertical forces and, consequently, the upward and downward force vectors are presented in parallel in the vector diagrams.

Figure 9.41 shows a sprinter in the set position of a sprint start, i.e. when the body is at rest and the resultant force acting on the body is zero. In this situation, five forces are acting on the body: body weight *W*, the forces *L* and *R* at the hands, and the forces *P* and *Q* at the feet. The force vectors are shown in Figure 9.41a and the corresponding vector chain is shown in Figure 9.41b. Since the resultant force acting on the sprinter is zero, the vector chain is a closed loop, i.e. irrespective of the order of the force vectors in the chain, the end of the last vector coincides with the start of the first vector. Figure 9.42a shows the sprinter just after the start as he accelerates forward under the action of the resultant force acting on his body, i.e. the resultant of his body weight and the forces acting on his feet. Figure 9.42b shows the corresponding vector chain and resultant force.

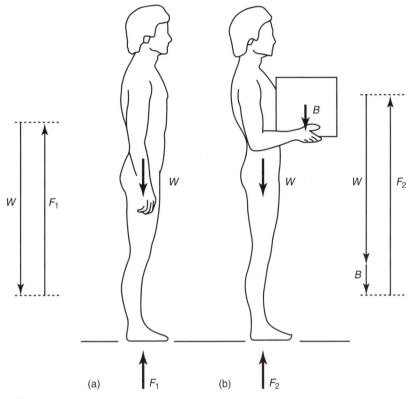

Figure 9.39 Forces acting on the human body. (a) Standing upright. (b) Standing upright with additional load, with corresponding vector chains. W, body weight; B, weight of object; F_1, F_2, ground reaction forces.

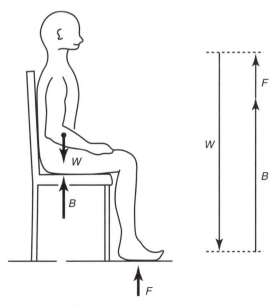

Figure 9.40 Forces acting on a man sitting on a chair and corresponding vector chain: W, body weight; F, combined upward force exerted on both feet; B, upward force exerted by the chair.

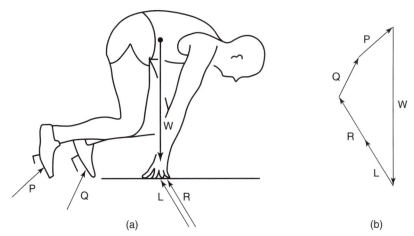

Figure 9.41 (a) Forces acting on sprinter in set position of sprint start. (b) Corresponding vector chain. W, body weight = 70 kgf; P, force on right foot = 21.5 kgf at 40.6° to the horizontal; Q, force on left foot = 18.5 kgf at 63.1° to the horizontal; L, force on left hand = 23.3 kgf at 58.0° to the horizontal; R, force on right hand = 23.3 kgf at 58.0° to the horizontal; scale, 1 cm = 10 kgf.

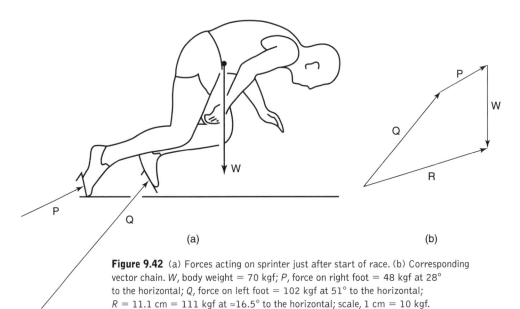

Figure 9.42 (a) Forces acting on sprinter just after start of race. (b) Corresponding vector chain. W, body weight = 70 kgf; P, force on right foot = 48 kgf at 28° to the horizontal; Q, force on left foot = 102 kgf at 51° to the horizontal; R = 11.1 cm = 111 kgf at ≈16.5° to the horizontal; scale, 1 cm = 10 kgf.

Trigonometry of a right-angled triangle

Whereas the vector chain and parallelogram of vectors methods of determining the resultant of a number of component vectors are very useful, it is often more practical to use trigonometry, especially when there is a large number of vectors. Trigonometry is the branch of mathematics that deals with the relationships between the lengths of the sides and the sizes of the angles in a triangle. Figure 9.43 shows a right-angled triangle in which one angle (between sides a and b) is 90°. The angles between sides a and c, and sides b and c, are α and θ, respectively.

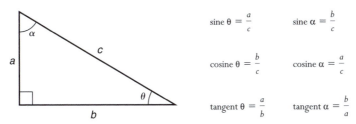

$$\text{sine } \theta = \frac{a}{c} \qquad \text{sine } \alpha = \frac{b}{c}$$

$$\text{cosine } \theta = \frac{b}{c} \qquad \text{cosine } \alpha = \frac{a}{c}$$

$$\text{tangent } \theta = \frac{a}{b} \qquad \text{tangent } \alpha = \frac{b}{a}$$

Figure 9.43 Definition of sine, cosine and tangent in a right-angled triangle.

In a right-angled triangle, the two angles less than 90° (α and θ in Figure 9.43) can be specified by the ratio between the lengths of any two sides of the triangle. The three most common ratios are sine, cosine and tangent, and they are defined in relation to the particular angle under consideration. For example, in relation to angle θ in Figure 9.43, side a is referred to as the opposite side, side b is referred to as the adjacent side, and side c is the hypotenuse, the side of the triangle opposite the right angle.

The sine of θ is defined as the ratio of the opposite side to the hypotenuse, i.e.

$$\text{sine } \theta = \frac{\text{opposite side}}{\text{hypotenuse}} = \frac{a}{c}.$$

The cosine of θ is defined as the ratio of the adjacent side to the hypotenuse, i.e.

$$\text{cosine } \theta = \frac{\text{adjacent side}}{\text{hypotenuse}} = \frac{b}{c}.$$

The tangent of θ is defined as the ratio of the opposite side to the adjacent side, i.e.

$$\text{tangent } \theta = \frac{\text{opposite side}}{\text{adjacent side}} = \frac{a}{b}.$$

Most electronic calculators provide a range of trigonometric ratios, including sine (sin), cosine (cos) and tangent (tan). Alternatively, tables of sine, cosine and tangent (for angles between 0° and 90°) can be obtained in publications such as Castle (1969). The lengths of sides and sizes of angles in right-angled triangles can be calculated using sine, cosine and tangent functions, provided that two sides or one side and one other angle are known. With reference to Figure 9.43, for example, if $c = 10$ cm and $\theta = 30°$, the lengths of sides a and b and the size of angle α can be determined as follows:

Calculation of the length of side a

$$\frac{a}{c} = \sin \theta,$$

$$a = c \sin \theta \text{ (i.e. c multiplied by sin } \theta),$$

$$a = c \sin 30°.$$

From sine tables, $\sin 30° = 0.5$ (i.e., the ratio of the length of side a to the length of side c is 0.5). Since $c = 10$ cm and $\sin 30° = 0.5$, it follows that

$a = 10$ cm $\times 0.5$

$a = 5$ cm.

Calculation of the length of side b

$\dfrac{b}{c} = \cos θ,$

$b = c \cos θ$ (i.e. c multiplied by $\cos θ$),

$b = c \cos 30°.$

From cosine tables, $\cos 30° = 0.866$ (i.e., the ratio of the length of side b to the length of side c is 0.866). Since $c = 10$ cm and $\cos 30° = 0.866$, it follows that

$b = 10$ cm $\times 0.866$

$b = 8.66$ cm.

Calculation of angle α

Angle α can be determined in a number of ways:

1. The sum of the three angles in any triangle (with or without a right angle) is 180°. As the sum of $θ$ and the right angle is 120°, it follows that $\alpha = 180° - 120° = 60°$.
2. The lengths of all three sides of the triangle are known: $a = 5$ cm, $b = 8.66$ cm and $c = 10$ cm. Consequently, α can be determined by calculating the sine, cosine or tangent of the angle:

$\sin \alpha = \dfrac{b}{c} = \dfrac{8.66 \text{ cm}}{10 \text{ cm}} = 0.866,$

$\alpha = 60°.$

$\cos \alpha = \dfrac{a}{c} = \dfrac{5 \text{ cm}}{10 \text{ cm}} = 0.5,$

$\alpha = 60°.$

$\tan \alpha = \dfrac{b}{a} = \dfrac{8.66 \text{ cm}}{5 \text{ cm}} = 1.732,$

$\alpha = 60°.$

Pythagoras' theorem

Pythagoras, a Greek mathematician (c. 570–495 BC), showed that in a right-angled triangle the square of the hypotenuse is equal to the sum of the squares of the other two sides. Therefore, with respect to Figure 9.43,

$$c^2 = a^2 + b^2,$$

$$c = \sqrt{(a^2 + b^2)}.$$

This can be demonstrated with the data from the above example, where $a = 5$ cm, $b = 8.66$ cm and $c = 10$ cm: $a^2 = 25$, $b^2 = 75$ and $c^2 = 100$.

Resolution of a vector into component vectors

Just as the resultant of any number of component vectors can be determined, any single vector can be replaced by any number of component vectors that have the same effect as the single vector. The process of replacing a vector by two or more component vectors is referred to as the resolution of a vector. In analysing human movement, displacement, velocity and force vectors are frequently resolved into vertical and horizontal components using trigonometry. The example of the sprinter in Figure 9.42 will be used to illustrate how the resolution of forces by trigonometry is used to determine the resultant force acting on the sprinter. There are three steps in the process.

1. Resolve all of the forces into their vertical and horizontal components

Figure 9.44a shows the forces acting on the sprinter: body weight W, the force P on the right foot and the force Q on the left foot. In Figure 9.44b, P and Q have been replaced by their vertical (P_V and Q_V) and horizontal (P_H and Q_H) components. Figure 9.45 shows the calculation of P_V and P_H. Figure 9.46 shows the calculation of Q_V and Q_H.

2. Calculate the vertical component R_V and horizontal component R_H of the resultant force R acting on the sprinter

$$R_V = P_V + Q_V - W,$$

$$R_V = 22.5 \text{ kgf} + 79.3 \text{ kgf} - 70 \text{ kgf} = 31.8 \text{ kgf}.$$

$$R_H = P_H + Q_H,$$

$$R_H = 42.4 \text{ kgf} + 64.2 \text{ kgf} = 106.6 \text{ kgf}.$$

3. Calculate R and the angle θ of R with respect to the horizontal

R, R_V and R_H are shown in Figure 9.47. From Pythagoras' theorem,

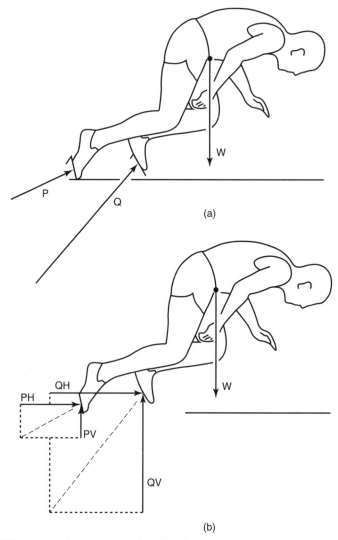

Figure 9.44 (a) The forces acting on a sprinter just after the start of a race and (b) the vertical and horizontal components of the forces. $W = 70$ kgf; $P = 48$ kgf at $28°$ to the horizontal; $Q = 102$ kgf at $51°$ to the horizontal.

$$R^2 = R_V^2 + R_{H}^2,$$
$$R^2 = 12\ 374.8,$$
$$R\ = 111.2\ \text{kgf},$$

$$\tan \theta = \frac{R_V}{R_H} = 0.2983,$$

$$\theta = 16.6°.$$

As expected, R and θ are the same as in the vector chain solution in Figure 9.42.

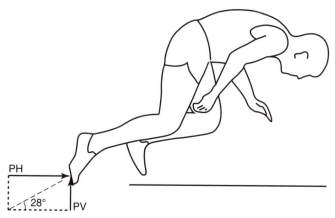

Figure 9.45 Calculation of the vertical and horizontal components of the force acting on the right foot of a sprinter just after the start of a race:

P_V = vertical component of P

P_H = horizontal component of P

$P_V/P = \sin 28°$

$P_V = P \times \sin 28° = 48$ kgf $\times$ 0.4695 = 22.5 kgf

$P_H/P = \cos 28°$

$P_H = P \times \cos 28° = 48$ kgf $\times$ 0.8829 = 42.4 kgf.

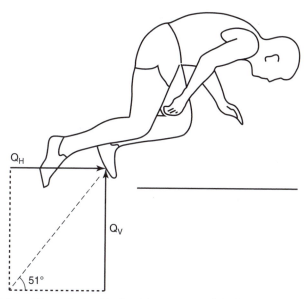

Figure 9.46 Calculation of the vertical and horizontal components of the force acting on the left foot of a sprinter just after the start of a race:

Q_V = vertical component of Q

Q_H = horizontal component of Q

$Q_V/Q = \sin 51°$

$Q_V = Q \times \sin 51° = 102$ kgf $\times$ 0.7771 = 79.3 kgf

$Q_H/Q = \cos 51°$

$Q_H = Q \times \cos 51° = 102$ kgf $\times$ 0.6293 = 64.2 kgf.

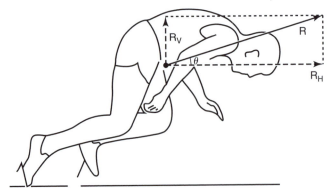

Figure 9.47 Resultant force acting on a sprinter just after the start of a race: R = resultant force; R_V = vertical component of R; R_H = horizontal component of R; R and θ are calculated in the text.

> Any single vector can be replaced by any number of component vectors that have the same effect as the single vector. The process of replacing a vector by two or more component vectors is referred to as the resolution of a vector.

CYCLE LENGTH, CYCLE RATE AND SPEED OF MOVEMENT IN HUMAN LOCOMOTION

Human locomotion refers to all forms of self-propelled transportation of the human body with or without the use of equipment. Human locomotion occurs mainly on land, such as walking, running and cycling, and in water, such as swimming, canoeing and rowing. All forms of human locomotion involve cycles of movement of the body in which each cycle of movement moves the body a certain distance. The distance achieved in each cycle of movement, referred to as the cycle length, and the number of cycles per unit of time, referred to as the cycle rate, determine the speed of movement. For example, when cycle length is measured in m/cycle and cycle rate in Hz, speed is in m/s, i.e.

speed (m/s) = cycle length (m/cycle) × cycle rate (Hz).

Stride parameters and stride cycle in walking and running

In walking and running, cycle length and cycle rate are usually referred to as stride length and stride rate, respectively. Each cycle of movement from heel-strike to heel-strike of the same foot moves the body forward one stride (Figure 9.48a). One stride consists of two consecutive steps. The stride cycle refers to the movement of the body during a single stride. In walking, the stride cycle of the right leg begins with a right heel-strike (contact of the ground with the right heel or, more often, the posteriolateral part of the heel) which initiates the stance phase of the right leg, i.e. the period of the stride cycle when the right leg is in contact with the ground. The first part of the stance phase is a period of double support, i.e.

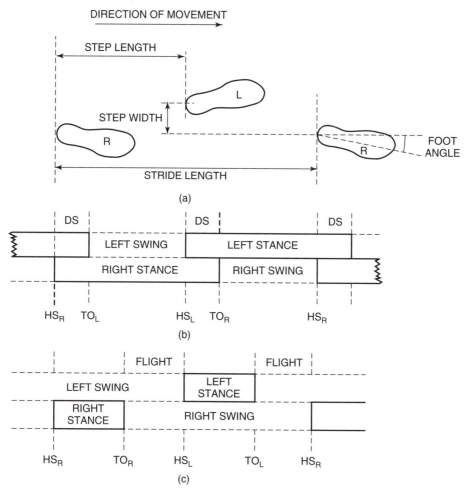

Figure 9.48 (a) Stride parameters. (b,c) Stride cycle in (b) walking and (c) running: HS_L = heel-strike left; HS_R = heel-strike right; TO_L = toe-off left; TO_R = toe-off right.

when both feet are in contact with the ground (Figure 9.48b). This period of double support lasts for approximately 10% of the cycle, at which point the left foot leaves the ground (referred to as toe-off) and the left leg swings forward. During the swing phase of the left leg, the right leg supports the body on its own; this period lasts for approximately 40% of the cycle and is referred to as the single-support phase of the right leg. At the end of the swing phase of the left leg, the left foot contacts the ground and another period of double support ensues. At approximately 60% into the cycle, the right foot leaves the ground to begin its swing phase, while the left leg experiences a period of single support. The cycle is completed by the heel-strike of the right foot. As the speed of walking increases, the duration of the periods of double support decreases until there is a sudden change from walking to running. The change is characterised by the absence of periods of double support and the presence of flight phases (when both feet are off the ground) between the single-support phases of each leg (Figure 9.48b,c).

Effect of speed of walking and running on stride length and stride rate

Figure 9.49 shows the relationships between stride length (SL), stride rate (SR) and speed (S) of walking and running for a male student (Hay 2002). The SL–S and SR–S graphs are based on data obtained from five walking trials and ten running trials. In the walking trials, the student was requested to walk at a constant speed in each trial, but at a slightly faster pace in each successive trial. All trials were recorded on video at 60 Hz and the stride length and rate in each trial (during a period of constant speed) were obtained by frame-by-frame playback using appropriate distance reference markers. A similar procedure was used in the running trials. Stride length and rate data were obtained for five speeds of walking over the range 1.5 m/s to 2.6 m/s (moderate to fast pace) and ten speeds of running over the range 2.1 m/s to 8.2 m/s (very slow to fast pace). The SL–S and SR–S graphs are the lines of best fit, reflecting the smooth changes in stride length and rate that normally occur with increasing speed of walking and running for a given individual. Most people will naturally change from walking to running at about 2.3 m/s because it is more economic in terms of energy expenditure to do so (Alexander 1992). This change in form of locomotion is reflected in the distinct SL–S and SR–S graphs for walking to running. However, the shapes of the SL–S and SR–S graphs for walking and running are very similar. In particular, the SL–S graphs are concave downward and the SR–S graphs are concave upward. In addition, stride length makes the greatest contribution to increase in speed in the lower half of the speed range and stride rate

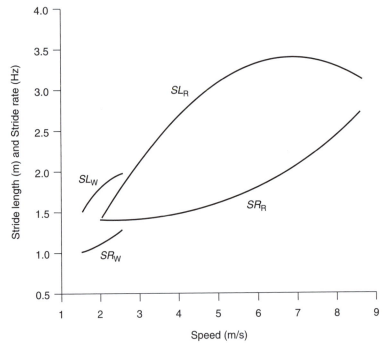

Figure 9.49 Stride length–speed and stride rate–speed graphs for a male student, walking and running: SL_W = stride length walking; SR_W = stride rate walking; SL_R = stride length running, SR_R = stride rate running.

makes the greatest contribution to increase in speed in the upper half of the speed range. Hay (2002) demonstrated that these relationships hold true for most forms of human locomotion, including walking, running, hopping, wheelchair racing, swimming, canoeing and kayaking.

Optimal stride length

Running economy, i.e. the rate of energy expenditure (oxygen uptake) for a given submaximal running speed, depends upon a number of biomechanical and physiological variables, but the interaction between the variables appears to be very complex (Williams and Cavanagh 1987; Kyrolainen *et al.* 2001). In any given situation, the stride length–stride rate combination adopted by a runner will depend upon the runner's personal anthropometric, anatomical and physiological characteristics and the environmental demands on the runner. For example, if the runner develops an injury, he is likely to alter his stride length and rate in order to minimise pain. Similarly, if the terrain is uneven or slippery, it is likely that the runner will adopt a combination of stride length and rate that reduces the risk of falling. However, when there are no particular constraints, most runners naturally tend to adopt a stride length–stride rate combination that is optimal in terms of energy expenditure (Cavanagh and Williams 1982; Heinert *et al.* 1988). Figure 9.50 shows the relationship between oxygen uptake (energy expenditure) and stride length for a male distance runner running on a treadmill at 3.83 m/s (7 min/mile) at different stride length–stride rate combinations, including the runner's preferred combination. The graph indicates that the most economical stride length would be approximately 2.53 m, corresponding to a stride rate of 1.51 Hz. This was very close to the runner's preferred combination. Running at stride lengths longer or shorter than the optimal resulted in an increase in energy expenditure.

A number of researchers have investigated the relationship between stride length, height and leg length (Cavanagh *et al.* 1977; Elliot and Blanksby 1979). Figure 9.51 shows the average stride length and average stride rate for ten male and ten female well-practised recreational runners running at 2.5 m/s, 3.5 m/s, 4.5 m/s and 5.5 m/s (Elliot and Blanksby 1979). The average heights and leg lengths of the men and women were 178.1 cm and 89.5 cm, 166.0 cm

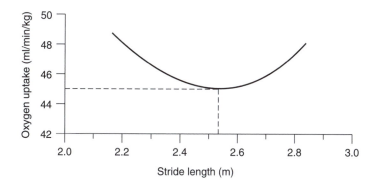

Figure 9.50 Relationship between stride length and oxygen uptake (energy expenditure) for a distance runner running on a treadmill at 3.83 m/s at different stride length–stride rate combinations: the most economical combination was a stride length of 2.53 m and a stride rate of 1.51 Hz.

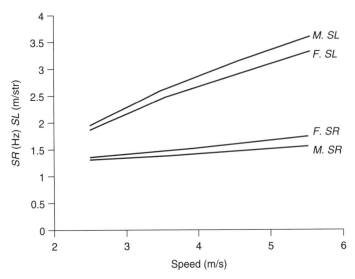

Figure 9.51 Average stride length and average stride rate for groups of male and female recreational runners running at 2.5 m/s, 3.5 m/s, 4.5 m/s and 5.5 m/s on a treadmill.

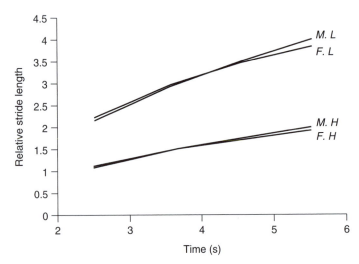

Figure 9.52 Relative stride length for groups of male (M) and female (F) recreational runners running at 2.5 m/s, 3.5 m/s, 4.5 m/s and 5.5 m/s on a treadmill: H, stride length divided by height; L, stride length divided by leg length.

and 83.1 cm, respectively. At each speed, the women had a shorter average stride length and a higher average stride rate than the men. However, the average relative stride lengths (stride length divided by height and stride length divided by leg length) at each speed were very similar for both groups (Figure 9.52). This may reflect a subconscious optimisation of personal and environmental constraints, common to men and women, that results in an optimum stride length–stride rate combination for constant-speed running, especially in well-practised runners.

In Practical Worksheet 2, students use a treadmill to investigate the effect of increase in running speed on stride rate, stride length and relative stride length.

Trajectory of the centre of gravity in walking

During walking, the movement of the body as a whole is reflected in the movement of the whole body centre of gravity which tends to follow a fairly smooth up-and-down and side-to-side trajectory. When viewed from the side, as shown in the upper part of Figure 9.53, the centre of gravity moves up and down twice during each stride with the low points of the trajectory occurring close to the mid-points of the double-support phases and the high points of the trajectory occurring close to the mid-points of the single-support phases. When viewed from overhead, as shown in the lower part of Figure 9.53, the trajectory of the centre of gravity follows the support phases, moving right during the period from the mid-point of single support of the left leg to the mid-point of single support of the right leg and moving left during the period from the mid-point of single support of the right leg to the mid-point of single support of the left leg. The vertical excursion (up–down range of motion) of the centre of gravity during walking increases with increasing walking speed and ranges from approximately 2.7 cm at 0.7 m/s (slow walk: 1.57 mph) to approximately 4.8 cm at 1.6 m/s (moderate walking speed: 3.58 mph) (Dagg 1977; Orendurff et al. 2004). In contrast, the mediolateral excursion (side-to-side range of motion) of the centre of gravity during walking

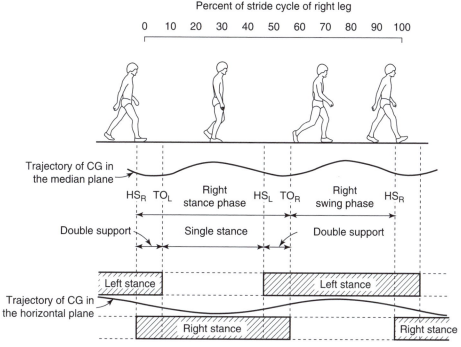

Figure 9.53 Stride cycle in walking: CG, centre of gravity; HS_L, heel-strike left; HS_R, heel-strike right; TO_L, toe-off left; TO_R, toe-off right.

decreases with increasing walking speed and ranges from approximately 7.0 cm at 0.7 m/s to approximately 3.8 cm at 1.6 m/s.

GROUND REACTION FORCE IN WALKING

The trajectory of the centre of gravity reflects the magnitude and direction of the ground reaction force. When standing upright, the ground reaction force is equal in magnitude but opposite in direction to body weight, i.e. the resultant force acting on the body is zero (Figure 9.54a). To start walking or running (or move horizontally by any other type of movement, such as jumping or hopping) the body must push or pull against something to provide the necessary resultant force to move it in the required direction. In walking and running, forward movement is achieved by pushing obliquely downward and backward against the ground. Provided that the foot does not slip, the leg thrust results in a ground reaction force directed obliquely upward and forward, which moves the body forward while maintaining an upright posture (Figure 9.54b). To understand the effect of the ground reaction force it is useful to resolve it into its vertical and horizontal components (Figure 9.54c). The vertical component counteracts body weight, i.e. the resultant vertical force acting on the body remains close to zero, and the horizontal component (resultant horizontal force) results in forward movement.

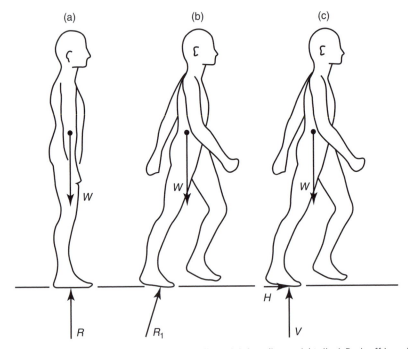

Figure 9.54 Ground reaction force in standing and walking. (a) Standing upright. (b,c) Push-off in walking. W, body weight; R, ground reaction force while standing; R_1, ground reaction during push-off; H, horizontal component of R_1; V, vertical component of R_1.

Components of the ground reaction force

Figure 9.55 shows the ground reaction force (F) and the anteroposterior (F_X), vertical (F_Y) and mediolateral (F_Z) components of the ground reaction force at one point in the single-support phase of the right leg. When walking straight forward, the mediolateral component is normally very small, resulting in little side-to-side movement of the body. Figure 9.56 shows the F_X, F_Y and F_Z components of the ground reaction force (force–time curves) exerted on each leg during one stride of the right leg (one heel-strike of the right foot to the next heel-strike of the right foot). The movement of the centre of gravity during walking (as in any movement) is determined by the resultant force acting on the body. During a period of single support, the resultant force acting on the body is determined by the body weight and the ground reaction force exerted on the grounded foot. During a period of double support, the resultant force acting on the body is determined by body weight and the ground reaction forces exerted on both feet.

The vertical component of the ground reaction force exerted on each leg is characteristically dominated by two smooth peaks, with the rise and fall of each peak taking up about half of the stance phase (Figure 9.56). The rise and fall of the first peak roughly corresponds to the period from heel-strike to heel-off and the rise and fall of the second peak roughly corresponds to the period from heel-off to toe-off.

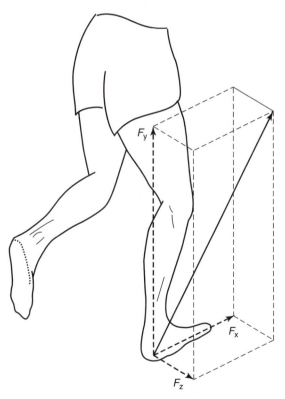

Figure 9.55 Anteroposterior (F_X), vertical (F_Y) and mediolateral (F_Z) components of ground reaction force F.

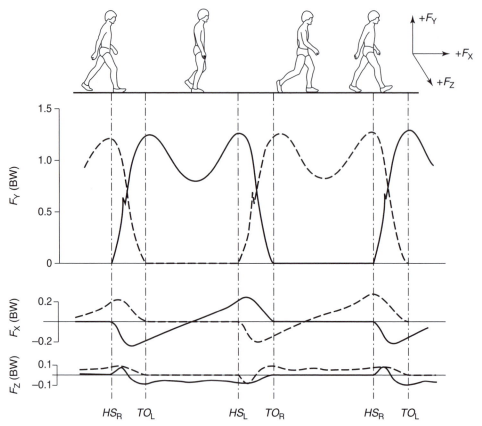

Figure 9.56 Anteroposterior (F_X), vertical (F_Y) and mediolateral (F_Z) components of the ground reaction force during the walking stride cycle of the right leg: BW, body weight; HS_L, heel-strike left; HS_R, heel-strike right; TO_L, toe-off left; TO_R, toe-off right; solid line, right leg; dotted line, left leg.

Like the vertical component, the anteroposterior component is normally characteristically dominated by two smooth peaks, whose rise and fall correspond to the rise and fall of the two peaks of the vertical component. The resultant anteroposterior component of force acts backward from the mid-point of double support to heel-off (a braking force), indicating deceleration of the centre of gravity, i.e. the forward speed of the body is decreased. In the heel-off to toe-off period, the resultant anteroposterior component acts forward, indicating forward acceleration of the centre of gravity, i.e. the forward speed of the body is increased.

The resultant mediolateral component of force acts medially during single stance and changes direction during double support, i.e. from medial on right foot to medial on left foot during the left heel-strike to right toe-off period (Figure 9.56).

In addition to the characteristic smooth phases of the vertical, anteroposterior and mediolateral components of the ground reaction force, all three components are often characterised by single or multiple transient spikes soon after heel-strike, which reflect the impact of the heel with the ground (see F_Y in Figure 9.56). Shock absorbing footwear will reduce or eliminate these transient spikes (Czerniecki 1988).

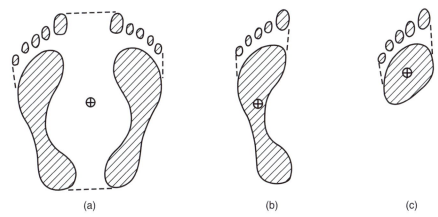

(a)   (b)   (c)

Figure 9.57 Location of centre of pressure. (a) Standing upright on both feet. (b) Standing on the left foot. (c) Standing on the left foot with the heel off the floor.

Centre of pressure

The ground reaction force is distributed across the whole of the area of contact between the feet and the floor. Figure 9.57a shows the contact area when standing barefoot on both feet; the contact area is much smaller than the area of the base of support. Figure 9.57b shows the contact area when standing on one foot and Figure 9.57c shows the contact area when standing on one foot with the heel raised off the ground. In Figures 9.57b and c, the contact area is very similar to the base of support. Whereas the ground reaction force is distributed across the whole of the contact area, the effect of the ground reaction force on the movement of the body is as if the ground reaction force acts at a single point, which is referred to as the centre of pressure (just as the whole weight of the body appears to act at the whole body centre of gravity, in terms of the effect of body weight on the movement of the body). With respect to Figure 9.57, the centre of pressure is at the point of intersection of the line of action of body weight with the base of support.

Path of centre of pressure in walking

As indicated in Figure 9.56, the magnitude and direction of the ground reaction force change continuously during walking. Figure 9.58a shows the change in the resultant (F_{XY}) of the anteroposterior (F_X) and vertical (F_Y) components. Because of the dominance of F_Y, the change in F_{XY} from heel-strike to toe-off reflects the double-peaked F_Y component in Figure 9.56. F_Y always acts upward so that the progressive change in direction of F_{XY} from upward and backward at heel-strike, through more or less vertical at heel-off, to upward and forward at toe-off is due to the change in the direction of F_X from backward (heel-strike to heel-off) to forward (heel-off to toe-off) (Figure 9.56).

During the stance phase, the foot essentially rolls forward from heel to toe such that the contact area between foot and ground and, consequently, the centre of pressure of the ground reaction force on each foot, change continuously, as shown in Figures 9.58b to f.

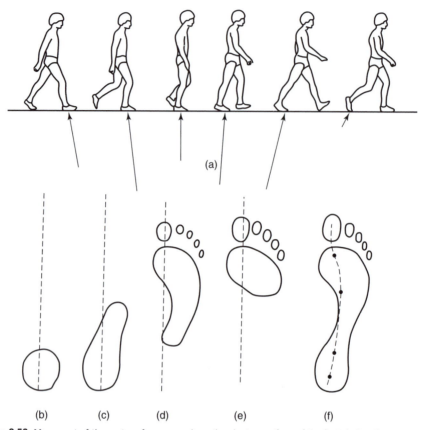

Figure 9.58 Movement of the centre of pressure along the plantar surface of the foot during the stance phase of the right foot. (a) Change in the magnitude and direction of F_{xy}. (b–e) Plantar contact area (b) just after HS_{R}; (c) at the middle of double support; (d) at HO_{R}; (e) at HS_{L}. (f) Path of the centre of pressure and location of the centre of pressure at the points corresponding to (b), (c), (d) and (e), respectively.

> The effect of the ground reaction force on the movement of the body is as if the ground reaction force acts at a single point, which is referred to as the centre of pressure.

In Practical Worksheet 3, students use a force platform to record and then analyse the antero-posterior and vertical components of the ground reaction force acting on a subject while walking.

GROUND REACTION FORCE IN RUNNING

The stride rate–speed and stride length–speed graphs in Figure 9.49 are based on the performance of a single male student as reported by Hay (2002). However, the relationships between stride rate, stride length and speed shown in the graphs are typical of men and women at all levels of performance (Hay 2002). Figure 9.49 shows that stride rate progressively increases throughout the upper half of the speed range. In contrast, stride length increases slightly and then decreases by about the same amount as maximum speed is achieved. Consequently, stride rate and, therefore, step rate, is largely responsible for increase in speed in the upper half of the speed range. The increase in step rate (steps per second) depends upon a decrease in step time (seconds per step), i.e. the shorter the step time, the higher the step rate. The step time for each leg is the sum of contact time (the time that the foot is in contact with the ground) and flight time (the time from toe-off of the foot to touch-down of the other foot). The decrease in step time (and increase in step rate) that occurs with increase in sprinting speed in the upper half of the speed range is due to a progressive decrease in contact time with little or no change in flight time (Weyand et al. 2000). To reduce contact time and maintain the same flight time, the average magnitude of the resultant upward force acting on the sprinter during contact time must increase. Consequently, the average magnitude of the vertical component F_Y of the ground reaction force must increase. In general, the faster the sprinting speed, the greater the average magnitude of F_Y. This is reflected in Figure 9.59, which shows typical ground reaction force–time graphs (vertical component) for physically active adults walking at 1.0 m/s and running at 3.0 m/s, 6.0 m/s and 9.0 m/s; the shorter the contact time, the higher the peak and average F_Y (Weyand et al. 2000). The world's fastest 100 m male sprinters have contact times of approximately 80 ms during the peak velocity phase (11.6 m/s to

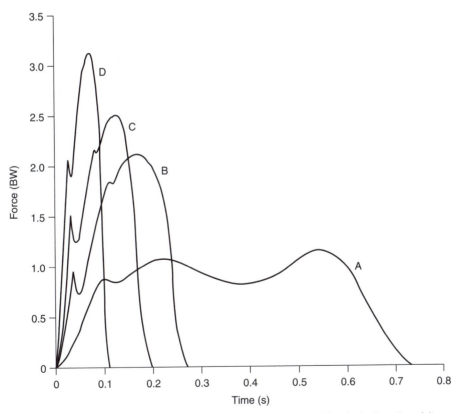

Figure 9.59 Typical ground reaction force–time graphs (vertical component) for physically active adults walking at 1.0 m/s (A) and running at 3.0 m/s (B), 6.0 m/s (C) and 9.0 m/s (D): BW, body weight.

11.8 m/s) (Moravec *et al.* 1988) and produce ground reaction forces (vertical component) in excess of three times body weight on one leg (Mero and Komi, 1986). Consequently, world-class sprinting requires great strength of the leg extensor muscles.

Approximately 80% of runners and joggers are rear-foot strikers, i.e. they contact the ground initially with the posteriolateral aspect of the shoe (Kerr *et al.* 1983). The remaining 20% of runners and joggers contact the ground initially with either the middle of the foot (mid-foot strikers) or the front part of the foot (forefoot strikers). Figure 9.60 shows the anteroposterior, vertical and mediolateral components of the ground reaction force acting on the right foot of a well-practised rear-foot striker while running at about 4.5 m/s. Contact time is 205 ms. The graphs are typical of well-practised middle-distance and long-distance rear-foot strikers over the middle-to-long-distance speed range (Cavanagh and Lafortune 1980). The anteroposterior component F_X is responsible for changes in forward velocity. The anteroposterior component exhibits two distinct phases, with each phase taking up about half of contact time. In the first phase (48% of contact time) F_X is negative with a single smooth peak of 0.41 body weight (BW) after 45 ms (22% of contact). Consequently, forward velocity decreases during this negative phase. In the second part of contact (52% of contact time), F_X is positive with a single smooth peak of 0.47 BW after 142 ms (69% of contact). Consequently, forward velocity increases during this positive phase. The negative phase is referred to as the absorption (braking) phase and the positive phase is referred to as the propulsion (accelera-tion) phase. In constant-speed running at 4.5 m/s, forward velocity decreases about 0.2 m/s in the absorption phase and increases about 0.2 m/s in the propulsion phase.

The vertical component F_Y is responsible for changes in vertical velocity. The downward vertical velocity of the body at foot-strike is reduced to zero during the absorption phase. In the propulsion phase, the upward velocity progressively increases. F_Y exhibits two peaks, with a first peak of 2.2 BW occurring after 32 ms (16% of contact time). A second peak, of 2.9 BW after 93 ms (45% of contact time), indicates maximum vertical compression of the leg (as vertical velocity is reversed) and corresponds closely with the end of the absorption phase. In constant-speed running at 4.5 m/s, the vertical velocity decreases about 1.6 m/s in the absorption phase and increases about 1.6 m/s in the propulsion phase. The change in vertical velocity of the body during the contact time is reflected in the vertical displacement of the centre of gravity (down during absorption, up during propulsion), as shown in the picture sequence in Figure 9.60.

The mediolateral component F_Z is responsible for changes in mediolateral velocity. The mediolateral component is very small (a maximum of 0.1 BW) relative to the anteroposterior and vertical components. It is negative for most of the contact time, indicating a small medi-ally directed force.

Active and passive loading

In most activities of everyday life, the magnitude and direction of the ground reaction force is determined by muscular activity under conscious control. In these circumstances, when the ground reaction force, or any other external load (apart from body weight), is completely controlled by conscious muscular activity, the load is called an active load. Because they are under conscious control, active loads are unlikely to be harmful under normal circumstances.

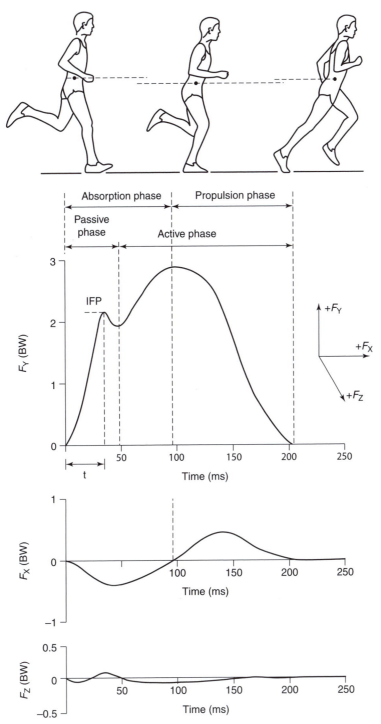

Figure 9.60 Anteroposterior (F_x), vertical (F_y) and mediolateral (F_z) components of the ground reaction force acting on the right foot of a well-practised rear-foot striker while running at about 4.5 m/s: BW, body weight; IFP, impact force peak, t, time to impact force peak.

In everyday situations, the muscles respond to changes in external loading to ensure that the body is not subjected to harmful loads.

However, it takes a finite time for muscles to respond fully (in terms of appropriate changes in the magnitude and direction of muscle forces) to changes in external loading; this time lag is referred to as muscle latency. Muscle latency varies between approximately 30 ms and 75 ms in adults (Nigg *et al.* 1984; Watt and Jones 1971). Consequently, muscles cannot fully respond to changes in external loading that occur within the latency period of the muscles. In these circumstances, the body is forced to respond passively (by passive deformation) to the external load; this type of load is a passive load. The body is unable to control passive loads and is vulnerable to injury from high passive loads.

The body is subjected to passive loading during the period of muscle latency following heel-strike in walking and running. Consequently, during the absorption phase, the ground reaction force is initially a passive load and then an active load (Figure 9.60). The period of muscle latency following heel-strike is referred to as the passive phase of ground contact and roughly corresponds to the period between heel-strike and foot-flat (when the fore-foot contacts the floor). During the remainder of ground contact, i.e. from foot-flat to toe-off, the ground reaction force is an active load and this period is referred to as the active phase of ground contact (Figure 9.60).

The passive phase of ground contact in walking and running is characterised by a rapid rise in the vertical component of the ground reaction force, resulting in a relatively sharp peak, referred to as the impact force peak, within the first 30–50 ms after impact (Figures 9.56 and 9.60). The force then declines slightly before rising again at the start of the active phase of ground contact.

The slope of the vertical component of the ground reaction force during the passive phase reflects the rate of loading (impact force peak divided by the time to impact force peak); the steeper the slope, the higher the rate of loading. The higher the rate of loading, the higher the strain on the system of materials subjected to the passive load, i.e. the support surface, the shoe (including insole and sock) and the human body, especially the ankle and foot. The higher the strain, the greater the risk of damage or injury. The rate of loading depends upon the stiffness of the system; the greater the stiffness, the higher the rate of loading. As described in Chapter 6, stiffness refers to the resistance of a material (or combination of materials) to deformation; the greater the resistance, the stiffer the material.

Muscles cannot fully respond to changes in external loading that occur within the latency period of the muscles. In these circumstances, the body responds passively and is vulnerable to injury from high passive loads.

Effect of shoes on rate of loading

Figure 9.61 shows the ground reaction force–time graphs (vertical component) for the same male subject running at approximately 4 m/s barefoot (Figure 9.61a) and in running shoes (Figure 9.61b). The duration of ground contact time is similar in both conditions, as is the

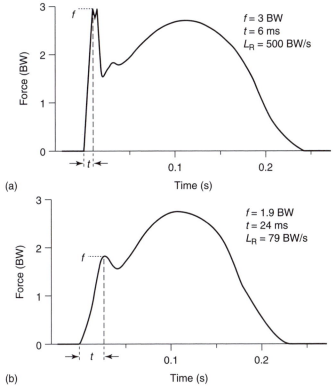

Figure 9.61 Ground reaction force–time curves (vertical component) for a male rear-foot striker running at approximately 4 m/s. (a) Barefoot. (b) In running shoes. BW, body weight; f, impact force peak; t, time to impact force peak L_R = rate of loading = f/t.

force–time curve in the active phase, but the force–time curve during the passive phase is different. The impact force peak in the barefoot condition is approximately 3 BW compared with approximately 1.9 BW with shoes. However, the most noticeable differences between the two conditions are the time to impact force peak and the rate of loading prior to impact force peak. The time to impact force peak when barefoot is approximately 6 ms compared with 24 ms when wearing shoes. The large difference in time to impact force peak is mainly responsible for the large difference in rate of loading; 500 BW/s (body weights per second) barefoot and 79 BW/s with shoes. The very high rate of loading in the barefoot condition may result in injury.

Figure 9.62 shows the ground reaction force–time graphs (vertical component) for another male subject running at 5 m/s in two types of running shoe, one with a hard (high-stiffness) sole and one with a soft (moderate-stiffness) sole. The hard-soled shoe results in a higher impact force peak and a higher rate of loading than the softer-soled shoe. Whereas soft-soled shoes reduce the rate of loading more than harder soled shoes, there is a limit to how soft a shoe can be if it is to be effective in reducing rate of loading to an acceptable level. If the shoe material is too soft it can bottom out quickly, such that rate of loading is largely determined by other parts of the system.

277

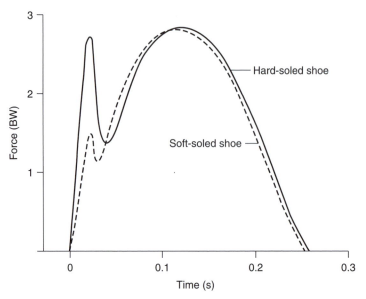

Figure 9.62 Ground reaction force–time curves (vertical component) for a male rear-foot striker running at 5 m/s in hard- and soft-soled shoes: BW, body weight.

Effect of leg and foot alignment on rate of loading

At foot-strike the alignment of the upper leg, lower leg and foot in relation to the line of action of the ground reaction force affects the leg's stiffness. The closer the line of action of the ground reaction force to the hip, knee and ankle joints, the stiffer the leg will tend to respond to foot-strike and, consequently, the higher the rate of loading. This is typical of a rear-foot striker, where the line of action of the ground reaction force passes close to the joint centres of the ankle and knee (Figure 9.63a).

When the knee is slightly flexed at foot-strike, the leg is more likely to respond like a spring, resulting in flexion of the hip, knee and ankle. This is typical of a fore-foot striker, where the line of action of the ground reaction force dorsiflexes the ankle and flexes the knee (Figure 9.63b). The stiffness of the spring depends considerably on the degree of activation of the muscles controlling the joints. Whereas muscle latency limits the speed with which a muscle can fully respond to a change in external loading, the muscles can still influence the rate of loading by setting the rotational stiffness of the joints prior to foot-strike. The greater the tension in the muscles, the greater the degree of rotational stiffness of the joints. A certain amount of rotational stiffness of the joints is necessary to prevent the spring from bottoming out too quickly. In general, the more the leg behaves like a spring at foot-strike, the lower the rate of loading. Striking the ground with the mid-foot or fore-foot is generally effective in preventing a high rate of loading following foot-strike, such that most mid-foot and fore-foot strikers do not exhibit a discernible impact force peak (Cavanagh *et al*. 1984) (Figure 9.63c).

In Practical Worksheet 4, students use a force platform to record and then analyse the anteroposterior and vertical components of the ground reaction force acting on a subject while running.

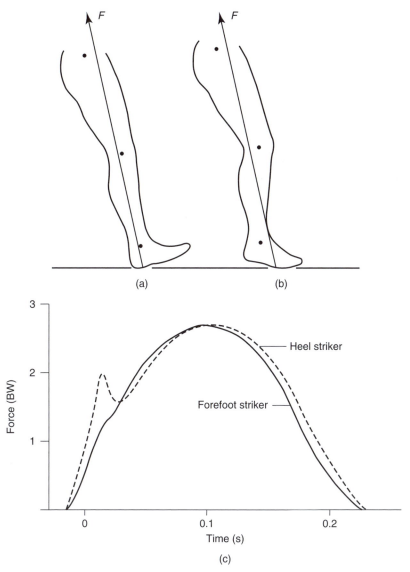

Figure 9.63 Effect of the alignment of the upper leg, lower leg and foot at foot-strike on the line of action of the ground reaction force (F), impact force peak and rate of loading. (a) Rear-foot striker. (b) Fore-foot striker. (c) Ground reaction force–time curves for a rear-foot striker and a fore-foot striker.

LINEAR MOMENTUM

In terms of linear motion (angular motion is considered in Chapter 10), the inertia of a body at rest, i.e. its reluctance to move, depends entirely on its mass; the larger the mass, the greater the inertia, and the greater the force that is needed to move it. The inertia of a moving body, i.e. the reluctance of the body to change its speed or direction of movement, depends upon its mass and linear velocity. The product of a body's mass and linear velocity is referred to as the linear momentum of the body. A cricket ball of mass 0.156 kg moving with a linear velocity of 40 m/s (about 90 mph) has a linear momentum of 6.27 kg·m/s, i.e.

$$\text{linear momentum of ball} = 0.156 \text{ kg} \times 40 \text{ m/s}$$

$$= 6.24 \text{ kg·m/s (kilogram metres per second)}.$$

Anyone who has ever been hit by a rapidly moving cricket ball or hockey ball will appreciate that the ball exhibited a great reluctance to change its speed and direction; this is reflected in the force exerted by the ball on impact.

In sports, the mass of a player during a game is fairly constant, if the loss of mass due to the exercise is discounted. Consequently, the linear momentum of a player will vary directly with his or her linear velocity; the greater the linear velocity, the greater the linear momentum and the greater the force that will be needed to change speed and direction. In rugby, a well-used ploy is to set up a situation in which the ball can be passed to a player who is moving rapidly forward close to the opposition goal line. The greater the linear momentum of the player when he receives the ball, the more difficult it will be for opposition to stop him going over the goal line. For example, a player of mass 70 kg moving with a linear velocity of 5 m/s has a linear momentum of 350 kg·m/s, i.e.

$$\text{linear momentum of player} = 70 \text{ kg} \times 5 \text{ m/s}$$

$$= 350 \text{ kg} \cdot \text{m/s}.$$

To stop the player dead in his tracks, the defending team would have to tackle the player with a linear momentum of the same magnitude but opposite in direction. This would be difficult to achieve due to the difference in speed of movement of the attacking player and the tacklers.

Further reference to velocity and momentum in this chapter, unless specified, will refer to linear velocity and linear momentum. Angular velocity and angular momentum are covered in Chapter 10.

NEWTON'S LAWS OF MOTION AND GRAVITATION

Irrespective of the number of forces acting on a body, the resultant force acting on a body at rest is zero. A body at rest will only begin to move when the resultant force acting on it becomes greater than zero. Similarly, the resultant force acting on a body that is moving with uniform linear velocity, i.e. in a straight line with constant speed, is also zero. It will only change direction, accelerate or decelerate when the resultant force acting on it becomes greater than zero. Furthermore, the amount of change in speed or direction that occurs will depend upon the magnitude and direction of the resultant force, i.e. there is a direct relationship between change of resultant force and change in movement. Isaac Newton described this relationship in what have come to be known as Newton's laws of motion. There are three laws of motion, sometimes referred to as the law of inertia (first law), the law of momentum (second law) and the law of interaction (third law). In addition to the three laws of motion, Newton's law of gravitation (law of attraction) describes the naturally occurring force of attraction that is always present between any two bodies. A body falls to the ground because of the gravitational attraction between the body and the earth, and the planets are maintained in their orbits round the sun by the gravitational attraction between the planets and the sun.

Newton's first law of motion

The first law of motion incorporates the fundamental principle that a change in resultant force is necessary to bring about a change in movement. The law may be expressed as follows:

> The resultant force acting on a body at rest or moving with uniform linear velocity is zero and the body will remain at rest or continue to move with uniform linear velocity unless the resultant force acting on it becomes greater than zero.

For example, at the start of a soccer match, a player kicks the ball (changes the resultant force acting on the ball) to get the ball moving. Similarly, the speed of a passenger travelling on a bus will be the same as that of the bus. If the speed of the bus is suddenly reduced by braking or a collision, the passenger, unless suitably restrained, will be thrown forward, as she will tend to move forward with the speed that she possessed before the bus braked. Seat belts are usually worn by passengers in motor vehicles in order to reduce the risk of injury due to sudden changes in speed.

Not all forces produce or bring about a change in movement. Whether a particular force has any effect on the movement of a body depends upon the size of the force in relation to the inertia of the body. For example, in order to lift a barbell, the lifter must exert an upward force that is greater than the weight of the barbell; otherwise the barbell will not move.

Newton's law of gravitation: gravity and weight

It is alleged that Newton was sitting under an apple tree one day when he saw an apple fall from the tree and that this observation led to the formulation of Newton's law of gravitation. The truth of the allegation cannot be confirmed, but the phenomenon of the natural force of attraction between bodies is a fundamental characteristic of the physical world. The law of gravitation may be expressed as follows:

> Every body attracts every other body with a force that varies directly with the product of the masses of the two bodies and inversely with the square of the distance between them.

Thus, the force of attraction F between two objects of masses m_1 and m_2 at a distance d apart is given by,

$$F = \frac{G \cdot m_1 \cdot m_2}{d^2}, \tag{9.2}$$

where G is a constant referred to as the gravitational constant and d is the distance between the centres of mass of the two bodies. The law of gravitation means that the force of attraction between any two bodies will be greater the larger the masses of the bodies and the closer they are together. It is, perhaps, hard to appreciate that a force of attraction exists between any two bodies. However, the force of attraction between bodies is normally minute and has no effect on the movement of the bodies. For example, the force of attraction between two men, each of mass 70 kg, standing 0.5 m apart is approximately one ten-millionth of a kilogram force (10^{-7} kgf). This force of attraction becomes even smaller the farther apart the men move.

There is, however, one body that results in a significant force of attraction between itself and other bodies, i.e. the earth. In relation to the law of gravitation, the earth is simply a massive body (radius 6.37×10^3 km; Elert 2000) with a huge mass (5.98×10^{24} kg; Elert 2000). Even though the distance between the centre of the earth (assumed to be the centre of mass of the earth) and any body on the surface of the earth (or in space close to the surface of the earth) is extremely large, the force of attraction between the earth and any other body is much larger than that which exists between any two bodies on or close to the earth's surface. This is due to the huge mass of the earth. The force of attraction between the earth and any other body is not large enough to have any effect on the movement of the earth, but it is certainly large enough to pull any body toward the earth. For example, consider two light bulbs hanging from separate flexes a few feet apart on the same ceiling. By the law of gravitation there will be a force of attraction exerted between each light bulb and the earth, such that each light bulb and flex hangs vertically. There will also be a force of attraction exerted between the two light bulbs. However, the magnitude of this force is insignificant and the light bulbs continue to hang vertically rather than at an angle toward each other.

The force of attraction between the earth and any body is referred to as the weight of the body. This is the force of attraction that keeps us in contact with the earth or brings us back to the surface of the earth very quickly should we momentarily leave it as, for example, when jumping off the ground. By the law of gravitation, the weight W of an object B may be expressed as,

$$W = \frac{G \cdot m_B \cdot m_e}{d_e^2},$$

(9.3)

where: G = gravitational constant = $6.673 \times 10^{-11} \cdot m^3 \cdot kg^{-1} \cdot s^{-2}$ (Elert 2000),

m_B = mass of the object,

m_e = mass of the earth = 5.98×10^{24} kg,

d_e = radius of the earth = 6.37×10^3 km.

Since G and m_e are constants, the term $G \cdot m_e / d_e^2$ is constant for any point on the earth's surface, i.e.

$$W = m_B \cdot g,$$

(9.4)

where $g = \dfrac{G \cdot m_e}{d_e^2},$

(9.5)

and g, not to be confused with G, is gravity. The earth is not a perfect sphere, d being slightly greater at the equator than at the poles. Since g varies inversely with the square of d, g is slightly greater at the poles than at the equator. It follows that the weight of an object will be slightly greater at the poles than at the equator. The law of gravitation applies to all bodies, including all of the planets. As the masses and radii of the planets and their satellites differ from each other, it follows that the weight of an object on a particular planet (the force of attraction between the object and a particular planet) will be different from its weight on every other planet, or satellite. For example, the mass of the moon ($0.073\,483 \times 10^{24}$ kg; Elert 2000) is approximately 1/81 of that of the earth and the radius of the moon (1.74×10^3 km; Elert 2000) is approximately 7/25 of that of the earth. Consequently, the weight of the object B on the moon can be expressed as

$$W_m = \frac{G \cdot m_B \cdot m_m}{d_m^2}, \tag{9.6}$$

where: W_m = weight of the object on the moon,
          G = gravitational constant,
         m_B = mass of the object,
        m_m = mass of the moon = $0.073\,483 \times 10^{24}$ kg,
        d_m = radius of the moon = 1.74×10^3 km.

As $m_m = 0.0123 m_e$ and $d_m = 0.2731 d_e$, substitution for m_m and d_m in Equation 9.6 results in

$$W_m = \frac{0.0123 G \cdot m_B \cdot m_e}{0.0746 d_e^2}$$

$$= \frac{0.1649 G \cdot m_B \cdot m_e}{d_e^2}$$

$$\approx \frac{G \cdot m_B \cdot m_e}{6 d_e^2} \tag{9.7}$$

Since $$W_e = \frac{G \cdot m_B \cdot m_e}{d_e^2}, \tag{9.8}$$

where W_e = weight of the object on earth, it follows from Equations 9.7 and 9.8 that

$$W_m \approx \frac{W_e}{6},$$

i.e. the weight of the object on the moon is approximately one-sixth of its weight on earth.

Since the mass of the object is constant, it follows that the moon's gravity is approximately one-sixth of the earth's gravity. This can be clearly demonstrated by manipulating Equation 9.7, i.e.

$$W_m = \frac{m_B \cdot G \cdot m_e}{6 d_e^2} = m_B \cdot g_m,$$

where g_m = the moon's gravity = $\dfrac{G \cdot m_e}{6 d_e^2}$. \hfill (9.9)

From Equations 9.5 and 9.9, it follows that $g_m = g/6$, where g is the earth's gravity.

The reduced gravity on the moon has two main effects on the movement of astronauts on the surface of the moon. Firstly, the strength of a particular astronaut on the moon would be the same as on earth, but his weight on the moon would be approximately one-sixth of his weight on earth. Therefore, he would be able project himself off the surface of the moon far more easily than he could on earth. Secondly, the astronaut would be attracted back to the surface of the moon by a force of approximately one-sixth of the attraction force on earth. Consequently, he would appear to float down to the surface of the moon rather than fall rapidly, as on earth.

Newton's second law of motion: the impulse of a force

From Newton's first law of motion, the resultant force acting on a body must be greater than zero in order to alter the motion of the body. A change in the velocity of a body will result in a simultaneous change in the momentum of the body (momentum = mass × velocity). When the resultant force acting on a body is greater than zero, the change in momentum, increase or decrease, experienced by the body depends upon the magnitude and direction of the resultant force and the length of time that the resultant force acts on the body. It was this realisation that led Newton to formulate his second law of motion. The law may be expressed as follows:

> When a force (resultant force greater than zero) acts on a body, the change in momentum experienced by the body takes place in the direction of the force and is directly proportional to the magnitude of the force and the length of time that the force acts.

The law can be expressed algebraically as follows:

$$F \cdot t \propto m \cdot v - m \cdot u \tag{9.10}$$

where: F = magnitude of the resultant force,
t = duration of force application,
m = mass of the object,
u = velocity of the object at the start of force application,
v = velocity of the object at the end of force application.

The term $F \cdot t$ (the product of the force F and the duration of force application t) is referred to as the impulse of the force. The term $m \cdot v - m \cdot u$ is the change in momentum experienced by the object as a result of the impulse of the force. When v is greater than u, i.e. there is an increase in momentum, F is an accelerating force. When v is less than u, i.e. there is a decrease in momentum, F is a decelerating or braking force.
From Equation 9.10,

$$F \propto \frac{m \cdot v - m \cdot u}{t}. \tag{9.11}$$

The right side of the equation indicates the rate of change of momentum. Newton's second law is often expressed in terms of Equation 9.11, i.e.

When a force (a resultant force greater than zero) acts on a body, the rate of change of momentum experienced by the body is directly proportional to the magnitude of the force and takes place in the direction of the force.

From Equation 9.11,

$$F \propto \frac{m(v-u)}{t}. \tag{9.12}$$

$$\text{As} \quad a = \frac{(v-u)}{t},$$

where a = the average acceleration of the body during time t, it follows from Equation 9.12 that

$$F \propto m \cdot a. \tag{9.13}$$

The second law is often expressed in terms of Equation 9.13, i.e.

When a force (resultant force greater than zero) acts on a body, the acceleration experienced by the body is directly proportional to the magnitude of the force and takes place in the direction of the force.

Since mass is constant, it is clear from Equation 9.13 that there is a direct relationship between F and a, i.e. the constant of proportionality between F and a is 1. Consequently,

$$F = m \cdot a. \tag{9.14}$$

Newton's second law of motion is often expressed as Equation 9.14, but the impulse–momentum expression is more widely used in the context of sport, i.e.

$$F \cdot t = m \cdot v - m \cdot u. \tag{9.15}$$

Newton's second law of motion is sometimes referred to as the impulse–momentum relationship or impulse–momentum principle. It has wide application in sport, as performance in many sports is concerned with increasing and decreasing speed of movement (and, therefore, changes in momentum) of the human body or associated implements, such as bats and balls. The principle has directly or indirectly led to the development or modification of some sports techniques. For example, in the shot put, the velocity of the shot as it leaves the thrower's hand is determined by the impulse of the force exerted on it by the thrower. The force exerted by the thrower depends largely on his strength; in general, the stronger the thrower, the greater the amount of force that he will be able to apply to the shot. The length of time that the thrower can apply force to the shot depends upon his/her technique, i.e. the movement pattern (the way the body segments move in relation to each other) during the whole putting action.

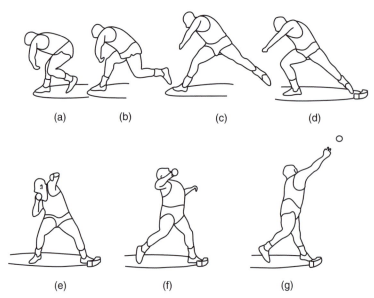

Figure 9.64 Glide (O'Brien) shot put technique.

Originally, shot put technique consisted largely of a standing put (Figure 9.64e–g). In a standing put the (right-handed) thrower stands sideways to the intended direction of the shot with the left foot against the stop-board and the right foot close to the centre of the 2.135 m (7 ft) diameter shot put circle. The thrower then rotates the trunk and flexes the right leg to obtain a position (Figure 9.64e) from which a powerful thrusting action can be made (Figure 9.64e–g). Development of the technique resulted from attempts to utilise the rear part of the circle in order to apply force to the shot for a longer period of time (and over a greater distance, see Chapter 11) and, thereby, increase the impulse applied to the shot. The greater the impulse, the greater the release velocity of the shot and, other things being equal, such as the height and angle of release, the greater the distance achieved. At the 1952 Olympic Games in Helsinki, the winner of the men's shot put (Parry O'Brien, USA) demonstrated a new technique, which is still the most popular technique. In the O'Brien or glide technique, as it is called, the thrower takes up a starting position in the rear of the circle, facing in the opposite direction to that of the intended direction of the shot, with the toe of the right foot (for a right-handed thrower) against the inner side of the circle. The thrower then flexes his hips and knees, such that the shot may actually be outside the circle (Figure 9.64a). From this position, the movement across the circle is initiated by an explosive extension of the left leg closely followed by and in association with extension of the right leg (Figure 9.64b). The purpose of this movement is to generate velocity of the shot in the direction of the put. Prior to landing with the left foot close to the stop-board, the thrower flexes the right knee and moves the right foot underneath his body, such that it lands about halfway across the circle (Figure 9.64c–d). At this stage, the thrower is close to a position from which the final thrusting movement, basically a standing put, can be made (Figure 9.64d–g). The advantage of the O'Brien technique is that, as a result of the impulse of the force applied to the shot during the movement across the

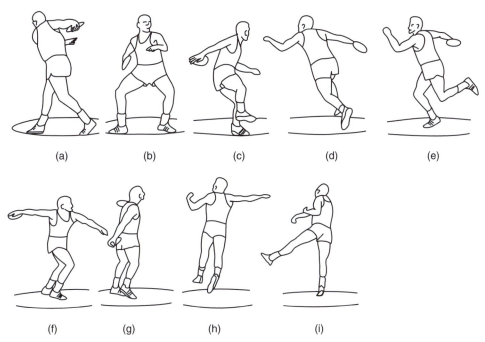

(a)　　　　(b)　　　　(c)　　　　(d)　　　　(e)

(f)　　　　(g)　　　　(h)　　　　(i)

Figure 9.65 One and three-quarter turn discus throw technique.

circle, the shot will already be moving in the direction of the put before the final putting action is initiated. Consequently, the total impulse applied to the shot during the complete sequence of movements will be greater than that applied in a standing put, resulting in a greater release velocity.

The technique of discus throwing originally consisted of a standing throw, i.e. half a turn that was made from the front of the 2.5 m (8 ft 2½ in) diameter discus circle (Figure 9.65f–i). The most popular technique now involves one and three-quarter turns from a starting position in the back of the circle with the thrower facing the opposite direction to that of the throw. The (right-handed) thrower starts the turning movement from a position with the shoulders turned as far as possible to the right (Figure 9.65a). The thrower then turns to the left and performs a fast rotating-stepping movement across the circle into a position from which the final slinging action can be initiated. The impulse of the force applied to the discus using the one and three-quarter turns technique is greater than that in a half turn standing throw and, consequently, results in a greater release velocity. Some shot putters use a one and three-quarter turn technique (rotational shot put technique), similar to that used in discus (Figure 9.66).

Newton's second law of motion is sometimes referred to as the impulse–momentum relationship or impulse–momentum principle. It has wide application in sport, as performance in many sports is concerned with increasing and decreasing speed of movement of the human body or associated implements, such as bats and balls.

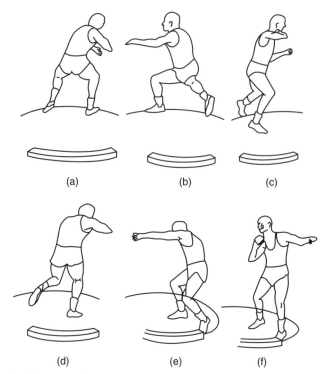

Figure 9.66 Rotational shot put technique.

Units of force

From Newton's second law of motion, the relationship between the acceleration a experienced by a mass m when acted upon by a resultant force F is given by Equation 9.14, i.e. $F = m \cdot a$. In the SI system, the unit of force is the newton (N). In accordance with Equation 9.14, a newton is defined as the force acting on a mass of 1 kg that accelerates it by 1 m/s², i.e.

$$1\,\text{N} = 1\,\text{kg} \times 1\,\text{m/s}^2 \ (\text{i.e. } 1\,\text{N} = 1\,\text{kg·m/s}^2). \tag{9.16}$$

From Newton's law of gravitation,

$$W = m \cdot g, \tag{9.17}$$

where W = weight of the mass m and g = gravity. It follows from Equations 9.14 and 9.17 that gravity is an acceleration. The magnitude of gravity varies slightly at different points on the earth's surface (see earlier section on Newton's law of gravitation) with an average value of 9.81 m/s², i.e. in the absence of air resistance, an object falling freely close to the earth's surface will accelerate at 9.81 m/s² (and decelerate at 9.81 m/s² if thrown vertically upward). From Equation 9.17, the weight of a mass of 1 kg, referred to as 1 kgf (kilogram force, see Table 8.1) is 9.81 N, i.e.

$1 \text{ kgf} = 1 \text{ kg} \times 9.81 \text{ m/s}^2 = 9.81 \text{ N.}$

The kgf is referred to as a gravitational unit of force. Most weighing machines in everyday use, such as kitchen scales and bathroom scales, are graduated in kgf or lbf (pounds force). Thus the weight of a man of mass 70 kg can be expressed as 70 kgf or 686.7 N, i.e.

$70 \text{ kgf} = 70 \text{ kg} \times 9.81 \text{ m/s}^2 = 686.7 \text{ N.}$

In calculations using SI units, the unit of force is the newton and all forces, including weights, must be expressed in newtons. For example, consider the sprinter in Figure 9.47. If the resultant force acting on the sprinter is 111.2 kgf and his mass is 70 kg, it follows from Equation 9.14 that the acceleration a of the sprinter in the direction of the resultant force at the instant shown in the figure is given by

$$a = \frac{F}{m},$$

where $F = 111.2$ kgf and $m = 70$ kg. To complete the calculation, F (equivalent to the weight of a mass of 111.2 kg) must be expressed in newtons, i.e.

$$F = 111.2 \text{ kgf} = 111.2 \text{ kg} \times 9.81 \text{ m/s}^2 = 1090.9 \text{ N.}$$

Therefore $a = \dfrac{1090.9 \text{ N}}{70 \text{ kg}} = 15.58 \text{ m/s}^2.$

Average force on a soccer ball during a place kick

Consider the average force exerted on a soccer ball of mass 0.45 kg during a kick. In Figure 9.67a the ball is at rest and in Figure 9.67b the ball has just separated from the player's boot following the kick. If the time of contact between the player's boot and the ball is 0.05 s

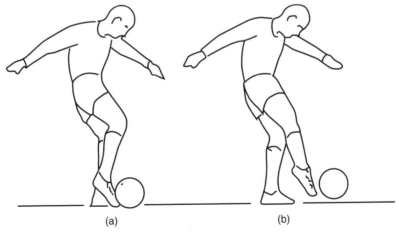

(a)　　　　　　　　　　　　　(b)

Figure 9.67 Soccer player kicking a ball. (a) Ball at rest as the foot contacts the ball. (b) Instant of separation of the ball from the player's foot following the kick.

and the velocity of the ball following the kick is 30 m/s (67.1 mph), the average force F exerted on the ball during the kick can be determined by using the impulse–momentum form of Newton's second law of motion (Equation 9.15), i.e.

$$F \cdot t = m \cdot v - m \cdot u.$$

$$\text{and} \quad F = \frac{m(v - u)}{t},$$

where $t = 0.05$ s, $m = 0.45$ kg, $u = 0$ and $v = 30$ m/s.
Therefore,

$$F = \frac{0.45 \text{ kg} \ (30 \text{ m/s} - 0 \text{ m/s})}{0.05 \text{ s}}$$

$$F = \frac{13.5 \text{ kg} \cdot \text{m/s}}{0.05 \text{ s}} = 270 \text{ N}.$$

As   1 kgf $= 9.81$ N,

then $F = \dfrac{270 \text{ N}}{9.81} = 27.52$ kgf.

In this example, the change in momentum of the ball as a result of the kick was 13.5 kg·m/s, i.e.

$$\text{change in momentum} = m \cdot v - m \cdot u$$

$$= 0.45 \text{ kg} \times 30 \text{ m/s} - 0.45 \text{ kg} \times 0$$

$$= 13.5 \text{ kg} \cdot \text{m/s}.$$

The change in momentum of the ball was produced by the impulse of a force of 270 N (average force) acting on the ball for a period of 0.05 s, i.e.

$$\text{impulse of force} = F \cdot t$$

$$= 270 \text{ N} \times 0.05 \text{ s} = 13.5 \text{ N} \cdot \text{s}.$$

It follows that the unit of measurement of impulse, newton seconds (N·s), and the unit of measurement of momentum, kilogram metres per second (kg·m/s), are equivalent. This can be demonstrated as follows:

From Equation 9.16, 1 N $= 1$ kg·m/s²,
therefore,   N·s $=$ kg·m/s² $\times$ s $=$ kg·m/s.

Average force on a golf ball during a drive

The average force exerted on a golf ball during a drive can be calculated in the same way as in the preceding example. For example, if F is the average force exerted on the ball, the mass of the ball $m = 0.046$ kg (1.62 ounces), $u = 0$, $v = 70$ m/s (156.6 mph) and t (time of contact between club-head and ball) $= 0.0005$ s, then

$$F = \frac{m(v - u)}{t}$$

$$F = \frac{0.046 \text{ kg} (70 \text{ m/s} - 0 \text{ m/s})}{0.0005 \text{ s}}$$

$$F = 6440 \text{ N} = 656 \text{ kgf}.$$

Since 1 tonf $= 1016$ kgf, then $F = 0.64$ tonf.

Free body diagram

A diagram showing, in vector form, all of the forces acting on a body as if isolated from its surroundings is called a free body diagram. The forces represented may be contact forces, such as pulls, pushes, support forces, wind resistance and buoyancy forces, or attraction forces, such as weight. The only forces acting on the man in Figure 9.68a are his weight W and the ground reaction force R. In a free body diagram, the point of application of a force may be indicated by either the tail end or the arrow tip of the vector. In Figure 9.68a the point of application of R is indicated by the tail of the vector and in Figure 9.68b the point of application of R is indicated by the arrow tip of the vector. In Figure 9.68a and b the point of application of W is the whole body centre of mass. When only the linear effect of the forces acting on a body are considered (rather than linear and angular), the free body diagram may be simplified by representing the body as a point from which the forces arise, as in Figure 9.68c.

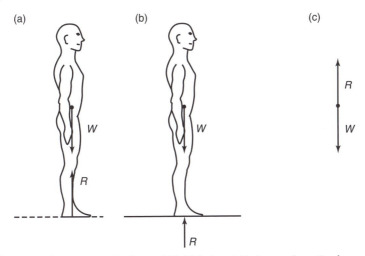

(a)   (b)   (c)

Figure 9.68 Forces acting on a man standing upright: W, body weight; R, ground reaction force.

Resultant force and equilibrium

When the resultant force acting on an object is zero, the body is described as being in a state of equilibrium. Consequently, Newton's first law of motion can be expressed as follows:

> A body will remain in a state of equilibrium (at rest or moving with uniform linear velocity) until the resultant force acting on it becomes greater than zero.

The motion of a skydiver and a person travelling in a lift will be described to illustrate the concept of equilibrium.

Skydiver

When a skydiver jumps out of an aeroplane, she will be accelerated toward the earth by the force of her body weight W (weight of skydiver, parachute and clothing) (Figure 9.69a). For the first few seconds of the fall, she will experience uniform downward acceleration, i.e. gravity. However, as her downward velocity increases, so will the air resistance R, i.e. the upward force exerted by the air on the underside of her body. After about 5 seconds, when downward velocity is approximately 50 m/s (112 mph), R will be equal in magnitude but opposite in direction to W (Figure 9.69b). Consequently, the resultant force on the skydiver will be zero and provided that the orientation and shape of her body does not change, she will continue to fall with a uniform velocity of about 50 m/s (Figure 9.70a,b). The skydiver will therefore be in a state of equilibrium. To land safely, the skydiver must reduce her downward velocity to about 10 m/s (22 mph). This is achieved by opening the parachute, which suddenly presents a massive area to the air and greatly increases the air resistance. So great is the increase in air resistance, that for about 2 seconds the air resistance is greater than the weight of the skydiver, i.e. $R > W$. Therefore, during this short period of time, there will be a resultant upward force acting on the skydiver. Consequently, she will decelerate and her downward velocity will be rapidly reduced to around 10 m/s (Figure 9.70). As she decelerates, the magnitude of the air resistance quickly decreases to again equal body weight, i.e. $R = W$. Consequently, a new state of equilibrium is established which continues until the skydiver lands on the ground.

It is possible to estimate the average magnitude of air resistance acting on the skydiver during the period of deceleration by applying Newton's second law of motion. However, it is important to ensure that each of the relevant vector quantities is afforded its correct direction

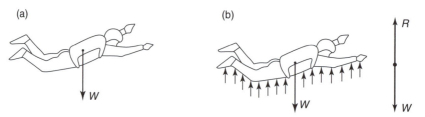

Figure 9.69 Forces acting on a skydiver. (a) Immediately after jumping from the aeroplane, the skydiver experiences downward acceleration due to gravity. (b) Air resistance increases to equal body weight in about 5 seconds. W, weight of skydiver, clothing and parachute; R, air resistance.

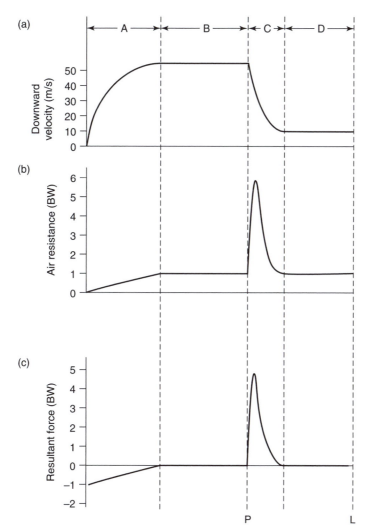

Figure 9.70 (a) Variation in downward velocity of a skydiver. (b) Corresponding air resistance. (c) Resultant force. A: period of acceleration after jumping out of the aeroplane. Downward velocity increases to a maximum at which point the magnitude of $R = W$. B: Period of free fall in equilibrium. P: Parachute opens. C: Period of deceleration. D: Period of equilibrium prior to landing (L).

in the impulse–momentum equation. In situations involving accelerating forces, such as the examples concerning the forces on a soccer ball and golf ball described in the earlier section on units of force, force and velocity are in the same direction and it is not necessary to designate a positive and a negative direction. However, in this example, the resultant force acting on the skydiver during the period of deceleration is in the opposite direction to the velocity of the skydiver. Consequently, it is necessary to define a positive and a negative direction and give each vector quantity its correct sign in the impulse–momentum equation. It does not matter which direction is regarded as positive, so long as all variables are given their correct sign. The positive direction is usually regarded as the direction of the resultant force. In the example of the skydiver, the resultant force during the period of deceleration is upward. Consequently,

293

in the worked example that follows, upward is positive and downward negative, i.e. R is positive because its direction is upward and W, u and v are all negative because their direction is downward. From Newton's second law of motion,

$$F = \frac{m(v - u)}{t},$$

where: $F = R - W$ = average resultant force acting on the skydiver during the period of deceleration,

m = mass of the skydiver, clothing and parachute = 70 kg,

u = velocity of skydiver before parachute opens = -50 m/s,

v = velocity of skydiver at the end of the period of deceleration = -10 m/s,

$t = 2$ s,

$$R - W = \frac{70 \text{ kg} \left(-10 \text{ m/s} - (-50 \text{ m/s})\right)}{2 \text{ s}}$$

$$R - W = \frac{70 \text{ kg} \left(-10 \text{ m/s} + 50 \text{ m/s}\right)}{2 \text{ s}}$$

$$R - W = \frac{70 \text{ kg} \left(+40 \text{ m/s}\right)}{2 \text{ s}}$$

$$R - W = 1400 \text{ N}$$

$$R = 1400 \text{ N} + W$$

$$R = 1400 \text{ N} + 686.7 \text{ N}$$

$$R = 2086.7 \text{ N} = 3.04 \text{ BW},$$

i.e. the average magnitude of the air resistance acting on the skydiver during the period of deceleration would be about three times the weight (BW) of the skydiver.

Travelling in a lift

Whether or not the lift is moving, there will be two forces acting on a man standing in a lift, his weight W and the ground reaction force R exerted by the floor of the lift on his feet (Figure 9.71).

When the lift and, therefore, the man is at rest, $R = W$, i.e. the resultant force acting on the man will be zero. He will be in equilibrium and experience a force at his feet equal to his body weight. As the lift starts to accelerate upward from rest, there will be a resultant upward force acting on the man, i.e. $R > W$. Therefore, during the period of acceleration the man will feel heavier than normal, since the force R acting on his feet will be greater than W. At the end of the period of acceleration, i.e. when the lift moves upward with uniform velocity, the force R will again be equal to W and equilibrium will be restored. When the lift starts to decelerate (as the upward velocity of the lift is reduced to zero) there will be a resultant downward force

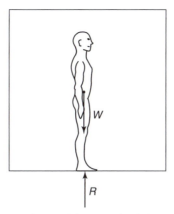

Figure 9.71 Forces acting on a man standing in a lift: W, weight of the man; R, ground reaction force.

acting on the man, i.e. $W > R$. Therefore, during the period of deceleration, the man will feel lighter than normal, since the force R will be less than W. As the lift starts to accelerate downward there will be a resultant downward force acting on the man, i.e. $W > R$, such that he will feel lighter than normal. At the end of the period of acceleration, i.e. when the lift moves downward with uniform velocity, the force R will again be equal to W and equilibrium will be restored. When the lift starts to decelerate (as the downward velocity of the lift is reduced to zero), there will be a resultant upward force acting on the man, i.e. $R > W$, such that he will feel heavier than normal. Figure 9.72 shows the relationship between the resultant force acting on the man and his velocity as the lift moves upward and downward from rest. You can easily verify these observations by travelling in a lift while standing on a set of bathroom scales.

The amount by which a person feels heavier or lighter during periods of acceleration and deceleration in a lift can be estimated by applying Newton's second law of motion. For example, consider a man of mass 70 kg standing in a lift, which accelerates upward from rest at 0.6 m/s^2. During the period of acceleration, there will be a resultant upward force acting on the man, i.e. $R > W$. From Newton's second law of motion,

$$F = m \cdot a,$$

where: $F = R - W =$ resultant upward force acting on the man during the period of upward acceleration,

   $m =$ mass of the man $= 70$ kg,
   $a =$ acceleration of the man $= 0.6 \text{ m/s}^2$.

$R - W = 70 \text{ kg} \times 0.6 \text{ m/s}^2$

$R - W = 42 \text{ N}$

$R = 42 \text{ N} + W$

$R = 42 \text{ N} + 686.7 \text{ N}$

$R = 728.7 \text{ N} = 1.06 \text{ BW}.$

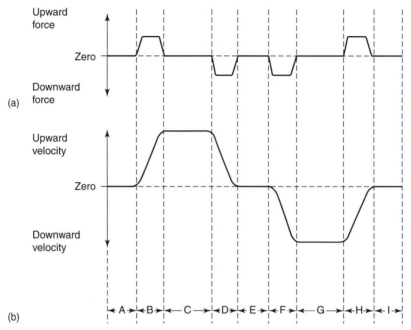

(a)

(b)

Figure 9.72 (a) Resultant force acting on a man standing in a lift. (b) His velocity as the lift moves up and down. A: Lift at rest, $R = W$; resultant force on the man is zero. B: Lift accelerating upward, $R > W$; resultant upward force on the man and velocity upward increasing. C: Lift moving upward with uniform velocity, $R = W$; resultant force is zero. D: Lift decelerating, $W > R$; resultant downward force, upward velocity decreasing. E: Lift at rest, $R = W$; resultant force is zero. F: Lift accelerating downward, $W > R$; resultant downward force, downward velocity increasing. G: Lift moving downward with uniform velocity, $R = W$; resultant force is zero. H: Lift decelerating downward, $R > W$; resultant upward force, downward velocity decreasing. I: Lift at rest, $R = W$; resultant force is zero.

Therefore, during the period of upward acceleration, the man would feel heavier than normal by about 4.28 kgf (42 N). The greater the upward acceleration, the heavier the man would feel. For example, when a rocket lifts off from its launching pad, the acceleration is so great that the upward force exerted on an astronaut inside the rocket is many times the body weight of the astronaut, i.e. the acceleration is many times the acceleration due to gravity but in an upward direction. Consequently, during the period of acceleration, the astronaut will feel many times heavier than normal.

If the lift in the example accelerated downward at 0.6 m/s², there would be a resultant downward force acting on the man, i.e. $W > R$. From Newton's second law of motion,

$$F = m \cdot a,$$

where: $F = W - R = $ resultant downward force acting on the man during the period of
               downward acceleration,
          $m = $ mass of the man $= 70$ kg,
          $a = $ acceleration of the man $= 0.6$ m/s²,

$$W - R = 70 \text{ kg} \times 0.6 \text{ m/s}^2$$

$W - R = 42$ N

$R = W - 42$ N

$R = 686.7$ N $- 42$ N

$R = 644.7$ N $= 0.94$ BW.

Therefore, during the period of downward acceleration, the man would feel lighter than normal by about 4.28 kgf (42 N). The greater the downward acceleration, the lighter the man would feel.

Newton's third law of motion

When a soccer player kicks a ball, there is a period of time in which the ball and the player's boot are in contact. During contact, the player exerts a force on the ball and simultaneously experiences a force exerted by the ball on his foot (Figure 9.73). Furthermore, the greater the force exerted by the player on the ball, the greater the force exerted by the ball on his foot. Similarly, the greater the force exerted by a shot putter on the shot, the greater the force exerted by the shot on the putter's hand (Figure 9.74). These examples indicate that whenever body A exerts a force on body B, then body B will simultaneously exert a force on body A. What is not so evident is that the forces are equal in magnitude and opposite in direction. This phenomenon is the basis of Newton's third law of motion. The law may be expressed as follows:

Whenever one body A exerts a force on another body B, body B simultaneously exerts an equal and opposite force on body A.

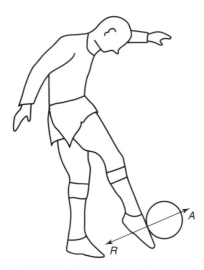

Figure 9.73 The force A exerted by a soccer player on a ball when kicking the ball and the simultaneous equal and opposite force R exerted by the ball on the kicker's foot.

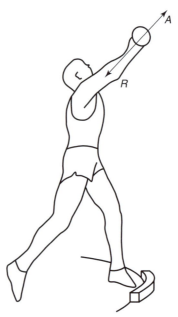

Figure 9.74 The force A exerted by a shot putter on a shot during a putting action and the simultaneous equal and opposite force R exerted by the shot on the putter's hand.

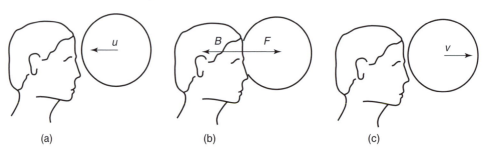

(a) (b) (c)

Figure 9.75 Heading a soccer ball. (a) The direction of the ball just prior to contact with the player's head. (b) The force F exerted by the player's head on the ball and the equal and opposite force B exerted by the ball on the player's head. (c) The direction of the ball just as it leaves the player's head.

Consider the force exerted by and, therefore, on the head of a soccer player when heading a ball (Figure 9.75). Assume that the ball travels horizontally just before and just after contact with the player's head and that the direction of the ball as it contacts the player's head (Figure 9.75a) is opposite to that at which it leaves the player's head (Figure 9.75c). From Newton's second law of motion,

$$F = \frac{m(v-u)}{t},$$

where: F = average force exerted on the ball during contact with the player's head,
  m = mass of the ball = 0.45 kg,

u = velocity of the ball as it comes into contact with the player's head $= -20$ m/s
(65.6 mph) (u is negative because its direction is opposite to F),

v = velocity of the ball as it leaves the player's head $= 15$ m/s (49.2 mph),

t = contact time between the ball and the player's head $= 0.05$ s,

$$F = \frac{0.45 \text{ kg} \left(15 \text{ m/s} - (-20 \text{ m/s})\right)}{0.05 \text{ s}}$$

$$F = \frac{0.45 \text{ kg} \left(15 \text{ m/s} + 20 \text{ m/s}\right)}{0.05 \text{ s}}$$

$$F = \frac{0.45 \text{ kg} \left(+ 35 \text{ m/s}\right)}{0.05 \text{ s}}$$

$$F = 315 \text{ N} = 32.1 \text{ kgf.}$$

Consequently, the average force acting on the ball and, therefore, on the player's head during contact would be approximately 32 kgf (about 46% of body weight for a player of mass 70 kg). The values of u, v, m and t used in this example are fairly typical of those that occur during the game (Asken and Schartz 1998). The average force and, consequently, the peak force acting on the head when heading the ball may be considerably greater than 32 kgf, especially when the ball is travelling very quickly. Considering that some players, particularly those who play in defensive positions, may be required to head the ball many times during a game, it is not surprising that they may suffer concussion during or after certain games.

There are many occasions when it is necessary to reduce the magnitude of forces acting on the human body in order to prevent injury. Such occasions occur largely during the performance of two types of movement:

- Stopping a moving object, such as catching a cricket ball, trapping a soccer ball on the chest or riding a punch in boxing;
- Stopping the human body, such as landing from a jump and falling in judo, wrestling and skateboarding.

The purpose of these movements is to reduce the momentum of the human body or that of the moving object to zero. In doing so, the deceleration force, as in landing from a jump (the ground reaction force), or the reaction to the deceleration force, as in catching a cricket ball (the force exerted on the hands), will be exerted on the body tissues, i.e. skin, muscles, ligaments and bones. If the moving object slows down very quickly, i.e. if the decelerating force applied to the object is very large, the body tissues may not be able to withstand the force and injury will occur. The underlying mechanical principle involved is still Newton's second law of motion, but the technical emphasis in the movement pattern employed is on how to exert sufficient impulse to reduce the momentum of the moving object to zero without injuring the body (momentum–impulse) rather than on trying to increase impulse in order to increase velocity (impulse–momentum). From Newton's second law of motion, the greater the length of time over which the momentum of a moving object is dissipated, the smaller will be the average force required to bring the object to rest and, consequently, the lower the risk of damage to the person or object providing the stopping force. This will be illustrated with respect to catching a cricket ball and landing from a fall.

Catching a cricket ball

When catching a ball, the hands exert a force on the ball, referred to as the action force, and simultaneously experience an equal and opposite force, referred to as the reaction force. If the player holds his arms and hands fairly stiff in readiness for the catch, the ball will tend to decelerate rapidly (high action force) on impact with the hands and rebound out of the hands before the fingers have chance to grasp it. At the same time, the reaction force may injure the hands. However, if the arms and hands are held fairly loosely in readiness for the catch, with the wrists slightly extended and the elbows and fingers slightly flexed, the impact of the ball on the hands will tend to flex the elbows, rather like compressing a spring, so that the hands move with the ball toward the chest (Figure 9.76). The movement of the hands in the direction of the ball allows the fingers sufficient time to grasp the ball; and since the momentum of the ball is dissipated over a longer period of time, the average size of the action force and, therefore, the reaction force on the hands is considerably reduced. The deceleration period of the ball can be lengthened even further with corresponding further reduction in the action

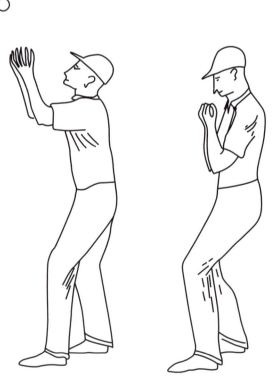

Figure 9.76 Catching a cricket ball.

and reaction forces by moving the trunk in the direction of the ball, i.e. downward and backward. A slip fielder may be seen to fall or roll backward in the process of taking a catch. Trapping a soccer ball on the chest is a similar action to catching a ball. As the ball contacts the chest, the trunk is moved backward, thereby dissipating the momentum of the ball over a longer period of time and reducing the force exerted on the ball and chest, with the result that the ball drops at the player's feet rather than bouncing away.

Landing from a jump or fall

Many court sports, including basketball, volleyball, badminton and tennis involve jumping and landing. Players usually try to land on their feet in order to control the landing and be in a position to move off quickly for the next phase of play. When landing from a vertical jump, the downward momentum of the body has to be dissipated. This is achieved by the player pushing against the floor with his feet; this results in an equal and opposite force exerted by the floor against his feet, i.e. the ground reaction force. A stiff-leg landing will decelerate the body very quickly, but only at the expense of a very large ground reaction force, which may result in injury. Good landing technique involves controlled flexion of the hips, knees and ankles; this significantly increases the period of deceleration and, consequently, reduces the average and peak ground reaction force (Figure 9.77a,b).

Figure 9.78 shows a volleyball player landing following a spike jump. During the landing period, the body is acted on by two forces, the ground reaction force R and body weight W.

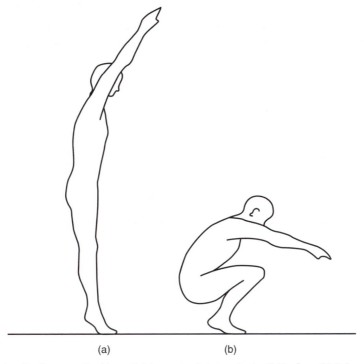

(a)   (b)

Figure 9.77 Landing from a vertical jump. (a) Legs extended at contact with the floor. (b) Subsequent controlled flexion of the hips, knees and ankles.

301

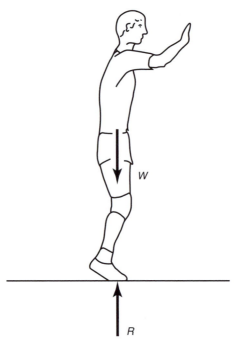

Figure 9.78 Forces acting on a volleyball player landing from a spike jump: W, body weight; R, ground reaction force.

If the downward velocity of the player when he contacts the floor is 3.4 m/s (after falling a distance of 0.6 m) and he lands fairly heavily (very little flexion of the hips, knees and ankles), his deceleration will be rapid and he will come to rest very quickly in about 0.1 s. During the period of deceleration there will be a resultant upward force acting on the player, i.e. $R > W$. From Newton's second law of motion,

$$F = \frac{m(v - u)}{t},$$

where: $F = R - W =$ average resultant force acting on the player during the period of
           deceleration,

       $m =$ mass of the player $= 70$ kg,

       $u =$ velocity of the player on contact with the floor $= -3.4$ m/s (u is negative
           because its direction is opposite to that of the resultant force),

       $v = 0$,

       $t = 0.1$ s,

i.e. $R - W = \dfrac{70 \text{ kg } (0 \text{ m/s} - (-3.4 \text{ m/s}))}{0.1 \text{ s}}$

         $R - W = 2380$ N

         $R = 2380$ N $+ W$

$$R = 2380 \text{ N} + 686.7 \text{ N}$$

$$R = 3066.7 \text{ N} = 4.46 \text{ BW},$$

i.e. the average magnitude of R during the period of deceleration would be about 4.5 times the body weight of the player. Consequently, the peak of R would be much larger than 4.5 BW and could result in injury. If the player landed relatively softly, by flexing his hips, knees and ankles to cushion the impact, the period of deceleration could be increased to approximately 0.3 s which would considerably reduce the average and peak levels of R, i.e.

$$R - W = \frac{70 \text{ kg } (0 \text{ m/s} - (-3.4 \text{ m/s}))}{0.3 \text{ s}}$$

$$R - W = 793 \text{ N}$$

$$R = 793 \text{ N} + W$$

$$R = 793 \text{ N} + 686.7 \text{ N}$$

$$R = 1479.7 \text{ N} = 2.15 \text{ BW}.$$

In both of these examples, the momentum of the player on contact with the floor was 238 kg·m/s (70 kg × 3.4 m/s). Consequently, the impulse of F (the average resultant force acting on the player during the period of deceleration) would need to be 238 N·s. In the hard landing this was achieved with an average resultant force $F = 2380$ N over a period of 0.1 s (2380 N × 0.1 s = 238 N·s) and in the soft landing it was achieved with an average resultant force $F = 793$ N over a period of 0.3 s (793 N × 0.3 s = 238 N·s). Figure 9.79 shows the resultant force–time graphs of the two types of landing. In each type of landing, the area between the force–time graph and the time axis represents the impulse of the resultant force. Each graph has a short negative period just after contact with the floor (approximately 16 ms and 47 ms in the hard and soft landings respectively), i.e. before the resultant force begins to decelerate the downward velocity of the player. The sums of the negative and positive areas of each graph are the same, i.e. 238 N·s.

Protective clothing and equipment

Special clothing and equipment is used in many sports to reduce the risk of injury from impact forces. In sports that involve a lot of jumping and landing, such as basketball and volleyball, the players usually wear fairly thick-soled shoes and thick socks in order to cushion landings. In sports such as gymnastics and judo, mats are used to decrease the forces on the body arising from landing and falling. In athletics, very deep landing areas are needed in order to prevent injury in the high jump and pole vault. Helmets are worn to reduce the risk of head injury in a range of sports, including cycling, skateboarding, canoeing, American football, cricket and rock climbing. Volleyball players and skateboarders wear knee pads and elbow pads. Batsmen and wicket keepers in cricket wear gloves and leg pads. In the days of prize fighting, when

303

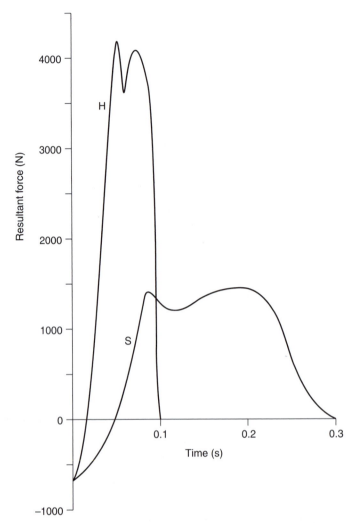

Figure 9.79 Resultant force–time graphs of hard (H) and soft (S) landings from a spike jump: Body weight, 686.7 N (70 kgf).

contestants fought without gloves, the injuries sustained were often very serious. In modern professional boxing, the boxers wear gloves of a prescribed weight and structure, which reduces impact forces. In amateur boxing, headguards are compulsory; professional boxers wear headguards in training.

From Newton's second law of motion, the greater the length of time over which the momentum of a moving object is dissipated, the smaller will be the average force required to bring the object to rest and, consequently, the lower the risk of damage to the person or object providing the stopping force.

The importance of the free body diagram in the solution of mechanical problems

Students sometimes have difficulty in understanding the operation of Newton's third law of motion. For example, consider a man pushing a large box across a level floor (Figure 9.80). From Newton's third law of motion, the force A exerted by the man on the box will be equal and opposite to the force R exerted by the box on the man. The question often asked is, 'If the force on the box is the same as that on the man's hands, how it is possible to move the box forward?' The misunderstanding arises from not taking into consideration all of the forces acting on the man and on the box. An object at rest will start to move only when the resultant force acting on the object is greater than zero. To determine the resultant force acting on an object it is necessary to consider all of the individual forces acting on the object by means of a free body diagram. An understanding of the free body diagram is the key to understanding mechanics. Mechanical problems concerning resultant forces usually involve two or more objects in contact with each other. The first step in solving such a problem should be to draw a complete free body diagram for each object.

Figure 9.81a shows a free body diagram of the forces acting on the box. The only horizontal forces acting on the box, i.e. the only forces that determine whether the box moves horizontally across the floor, are A and F_B (Figure 9.81b). It follows that the box will move forward if the force exerted by the man on the box is greater than the friction between the box and the floor, i.e. if $A > F_B$.

The forces acting on the man pushing the box are shown in Figure 9.82a. The only horizontal forces acting on the man are R and F_M (Figure 9.82b). Consequently, the box will move forward if the frictional force at the man's feet is greater than the resistance of the box, i.e.

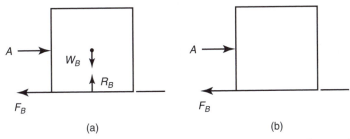

Figure 9.80 Equal and opposite forces exerted by a man on a box (A) and the box on the man (R).

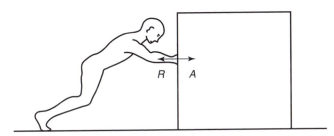

Figure 9.81 Free body diagrams. (a) The forces acting on the box. (b) The horizontal forces acting on the box. W_B, weight of the box; R_B, reaction force exerted by the floor on the box; A, force exerted by the man on the box; F_B, friction force between the box and the floor.

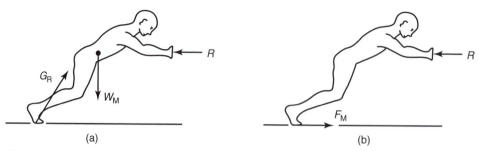

Figure 9.82 Free body diagrams. (a) The forces acting on the man. (b) The horizontal forces acting on the man. W_M, weight of the man; G_R, ground reaction force on the man; R, force exerted by the box on the man; F_M, friction force between the man and the floor.

if $F_M > R$. As R is equal in magnitude to A, the box will move forward if $F_M > A$. As the box will move forward if $F_M > A$ and $A > F_B$, it follows that the box will move forward if $F_M > F_B$, i.e. if the friction between the man's feet and the floor is greater than the friction between the box and the floor.

CONSERVATION OF LINEAR MOMENTUM

When two bodies collide, such as a club-head hitting a golf ball, they exert equal and opposite forces on each other for the same length of time, i.e. the two bodies experience equal and opposite impulses. Since the impulses are equal and opposite, the change in the linear momentum of each body must be equal and opposite. Consequently, the sum of the momentum of the two bodies after the collision will be the same as before the collision, i.e. there will have been a transfer of linear momentum from one body to the other, but no loss or gain in the combined momentum of the two bodies. This phenomenon is referred to as conservation of linear momentum. The principle of conservation of linear momentum may be expressed as follows:

> If no external force acts on a system of colliding objects, the total amount of linear momentum in the system remains constant, i.e. the sum of the linear momentum of the colliding objects remains constant.

Algebraically, the principle can be expressed as follows:

$$m_1 \cdot u_1 + m_2 \cdot u_2 = m_1 \cdot v_1 + m_2 \cdot v_2, \qquad (9.18)$$

where: m_1 and m_2 = the masses of the colliding bodies,
  u_1 = velocity of m_1 before the collision,
  u_2 = velocity of m_2 before the collision,
  v_1 = velocity of m_1 after the collision,
  v_2 = velocity of m_2 after the collision.

Practically, it is difficult to demonstrate the principle of the conservation of linear momentum, since the weights of the colliding objects will affect their motion in addition to the impulse of the impact force. However, when the contact time is very small and the impact force very large in relation to the weights of the colliding objects, as in driving a golf ball off a tee, conservation of linear momentum of the colliding bodies may be demonstrated experimentally. For example, high-speed film analysis of a golf drive has shown that if a club-head of mass 0.2 kg with a velocity of approximately 50 m/s hits a stationary ball of mass 0.046 kg, the resulting velocity of the ball is approximately 70 m/s (Daish 1972). From Equation 9.18, the linear momentum of the club-head and ball before impact is equal to $m_1 \cdot u_1 + m_2 \cdot u_2$, where:

m_1 = mass of club-head = 0.2 kg,
m_2 = mass of the ball = 0.046 kg,
u_1 = velocity of m_1 before the collision = 50 m/s,
u_2 = velocity of m_2 before the collision = 0,

i.e. $m_1 \cdot u_1 + m_2 \cdot u_2 = (0.2 \text{ kg} \times 50 \text{ m/s}) + (0.046 \text{ kg} \times 0) = 10.0 \text{ kg·m/s}$.

The linear momentum of the club-head and ball after impact is equal to $m_1 \cdot v_1 + m_2 \cdot v_2$, where:

v_1 = velocity of m_1 after the collision,
v_2 = velocity of m_2 after the collision = 70 m/s,

i.e. $m_1 \cdot v_1 + m_2 \cdot v_2 = (0.2 \text{ kg} \times v_1) + (0.046 \text{ kg} \times 70 \text{ m/s}) = 0.2 \text{ kg·} v_1 + 3.22 \text{ kg·m/s}$.

In accordance with the principle of the conservation of linear momentum, the total linear momentum after impact is equal to the total linear momentum before impact, i.e.

$$0.2 \text{ kg} \cdot v_1 + 3.22 \text{ kg·m/s} = 10.0 \text{ kg·m/s}$$

$$0.2 \text{ kg} \cdot v_1 = 10.0 \text{ kg·m/s} - 3.22 \text{ kg·m/s} = 6.78 \text{ kg·m/s}$$

$$v_1 = \frac{6.78 \text{ kg·m/s}}{0.2 \text{ kg}} = 33.9 \text{ m/s},$$

i.e. the velocity of the club-head after impact is 33.9 m/s, a reduction of 16.1 m/s. Theoretically, the impulse responsible for the reduction in the velocity of the club-head from 50 m/s to 33.9 m/s should be the same as the impulse responsible for increasing the velocity of the ball from zero to 70 m/s. The momentum of the ball after the impact = 3.22 kg·m/s (i.e. 0.046 kg × 70 m/s). Consequently, the impulse exerted on the ball during the impact = 3.22 N·s. It follows that the club-head would have experienced an equal and opposite impulse of 3.22 N·s during the impact, which would have reduced its velocity by:

$$\text{change in velocity of club-head} = \frac{\text{impulse on club-head}}{\text{mass of club-head}} = \frac{3.22 \text{ N·s}}{0.2 \text{ kg}} = 16.1 \text{ m/s}.$$

The reduction of 16.1 m/s is exactly the same as that obtained by applying the principle of conservation of linear momentum.

UNIFORMLY ACCELERATED MOTION

Acceleration is the rate of change of speed, i.e.

$$a = \frac{v - u}{t_2 - t_1},$$

where: a = average acceleration,
u = speed at t_1,
v = speed at a later time t_2,

i.e. $a = \dfrac{v - u}{t}$,   (9.19)

where $t = t_2 - t_1$.

From Equation 9.19,

$$v = u + a \cdot t.$$ (9.20)

Equation 9.20 shows how the speed v of an object with an initial speed of u changes with time when it experiences a uniform (constant) acceleration a. For example, consider the motion of a stone that is dropped from rest from a height of 200 m. Assuming that the effect of air resistance on the stone is negligible, the acceleration of the stone will be constant and the speed of the stone can be calculated using Equation 9.20, where $u = 0$ and a = gravity = 9.81 m/s^2. Table 9.9 shows the speed of the stone after each second in the first six seconds after release. Figure 9.83 shows the corresponding speed–time graph. As acceleration is constant, the speed–time graph is a straight line.

In any speed–time graph, the area between the speed–time graph and the time axis is equivalent to the distance travelled by the object during the period of time under consideration. For example, the distance fallen by the stone in the first 3 seconds after release is represented by the shaded area A in Figure 9.83. The average speed of the stone during this period is equal to $(u + v)/2$, where $u = 0$ (speed at $t = 0$) and $v = 29.43$ m/s (speed at $t = 3$ s),

Table 9.9 Distance fallen and speed of a stone after each second during the first six seconds after being dropped from rest from a height of 200 m.

Time (s)	Speed (m/s)	Distance (m)
0	0	0
1	9.81	4.90
2	19.62	19.62
3	29.43	44.14
4	39.24	78.48
5	49.05	122.62
6	58.86	176.58

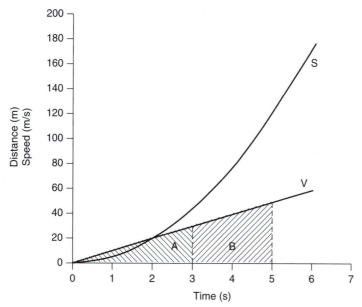

Figure 9.83 Distance–time (S) and speed–time (V) graphs of a falling stone during the first 6 seconds after release.

i.e.   average speed $= \dfrac{0 + 29.43 \text{ m/s}}{2} = 14.71 \text{ m/s.}$

As distance = average speed × time, the distance fallen in the first 3 seconds after release (s_{0-3}) is 44.14 m (s is the traditional symbol for distance), i.e.

$$s_{0-3} = 14.71 \text{ m/s} \times 3 \text{ s} = 44.14 \text{ m.}$$

Similarly, the distance fallen by the stone during the period 3–5 seconds after release (s_{3-5}) is 78.48 m, i.e.

$$s_{3-5} = \dfrac{u + v}{2} \times 2s,$$

where $u = 29.43 \text{ m/s}$ (speed at $t = 3$ s) and $v = 49.05 \text{ m/s}$ (speed at $t = 5$ s), i.e.

$$s_{3-5} = \dfrac{29.43 \text{ m/s} + 49.05 \text{ m/s}}{2} \times 2s = 78.48\,\text{m.}$$

This is represented by the shaded area B in Figure 9.83. The distance fallen during the first 5 seconds after release is the sum of areas A and B, i.e.

$$s_{0-5} = s_{0-3} + s_{3-5} = 44.14 \text{ m} + 78.48 \text{ m} = 122.62 \text{ m.}$$

309

Table 9.9 shows the cumulative distance fallen by the stone after each second in the first 6 seconds after release. Figure 9.83 shows the corresponding distance–time graph.

For an object moving with uniform acceleration, the distance s travelled by the object is given by,

$$s = \frac{u + v}{2} \cdot t,$$

(9.21)

where: $u =$ speed at t_1,

              $v =$ speed at a later time t_2,

              $t = t_2 - t_1$.

Substituting v from Equation 9.20 in Equation 9.21 gives,

$$s = \frac{(u + (u + a \cdot t))}{2} \cdot t$$

$$s = \frac{(2u + a \cdot t)}{2} \cdot t$$

$$s = u \cdot t + \frac{a \cdot t^2}{2}.$$

(9.22)

From Equation 9.21,

$$t = \frac{2s}{(u + v)}.$$

Substituting this expression for t in Equation 9.20 gives,

$$v = u + \frac{a \cdot 2s}{(u + v)}$$

$$v(u + v) = u(u + v) + 2a \cdot s$$

$$v^2 - u^2 = 2a \cdot s.$$

(9.23)

Equations 9.20 to 9.23 are collectively referred to as the equations of motion for an object moving with uniform acceleration. The equations, summarised in Table 9.10, show the rela-

Table 9.10 Equations of motion for an object moving with uniform acceleration.

	s	u	v	a	t
$v = u + a \cdot t$		✓	✓	✓	✓
$s = \dfrac{(u + v) \cdot t}{2}$	✓	✓	✓		✓
$s = u \cdot t + \dfrac{a \cdot t^2}{2}$	✓	✓		✓	✓
$v^2 - u^2 = 2a \cdot s$	✓	✓	✓	✓	

tionships between distance travelled, speed, acceleration and time that describe the motion of the object.

Air resistance

In everyday life, including sport, the human body is always surrounded by air or water, or a combination of air and water, which presses on the body and affects its movement. The amount of pressure exerted by air or water, usually referred to as air resistance and water resistance, depends upon a number of factors, including the shape and speed of the body and the density of air and water. Whereas water resistance has a considerable effect on movement of the human body, the effect of air resistance is usually negligible. Nevertheless, the constant presence of surrounding air means that the human body is unlikely to experience uniform acceleration, since the resultant force acting on the human body during movement is unlikely to be constant, even for a very short period of time.

In mechanics, air and water are both regarded as fluids, as the factors that determine air resistance and water resistance are the same. Fluid mechanics (the study of the forces that act on bodies moving through fluids and the effects of the forces on the movement of the bodies) is covered in some detail in Chapter 12.

Air resistance and water resistance are examples of drag, i.e. the force exerted by a fluid on a body moving through the fluid that opposes the movement of the body. The magnitude of drag depends upon the coefficient of drag, the density of the fluid, the area of the body presented to the fluid (perpendicular to the direction of movement) and the speed of the body relative to the speed of the fluid. Drag is expressed algebraically as follows:

$$F_D = \frac{C_D \cdot \rho \cdot A \cdot v^2}{2},$$

(9.24)

where F_D = drag (N),
  C_D = coefficient of drag,
  ρ = density of fluid (kg/m^3) (ρ = Greek letter rho),
  A = area (m^2),
  v = relative speed (m/s).

Coefficient of drag: The coefficient of drag is a dimensionless number, i.e. a number without units, which reflects the interaction of the shape, surface texture and speed of movement of the body. Its approximate range is 0–2.3 (Filippone 2005).

Density: The density of air is approximately 1.25 kg/m^3 and the density of water is approximately 1000 kg/m^3 (Cutnell and Johnson 1995). Consequently, for equivalent C_D, A and v, water resistance is about 800 times greater than air resistance.

Area: When standing upright in the anatomical position, the frontal area of an adult male is approximately 0.62 m^2 (Kubaha *et al.* 2003). In running, the frontal area of an adult man is approximately 0.45 m^2 (Davies 1980).

Relative speed: In still air (no wind), the speed of the body relative to the air is the same as the speed of the body. For example, if a sprinter is running at 10 m/s through still air, his speed relative to the air is 10 m/s. If the sprinter is running at 10 m/s with a tailwind (in the same direction as the runner) of 1 m/s, the speed of the sprinter relative to the air is 9 m/s (10 m/s − 1 m/s). If the sprinter is running at 10 m/s into a headwind (in the opposite direction to that of the sprinter) of 1 m/s, the speed of the sprinter relative to the air is 11 m/s (10 m/s −(−1 m/s)). Drag increases with the square of the relative speed, i.e. a two-fold increase in relative speed results in a four-fold increase in drag.

All bodies moving through fluids experience drag. Some bodies, owing to their shape (such as a discus, javelin and aeroplane wing) or speed of rotation (such as topspin on a tennis ball or sidespin on a soccer ball) also experience a force at right angles to the drag force. This force is referred to as hydrodynamic lift. Hydrodynamic lift is covered in some detail in Chapter 12. For the remainder of this section, it is assumed that the motion of the objects described is not affected by hydrodynamic lift.

Table 9.11 shows the estimated drag (based on Equation 9.24) acting on an adult man

Table 9.11 Drag on an adult male walking, an elite male sprinter at maximum speed, an elite male long jumper at take-off, a shot just after release by an elite female shot putter, and six different types of ball moving at the speeds indicated in still air.

	Mass (g)	Radius (cm)	Coefficient of drag	Density (kg/m^3)[1]	Area (cm^2)*	Speed (m/s)	Drag (N)	Deceleration (m/s^2)
Walking[2][3]	85 000		0.6	1.25	4500	1.5	0.3797	0
Sprinting[2][3][4]	85 000		0.6	1.25	4500	11.7	23.1019	0.27
Long jump[2][3][5]	85 000		0.6	1.25	4500	9	13.6688	0.16
Shot[6][7]	4000	5.12	0.45	1.25	82.51	10	0.2321	0.06
Cricket ball[7][8]	157	3.58	0.45	1.25	40.29	10	0.1133	0.72
Baseball[7][8]	144	4.50	0.45	1.25	63.62	10	0.1789	1.24
Tennis ball[7][8]	57	3.25	0.45	1.25	33.18	10	0.0933	1.64
Golf ball[7][8]	46	2.20	0.45	1.25	15.20	10	0.0428	0.93
Squash ball[8]	24	2.03	0.45	1.25	12.97	10	0.0365	1.52
Table-tennis ball[7][8]	2.7	2.0	0.45	1.25	12.57	10	0.0354	13.11

The data for mass, radius and area are presented in grams, centimetres and square centimetres respectively. For the calculations of drag, the areas have to be converted to square metres (see Equation 9.24). Similarly, for the calculations of acceleration (drag divided by mass), the masses have to be converted to kilograms (see Equations 9.14 and 9.16).

[1] Density of air: Cutnell and Johnson 1995;
[2] Coefficient of drag: Linthorne 1994;
[3] Area: Davies 1980;
[4] Speed: Wagner 1998;
[5] Speed: Hay *et al*. 1986;
[6] Mass and radius of shot: IAAF 1984;
[7] Coefficient of drag: Daish 1972;
[8] Mass and radius: http://en.wikipedia.org/

* Area of shot and all of the balls = $\pi \cdot r^2$, where r = radius.

Table 9.12 Mass, radius, volume, density and deceleration of a shot and six types of ball all moving in air at 10 m/s.

	Mass (g)	Radius (cm)	Volume (cm³)*	Density (g/cm³)	Deceleration (m/s²)
Shot	4000	5.12	562.2	7.11	0.06
Cricket ball	157	3.58	192.2	0.82	0.72
Baseball	144	4.50	381.7	0.38	1.24
Tennis ball	57	3.25	143.8	0.40	1.64
Golf ball	46	2.20	44.6	1.03	0.93
Squash ball	24	2.03	35.04	0.68	1.52
Table tennis ball	2.7	2.0	33.51	0.08	13.11

* Volume = $4\pi \cdot r^3/3$ where r = radius.

when walking at 1.5 m/s, sprinting at 11.7 m/s (the maximum speed of an elite male sprinter in a 100 m race) and just after take-off in a long jump (horizontal component of velocity at take-off for an elite male athlete is about 9 m/s). In elite shot putting (men and women), the horizontal component of velocity of the shot at release is about 10 m/s. Table 9.11 shows the estimated drag on a shot just after release by an elite female athlete. Like a shot, most balls used in sports are spherical. Table 9.11 shows the estimated drag on a number of different balls (tennis, baseball, cricket, table tennis, squash and golf) moving through air at 10 m/s.

Air resistance slows down or tends to slow down the moving object. Consequently, the effect of air resistance on the movement of an object is reflected in the deceleration that would be produced if the air resistance was the resultant force acting on the object. From Newton's second law (Equation 9.14), for a given amount of air resistance F, the greater the mass m of the object, the smaller the deceleration a produced ($a = F/m$), i.e. the smaller the effect of the air resistance on the movement of the object. This is reflected in the final column of Table 9.11. A direct comparison of the effect of air resistance on the shot and the six types of ball (all spherical and all moving at 10 m/s) can be made by investigating the relationship between the density and deceleration of the objects (Table 9.12). In general, the greater the density, the smaller the deceleration.

> The magnitude of drag experienced by a body depends upon the coefficient of drag, the density of the fluid, the area of the body presented to the fluid and the speed of the body relative to the speed of the fluid.

As shown in Table 9.11, air resistance on the human body during self-propelled movement is usually very small. At natural walking speed (1.5 m/s), air resistance is extremely small (approximately 0.4 N, resulting in an equivalent deceleration of zero to two decimal places) and certainly imperceptible to the individual. Air resistance is perceptible at maximum sprinting speed (approximately 23 N, resulting in an equivalent deceleration of approximately 0.27 m/s²), but not likely to have a significant effect on performance (Mureika 2001). In the long jump, air resistance (approximately 14 N, resulting in an equivalent deceleration

313

of approximately 0.16 m/s^2) may reduce horizontal distance during the flight phase of the jump by approximately 0.06 m in an 8.79 m jump. Similarly, in shot put, air resistance (approximately 0.23 N resulting in an equivalent deceleration of approximately 0.06 m/s^2) may reduce horizontal distance by approximately 0.11 m in a 19.85 m put. However, the effect of air resistance on the movement of a shot during flight and on human movement during the flight phase of a jumping action is usually small enough to be regarded as negligible. Consequently, during flight, a shot and the human body experience more-or-less uniform acceleration (gravity) and their movement can be very accurately described by applying the equations of uniformly accelerated motion (Equations 9.20 to 9.23).

PROJECTILES

In mechanics, a projectile is an object with no means of self-propulsion that is thrown (e.g. a ball or stone), thrust (e.g. a shot) or in some other way launched into the air. If the effect of air resistance on the movement of a projectile may be regarded as negligible, the only force acting on the projectile during flight is its weight, which acts vertically downward. Consequently, the vertical motion of the projectile will be subject to the uniform acceleration of gravity, i.e. following release, the upward velocity of the projectile will decrease at 9.81 m/s^2 until it reaches its maximum height, at which point its vertical velocity will be zero. It will then accelerate downward at 9.81 m/s^2 until it hits the ground. In contrast, as there are no horizontal forces acting on the projectile (resultant horizontal force = 0), its horizontal velocity will remain constant during flight. The time of flight and maximum height of the projectile can be determined by considering the vertical motion of the projectile. The horizontal range (horizontal distance from release to landing) can then be determined by considering the horizontal motion of the projectile. The basic equations (based on Equations 9.20 to 9.23) will be derived and then applied in a number of real examples.

Vertical and horizontal components of velocity of the projectile at release

As shown in Figure 9.84, if a projectile is released with a velocity v and angle of release θ, then the vertical and horizontal components of velocity are $v \cdot \sin \theta$ and $v \cdot \cos \theta$, respectively.

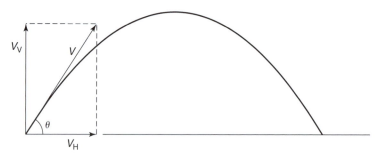

Figure 9.84 Vertical and horizontal components of release velocity of a projectile: V, release velocity; V_V, vertical component of release velocity; V_H, horizontal component of release velocity. $V_V/V = \sin \theta$, i.e. $V_V = V \cdot \sin \theta$; $V_H/V = \cos \theta$, i.e. $V_H = V \cdot \cos \theta$.

Flight time for a projectile that lands at the same level as the release point (as in Figure 9.84)

Consider vertical motion from release to landing:

$$s = u \cdot t + \frac{a \cdot t^2}{2},$$ (9.22)

where: $t =$ flight time,
$u = v_0 \cdot \sin \theta$ (where $v_0 =$ release velocity),
$a = -g$ (g is negative with respect to u),
$s =$ resultant vertical displacement $= 0$.

The projectile lands at the same level as the release point, i.e. even though the projectile may cover a large distance in rising to its maximum height and then falling back to the ground, its resultant vertical displacement from release to landing is zero, i.e. $s = 0$.

By substitution and rearrangement,

$$0 = v_0 \cdot \sin \theta \cdot t - \frac{g \cdot t^2}{2},$$

i.e. flight time $t = \dfrac{2v_0 \cdot \sin \theta}{g}$. (9.25)

From Equation 9.25, it is clear that for a given release velocity v_0, the maximum flight time occurs when $\sin \theta$ has its maximum value, i.e. when $\theta = 90°$. Consequently, maximum flight time is achieved by launching the projectile vertically upward.

Maximum height

Consider vertical motion from release to maximum height.

$$v^2 - u^2 = 2a \cdot s,$$ (9.23)

where $s = s_m =$ upward vertical distance from release to maximum height,
$u = v_0 \cdot \sin \theta$ (where $v_0 =$ release speed),
$v =$ vertical velocity at maximum height $= 0$,
$a = -g$.

By substitution and rearrangement,

$$0 - (v_0 \cdot \sin \theta)^2 = -2g \cdot s_m,$$

i.e. maximum height $s_m = \dfrac{v_0^2 \cdot \sin^2 \theta}{2g}$. (9.26)

315

From Equation 9.26, it is clear that for a given release velocity v_0, maximum height occurs when $\sin^2 \theta$ has its maximum value, i.e. when $\theta = 90°$. Consequently maximum height is achieved by launching the projectile vertically upward.

Range

Consider horizontal motion from release to landing.

$$s = u \cdot t + \frac{a \cdot t^2}{2},$$

$$(9.22)$$

where: $s = s_r = $ range

         $a = 0$

         $u = v_0 \cdot \cos \theta$ (where $v_0 = $ release velocity)

$$t = \text{flight time} = \frac{2v_0 \cdot \sin \theta}{g}.$$

$$(9.25)$$

By substitution,

$$s_r = v_0 \cdot \cos \theta \, \frac{2v_0 \cdot \sin \theta}{g} + 0,$$

i.e.   range $s_r = \dfrac{2v_0^2 \cdot \cos \theta \cdot \sin \theta}{g}.$

$$(9.27)$$

From Equation 9.27, it is clear that for a given release velocity v_0, the maximum range occurs when $\cos \theta \cdot \sin \theta$ has its maximum value, i.e. when $\theta = 45°$. Consequently, maximum range is achieved by launching the projectile at $45°$ to the horizontal.

Equations 9.25, 9.26 and 9.27 only apply to projectiles where the launch point and landing point are on the same level and where air resistance is negligible. However, even with air resistance (but no hydrodynamic lift force), maximum flight time and maximum height are achieved with $\theta = 90°$ and maximum range is achieved with $\theta = 45°$. The relationship between flight time, maximum height and release angle for a projectile (release velocity $= 50$ m/s) in the absence of air resistance is shown in Figure 9.85a. The relationship between flight time, range and release angle for a projectile (release velocity $= 50$ m/s) in the absence of air resistance is shown in Figure 9.85b. The data corresponding to the points in Figure 9.85a and b are shown in Table 9.13. It is clear from Figure 9.85a that maximum height increases as release angle increases. Figure 9.85b shows that range increases with increase in release angle between $0°$ and $45°$ and then decreases with increase in release angle between $45°$ and $90°$. Figure 9.85b also shows that flight time increases with release angle.

Trajectory of a projectile in the absence of air resistance

Figure 9.86a shows the typical trajectory (horizontal displacement–vertical displacement graph) of a projectile launched from ground level and landing at ground level in the absence of air resistance. In this particular example, the launch velocity of the projectile is 50 m/s

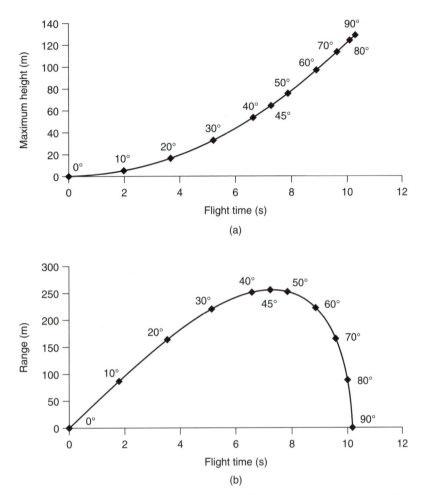

Figure 9.85 (a) Relationship between flight time, maximum height and release angle for a projectile (release velocity = 50 m/s) in the absence of air resistance. (b) Relationship between flight time, range and release angle for a projectile (release velocity = 50 m/s) in the absence of air resistance. The data corresponding to the points are shown in Table 9.13.

and launch angle is 70° to the horizontal. Figure 9.86b shows the corresponding vertical velocity–time and vertical displacement–time graphs and Figure 9.86c shows the corresponding horizontal velocity–time and horizontal displacement–time graphs. Table 9.14 shows the data (at 1 s intervals) used to plot the graphs in Figure 9.86.

Flight time

Flight time t is given by Equation 9.25, i.e.

$$t = \frac{2v_0 \cdot \sin \theta}{g},$$

where: v_0 = release velocity = 50 m/s,

Table 9.13 Flight time, maximum height and range for a projectile (release velocity = 50 m/s) without air resistance over the release angle range 0°–90°.

Angle (°)	Flight time (s)	Maximum height (m)	Range (m)
0	0	0	0
10	1.77	3.98	87.16
20	3.49	14.91	163.81
30	5.10	31.86	220.70
40	6.55	52.65	250.97
45	7.21	63.71	254.84
50	7.81	74.77	250.97
60	8.83	95.57	220.70
70	9.58	112.52	163.81
80	10.04	123.58	87.17
90	10.19	127.42	0

Flight time, calculated from Equation 9.25; maximum height, calculated from Equation 9.26; range, calculated from Equation 9.27.

$$\theta = \text{release angle} = 70°,$$
$$g = 9.81 \text{ m/s}^2,$$

i.e.   flight time $t = \dfrac{2 \times 50 \times 0.93969}{9.81} = 9.58 \text{ s.}$

Maximum height

Maximum height s_m is given by Equation 9.26, i.e.

$$\text{maximum height } s_m = \frac{v_0^2 \cdot \sin^2 \theta}{2g},$$

where:

$$v_0 = \text{release velocity} = 50 \text{ m/s},$$
$$\theta = \text{release angle} = 70°,$$
$$g = 9.81 \text{ m/s}^2,$$

i.e.   maximum height $s_m = \dfrac{2500 \times 08830}{19.62} = 112.51 \text{ m.}$

Range

Range s_r is given by Equation 9.27, i.e.

$$s_r = \frac{2v_0^2 \cdot \cos \theta \cdot \sin \theta}{g},$$

where: $v_0 = \text{release velocity} = 50 \text{ m/s}$

318

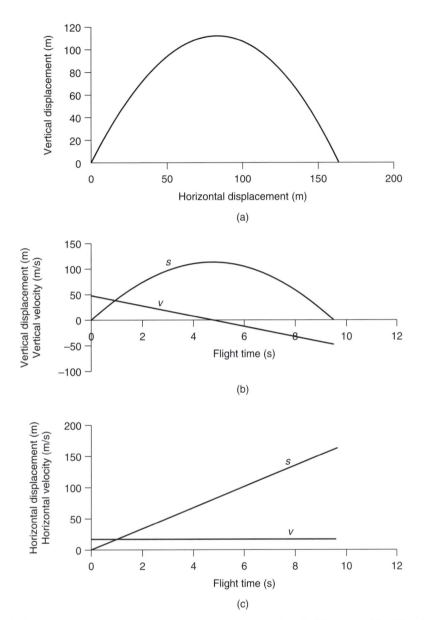

Figure 9.86 Trajectory of a projectile, in the absence of air resistance, launched from ground level, launch velocity = 50 m/s, launch angle = 70° to the horizontal, and landing at ground level. (a) Trajectory. (b) Vertical velocity–time (*v*) and vertical displacement–time (*s*) graphs. (c) Horizontal velocity–time (*v*) and horizontal displacement–time (*s*) graphs. The data used to plot the graphs are shown in Table 9.14.

θ = release angle = 70°,
g = 9.81 m/s²,

i.e. range $s_r = \dfrac{5000 \times 0.3421 \times 0.9397}{9.81} = 163.84$ m.

319

Table 9.14 Horizontal velocity, horizontal displacement, vertical velocity and vertical displacement of a projectile with release velocity of 50 m/s and release angle of 70° at one-second intervals from release to landing.

Time (s)	Horizontal velocity (m/s)	Horizontal displacement (m)	Vertical velocity (m/s)	Vertical displacement (m)
0	17.10	0	46.98	0
1	17.10	17.10	37.17	42.08
2	17.10	34.20	27.36	74.35
3	17.10	51.30	17.55	96.81
4	17.10	68.40	7.74	109.46
5	17.10	85.50	−2.06	112.30
6	17.10	102.61	−11.87	105.33
7	17.10	119.71	−21.68	88.55
8	17.10	136.81	−31.49	61.96
9	17.10	153.91	−41.31	25.56
9.58	17.10	163.81	−46.98	0

Flight time, calculated from Equation 9.22, by consideration of vertical motion; horizontal velocity, constant; horizontal displacement, calculated from Equation 9.22, by consideration of horizontal motion; vertical velocity, calculated from Equation 9.20 by consideration of vertical motion; vertical displacement, calculated from Equation 9.22 by consideration of vertical motion.

Time to maximum height t_m

Consider vertical motion from release to maximum height.

$$v = u + a \cdot t, \tag{9.20}$$

where: v = vertical velocity at maximum height = 0,
$a = -9.81 \text{ m/s}^2$,
θ = release angle = 70°,
u = vertical component of release velocity v_0,
$= v_0 \cdot \sin \theta,$
$= 50 \times 0.9397 = 46.98 \text{ m/s}.$

By substitution and rearrangement,

$$0 = 46.98 - 9.81 \times t_m$$

$$t_m = \frac{46.98}{9.81} = 4.79 \text{ s},$$

i.e. time to maximum height t_m = 4.79 s.

Horizontal displacement from release to maximum height s_h

Consider horizontal motion from release to maximum height.

$$s = u \cdot t + \frac{a \cdot t^2}{2},$$ (9.22)

where: t = time from release to maximum height = 4.79 s,

θ = release angle = 70°,

a = 0,

u = horizontal component of release velocity v_0,

  = $v_0 \cdot \cos \theta$,

  = 50 × 0.3420 = 17.10 m/s.

By substitution,

s_h = 17.10 × 4.79 = 81.92 m.

The time to maximum height (4.79 s) is exactly half of flight time (9.58 s) and the horizontal displacement from release to maximum height (81.92 m) is exactly half of the range (163.84 m). These results are to be expected, since the release and landing points are on the same level and the acceleration of the projectile is constant. Horizontal acceleration is zero. Therefore, horizontal velocity is constant and horizontal displacement increases at a constant rate, which is indicated by the straight line horizontal displacement–time graph (Figure 9.86c). Vertical acceleration is due to gravity, which results in constant deceleration upward of 9.81 m/s² and constant acceleration downward of 9.81 m/s²; this is reflected in the straight line vertical velocity–time graph (Figure 9.86b) and the equal and opposite vertical velocity at release and landing (Table 9.14). The results also reflect the main characteristic of the flight of a projectile in the absence of air resistance, i.e. the second half of the trajectory (from maximum height to landing) is a mirror image of the first half of the trajectory (from release to maximum height); see Figure 9.86a. Mathematicians refer to this type of curve as a parabola.

Trajectory of a shot

In shot put, the effect of air resistance on the trajectory of the shot is small enough to be regarded as negligible (Lichtenberg and Wills, 1978), i.e. the only force acting on a shot during flight may be considered to be its weight. Therefore, during flight, the horizontal acceleration of the shot may be considered to be zero and the horizontal velocity of the shot may be considered to be constant. Similarly, the vertical acceleration of the shot may be considered to be constant, i.e. the acceleration due to gravity. Provided that some details of the trajectory of the shot or the release conditions of the shot are known, the complete trajectory can be described by applying the equations of uniformly accelerated motion. The actual equations that are used depend upon the variables that need to be quantified. Sometimes only one step (using one equation) is necessary, whereas other calculations may require two or three steps. The guiding principle underlying each calculation is to ensure that the time period under consideration and the direction of motion during the time period are clearly defined at the outset.

The length of a shot put is measured from the inside of a 10 cm high stop-board at the front of the circle to the mark in the landing area closest to the circle (Figure 9.87). As the shot is normally released from a position outside the circle, referred to as the release distance s_d (horizontal displacement of the centre of the shot from the circle), the measured distance s_0 is the sum of s_d and the flight distance s_r (horizontal distance travelled during flight), i.e. $s_0 = s_d + s_r$. The maximum height of the shot during flight s_m (maximum height above the ground) is the sum of the release height s_1 (height of the shot at release) and the flight height s_f (vertical displacement of the shot between release and maximum height), i.e. $s_m = s_1 + s_f$.

The women's shot put at the 1999 World Athletics Championships was won by Astrid Kumbernuss, Germany with a put of 19.85 m. Playback of a video of the put at 25 Hz showed that the flight time was approximately 1.92 s (48 frames × 0.04 s), the release angle was approximately 39° and the release distance was approximately 0.25 m. Using this information, the complete trajectory can be described (Figure 9.87).

Calculate the horizontal component of velocity at release v_h

Consider horizontal motion during flight.

$$s = u \cdot t + \frac{a \cdot t^2}{2},$$
(9.22)

where: $s = s_r = s_0 - s_d = 19.85 \text{ m} - 0.25 \text{ m} = 19.60 \text{ m},$
$u = $ horizontal component of release velocity $= v_h,$
$a = $ horizontal acceleration $= 0,$
$t = $ flight time $= 1.92$ s.

By substitution and rearrangement,

$$19.60 \text{ m} = v_h \times 1.92 \text{ s},$$

i.e. $v_h = \dfrac{19.60 \text{ m}}{1.92 \text{ s}} = 10.21 \text{ m/s}.$

Calculate the vertical component of velocity at release v_v

From Figure 9.86,

$$\frac{v_v}{v_h} = \tan \theta,$$

where $v_h = 10.21$ m/s and $\theta = 39°$,
i.e. $v_v = v_h \cdot \tan \theta = 10.21 \text{ m/s} \times 0.8098 = 8.27 \text{ m/s}.$

Calculate release height s_l

Consider vertical motion during flight.

$$s = u \cdot t + \frac{a \cdot t^2}{2}.$$ (9.22)

where: $s = s_l$,

$u = v_v$ = vertical component of release velocity = 8.27 m/s,

a = vertical acceleration = -9.81 m/s^2,

t = flight time = 1.92 s.

By substitution and rearrangement,

$$s_l = (8.27 \times 1.92) + \frac{(-9.81 \times 1.92^2)}{2} = 15.87 - 18.08 = -2.21 \text{ m}.$$

The negative result indicates, as expected, that the point where the shot landed was below the release point, i.e. a vertical displacement of 2.21 m below the release point.

Calculate flight height s_f

Consider vertical motion from release to maximum height.

$$v^2 - u^2 = 2a \cdot s$$ (9.23)

where: $s = s_f$,

$u = v_v$ = vertical component of release velocity = 8.27 m/s,

v = vertical velocity at maximum height = 0,

a = vertical acceleration = -9.81 m/s^2.

By substitution and rearrangement,

$$0 - (8.27)^2 = -19.62 \times s_f$$

$$s_f = \frac{(8.27)^2}{19.62} = 3.48 \text{ m}.$$

Calculate maximum height s_m

$$s_m = s_l + s_f = 2.21 \text{ m} + 3.48 \text{ m} = 5.69 \text{ m}.$$

v_v, v_h and flight time were used to calculate the horizontal and vertical displacement of the shot at 0.2 s intervals (Table 9.15). These data were used to plot the trajectory of the shot shown in Figure 9.87.

For a projectile launched from ground level and landing at ground level, the optimum release angle to maximise range is 45° (Figure 9.85b). However, a shot is released from above

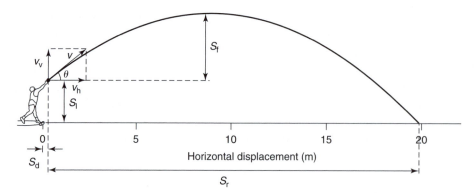

Figure 9.87 Trajectory of a shot put: s_d, release distance; s_i, release height; s_r, flight distance; s_f, flight height; v_i release velocity; v_h, horizontal component of release velocity; v_v, vertical component of release velocity; the data used to plot the trajectory are shown in Table 9.15.

Table 9.15 Horizontal velocity, horizontal displacement, vertical velocity and vertical displacement of a shot during flight at 0.2 s intervals: release velocity = 13.14 m/s; release angle = 39°; flight time = 1.92 s; release height = 2.21 m; release distance = 0.25 m.

Time (s)	Horizontal velocity (m/s)	Horizontal displacement (m)	Vertical velocity (m/s)	Vertical displacement (m)
0	10.21	0.25	8.27	2.21
0.2	10.21	2.29	6.31	3.67
0.4	10.21	4.33	4.35	4.73
0.6	10.21	6.38	2.38	5.41
0.8	10.21	8.42	0.42	5.69
1.0	10.21	10.46	−1.54	5.58
1.2	10.21	12.50	−3.50	5.07
1.4	10.21	14.54	−5.46	4.17
1.6	10.21	16.59	−7.43	2.89
1.8	10.21	18.63	−9.39	1.20
1.92	10.21	19.85	−10.56	0

Flight time, calculated from Equation 9.22, by consideration of vertical motion; horizontal velocity, constant; horizontal displacement, calculated from Equation 9.22 by consideration of horizontal motion; vertical velocity, calculated from Equation 9.20, by consideration of vertical motion; vertical displacement, calculated from Equation 9.22 by consideration of vertical motion.

ground level such that the optimal release angle is less than 45° (Lichtenberg and Wills 1978). Application of the equations of uniformly accelerated motion indicate that for a fixed release speed and fixed release height, the optimal release angle is approximately 42°. For example, Figure 9.88 shows the relationship between release angle, flight time and range for a release velocity of 13.14 m/s and release height of 2.21 m (as in the put by Astrid Kumbernuss in Figure 9.87). The data corresponding to Figure 9.88 are shown in Table 9.16. Figure 9.88 indicates that maximum range (19.68 m) would be achieved with a release angle of 42°. However, the predicted relationships in Figure 9.88 are based on the assumption that release

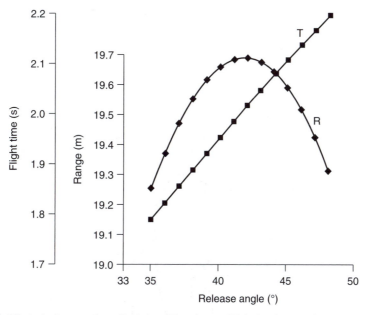

Figure 9.88 Effect of release angle on flight time (T) and range (R) in the absence of air resistance for a shot with release velocity of 13.14 m/s and release height of 2.21 m. The data used to plot the graphs are shown in Table 9.16.

Table 9.16 Effect of release angle on flight time and range for a shot with a release velocity of 13.14 m/s and release height of 2.21 m in the absence of air resistance.

Angle (°)	Flight time (s)	Range (m)
35	1.79	19.25
36	1.82	19.37
37	1.85	19.46
38	1.89	19.55
39	1.92	19.61
40	1.95	19.65
41	1.98	19.68
42	2.02	19.68
43	2.05	19.67
44	2.08	19.64
45	2.11	19.58
46	2.14	19.51
47	2.17	19.42
48	2.19	19.30

speed, release height and release angle are independent of each other, i.e. changing one variable will not change the others. However, analysis of actual puts by elite athletes has shown
that the three variables are not independent (Matheras 1998; Linthorne 2001). As the release
angle or release height are increased above the optimum (for maximum range) for an athlete,
the release speed that the athlete can produce decreases which results in reduced range.

The range of release angles exhibited by elite shot putters is 26°–45° with an average of
37° (Susanka and Stepanek 1988; Tsirakos *et al*; 1995). Release speed is the most important
determinant of range. It is reasonable to assume that through extensive training and practice, elite shot putters optimise their anthropometric (including height and arm length) and
musculoskeletal (including strength and power) attributes in order to maximise the impulse
of the propulsive thrust exerted on the shot and therefore maximise the release velocity of
the shot. For most athletes, this appears to be associated with a release angle in the region
of 37°.

Effect of air resistance on the range of a shot put

In the example of the shot put by Astrid Kumbernuss, the horizontal component of velocity
at release was estimated to be 10.21 m/s. Consequently, using Equation 9.24 and the data in
Table 9.11 for coefficient of drag (0.45), density of air (1.25 kg/m^3), area (82.51 cm^2), the
horizontal component of air resistance on the shot just after release is estimated to be 0.24 N,
resulting in a horizontal deceleration of the shot of approximately 0.06 m/s^2. The vertical
component of air resistance on the shot would retard the upward movement of the shot (from
release to maximum height) and would also retard the downward movement of the shot (from
maximum height to landing) such that the effect on flight time can be regarded as negligible.
Consequently, the effect of the horizontal component of air resistance on the range of the shot
can be estimated as follows.

Calculate the horizontal velocity of the shot on landing v₁

$$v = u + a \cdot t, \tag{9.20}$$

where: $v = v_1,$
u = horizontal velocity of the shot at release = 10.21 m/s,
$a = -0.06$ m/s^2,
t = flight time = 1.92 s.

By substitution,

$$v_1 = 10.21 - (0.06 \times 1.92) = 10.094 \text{ m/s}.$$

Calculate range

$$s = \frac{u + v}{2} \cdot t, \tag{9.21}$$

where: s = range

u = horizontal velocity of the shot at release = 10.21 m/s,

$v = v_1$ = horizontal velocity of the shot on landing = 10.094 m/s,

t = flight time = 1.92 s.

By substitution,

$$s = \frac{10.21 + 10.094}{2} \times 1.92 = 19.49 \text{ m.}$$

Consequently, air resistance is estimated to reduce the range of the shot by about 0.11 m (4¼ in) from 19.60 m (64 ft 3½ in) to 19.49 m (63 ft 11¼ in). This estimation is in agreement with Lichtenberg and Wills (1978), who estimated that air resistance reduces a 73 ft (22.25 m) shot put by a male athlete by about 6 in (0.15 m) in still air.

Variation in wind speed and direction will affect relative velocity and, therefore, the amount of air resistance acting on a shot during flight (Equation 9.24). Whereas the effect of such wind variation on the trajectory of a shot is likely to be very small, the result of a competition, which might be decided by a few centimetres, could, theoretically, be affected by marked differences in wind speed or direction between throws.

Trajectory of a long jumper

As in shot put, the effect of air resistance on the trajectory of the centre of gravity of a long jumper is likely to be very small, largely because the duration of flight is so short, i.e. less than one second (Ward-Smith 1985). A long jump is measured as the perpendicular distance from the front edge of the take-off board to the nearest mark in the sand made by the jumper on landing. The surface of the sand in the landing area should be level with the top of the take-off board. The centre of gravity of the jumper is usually in front of the front edge of the board at take-off, referred to as the take-off distance s_d, and behind the feet on landing, referred to as the landing distance s_l. Consequently, the measured distance s_0 is the sum of s_d, s_l and the flight distance s_r (horizontal distance travelled during flight), i.e. $s_0 = s_d + s_r + s_l$ (Figure 9.89). The maximum height of the centre of gravity during flight s_m is the sum of the take-off height s_t (height of the centre of gravity at take-off) and the flight height s_f (vertical displacement of the centre of gravity between take-off and maximum height), i.e. $s_m = s_t + s_f$. On landing, the centre of gravity is above as well as behind the heels. The height of the centre of gravity on landing is referred to as the landing height s_n. The relative height of the centre of gravity $s_v = s_t - s_n$, i.e. the vertical distance between the positions of the centre of gravity at take-off and landing.

The men's long jump at the 1983 USA Track and Field Championships was won by Carl Lewis with a jump of 8.79 m (Hay et al. 1986). The jump was made up of take-off, flight and landing distances of 0.46 m, 7.77 m and 0.56 m, respectively, and the vertical v_v and horizontal v_h components of velocity at take-off were 3.2 m/s and 9.5 m/s, respectively. The height of the centre of gravity at take-off s_t was 1.33 m. Using this information, the complete trajectory of the jump can be described, as shown in Figure 9.89.

327

Calculate flight time t_f

Consider horizontal motion during flight.

$$s = u \cdot t + \frac{a \cdot t^2}{2}.$$

(9.22)

where: $s = s_r = 7.77$ m,
  $u = v_h = 9.5$ m/s,
  $a =$ horizontal acceleration $= 0$,
  $t = t_f$.

By substitution,

$$7.77 = 9.5 \times t_f,$$

i.e.   flight time $t_f = \dfrac{7.77}{9.5} = 0.818$ s.

Calculate the landing height s_n

Consider vertical motion during flight.

$$s = u \cdot t + \frac{a \cdot t^2}{2}.$$

(9.22)

where: $s = s_v$,
  $u = v_v = 3.2$ m/s,
  $a = -9.81$ m/s^2,
  $t = t_f = 0.818$ s.

By substitution,

$$s_v = (3.2 \times 0.818) + \frac{(-9.81 \times 0.818^2)}{2}$$

$$s_v = 2.62 - 3.28 = -0.66 \text{ m}.$$

The negative result indicates, as expected, that the position of the centre of gravity on landing was below its position at take-off, i.e. there is a vertical displacement of 0.66 m below its position at the take-off point. As $s_v = s_t - s_n$, then,

$$s_n = s_t - s_v = 1.33 \text{ m} - 0.66 \text{ m} = 0.67 \text{ m},$$

i.e. the landing height $s_n = 0.67$ m.

Calculate flight height s_f

Consider vertical motion from take-off to maximum height.

$$v^2 - u^2 = 2a \cdot s, \tag{9.23}$$

where: $s = s_f$,

$u = v_v = 3.2$ m/s,

v = vertical velocity at maximum height = 0,

$a = -9.81$ m/s^2.

By substitution and rearrangement,

$$0 - 3.2^2 = -19.62 \times s_f$$

$$s_f = \frac{3.2^2}{19.62} = 0.52 \text{ m},$$

i.e. flight height $s_f = 0.52$ m.

Calculate maximum height s_m

$$s_m = s_t + s_f = 1.33 \text{ m} + 0.52 \text{ m} = 1.85 \text{ m}.$$

v_v, v_h and flight time were used to calculate the horizontal and vertical displacement of the centre of gravity at 0.1 s intervals (Table 9.17). These data were used to plot the trajectory of the centre of gravity shown in Figure 9.89.

The height of the centre of gravity of a long jumper at take-off is higher than on landing. Consequently, the optimal release angle for maximum range is less than 45° (Linthorne *et al.* 2005). Application of the equations of uniformly accelerated motion indicates that for a fixed take-off speed of 10.02 m/s and fixed relative height of −0.66 m, as in the jump by Carl Lewis

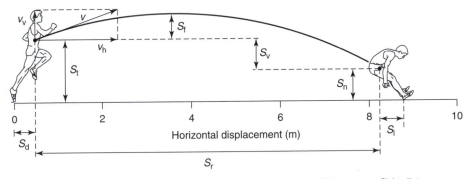

Figure 9.89 Trajectory of the centre of gravity of a long jumper: s_d, take-off distance; s_f, flight distance; s_l, landing distance; s_t, take-off height; s_f, flight height; s_n, landing height; v_i, take-off velocity; v_h, horizontal component of take-off velocity; v_v, vertical component of take-off velocity. The data used to plot the trajectory are shown in Table 9.17.

Table 9.17 Horizontal velocity, horizontal displacement, vertical velocity and vertical displacement of the centre of gravity of a long jumper during flight at 0.1 s intervals: take-off velocity = 10.02 m/s; take-off angle = 18.6°; flight time = 0.818 s; take-off height = 1.33 m; take-off distance = 0.46 m.

Time (s)	Horizontal velocity (m/s)	Horizontal displacement (m)	Vertical velocity (m/s)	Vertical displacement (m)
0	9.5	0.46	3.20	1.33
0.1	9.5	1.41	2.22	1.60
0.2	9.5	2.36	1.24	1.77
0.3	9.5	3.31	0.26	1.85
0.4	9.5	4.26	−0.72	1.82
0.5	9.5	5.21	−1.71	1.70
0.6	9.5	6.16	−2.69	1.48
0.7	9.5	7.11	−3.67	1.17
0.8	9.5	8.06	−4.65	0.75
0.818	9.5	8.23	−4.82	0.67

Flight time, calculated from Equation 9.22, by consideration of horizontal motion; horizontal velocity, constant; horizontal displacement, calculated from Equation 9.22, by consideration of horizontal motion; vertical velocity, calculated from Equation 9.20, by consideration of vertical motion; vertical displacement, calculated from Equation 9.22, by consideration of vertical motion.

in Figure 9.89, the optimal take-off angle is approximately 43°. However, the actual take-off angle by Carl Lewis was 18.6°. This is much lower than the predicted optimum angle, but consistent with the 15°–27° range of take-off angles exhibited by elite long jumpers (Hay *et al.* 1986; Lees *et al.* 1993, 1994). There are two main reasons why actual take-off angles are much smaller than predicted optimum angles.

First, release velocity is the most important determinant of flight distance in shot put and long jump (and most other projectiles). Consequently, any variation in technique that reduces take-off velocity will almost certainly reduce flight distance. In order for the take-off angle to be 45°, the vertical component of velocity at take-off would have to be the same as the horizontal component. Even a 43° take-off angle would require the vertical component to be 90% of the horizontal component. However, the maximum vertical velocity that elite long jumpers can achieve at take-off is approximately 3.6 m/s (Hay *et al.* 1986; Lees *et al.*1993). Even elite male high jumpers cannot generate more than about 4.3 m/s at take-off. A take-off angle of 43° with a vertical component of velocity v_v of 3.6 m/s would require a horizontal component v_h of 3.83 m/s and a resultant take-off velocity of 5.28 m/s. This combination of take-off velocity and take-off angle would result in a flight time of 0.88 s and a flight distance of 3.43 m, which is less than half that normally achieved by elite male jumpers. The difference, of course, is due to the much greater horizontal component of velocity generated by elite jumpers. Whereas the range of vertical velocity at take-off in elite long jumpers is approximately 2.4 m/s to 3.6 m/s in women and 3.0 m/s to 3.6 m/s in men, the range of horizontal velocity at take-off is approximately 7.2 m/s to 8.6 m/s in women and 8.5 m/s to 9.5 m/s in men (Hay *et al.* 1986; Lees *et al.* 1993). As the horizontal component is usually more than double the vertical component, the take-off angle is usually in the range 15°–27°. The small take-off angle is more than compensated for by the large horizontal component of velocity.

Second, at take-off, a long jumper would ideally like to maximise vertical velocity in order to maximise flight time and, simultaneously, maximise horizontal velocity in order to maximise flight distance. However, as in shot put, take-off velocity, take-off angle and take-off height in long jump are not independent of each other (Linthorne et al. 2005). As the take-off angle or take-off height are increased above the optimum (for maximum range) for a jumper, the take-off speed that the jumper can produce decreases, resulting in reduced range. It is reasonable to assume that through extensive training and practice, elite long jumpers optimise their anthropometric (including height and leg length) and musculoskeletal (including strength and power) attributes in order to achieve the optimal combination of take-off velocity and take-off height that, when properly executed, results in maximum flight distance. For most long jumpers, this appears to be associated with a take-off angle in the range 15°–27°.

Effect of air resistance on flight distance in the long jump

In the above example of the long jump by Carl Lewis, the horizontal component of velocity at take-off was 9.5 m/s. Consequently, using Equation 9.24 and the data in Table 9.11 for coefficient of drag (0.60), density of air (1.25 kg/m³), area (4500 cm²) and mass (85 kg), the horizontal component of air resistance on the jumper during flight is estimated to be 15.23 N, resulting in a horizontal deceleration of 0.18 m/s². The vertical component of air resistance on the jumper would retard upward movement (from take-off to maximum height) and would also retard downward movement (from maximum height to landing), such that the effect on flight time can be regarded as negligible. Consequently, the effect of the horizontal component of air resistance on the flight distance of the jumper can be estimated.

Calculate the horizontal velocity of the jumper on landing v_1

$$v = u + a \cdot t,$$ (9.20)

where: $v = v_1,$
u = horizontal velocity of the jumper at take-off = 9.5 m/s,
$a = -0.18$ m/s²,
t = flight time = 0.818 s.

By substitution,

$$v_1 = 9.5 - (0.18 \times 0.818) = 9.35 \text{ m/s}.$$

Calculate range s_r

$$s = \frac{u + v}{2} \cdot t,$$ (9.21)

331

where: $s = s_r = $ range,

$u = $ horizontal velocity of the jumper at take-off $= 9.5$ m/s,

$v = v_1 = $ horizontal velocity of the jumper on landing $= 9.3$ m/s,

$t = $ flight time $= 0.818$ s.

By substitution,

$$s_r = \frac{(9.5 + 9.35)}{2} \times 0.818 = 7.71 \, \text{m}.$$

Consequently air resistance is estimated to reduce flight distance by about 0.06 m (2½ in) from 7.77 m (25 ft 6 in) to 7.71 m (25 ft 3½ in). Variation in wind speed and direction will affect relative velocity and, therefore, the amount of air resistance acting on a jumper during flight (Equation 9.24). Whereas the effect of such wind variation on the trajectory of a long jumper is likely to be very small, the result of a competition, which might be decided by a few centimetres, could, theoretically, be affected by marked differences in wind speed or direction between jumps.

REVIEW QUESTIONS

Linear kinematics

1. Define or describe the following terms: force, mechanics, biomechanics, forms of motion, linear motion, rectilinear translation, curvilinear translation, distance, speed, linear displacement, linear velocity, linear acceleration, kinematics, kinetics.

2. With regard to human movement, give an example of rectilinear translation and an example of curvilinear translation.

3. A runner completes the first and second laps of an 800 m race (on a 400 m track) in 56 s and 52 s, respectively. Calculate the average speed of the runner in each lap and over the whole race. Record the time, distance and average speed data in Table 9Q.1.

4. Middle-distance runners often train on a treadmill by running at different speeds. Table 9Q.2 shows the leg length and time for 10 strides of an athlete running on a treadmill at speeds of 3.5 m/s and 5.5 m/s. Calculate the stride rate, stride length and relative stride length (with respect to leg length) of the athlete at the two speeds. Record the results in Table 9Q.2.

Table 9Q.1 Average speed in Laps 1 and 2 and in whole race.

Lap	Time (s)	Distance (m)	Average speed (m/s)
1			
2			
Total time			

Table 9Q.2 Leg length and stride parameters at 3.5 m/s and 5.5 m/s.

Leg length (m)	Speed (m/s)	Time for 10 strides (s)	Stride rate (strides/s)	Stride length (m/stride)	Relative stride length
0.9	3.5	6.94			
0.9	5.5	5.80			

5. London Marathon: 18th April 1999
   Women's race: Winners time = 2 h 23 min 21 s
   Men's race: Winner's time = 2 h 7 min 56 s
   Distance = 26 miles 385 yards
   1 mile = 1760 yd
   1 yd = 0.9144 m
   1 m = 1.0936 yd
   1 mile = 1609.34 m

5.1 Use the data provided to complete Tables 9Q.3 and 9Q.4 for distance, time and average speed in the units indicated. (The letter m is the symbol for miles in the British imperial system and for metres in the SI system.)

5.2 Calculate the average speed of the winner of the women's race as a percentage of the average speed of the winner of the men's race.

5.3 Calculate the average time in minutes to complete one mile and one kilometre by the winner of each race. Record the distance, time and average time data in Table 9Q.5.

Table 9Q.3 Distance, time and average speed for the winner of the women's race in different units (winner's time = 2 h 23 min 21 s).

Distance	Time	Average speed
miles (m)	hours (h)	mph
kilometres (km)	hours (h)	km/h
metres (m)	seconds (s)	m/s

Table 9Q.4 Distance, time and average speed for the winner of the men's race in different units (winner's time = 2 h 7 min 56 s).

Distance	Time	Average speed
miles (m)	hours (h)	mph
kilometres (km)	hours (h)	km/h
metres (m)	seconds (s)	m/s

Table 9Q.5 Average time per mile and average time per kilometre for the winners of the women's race and the men's race.

	Distance (miles)	Distance (km)	Winner's time (min)	Per mile (min)	Per km (min)
Women's race					
Men's race					

Table 9Q.6 Units and unit abbreviations.

Variable	Unit	Unit symbol
Force		
Time		
Impulse		
Mass		
Velocity		
Linear momentum		

Linear impulse and linear momentum

6. In Table 9Q.6, list the metric units and their symbols for the variables.

7. If a soccer ball of mass 0.35 kg is at rest and then kicked such that its velocity when it separates from the kicker's foot is 42 m/s (94 mph), calculate the average force exerted on the ball during the kick if the contact time between boot and ball is 0.05 s. Give the force in N, kgf and lbf (1 kgf = 2.2046 lbf).

8. If a golf ball of mass 0.06 kg is at rest on a tee and is then driven such that its velocity when it separates from the club-head is 72 m/s (161 mph), calculate the average force exerted on the ball if the contact time between club-head and ball is 0.0005 s. Give the force in N, kgf, lbf and tons (1 ton = 2240 lbf).

9. In a shot put, if the impulse of the force exerted on the shot (mass = 7.26 kg) in the direction of release velocity is 159.72 N·s, calculate the release velocity of the shot. Assume that the shot was initially at rest.

10. If a gymnast of mass 55 kg lands on the mat following a vault with a downward velocity of 6.2 m/s and comes to rest in 0.2 s, calculate the average vertical force exerted on the gymnast during the landing. Give the force in N, kgf, lbf and body weight (BW).

Vectors

11. Differentiate between vector and scalar quantities.

12. Define the terms sine, cosine and tangent, with respect to a right-angled triangle.

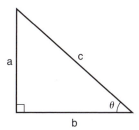

Figure 9Q.1 A right-angled triangle.

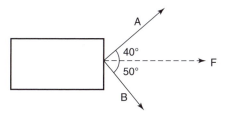

Figure 9Q.2 Resultant of two forces pulling on a box.

13. If the angle θ in Figure 9Q.1 = 40° and the length of side c = 20 cm, calculate the lengths of sides a and b given that cos40° = 0.766 and sin40° = 0.643.

14. In Figure 9Q.2, if the angle between the component force A and the resultant force F is 40° and the angle between the component force B and the resultant force F is 50°, calculate A and B, given that F = 200 N, cos40° = 0.766 and cos50° = 0.643.

15. In Figure 9Q.3, if the force B exerted by the biceps brachii (assuming that this is the only active elbow flexor) = 100 N, calculate the magnitude of the swing S and stabilisation T components, given that sin60° = 0.866 and cos60° = sin30° = 0.5. The swing and stabilisation components are at right angles to each other.

16. Figure 9Q.4 shows the ground reaction force F exerted on a runner at an instant during the propulsion phase together with the X, Y and Z components of F (F_X, F_Y, F_Z). If body weight W = 70 kgf, F_X = 0.8 BW, F_Y = 2.5 BW and F_Z = 0.4 BW, determine the magnitude and direction of:
    i. F_{XY} with respect to the horizontal;
    ii. F_{YZ} with respect to the horizontal;
    iii. F_{XZ} with respect to F_Z;
    iv. F with respect to F_{XZ}.

17. Figure 9Q.5 shows the anteroposterior F_X and vertical F_Y components of the ground reaction force F exerted on an athlete running at 5 m/s.
    i. Use the force–time curves to determine (approximately) the magnitude of F_X and F_Y in Frames 2 and 4 of the stick-figure sequence and record these values in Table 9Q.7. The point of application of the ground reaction force is indicated by the short vertical line underneath each frame.
    ii. Calculate the magnitude and direction (with respect to the horizontal) of the

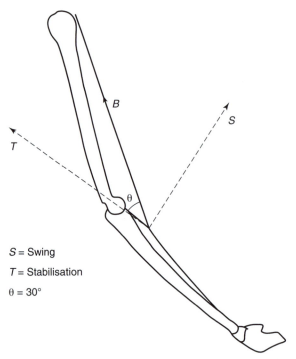

S = Swing

T = Stabilisation

$\theta = 30°$

Figure 9Q.3 Swing S and stabilisation T components of the biceps brachii muscle force.

resultant force F_{XY} (resultant of F_X and F_Y) in Frames 2 and 4. Record the results in Table 9Q.7.

iii. Using a scale of 2 cm = 1 BW (body weight), draw the resultant force F_{XY} in Frames 2 and 4 of the stick-figure sequence.

18. Figure 9Q.6a shows the anterior aspect of the right knee complex, in particular, the quadriceps muscle group. Figure 9Q.6b shows the force vectors for the vastus latera-lis (L), combined rectus femoris and vastus intermedius (F) and vastus medialis (M). Determine the resultant quadriceps force (magnitude and direction) by (i) vector chain method and (ii) calculation.

Ground reaction force

19. Define or describe the following terms: muscle latency, passive load, active load, passive phase, active phase, absorption phase, propulsion phase, stiffness and rate of loading.

20. Figure 9Q.7 shows the anteroposterior F_X and vertical F_Y force–time components of the ground reaction force acting on the right foot of a rear-foot striker (mass = 70 kg) during ground contact while running in running shoes at approximately 3.5 m/s.
    i.   Record the mass and weight of the subject in Table 9Q.8.
    ii. Use the graphs to determine the forces (N) and times (s) corresponding to the vari-ables 1–5 listed in Table 9Q.8. Record the forces and times in Table 9Q.8.

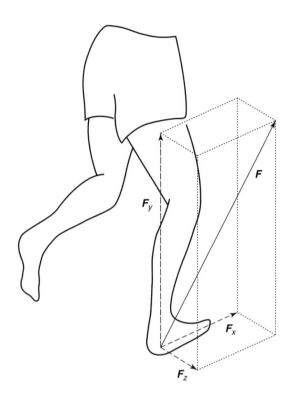

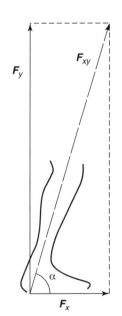

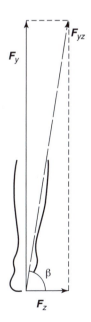

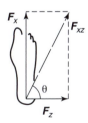

Figure 9Q.4 Ground reaction force components.

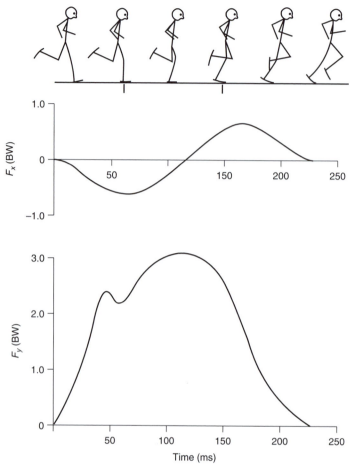

Figure 9Q.5 Force–time graphs of the anteroposterior F_X and vertical F_Y components of the ground reaction force with stick-figure sequence.

Table 9Q.7 Magnitude and direction of F_X, F_Y and F_{XY}.

	Frame 2	Frame 4
F_X (BW)		
F_Y (BW)		
F_{XY} (BW)		
F_{XY} (°)		

iii. Calculate the forces in units of body weight (BW) and record the forces in Table 9Q.8.

iv. Using the time data in Table 9Q.8 for points 1–5, calculate and record the time variables 6–10 in Table 9Q.8.

v. Calculate and record in Table 9Q.8 the rate of loading (L_R) during impact in N/s and BW/s.

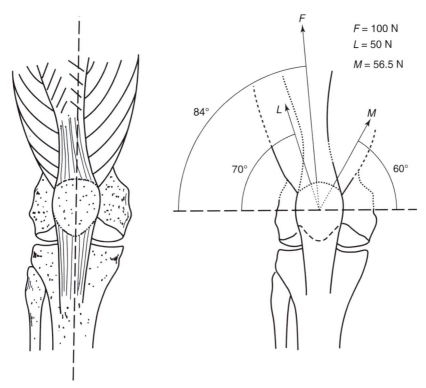

Figure 9Q.6 Force components of the quadriceps muscle group.

Uniformly accelerated motion

In all of the questions, assume that the effect of air resistance is negligible.

21. A high jumper takes off with an upward vertical velocity of 4.2 m/s. Calculate:
    i.   How high his centre of gravity rises from take-off to maximum height;
    ii. The length of time from take-off to the maximum height.

22. During the upward propulsion phase of take-off (upward velocity at the start of the propulsion phase = 0), the net upward impulse on a high jumper of mass 60 kg is 246 N·s. Calculate how high the jumper's centre of gravity rises from take-off to maximum height.

23. A stone is dropped from a height of 150 m. Calculate the time it takes for the stone to hit the ground and the velocity of the stone as it hits the ground.

24. A ball is thrown upward with a release velocity of 10 m/s from a release height of 2 m. Use the convention that upward is positive and downward is negative to:
    i.   Complete Table 9Q.9 to show the velocity and displacement of the ball at 0.2 s intervals and on landing.
    ii. Plot the displacement–time and velocity–time graphs of the motion of the ball.

339

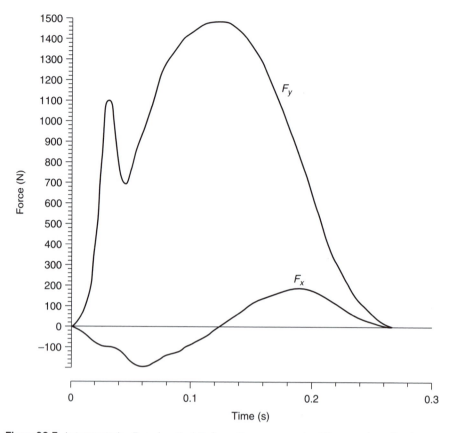

Figure 9Q.7 Anteroposterior F_x and vertical F_y force–time components of the ground reaction force acting on the right foot of a rear-foot striker.

(Suggestion: use a spreadsheet program such as Microsoft Excel to calculate and plot the data.)

25. A shot putter releases the shot from a height of 2.1 m with a velocity of 12.5 m/s at a release angle of 38° with respect to the horizontal. Calculate the range of the put, the maximum height of the shot during its trajectory and the impulse responsible for the release velocity.

Table 9Q.8 Analysis of the vertical component (F_Y–time) of the ground reaction force acting on the right foot of the subject during contact time in running.

Name of subject:			
		Mass (kg)	Weight (N)
Mass and weight of subject			

Key points on F_Y–time graph	Time (s)	Force (N)	Force (BW)
1. Heel contact (t_1, F_{Y1})		0	0
2. Impact force peak (t_2, F_{Y2})			
3. End of the passive phase (minimum force following impact force peak) (t_3, F_{Y3})			
4. End of absorption phase (t_4, F_{Y4}) (when $F_X = 0$)			
5. Toe-off (t_5, F_{Y5})		0	0

	Time (s)	Proportion of contact time (%)
6. Contact time ($t_5 - t_1$)		100
7. Time to impact force peak ($t_2 - t_1$)		
8. Duration of passive phase ($t_3 - t_1$)		
9. Duration of absorption phase ($t_4 - t_1$)		
10. Duration of propulsion phase ($t_5 - t_4$)		

	L_R (N/s)	L_R (BW/s)
Rate of loading (L_R) during impact ($F_{Y2}/(t_2 - t_1)$)		

Table 9Q.9 Displacement and velocity of a ball thrown upward with a release velocity of 10 m/s from a release height of 2 m.

Time into flight (s)	Velocity (m/s)	Displacement (m)
0	10.0	2.0
0.2		
0.4		
0.6		
0.8		
1.0		
1.2		
1.4		
1.6		
1.8		
2.0		
2.2		
2.222		

Angular motion

Newton's laws of motion apply to angular motion as well as linear motion. The purpose of this chapter is to describe the fundamental mechanical concepts underlying the study of angular motion, in particular, the turning effect of a force, angular impulse and angular momentum.

OBJECTIVES

After reading this chapter, you should be able to do the following:

1. Differentiate angular kinematics and angular kinetics.
2. Describe the various methods of determining the location of the centre of gravity of the human body.
3. Describe the relationship between muscle forces, external forces and joint reaction forces in human movements.
4. Differentiate centripetal force and centrifugal force.
5. Differentiate concentric force, eccentric force and couple.
6. Describe the relationship between angular impulse and angular momentum.
7. Describe the ways in which twist can be generated in aerial movements.

MOMENT OF A FORCE

Consider a rectangular block of wood resting on a table, as shown in Figure 10.1a. The centre of gravity of the block of wood is located at its geometric centre and the line of

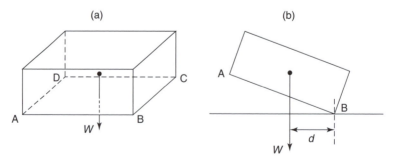

Figure 10.1 Turning moment of a force. (a) Block of wood at rest on base of support ABCD. (b) Turning moment $W \cdot d$ of the weight of the block W, tending to restore to the block to its original resting position after being tilted over on edge BC: d, moment arm of W about edge BC.

action of its weight intersects the base of support ABCD. If the block is tilted over onto one of the edges of the base of support, such as the edge BC, as in Figure 10.1b, the weight of the block W will tend to rotate the block about the supporting edge back to its original resting position in Figure 10.1a. The tendency to restore the block to its original position is the result of the moment (or turning moment) of W about the axis of rotation BC. The magnitude of the moment of W about the axis BC is equal to the product of W and the perpendicular distance d between the axis BC and the line of action of W (Figure 10.1b), i.e.

moment of W about axis BC $= W{\cdot}d$ (W multiplied by d).

If $W = 2$ kgf and $d = 0.1$ m, then

moment of W about axis BC $= 2$ kgf $\times 0.1$ m $= 0.2$ kgf·m.

As 2 kgf $= 19.62$ N, then

moment of W about axis BC $= 19.62$ N $\times 0.1$ m $= 1.962$ N·m.

The N·m (newton metre) is the unit of moment of force in the SI system (Table 8.1).

In general, when a force F acting on an object rotates or tends to rotate the object about some specified axis, the moment of F is defined as the product of F and the perpendicular distance d between the axis of rotation and the line of action of F, i.e. moment of $F = F{\cdot}d$. The axis of rotation is often referred to as the fulcrum and the perpendicular distance between the line of action of the force and the axis of rotation is usually referred to as the moment arm of the force. The moment of a force is sometimes referred to as torque. For a given moment of force, the greater the force, the smaller the moment arm of the force, and vice versa. For example, in trying to push open a heavy door, much less force will be required if the force is applied to the side of the door farthest away from the hinges, i.e. a large moment arm, than if the force is applied to the door close to the hinges, i.e. a small moment arm (Figure 10.2).

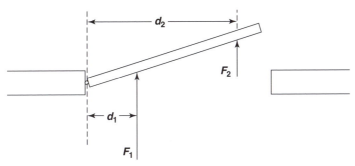

Figure 10.2 Effect of length of moment arm on magnitude of force needed to produce a particular moment of force to open a door. $F_1{\cdot}d_1 = F_2{\cdot}d_2$. If $d_2 = 3d_1$, then $F_1 = 3F_2$.

> The moment of a force is the product of the magnitude of the force and the perpendicular distance between the line of action of the force and the axis of rotation.

Clockwise and anticlockwise moments

When an object is acted upon by two or more forces that tend to rotate the object, the actual amount and speed of rotation that occurs will depend upon the resultant moment acting on the object, i.e. the resultant of all the individual moments. For example, consider two boys A and B sitting on a see-saw S, as shown in Figure 10.3. A see-saw is normally constructed so that its centre of gravity coincides with the fulcrum, i.e. in any position, the line of action of its weight will pass through the fulcrum and, therefore, the weight of the see-saw will not exert a turning moment on the see-saw, since the moment arm of its weight about the fulcrum will be zero. Consequently, in Figure 10.3 the only moments tending to rotate the see-saw will be those exerted by the weights of the two boys. The weight of A will exert an anticlockwise moment $W_A \times d_A$ and the weight of B will exert a clockwise moment $W_B \times d_B$. When $W_A \times d_A$ is greater than $W_B \times d_B$, there will be a resultant anticlockwise moment acting on the see-saw, such that B will be lifted as A descends. When $W_A \times d_A$ is equal to $W_B \times d_B$, i.e. when the clockwise moment is equal to the anticlockwise moment, the resultant moment acting on the see-saw will be zero and the see-saw will not rotate in either direction, but remain perfectly still in a balanced position. Consequently, if the weight of one of the boys is known, the weight of the other boy can be found by balancing the see-saw with one boy on each side of the fulcrum with both boys off the floor and then equating the clockwise and anticlockwise moments. For example, if $W_A = 40$ kgf and in the balanced position $d_A = 1.5$ m and $d_B = 2.0$ m, then by equating moments about the fulcrum,

anticlockwise moments (ACM) = clockwise moments (CM)

$$40 \text{ kgf} \times 1.5 \text{ m} = W_B \times 2.0 \text{ m}$$

$$W_B = \frac{40 \text{ kgf} \times 1.5 \text{ m}}{2.0 \text{ m}} = 30 \text{ kgf.}$$

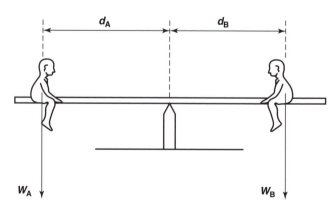

Figure 10.3 Two boys sitting on a see-saw: W_A, weight of boy A; W_B, weight of boy B; d_A, moment arm of W_A; d_B, moment arm of W_B.

> When an object is acted upon by two or more forces that tend to rotate the object, the amount and speed of rotation that occurs will depend upon the resultant moment.

The location of the joint centre of gravity of two masses

To balance an object on a knife-edge support, it is necessary to position the object so that its centre of gravity lies in the vertical plane through the knife-edge support. Therefore, in the example of the see-saw, when the see-saw is in a balanced position with both boys off the floor, the centre of gravity of the composite body consisting of the see-saw and the two boys must lie in the vertical plane through the fulcrum. However, as the centre of gravity of the see-saw coincides with the fulcrum in all positions of the see-saw, it follows that the joint centre of gravity of the two boys, i.e. the point at which the combined weight of the two boys can be considered to act, must also lie in the vertical plane through the fulcrum, otherwise the see-saw would rotate as a result of a non-zero resultant moment.

If boy A sat farther away from the fulcrum, such that $d_A = 2.25$ m, and boy B moved farther away from the fulcrum, in order to balance the see-saw, d_B could be found by equating the clockwise and anticlockwise moments as before, i.e.

$$W_A = 40 \text{ kgf}$$
$$W_B = 30 \text{ kgf}$$
$$d_A = 2.25 \text{ m}$$
$$ACM = CM$$
$$40 \text{ kgf} \times 2.25 \text{ m} = 30 \text{ kgf} \times d_B$$
$$d_B = \frac{40 \text{ kgf} \times 2.25 \text{ m}}{30 \text{ kgf}} = 3.0 \text{ m}.$$

In each of these examples, the see-saw was in a balanced position, i.e. the joint centre of gravity of the two boys was directly above the fulcrum when,

$$W_A \times d_A = W_B \times d_B$$

$$\frac{W_A}{W_B} = \frac{d_B}{d_A}.$$

Therefore, whatever the distance between the centre of gravity of boy A and the centre of gravity of boy B, the ratio of the moment arms of the weights of the two boys about their joint centre of gravity will remain constant. In the first example,

$$\frac{d_A}{d_B} = \frac{2.0}{1.5} = 1.333.$$

In the second example,

$$\frac{d_B}{d_A} = \frac{3.0}{2.25} = 1.333.$$

345

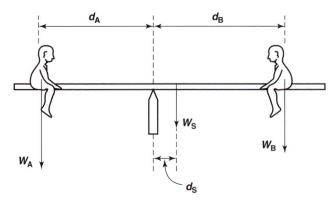

Figure 10.4 Two boys sitting on a see-saw in a balanced position with the centre of gravity of the see-saw located a distance to the right of the fulcrum: W_A, weight of boy A = 40 kgf; d_A, moment arm of W_A = 1.25 m; W_S, weight of see-saw = 20 kgf; d_S, moment arm of W_S = 0.25 m; W_B, weight of boy B; d_B, moment arm of W_B = 1.5 m.

For any two weights W_1 and W_2, the ratio of their moment arms d_1 and d_2 about their joint centre of gravity will be constant, i.e.

$$\frac{W_1}{W_2} = \frac{d_2}{d_1} = \text{a constant value.} \tag{10.1}$$

In these examples, it was not necessary to involve the weight of the see-saw in the calculations, as it had no moment about the fulcrum. However, provided that both the weight of the see-saw and the position of its centre of gravity are known, the weight of boy B could be found by balancing the see-saw, with one boy each side of the fulcrum, about any point on its length and then equating the clockwise and anticlockwise moments as before. For example, Figure 10.4 shows the see-saw in a balanced position with the centre of gravity of the see-saw located a distance of 0.25 m to the right of the fulcrum. By equating the anticlockwise and clockwise moments,

$$W_A \times d_A = (W_S \times d_S) + (W_B \times d_B),$$

where W_S = weight of the see-saw = 20 kgf
and d_S = moment arm of W_S about the fulcrum = 0.25 m.

If W_A = 40 kgf, d_A = 1.25 m and d_B = 1.5 m, then

$$40 \text{ kgf} \times 1.25 \text{ m} = (20 \text{ kgf} \times 0.25 \text{ m}) + (W_B \times 1.5 \text{ m})$$

$$50 \text{ kgf·m} = 5 \text{ kgf·m} + (1.5 \times W_B) \text{ kgf·m}$$

$$W_B = \frac{45 \text{ kgf·m}}{1.5 \text{m}} = 30 \text{ kgf.}$$

In this example, the total clockwise moment was the sum of two component moments, i.e. the moment of W_S and the moment of W_B. The total clockwise moment could be exerted by a

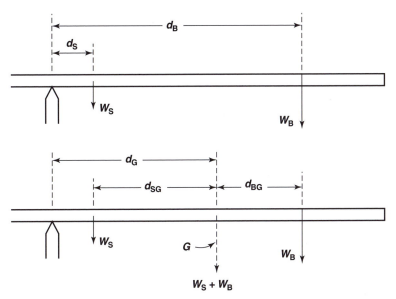

Figure 10.5 Location of joint centre of gravity of two masses: W_S, weight of see-saw; W_B, weight of boy B; G, vertical plane containing joint centre of gravity of see-saw and boy B; d_{SG}, moment arm of W_S about joint centre of gravity of see-saw and boy B; d_{BG}, moment arm of W_B about joint centre of gravity of see-saw and boy B; d_G, moment arm of joint centre of gravity of see-saw and boy B about fulcrum.

force equal to $W_S + W_B$ acting at the joint centre of gravity of S and B. For example, consider the plane containing the joint centre of gravity of S and B, as shown in Figure 10.5. From Equation 10.1,

$$\frac{W_S}{W_B} = \frac{d_{BG}}{d_{SG}},$$

where d_{BG} = moment arm of W_B about the joint centre of gravity of S and B,
d_{SG} = moment arm of W_S about the joint centre of gravity of S and B.

As $W_S = 20$ kgf and $W_B = 30$ kgf, it follows that

$$\frac{d_{BG}}{d_{SG}} = \frac{2}{3},$$

i.e. $d_{BG} = \dfrac{2 \times d_{SG}}{3}.$ (10.2)

From Figure 10.5,

$d_B = d_S + d_{SG} + d_{BG}$
i.e. $d_{SG} + d_{BG} = d_B - d_S = 1.5 \text{ m} - 0.25 \text{ m} = 1.25 \text{ m}$ (10.3)

From Equations 10.2 and 10.3,

$$d_{SG} + \frac{2 \times d_{SG}}{3} = 1.25 \text{ m},$$

i.e. $d_{SG} = 0.75$ m.

From Figure 10.5,

$$d_G = d_S + d_{SG} = 0.25 \text{ m} + 0.75 \text{ m} = 1.0 \text{ m}.$$

Therefore the joint moment of $W_S + W_B$ is given by

$$(W_S + W_B) \times d_G = 50 \text{ kgf} \times 1.0 \text{ m} = 50 \text{ kgf·m}.$$

This is the same as the sum of the moments of W_S and W_B, i.e.

$$(W_S \times d_S) + (W_B \times d_B) = (20 \text{ kgf} \times 0.25 \text{ m}) + (30 \text{ kgf} \times 1.5 \text{ m}) = 50 \text{ kgf·m}.$$

Therefore, the sum of the moments of W_S and W_B is equivalent to the moment exerted by a single force of magnitude $W_S + W_B$ acting at the joint centre of gravity of S and B. This is an illustration of the principle of moments, i.e. the moment of the resultant of any number of forces about any axis is equal to the algebraic sum of the moments of the individual forces about the same axis. When all of the forces are weights, such as the weights of the segments of the human body, the sum of the moments of the weights about any particular axis is equal to the moment of the total body weight acting at the whole body centre of gravity. As will be described shortly, this principle is used to determine the location of the whole body centre of gravity in biomechanical analysis.

Two conditions for a state of equilibrium

In the situations illustrated in Figures 10.3 and 10.4, the see-saw is in equilibrium, i.e. when in a balanced position, the resultant force on the see-saw is zero. Consequently, the resultant downward force on the see-saw, i.e. the weights of the see-saw and the two boys, must be counteracted by one or more forces whose resultant is equal and opposite to the weights of the see-saw and the two boys. In the case of the see-saw, the counteracting force is a single force R exerted by the see-saw support through the fulcrum. Figure 10.6 shows the free body diagrams for the see-saw in the situations illustrated in Figure 10.3 and Figure 10.4, respectively. As $W_A = 40$ kgf, $W_B = 30$ kgf and $W_S = 20$ kgf, then $R = W_A + W_B + W_S = 90$ kgf.

With regard to linear motion, an object is in equilibrium when the resultant force acting on the object is zero. With regard to angular motion, an object is in equilibrium when the resultant moment acting on the object is zero. Both conditions, zero resultant force and zero resultant moment, are illustrated in the see-saw examples in Figures 10.3 and 10.4.

When the resultant moment of the forces acting on an object is zero, the sum of the clockwise and anticlockwise moments will be zero with respect to any reference axis of rotation.

348

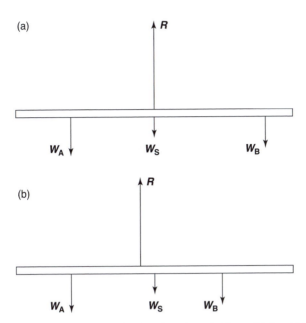

Figure 10.6 Free body diagrams of see-saw in the situations shown in Figures 10.3 and 10.4, respectively: W_A, weight of boy A; W_S, weight of see-saw; W_B, weight of boy B; R, force exerted by see-saw support on see-saw; in both cases, $R = W_A + W_S + W_B$.

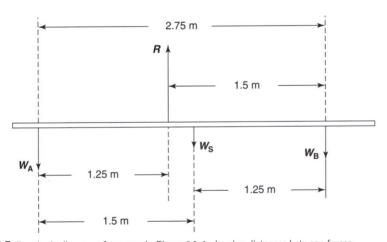

Figure 10.7 Free body diagram of see-saw in Figure 10.4, showing distances between forces.

For example, consider the forces acting on the see-saw, as shown in Figure 10.6b, and redrawn showing the distances between the individual forces in Figure 10.7. By taking moments about a horizontal axis (perpendicular to the plane of Figure 10.7) through the point of application of W_A,

CM = ACM

$(W_S \times 1.5 \text{ m}) + (W_B \times 2.75 \text{ m}) = R \times 1.25 \text{ m}$

As $W_S = 20$ kgf and $W_B = 30$ kgf, then

$$R = \frac{(20 \text{ kgf} \times 1.5 \text{ m}) + (30 \text{ kgf} \times 2.75 \text{ m})}{1.25 \text{ m}}$$

$$R = \frac{112.5 \text{ kgf} \cdot \text{m}}{1.25 \text{ m}} = 90 \text{ kgf.}$$

Alternatively, by taking moments about a horizontal axis (perpendicular to the plane of Figure 10.7) through the point of application of W_B,

CM = ACM

$R \times 1.5 \text{ m} = (W_S \times 1.25 \text{ m}) + (W_A \times 2.75 \text{ m})$

$$R = \frac{(20 \text{ kgf} \times 1.25 \text{ m}) + (40 \text{ kgf} \times 2.75 \text{ m})}{1.5 \text{ m}}$$

$$R = \frac{135 \text{ kgf} \cdot \text{m}}{1.5 \text{ m}} = 90 \text{ kgf.}$$

> The moment of the resultant of any number of forces about any axis is equal to the algebraic sum of the moments of the individual forces about the same axis. This is referred to as the principle of moments.

LOCATION OF THE CENTRE OF GRAVITY OF THE HUMAN BODY

In all movements, the movement of the centre of gravity of the body and, therefore, the movement of the body as a whole, is determined by the impulse of the resultant force acting on the body during the movement. For example, in a long jump, take-off velocity is determined by the velocity of the centre of gravity generated in the run-up and the impulse of the resultant force acting on the centre of gravity during the period from touch-down to take-off (Figure 10.8). Provided that the velocity of the jumper at the instance of touch-down is known and the components of the ground reaction force are recorded from touch-down to take-off, the take-off velocity of the jumper can be determined from the impulse of the resultant force acting on the jumper from touch-down to take-off. However, force platforms are not usually available. Furthermore, the position of the centre of gravity at take-off (take-off height and take-off distance in Figure 9.89) as well as the take-off velocity would be needed in order to describe the trajectory of the centre of gravity during flight. In such situations, the position of the centre of gravity (take-off height and take-off distance) and velocity of the centre of gravity at take-off are determined from the distance–time graph of the movement of the centre of gravity (as described in the section on linear kinematics of a 100 m sprint in Chapter 9). To produce a distance–time graph of the movement of the centre of gravity, it is necessary to locate the position of the centre of gravity in each video frame of the movement under consideration. There are two approaches to determining the position of the centre of gravity of the human body, the direct (whole body) approach, in which the body is considered

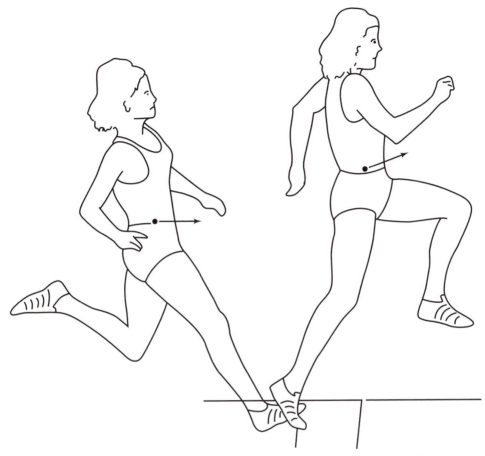

Figure 10.8 Position and velocity of whole body centre of gravity of female long jumper at touch-down and take-off: velocity vectors based on mean data in Lees *et al.* (1993).

as a whole and the indirect (segmental) approach, in which the body is considered to consist of a number of segments (Hay 1973). In both approaches, the position of the centre of gravity is determined from the intersection of three non-parallel planes that contain the centre of gravity.

Direct approach

There are, theoretically, three direct methods of determining the position of the centre of gravity of the human body: suspension, balancing and the use of a reaction board (equating the moment of the weight of the body about a horizontal support). The suspension method was described in Chapter 9 (Figures 9.18 and 9.19) and simply involves suspending the body from at least three points and noting the point of intersection of the lines of action of the weight of the body in the different positions. However, this method is impractical with regard to the human body, as it would be difficult to suspend the body from three or more positions while the subject maintained the required body posture.

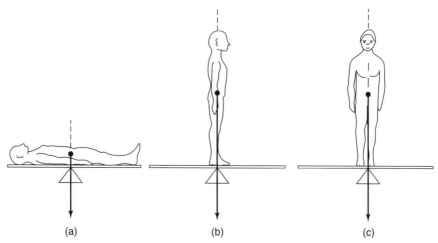

(a)   (b)   (c)

Figure 10.9 Method to determine position of centre of gravity of human body by balancing body on board.

Balancing the body on a knife-edge support is a more practical method than suspension. The position of the centre of gravity may be estimated by balancing the body on a plane wooden board, as shown in Figure 10.9a. Initially, it would be necessary to balance the board so that its centre of gravity (as in a see-saw) was located in the vertical plane through the knife-edge support. The subject could then lie down on the board and move his/her body up and down the board until it balanced. The centre of gravity of the body must then lie in the vertical plane through the knife-edge support. By repeating the procedure with the body in two other orientations, as in Figure 10.9b and c, the position of the centre of gravity of the body could be estimated by finding the point of intersection of the three planes.

Whereas the balancing method involves locating the position in which the weight of the body has no moment about the single knife-edge support, the position of the centre of gravity can also be determined by equating the moment of body weight while resting on a wooden board supported by two parallel knife-edge supports. This method is referred to as the reaction board method. Figure 10.10a shows a wooden board (approximately 2.5 m × 0.5 m) supported in a horizontal position by two parallel knife-edge supports, one of which rests on a set of weighing scales. Figure 10.10b shows a free body diagram of the board. The weight of the board can be measured by simply weighing it. By taking moments about knife-edge support A,

CM = ACM   (10.4)

$$W_B \times d_1 = S_1 \times l$$

i.e. $d_1 = \dfrac{S_1 \times l}{W_B}$,

where: W_B = weight of the board,
           l = distance the knife-edge supports,
           S_1 = vertical force exerted by the scales on knife-edge support B,
           d_1 = horizontal distance between knife-edge support A and vertical plane containing centre of gravity of the board.

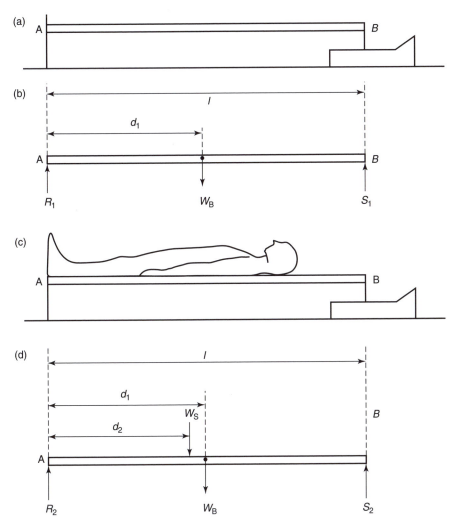

Figure 10.10 Reaction board method to determine position of centre of gravity of human body. (a) Wooden board supported horizontally by parallel knife-edge supports A and B, with edge B resting on a set of weighing scales. (b) Free body diagram of board. (c) Man lying on board with soles of feet coincident with vertical plane through knife-edge support A. (d) Free body diagram of board with man lying on it: W_B, weight of board; W_S, weight of man; l, distance between knife-edge supports; R_1, vertical force exerted by edge A on board without man; R_2, vertical force exerted by edge A on board with man lying on it; S_1, vertical force exerted by scales on knife-edge support B without man; S_2, vertical force exerted by scales on knife-edge support B with man lying on board; d_1, horizontal distance between knife-edge support A and vertical plane containing centre of gravity of board; d_2, horizontal distance between knife-edge support A and vertical plane containing centre of gravity of man.

Figure 10.10c shows a man lying on the board with the soles of his feet coincident with the vertical plane through knife-edge support A. Figure 10.10d shows a free body diagram of the board with the man lying on it. W_B, l and d_1 will be the same as before the man lay on the board, but the vertical force exerted by the scales on the board will increase due to the weight of the man. By taking moments about knife-edge support A,

353

CM = ACM

$$(W_B \times d_1) + (W_S \times d_2) = S_2 \times l$$

where: W_S = weight of the man,

S_2 = vertical force exerted by the scales on knife-edge support B,

d_2 = horizontal distance between knife-edge support A and vertical plane containing the centre of gravity of the man,

i.e. $W_S \times d_2 = (S_2 \times l) - (W_B \times d_1)$

$W_S \times d_2 = (S_2 \times l) - (S_1 \times l)$ (by substitution of $W_B \times d_1$ from Equation 10.4)

$$d_2 = \frac{l \times (S_2 - S_1)}{W_S}. \tag{10.5}$$

For example, if

S_1 = 10 kgf,
S_2 = 39.5 kgf,
W_S = 72 kgf,
l = 2.5 m,

then $d_2 = \dfrac{2.5 \text{ m} \times (39.5 \text{ kgf} - 10 \text{ kgf})}{72 \text{ kgf}}$

$d_2 = 1.024$ m.

Therefore, the vertical plane containing the centre of gravity of the man will be at a distance of 1.024 m from knife-edge support A. If the height of the man is 1.83 m (6 ft), his centre of gravity will be located in the transverse plane at 55.9% of his stature ((1.024 m / 1.83 m) × 100% = 55.9%) when standing upright. By repeating the procedure with the body in two other orientations, the position of the centre of gravity of the body can be estimated by finding the point of intersection of the three planes.

This method is referred to as the one-dimension reaction board method, since the orientation of the body has to be changed in order to locate each separate plane. By using a rectangular or triangular reaction board with three points of support and two sets of weighing scales, the location of the centre of gravity of the body in two planes can be determined in a single step. Figure 10.11 shows an overhead view of a triangular reaction board (the length of each side is approximately 2.5 m) supported in a horizontal position by separate point supports (such as the rounded head of a metal bolt) at each of the three corners of the board. The supports can be underneath the board close to the corners rather than at the corners, but the vertical planes containing the two supports on two sides of the board (AC and BC in Figure 10.11) must be marked on the upper surface of the board. If corners A and B rest on separate sets of weighing scales, the vertical line (intersection of two vertical planes) containing the centre of gravity of the subject lying on the board can be determined by equating moments about AC and BC respectively, using Equation 10.4, as shown in Figure 10.11.

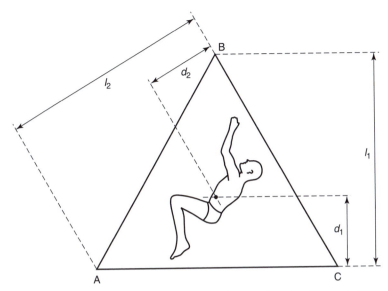

Figure 10.11 Reaction board method to determine position of centre of gravity of human body in two dimensions: W_S, weight of subject lying on board; A_1, vertical force exerted on support A without the subject; A_2, vertical force exerted on support A with subject lying on board; B_1, vertical force exerted on support B without subject; B_2, vertical force exerted on support B with subject lying on board; l_1, perpendicular distance between B and line AC; l_2, perpendicular distance between A and line BC; d_1, distance between vertical plane through AC and vertical plane containing centre of gravity of subject lying on board in one of the positions recorded on a video of the subject performing a back somersault, $d_1 = l_1 \times (B_2 - B_1)/W_S$; d_2, distance between vertical plane through BC and vertical plane containing centre of gravity of subject, $d_2 = l_2 \times (A_2 - A_1)/W_S$.

Whereas the suspension and reaction board methods are fairly accurate if carefully applied, they are of limited value for three main reasons:

- It is unlikely that the subject will be able to reproduce in a static position all of the positions obtained during the movement under consideration and displayed in the separate video frames of the movement.
- Unless photographs of the subject are taken at each stage of the procedure, it is difficult to map the position of the centre of gravity onto the video image.
- The methods are very time consuming, especially when there are a lot of video frames to be analysed.

In Practical Worksheet 5, students use a one-dimension reaction board to examine the effect of changes in body position on the position of the whole body centre of gravity.

Indirect approach

In the indirect approach, the human body is considered to consist of a number of segments linked by joints. Each segment has its own weight and centre of gravity. Provided that the weight of each segment and the position of the centre of gravity of each segment can be determined, the position of the whole body centre of gravity can be determined by application of the principle of moments, i.e. the sum of the moments of the weights of the segments about any particular axis is equal to the moment of the total weight. Figure 10.12 shows a female long jumper just before take-off with her body divided into nine segments: combined trunk, head and neck, left upper arm, combined left forearm and hand, right upper arm, combined right forearm and hand, left thigh, combined left shank (lower leg) and foot, right thigh, combined right shank and foot. The position of the centre of gravity of each segment is shown, together with the position of the whole body centre of gravity. The coordinates of the whole body centre of gravity with respect to any axis of rotation and any dimension can be determined by applying the principle of moments, as shown in Figure 10.12.

The method is fairly straightforward and has been incorporated into a range of commercially available video motion analysis software. However, the accuracy of the method depends largely on the accuracy with which the weights of the segments and the positions of their centres of gravity can be determined. A number of studies have been undertaken to provide these data. The main studies may be classified as cadaver studies, immersion studies and anthropomorphic models (Hay 1973; Spriging et al. 1987).

Cadaver studies

The earliest reported cadaver study appears to be that of Harless in 1860 (Hay 1973), who dissected two adult male cadavers. In 1889, Braune and Fischer (Hay 1973) dissected four adult male cadavers. Each cadaver was frozen solid with the joints of the upper and lower limbs in mid-range position. The segments were then separated by sawing through each joint in a plane that bisected the angle between the segments. Each segment was then weighed and the position of its centre of gravity determined by balancing or suspension. The most comprehensive and most frequently cited cadaver studies are those of Dempster (1955) and Clauser et al. (1969), who used very similar methods to those of Braune and Fischer. Dempster dissected eight white male cadavers (age range 52–83 years) and presented individual and average data on segmental weight (percentage of total weight), segmental centre of gravity position (as a proportion of the distance between defined segmental end points) and segment density. Loss of weight due to dismemberment, especially unknown quantities of body fluids, resulted in the sum of the average segment weights and, therefore, the sum of the average segmental percentages (97.2%) being less than the corresponding whole body data (which were recorded prior to dissection). Dempster indicated that the weight loss was proportional to the weight of the segments. In the average segmental weight data presented in Table 10.1, the 2.8% weight discrepancy has been distributed in proportion to the segmental percentages so that the total percentage is 100% rather than 97.2%. For example, the percentage weight of each upper arm is given as 2.73% which is equal to 2.65/97.2 × 100, where 2.65% is the average percentage weight of the upper arm reported by Dempster.

Clauser et al. (1969) dissected 13 adult male cadavers (age range 28–74 years), selected to closely approximate a wide range of body types. Care was taken to minimise tissue loss during dismemberment. The average data for segmental weight and segmental centre of gravity locus from the Clauser et al. study are shown in Table 10.1.

There do not appear to be any reported cadaver-based data on segment weights and segment centre of gravity loci in female cadavers.

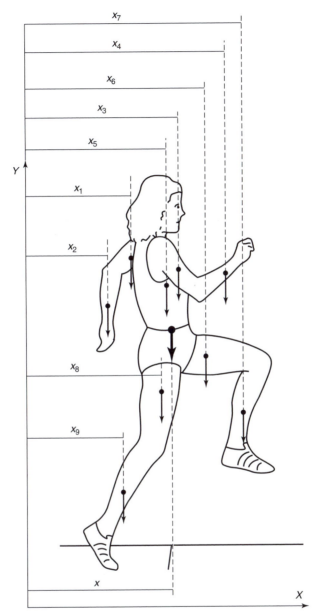

Figure 10.12 Determination of position of whole body centre of gravity by application of the principle of moments. By taking moments about the Z axis in the X dimension,

$W{\cdot}x = W_1{\cdot}x_1 + W_2{\cdot}x_2 + W_3{\cdot}x_3 + W_4{\cdot}x_4 + W_5{\cdot}x_5 + W_6{\cdot}x_6 + W_7{\cdot}x_7 + W_8{\cdot}x_8 + W_9{\cdot}x_9$, where: W = total weight of the body; x = moment arm of W = X coordinate of the whole body centre of gravity; W_1 = weight of the left upper arm; x_1 = moment arm of W_1; W_2 = weight of combined left forearm and hand; x_2 = moment arm of W_2; W_3 = weight of the right upper arm; x_3 = moment arm of W_3; W_4 = weight of combined right forearm and hand; x_4 = moment arm of W_4; W_5 = combined weight of trunk, head and neck; x_5 = moment arm of W_5; W_6 = weight of the left thigh; x_6 = moment arm of W_6; W_7 = weight of combined left shank and foot; x_7 = moment arm of W_7; W_8 = weight of the right thigh; x_8 = moment arm of W_8; W_9 = weight of combined right shank and foot; x_9 = moment arm of W_9; i.e. $x = (W_1 \cdot x_1 + W_2 \cdot x_2 + W_3 \cdot x_3 + W_4 \cdot x_4 + W_5 \cdot x_5 + W_6 \cdot x_6 + W_7 \cdot x_7 + W_8 \cdot x_8 + W_9 \cdot x_9)/W$.

Table 10.1 Mean segment weights (percentage of total weight) and centre of gravity locations (proportion of segment length in direction indicated) for adult men (Dempster 1955; *Clauser et al.* 1969; Plagenhoef et al. 1983).

Segment*	Dempster[1]		Clauser et al.[2]		Plagenhoef et al.[3]	
	Weight	CG locus	Weight	CG locus	Weight	CG locus
Upper arm	2.73	0.436[a]	2.6	0.513[a]	3.25	0.436[a]
Forearm	1.59	0.430[b]	1.6	0.390[b]	1.87	0.430[b]
Hand	0.62	0.506[c]	0.7	0.480[c]	0.65	0.468[c]
Forearm and hand	2.21	0.677[d]	2.3	0.626[d]	2.52	0.671[d]
Whole upper limb	4.94	0.512[e]	4.9	0.413[e]	5.77	0.500[e]
Thigh	9.93	0.433[f]	10.3	0.372[f]	10.50	0.433[f]
Shank	4.63	0.433[g]	4.3	0.371[g]	4.75	0.434[g]
Foot	1.44	0.429[h]	1.5	0.449[h]	1.43	0.500[h]
Shank and foot	6.07	0.434[i]	5.8	0.475[i]	6.18	0.605[i]
Whole lower limb	16.00	0.434[j]	16.1	0.382[j]	16.68	0.436[j]
Trunk, head and neck	58.13	0.604[k]	58.0	0.604[m]	55.10	0.566[k]
Trunk, head and neck	58.13	0.346[n]	58.0	0.346[p]	55.10	0.370[n]
Head and neck	8.13	0.433[q]	7.3	0.433[r]	8.26	0.450[q]
Head	7.00[s]	0.545[t]	7.0[s]	0.545[t]	7.0[s]	0.545[t]
Trunk	50.00	0.620[v]	50.7	0.620[w]	46.48	0.630[v]

* Segments in the anatomical position (Figure 9.4); [a], shoulder axis to elbow axis; [b], elbow axis to wrist axis; [c], wrist axis to first interphalangeal joint of the second finger; [d], elbow axis to styloid process of the ulna; [e], shoulder axis to styloid process of the ulna; [f], hip axis to knee axis; [g], knee axis to ankle axis; [h], intersection of line joining ankle axis and ball of the foot with vertical line perpendicular to sole of foot that divides foot in the ratio 0.429: 0.571 from heel to toe; [i], knee axis to medial malleolus; [j], hip axis to ankle axis; [k], top of head to hip axis with head, neck and trunk in normal upright posture; [m], top of head to hip axis with head, neck and trunk in normal upright posture (Dempster 1955); [n], shoulder axis to hip axis with trunk in normal upright posture; [p], shoulder axis to hip axis with trunk in normal upright posture (Dempster 1955); [q], top of head to centre of body of 7th cervical vertebra; [r], top of head to centre of body of 7th cervical vertebra (Dempster 1955); [s], data from Braune and Fischer (1889), reported by Hay (1973); [t], top of head to occipital–atlas joint, from Braune and Fischer (1889), reported by Hay (1973); [v], shoulder axis to hip axis; [w], shoulder axis to hip axis (Dempster 1955); [1], mean data from eight white male cadavers (age range 52–83 years); [2], mean data from 13 white male cadavers (age range 28–74 years); [3], mean weight data from 35 living college-age men using water immersion method and density data from Dempster (1955) and mean CG locus data from seven living college-age men using water immersion method.

Immersion studies

As mass is the product of volume and density, a number of studies have estimated segmental masses by measuring the volume of the segments by water displacement (carefully immersing each segment or segments in a tank of water and measuring the volume of water displaced) and multiplying the volume of the segment by the corresponding average segmental density reported by Dempster (1955). The most comprehensive immersion study carried out on living subjects would appear to be that of Plagenhoef *et al.* (1983). Segmental volumes of 135 college-age athletes (100 women and 35 men) were measured. The corresponding average

Table 10.2 Mean segment weights (percentage of total weight) and centre of gravity locations (proportion of segment length in direction indicated) for adult women (Plagenhoef et al. 1983).[†]

Segment*	Weight	CG locus
Upper arm	2.90	0.458[a]
Forearm	1.57	0.434[b]
Hand	0.50	0.468[c]
Forearm and hand	2.07	0.657[d]
Whole upper limb	4.97	0.486[e]
Thigh	11.75	0.428[f]
Shank	5.35	0.419[g]
Foot	1.33	0.500[h]
Shank and foot	6.68	0.568[i]
Whole lower limb	18.43	0.420[j]
Trunk, head and neck	53.20	0.603[k]
Trunk, head and neck	53.20	0.450[m]
Head and neck	8.20	0.450[n]
Head	7.00[p]	0.545[q]
Trunk	45.00	0.569[m]

* Segments in the anatomical position (Figure 9.4); [a], shoulder axis to elbow axis; [b], elbow axis to wrist axis; [c], wrist axis to first interphalangeal joint of second finger; [d], elbow axis to styloid process of ulna; [e], shoulder axis to styloid process of ulna; [f], hip axis to knee axis; [g], knee axis to ankle axis; [h], intersection of line joining ankle axis and ball of foot with vertical line perpendicular with sole of foot that divides foot in ratio 0.429: 0.571 from heel to toe; [i], knee axis to medial malleolus; [j], hip axis to ankle axis; [k], vertex (top of head) to hip axis with head, neck and trunk in normal upright posture; [m], shoulder axis to hip axis with trunk in normal upright posture; [n], vertex (top of head) to centre of body of 7th cervical vertebra; [p], from Braune & Fischer (1889), reported by Hay (1973); [q], top of head to occipital–atlas joint, from Braune & Fischer (1889), reported by Hay (1973); [†], mean weight data from 100 living college-age women using water immersion method and density data from Dempster (1955) and mean CG locus data from nine living college-age women using water immersion method.

segmental weights are shown in Table 10.1 for men and Table 10.2 for women. Segmental centre of gravity loci were estimated using seven men and nine women (from the group of 135 subjects) using the immersion method described by Clauser et al. (1969); this involves immersing the segment to a proportion of its volume (using average data presented by Clauser at al.) that corresponds to the plane of the segmental centre of gravity. The average segmental centre of gravity loci from the Plagenhoef et al. study (1983) are shown in Table 10.1 for men and Table 10.2 for women. The studies referred to in Tables 10.1 and 10.2 did not all report data for the same segments. Consequently, to complete the data sets in Tables 10.1 and 10.2, data have been included from other studies, as indicated.

Anthropomorphic models

To personalise the determination of segment weights and segment centre of gravity positions for a particular subject, a number of anthropomorphic models have been developed; these include Whitsett (1963), Hanavan (1964), Hatze (1980) and Yeadon (1990). All of the models

359

are based on anthropometric measurements taken directly from the subject. The measurements are used to construct geometric representations of the body segments. The masses of segments are estimated from segment volume and average density and the positions of segmental centres of gravity are estimated by mathematical methods on the basis of the geometry of the segment shapes. The main disadvantages of anthropomorphic models are that anthropometric measurements have to be taken directly from the subject and the time required to take all the measurements may be considerable. For example, the time required to take the 242 measurements required for applying the Hatze (1980) model is about 80 minutes per subject (Spriging et al., 1987).

It is reasonable to expect that a personalised model would be more accurate than the application of average percentage data from cadaver and immersion studies. However, the amount of comparative data currently available is meagre (Spriging et al. 1987) and seems to indicate that the difference in the results of the different methods (in the estimated position of the whole body centre of gravity) is unlikely to be significant in the analysis of whole body movement.

The major advantage of using percentage data for segment weight and segment centre of gravity position is that the position of the whole body centre of gravity of the subject can be determined from a video image without the need for any anthropometric information about the subject. Not surprisingly, the application of percentage data for segment weight and segment centre of gravity position is the preferred method in most biomechanical analyses, especially those based on video analysis.

Determination of the whole body centre of gravity by the application of the principle of moments

In undertaking segmental analysis, the analyst has to decide the number of segments that will comprise the segmental model. The more segments in the model, the greater the number of segmental end points and, therefore, the greater the time needed to digitise each video frame. Digitisation refers to the process of identifying and recording the coordinates of each point in the segmental model, as well as reference points for the origin and axes of the reference axis system upon which the analysis will be based (Figure 10.13). The number of segments in the model will largely depend on the purpose of the analysis. For example, if the description of ankle movement is an important objective, it will be necessary to have separate shank and foot segments for each leg. However, the weight of each foot is small relative to total body weight and the effect of movement of the foot relative to the shank on the position of the whole body centre of gravity is likely to be insignificant. Consequently, if the main objective of the analysis is the movement of the whole body centre of gravity, the analyst may decide to regard the shank and foot as a single segment. Similarly, the forearm and hand may be regarded as a single segment. In detailed biomechanical analyses of elite long jumpers, researchers have used a number of segmental models ranging from an 11-segment model (Lees et al. 1993) to a 16-segment model (Linthorne et al. 2005).

Figure 10.13 shows the image of a female long jumper just before take-off taken from a video frame and superimposed, for the purpose of analysis, onto a one-centimetre grid. The segment end points defining a 9-segment model (defined in Figure 10.12) are shown. The first

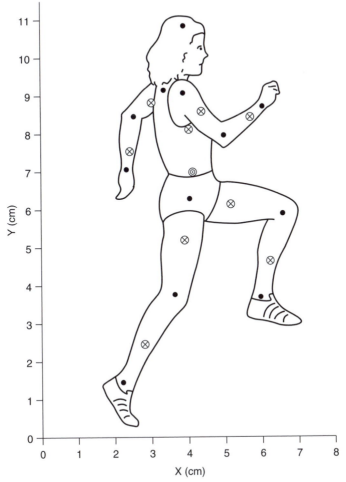

Figure 10.13 Segment end points (●) defining a 9-segment model and the corresponding positions of the segment centres of gravity (⊗) and whole body centre of gravity (⊙).

two columns of Table 10.3 show the x and y coordinates of the segment end points. Column 6 of Table 10.3 shows the corresponding x and y coordinates of the segment centres of gravity. These points are shown in Figure 10.13. Table 10.4 shows the coordinates of the segment centres of gravity and the coordinates of the whole body centre of gravity, determined by application of the principle of moments. In applying the principle of moments, it is not necessary to know the actual body weight of the subject. Use of the segment weight proportions rather than the segment weights in the calculation of segment and body weight moments will give the same result. However, as proportion has no unit (it is simply a number because it is the ratio of two weights), the units of the calculated moments will be cm rather than N·cm. This may be confusing to some students and so a nominal body weight of 63 kgf (618 N) has been used in the illustration in Table 10.4.

In Practical Worksheet 6, students use a one-dimension reaction board to compare the direct and indirect (segmental) methods of determining the position of the whole body centre

Table 10.3 Coordinates of the segment end points and segment centres of gravity of the female long jumper shown in Figure 10.13.

Segment	Coordinates (cm)[1]		Length (cm)[2]	CG_P [3]	CG_S (cm)[4]	CG_0 (cm)[5]
	a	b			c	
Right upper arm	Shoulder	Elbow				
x	3.8	4.9	1.1	0.458	0.50	4.30
y	9.0	7.9	−1.1	0.458	−0.50	8.50
Right forearm and hand	Elbow	Wrist				
x	4.9	5.9	1.0	0.657	0.66	5.56
y	7.9	8.6	0.7	0.657	0.46	8.36
Left upper arm	Shoulder	Elbow				
x	3.3	2.5	−0.8	0.458	−0.37	2.93
y	9.1	8.4	−0.7	0.458	−0.32	8.78
Left forearm and hand	Elbow	Wrist				
x	2.5	2.3	−0.2	0.657	−0.13	2.37
y	8.4	7.0	−1.4	0.657	−0.92	7.48
Trunk, head and neck	Vertex	Right hip*				
x	3.8	4.0	0.2	0.603	−0.12	3.92
y	10.8	6.2	−4.6	0.603	−2.77	8.03
Right thigh	Hip	Knee				
x	4.0	3.6	−0.4	0.428	−0.17	3.83
y	6.2	3.7	−2.5	0.428	−1.07	5.13
Right shank and foot	Knee	Ankle				
x	3.6	2.2	−1.4	0.568	−0.79	2.81
y	3.7	1.4	−2.3	0.568	−1.31	2.39
Left thigh	Hip	Knee				
x	4.0	6.5	2.5	0.428	1.07	5.07
y	6.2	5.8	−0.4	0.428	−0.17	6.03
Left shank and foot	Knee	Ankle				
x	6.5	5.9	−0.6	0.568	−0.34	6.16
y	5.8	3.6	−2.2	0.568	−1.25	4.55

* In this example, the coordinates of the left hip joint and right hip joint are the same. If the coordinates of the left hip and right hip had been different from each other, it would have been necessary to find the midpoint of the line linking the two joints as the hip reference point for determining the position of the centre of gravity of the trunk, head and neck segment.

[1], x and y coordinates of segment end points a and b; [2], length of segment in the dimension = b − a; [3], position of segmental centre of gravity as a proportion of segment length in direction a to b (from Table 10.2); [4], position of segmental centre of gravity in the dimension in relation to a; [5], coordinates of the position of the centre of gravity of the segment = a + c.

Table 10.4 Coordinates of the segment centres of gravity and whole body centre of gravity (determined by the principle of moments) of the female long jumper shown in Figure 10.13.

Segment	Coordinates (cm)[1]		Weight[2]	Weight (N)[3]	Moment x [4] (N·cm)	Moment y [5] (N·cm)
	x	y				
Right upper arm	4.30	8.50	0.0290	17.92	77.06	152.32
Right forearm and hand	5.56	8.36	0.0207	12.79	71.13	106.92
Left upper arm	2.93	8.78	0.0290	17.92	37.47	157.34
Left forearm and hand	2.37	7.48	0.0207	12.79	30.31	95.67
Trunk, head and neck	3.92	8.03	0.5320	328.78	1288.80	2640.07
Right thigh	3.83	5.13	0.1175	72.61	278.11	372.51
Right shank and foot	2.81	2.39	0.0668	41.28	116.00	98.66
Left thigh	5.07	6.03	0.1175	72.61	368.13	437.84
Left shank and foot	6.16	4.55	0.0668	41.28	254.28	187.82
Coordinates of CG [6]	4.08	6.87				
Totals				618.00	2521.29	4249.15

[1], x and y coordinates of the segmental centres of gravity from Table 10.3 (cm); [2], weight of segments as a proportion of total body weight (from Table 10.2); [3], weight of segments in newtons (total body weight = 63 kgf = 618 N); [4], moments of segmental weights about Z axis with respect to X dimension (N·cm); [5], moments of segmental weights about Z axis with respect to Y dimension (N·cm); [6], Moment of body weight = sum of moments of segments, i.e.:

$W·x_G$ = sum of moment X,
where W = body weight = 618 N and x_G = X coordinate of CG,

i.e. $x_G = \dfrac{\text{sum of moment X}}{W} = \dfrac{2521.29 \text{ N}\cdot\text{cm}}{618 \text{ N}} = 4.08$ cm.

Similarly, $y_G = \dfrac{\text{sum of moment Y}}{W} = \dfrac{4249.15 \text{ N}\cdot\text{cm}}{618 \text{ N}} = 6.87$ cm,

where y_G = Y coordinate of CG.

of gravity of the human body. In Practical Worksheet 7, students record a video of a standing long jump and analyse the video to determine take-off distance, flight distance and landing distance.

There are two approaches to determining the position of the centre of gravity of the human body, the direct (whole body) approach and the indirect (segmental) approach.

LEVERS

Whereas weight forces are always vertical, other external forces acting on a body are likely to be oblique. For example, consider using a claw hammer to pull out a nail from a piece of wood, as shown in Figure 10.14a. In this example, the line of contact between the claw of the

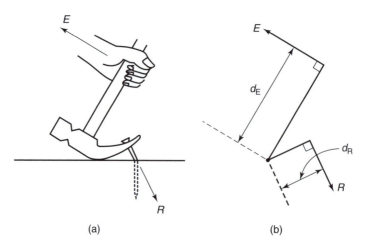

Figure 10.14 (a) Pulling a nail out of a piece of wood using a claw hammer. (b) Corresponding force–moment arm diagram. E, force exerted on hammer handle; d_E, moment arm of E; R, resistance force exerted by nail; d_R, moment arm of R.

hammer and the surface of the wood constitutes the fulcrum. E is the force exerted on the handle of the hammer and R is the resistance of the nail. Figure 10.14b shows a force–moment arm diagram, i.e. the forces E and R and their moment arms d_E and d_R are shown in relation to the fulcrum, to illustrate the turning effects of the forces more clearly. The nail will be pulled out if the anticlockwise moment exerted by E is greater than the clockwise moment exerted by R, i.e. if $E \cdot d_E > R \cdot d_R$.

In this situation, the hammer is being used as a lever, a rigid or quasi-rigid object that can be made to rotate about a fulcrum in order to exert a force on another object. As in the example of the hammer, a lever encounters a resistance force R in response to an effort force E. The simplest form of lever, which is actually the simplest form of machine, i.e. a powered mechanism designed to apply force (Dempster 1965), is exemplified by a crowbar, as shown in Figure 10.15. In this case, the power is supplied by the person using the crowbar. The greater the moment arm of E (d_E), i.e. the greater the leverage of the crowbar, the smaller will be the effort required to overcome the moment of the resistance force.

Lever systems

Levers are classified into three systems, depending on the location of the points of application of the E and R forces in relation to the fulcrum. A lever can be any shape, as will be demonstrated in the section on lever systems in the human musculoskeletal system. However, in describing the different classes of levers, it is usual to represent the lever as a straight line and the fulcrum as the vertex of small triangle, as shown in Figure 10.16a.

In a first-class lever system, the fulcrum is between the E and R forces (Figure 10.16a). The use of a crowbar is an example of a first-class lever system (Figure 10.15), as is a see-saw (Figure 10.3). Scissors are a pair of first-class levers that share the same fulcrum (Figure 10.16b).

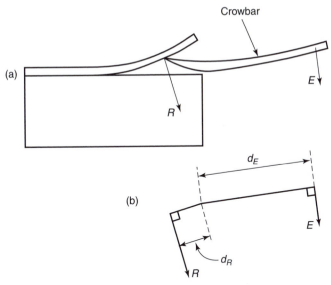

Figure 10.15 (a) Use of crowbar to open a box. (b) Corresponding force–moment arm diagram. E, force exerted on crowbar; d_E, moment arm of E; R, resistance force exerted on crowbar by box lid; d_R, moment arm of R.

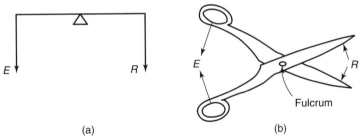

Figure 10.16 (a) First-class lever system. (b) Scissors are a pair of first-class levers that share the same fulcrum. E, effort force; R, resistance force.

In a second-class lever system, the R force is between the fulcrum and the E force as in, for example, a wheelbarrow (Figure 10.17a,b). A crowbar may also take the form of a second-class lever (Figure 10.17c). In a third-class lever system, the E force is between the fulcrum and the R force as, for example, when holding a fishing rod (Figure 10.18a,b). Tongs consist of a pair of third-class levers that share the same fulcrum (Figure 10.18c).

A lever is an object that can be made to rotate about a fulcrum in order to exert a force on another object.

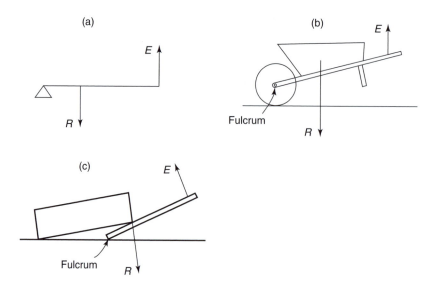

Figure 10.17 (a) Second-class lever system. (b) A wheelbarrow is a second-class lever system. (c) A crowbar can take the form of a second-class lever system. E, effort force; R, resistance force.

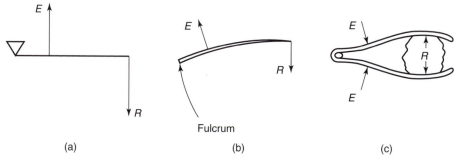

Figure 10.18 (a) Third-class lever system. (b) A fishing rod is a third-class lever system. (c) Tongs consist of a pair of third-class levers that share the same fulcrum. E, effort force; R, resistance force.

Mechanical advantage

The mechanical advantage (MA) of a lever system is a measure of its efficiency in terms of the amount of effort needed to overcome a particular resistance, i.e.

$$\text{MA} = \frac{\text{magnitude of resistance}}{\text{magnitude of effort}} = \frac{R}{E}$$

$$= \frac{\text{length of moment arm of } E}{\text{length of moment arm of } R} = \frac{d_E}{d_R}.$$

Any machine with a mechanical advantage greater than 1.0 is regarded as very efficient. A first-class lever may have a mechanical advantage greater than 1.0 or less than 1.0. The first-class lever system in Figure 10.15 has a mechanical advantage much greater than 1.0, since d_E is much greater than d_R. All second-class lever systems have mechanical advantages greater than 1.0, as d_E is always larger than d_R. All third-class lever systems have mechanical advantages less than 1.0, as d_E is always smaller than d_R. In all three lever systems, the greater the length of d_E in relation to the length of d_R, the greater the leverage of the system.

Lever systems in the human musculoskeletal system

The bones of the skeleton are essentially levers and each joint constitutes a fulcrum. The muscles pull on the bones to control the movement of the joints. The resistance to movement exerted by a body segment is in the form of the segment's weight and any other external loads attached to the segment. Most, if not all, of the skeletal muscles of the body operate in first-class or third-class lever systems. Like the third-class lever systems, most of the first-class lever systems have mechanical advantages less than 1.0 because the tendons of the muscles that operate within them tend to be inserted close to the joints they control and, as such, have shorter moment arms than the resistance forces they counteract.

External and internal forces

Figure 10.19a shows the position of the head in normal upright standing. In this position the line of action of the weight of the head passes in front of the vertebral column and, as such,

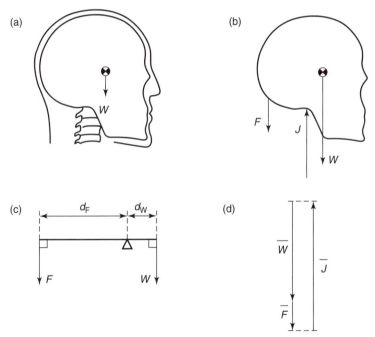

Figure 10.19 Forces acting on head when standing upright. (a) Location of centre of gravity of head. (b) Free body diagram of head. (c) Force–moment arm diagram of forces acting on head. (d) Vector chain of forces acting on head. W, weight of head; d_W, moment arm of W; F, force exerted by neck extensor muscles; d_F, moment arm of F; J, joint reaction force exerted by atlas on occipital bone.

367

exerts a clockwise moment that tends to rotate the head forward and downward about a mediolateral axis through the fulcrum, i.e. the joint between the occipital bone (at the base of the skull) and the atlas (the first cervical vertebra). The tendency of the weight of the head W to rotate the head forward and downward is counteracted by the neck extensor muscles.

Figure 10.19b shows a free body diagram of the head, where F is the force exerted by the neck extensor muscles and J is the force exerted at the fulcrum, i.e. the joint reaction force exerted by the atlas on the occipital bone. Figure 10.19c shows the corresponding force–moment arm diagram. F and W constitute a first-class lever system. In this example, it is assumed that F acts vertically downward. The weight of the head of an adult is approximately 7.0% of total body weight (Table 10.1). Consequently, if total body weight is 70 kgf, the weight of the head will be approximately 4.9 kgf. The moment arms of W and F will be approximately 2 cm and 7 cm, respectively. As the head is in equilibrium, the resultant moment acting on the head will be zero and the resultant force acting on the head will be zero. Consequently, the forces F and J can be determined by equating moments and then equating forces as follows:

Equating moments:

$$W \cdot d_W = F \cdot d_F,$$

where: W = 4.9 kgf,
  d_W = moment arm of W = 2 cm,
  F = force exerted by the neck extensor muscles,
  d_F = moment arm of F = 7 cm,

$$F = \frac{W \cdot d_W}{d_F} = \frac{4.9 \text{ kgf} \times 2 \text{ cm}}{7 \text{ cm}} = 1.4 \text{ kgf.}$$

Equating forces: As F and W are vertical forces, J must also be vertical and the resultant force must be zero. Using the convention that upward is positive and downward is negative, then

  resultant force $= J - F - W = 0$
  $J = F + W = 1.4 \text{ kgf} + 4.9 \text{ kgf}$
  $J = 6.3 \text{ kgf.}$

Consequently, to counteract W, an external force, the musculoskeletal system has to exert two internal forces, F and J. Force F is an active force, a muscle force, and J is a passive force, a joint reaction force. This example illustrates the relationship between the internal and external forces that act on the body; the musculoskeletal system exerts internal forces to counteract the effects of gravity on body segments.

In this example, all of the forces acting on the head were vertical forces and, as such, the vector chain of the forces is a straight line (Figure 10.19d). In most musculoskeletal lever systems, the internal and external forces are not usually parallel. For example, Figure 10.20a shows the head position of a person writing at a desk. In this situation, the head and trunk are tilted forward such that d_W will be greater than when the head is in the upright position

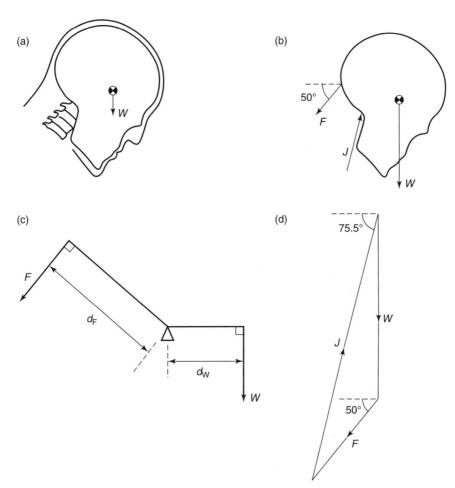

Figure 10.20 Forces acting on head when writing at a desk. (a) Location of centre of gravity of head. (b) Free body diagram of head. (c) Force–moment arm diagram of forces acting on head. (d) Vector chain of forces acting on head. W, weight of head; d_W, moment arm of W; F, force exerted by neck extensor muscles; d_F, moment arm of F; J, joint reaction force exerted by atlas on occipital bone.

(about 4 cm rather than 2 cm). d_F will be approximately the same as when the head is in the upright position, i.e. about 7 cm, but the line of action of F will be at approximately 50° to the horizontal. Figure 10.20b shows a free body diagram of the head and Figure 10.20c shows the corresponding force–moment arm diagram. By taking moments about the fulcrum,

$$W \cdot d_W = F \cdot d_{F,}$$

where: $W = 4.9$ kgf,
$d_W = 4$ cm,
$d_F = 7$ cm,

i.e. $F = \dfrac{W \cdot d_W}{d_F} = \dfrac{4.9 \text{ kgf} \times 4 \text{ cm}}{7 \text{ cm}} = 2.8$ kgf.

369

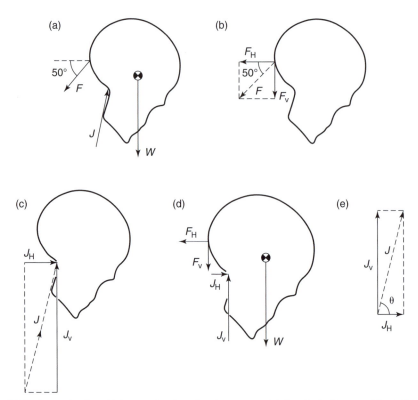

Figure 10.21 Determination of joint reaction force by trigonometry. (a) Free body diagram of head. (b) Horizontal and vertical components of F. (c) Horizontal and vertical components of J. (d) Free body diagram of head with forces resolved into their horizontal and vertical components. (e) Angle of J (θ) with respect to the horizontal.

The joint reaction force J can be found in two ways: constructing the vector chain and calculation by trigonometry. Figure 10.20d shows the vector chain solution: J has a magnitude of approximately 7.25 kgf and acts at an angle of approximately 75.5° to the horizontal. Figure 10.21 shows the solution by trigonometry. Figure 10.21a shows a free body diagram of the head (same as Figure 10.20b). Figure 10.21b shows the force F resolved into its horizontal and vertical components, and Figure 10.21c shows the force J resolved into its horizontal and vertical components. Figure 10.21d shows the forces acting on the head in terms of their horizontal and vertical components. Since the head is in equilibrium, the resultant force on the head will be zero. Consequently, the resultant of the horizontal forces will be zero and the resultant of the vertical forces will be zero. Using the convention that forces acting to the right or upward are positive and that forces acting to the left or downward (with respect to Figure 10.21) are negative, it follows that with regard to the horizontal forces,

$$J_H - F_H = 0$$

where: J_H = horizontal component of J,
   F_H = horizontal component of F,

i.e. $\quad J_H = F_H$
$\qquad J_H = F \cdot \cos 50° = 2.8 \text{ kgf} \times 0.6428$
$\qquad J_H = 1.8 \text{ kgf}.$

With regard to the vertical forces,

$\quad J_V - F_V - W = 0,$

where: $\quad J_V = $ vertical component of J,
$\qquad F_V = $ vertical component of F,

i.e. $\quad J_V = F_V + W$
$\qquad J_V = F \cdot \sin 50° + W$
$\qquad J_V = 2.8 \text{ kgf} \times 0.7664 + 4.9 \text{ kgf}$
$\qquad J_V = 2.15 \text{ kgf} + 4.9 \text{ kgf}$
$\qquad J_V = 7.05 \text{ kgf}.$

As J_V and J_H are at right angles to each other, the magnitude of their resultant J can be found by applying Pythagoras' theorem, i.e.

$$J^2 = J_V^2 + J_H^2 = (7.05^2 + 1.8^2) \text{ kgf}^2$$
$$J^2 = 52.94 \text{ kgf}^2$$
$$J = 7.27 \text{ kgf}.$$

If J makes an angle of θ with respect to the horizontal (Figure 10.21e), then

$\quad \tan \theta = J_V/J_H = 7.05/1.8 = 3.914$
$\qquad \theta = 75.7°.$

As expected, the vector chain method and calculation by trigonometry method produce almost exactly the same result for the magnitude and direction of J.

Most of the skeletal muscles of the human body operate in first-class or third-class lever systems with mechanical advantages less than 1.

Effect of increasing the moment arm of external forces on the magnitude of internal forces

The examples of the forces acting on the head in the upright (Figure 10.19) and writing positions (Figure 10.20) show that an increase in the moment arm of an external force results in an increase in the magnitude of the counteracting muscle forces, which, in turn, results in an increase in the associated joint reaction forces. This is illustrated in Figure 10.22, which shows a 6 m long beam of wood of weight W balanced in three positions on a knife-edge support.

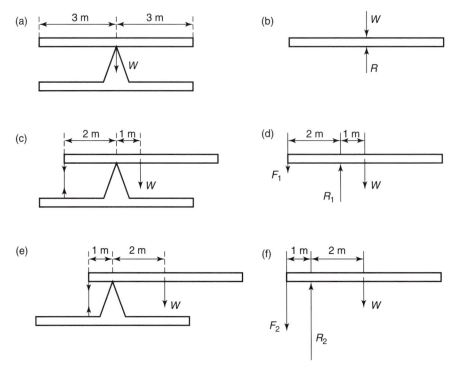

Figure 10.22 Effect of increasing moment arm of weight W of a beam on magnitude of restraining forces needed to maintain equilibrium. (a) Beam balanced with line of action of W acting through fulcrum. (b) Free body diagram of beam in (a). (c) Beam in equilibrium with line of action of W displaced 1 m to the right. (d) Free body diagram of beam in (c). (e) Beam in equilibrium with line of action of W displaced 2 m to the right, (f) Free body diagram of beam in (e).

In Figure 10.22a, the beam is balanced with the line of action of its weight passing through the knife-edge support, i.e. the moment of W about the fulcrum is zero. In this situation, the reaction force R is sufficient to counteract W and maintain equilibrium; Figure 10.22b shows a free body diagram of the beam. In Figure 10.22c, the beam has been displaced 1 m to the right, such that W exerts a clockwise turning moment on the beam of $W \times 1$ m. The beam is held in equilibrium by the reaction force R_1 and a force F_1 exerted by a tie that attaches the left end of the beam to the base of support. If it is assumed that F_1 acts vertically, R_1 will also act vertically. Figure 10.22d shows a free body diagram of the beam. By equating moments about the fulcrum,

$$W \times 1 \text{ m} = F_1 \times 2 \text{ m},$$

$$\text{i.e.} \quad F_1 = \frac{W \times 1 \text{ m}}{2 \text{ m}} = 0.5W.$$

By equating the forces,

$$R_1 = F_1 + W = 0.5W + W = 1.5W.$$

In Figure 10.22e, the beam has been displaced 2 m to the right with respect to its original position, such that W exerts a clockwise turning moment on the beam of $W \times 2$ m. The beam is held in equilibrium by the reaction force R_2 and a force F_2 exerted by the tie. Assuming that F_2 and, consequently, R_2 act vertically, Figure 10.22f shows a free body diagram of the beam. By equating moments about the fulcrum,

$$W \times 2 \text{ m} = F_2 \times 1 \text{ m},$$

i.e. $F_2 = \dfrac{W \times 2 \text{ m}}{1 \text{ m}} = 2W.$

By equating the forces,

$$R_2 = F_2 + W = 2W + W = 3W.$$

Forces at the hip in single-leg stance

The distribution of load on the beam in Figure 10.22e is similar to that on the pelvis during single-leg support during standing or walking (Figure 10.23a–c). In this position, the pelvis acts as a first-class lever and rotates about the hip joint under the action of the weight of the body and the force exerted by the hip abductor muscles. Figure 10.23c shows a free body diagram of the pelvis in this situation and Figure 10.23d shows the corresponding force–moment arm diagram. W is the weight of the body less the weight of the grounded leg. For a man of total body weight of 70 kgf, W is approximately 59 kgf (84% of total body weight; see Dempster data in Table 10.1). A is the force exerted by the hip abductor muscles. W will tend to rotate the pelvis clockwise about the hip joint and A will normally maintain the pelvis in a horizontal position by exerting an equal and opposite moment. Force J is the joint reaction force, that is, the force exerted by the head of the femur on the pelvis via the acetabulum. When the pelvis is in equilibrium, the resultant of W, A and J will be zero. The line of action of A will be approximately 80° to the horizontal. The moment arms of A and W with respect to the hip joint axis of rotation will be approximately 6 cm and 11 cm, respectively. By taking moments about the fulcrum (the point of application of J),

$$W \cdot d_W - A \cdot d_A = 0,$$

where: $W = 59$ kgf,

$\qquad d_W = 11$ cm,

$\qquad d_A = 6$ cm,

i.e. $A = \dfrac{W \cdot d_W}{d_A} = \dfrac{59 \text{ kgf} \times 11 \text{ cm}}{6 \text{ cm}} = 108$ kgf.

The vector chain determination of J is shown in Figure 10.23e; $J = 166$ kgf at an angle of 83° to the horizontal. The determination of J by trigonometry is shown in Figure 10.23f and g; $J = 166.4$ kgf at an angle of 83.5° to the horizontal. The results show that the joint reaction force in one-legged stance is in the region of 2.4 times body weight.

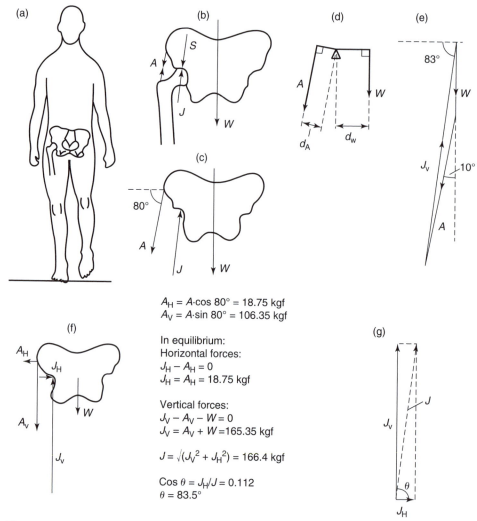

(a)

(b)

(d)

(e)

(c)

$A_H = A \cdot \cos 80° = 18.75$ kgf
$A_V = A \cdot \sin 80° = 106.35$ kgf

In equilibrium:
Horizontal forces:
$J_H - A_H = 0$
$J_H = A_H = 18.75$ kgf

Vertical forces:
$J_V - A_V - W = 0$
$J_V = A_V + W = 165.35$ kgf

$J = \sqrt{(J_V^2 + J_H^2)} = 166.4$ kgf

$\cos \theta = J_H/J = 0.112$
$\theta = 83.5°$

(f)

(g)

Figure 10.23 Forces at hip in single-leg stance. (a) Single-leg support on right leg during walking cycle. (b) Forces on pelvis and hip joint. (c) Free body diagram of pelvis. (d) Force–moment arm diagram. (e) Vector chain determination of hip joint reaction force, (f,g) Determination of hip joint reaction force by trigonometry (where forces are in equilibrium)

The force S exerted by the pelvis on the head of the femur, is equal and opposite to that of J (Figure 10.23b). When someone is recovering from a serious leg injury, such as a broken femur, it is necessary to reduce S during weight-bearing activities, such as standing and walking, by using crutches and walking sticks. Figure 10.24a shows a man walking with the aid of a stick in his left hand. During the right leg single-support phase of the walking cycle, the stick helps to support the weight of the body and, therefore, reduces the load on the right leg. In this situation, the stick is, in effect, an extension of the left arm, enabling the left arm to support the weight of the body by pushing against the floor. In this example, the left arm can

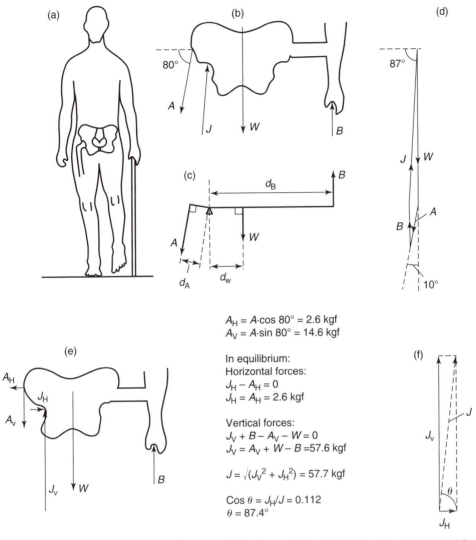

$A_H = A \cdot \cos 80° = 2.6$ kgf
$A_V = A \cdot \sin 80° = 14.6$ kgf

In equilibrium:
Horizontal forces:
$J_H - A_H = 0$
$J_H = A_H = 2.6$ kgf

Vertical forces:
$J_V + B - A_V - W = 0$
$J_V = A_V + W - B = 57.6$ kgf

$J = \sqrt{(J_V{}^2 + J_H{}^2)} = 57.7$ kgf

$\text{Cos } \theta = J_H/J = 0.112$
$\theta = 87.4°$

Figure 10.24 Forces at the hip in single-leg stance while using a walking stick. (a) Single-leg support on right leg during walking cycle. (b) Forces on pelvis and hip joint. (c) Free body diagram of pelvis. (d) Force–moment arm diagram. (e) Vector chain determination of hip joint reaction force. (f,g) Determination of hip joint reaction force by trigonometry (where forces are in equilibrium)

be considered to be a lateral extension of the pelvis, and the free body diagram of the pelvis can be represented as in Figure 10.24b. The corresponding force–moment arm diagram is shown in Figure 10.24c.

When walking without a stick, as in Figure 10.23, the moment of W is counteracted by the moment of A on its own. When walking with a stick, the moment of W is counteracted by the combined moment of A and the force B exerted by the stick on the man's left hand. When the pelvis is in equilibrium, the resultant of W, A, B and J will be zero. For a man of total body weight 70 kgf, B will be about 16 kgf with a moment arm of approximately 35 cm with respect to the hip joint axis of rotation; it is assumed that B acts vertically. By taking moments about the fulcrum,

$$W \cdot d_W - A \cdot d_A - B \cdot d_B = 0$$

where: $\quad W = 59$ kgf,
$\qquad d_W = 11$ cm,
$\qquad B = 16$ kgf,
$\qquad d_B = 35$ cm,
$\qquad d_A = 6$ cm,

i.e. $\quad A = \dfrac{W \cdot d_W - B \cdot d_B}{d_A}$

$$A = \frac{(59 \text{ kgf} \times 11 \text{ cm}) - (16 \text{ kgf} \times 35 \text{ cm})}{6 \text{ cm}} = 14.8 \text{ kgf.}$$

The vector chain determination of J is shown in Figure 10.24d; $J = 57.5$ kgf at an angle of $87°$ to the horizontal. The determination of J by trigonometry is shown in Figure 10.24 e and f; $J = 57.6$ kgf at an angle of $87.4°$ to the horizontal. The results indicate that using a walking stick considerably reduces the force exerted by the hip abductor muscles in single-leg stance (108 kgf to 14.8 kgf) which, in turn, considerably reduces the hip joint reaction force (166 kgf to 57.5 kgf).

Forces at the knee in knee extension from a sitting position

Many of the muscles of the body, especially those in the limbs, operate in third-class lever systems. A typical example of a third-class lever system in the leg is the action of the quad-riceps in extending the knee. The distal ends of the quadriceps muscles all insert onto the quadriceps tendon. The quadriceps tendon encloses the anterior surface of the patella and is continuous with the patellar ligament, which inserts onto the tibial tuberosity. When the quadriceps muscles contract, the force is transmitted to the tibia which tends to extend the knee. The patella increases the moment arm of the quadriceps tendon about the axis of knee flexion and extension and, as such, increases the moment of the quadriceps muscle force. During knee flexion or extension, the posterior aspect of the patella slides on the patellar surface of the femur. The contact force between the patella and femur is referred to as the patellofemoral joint reaction force. The contact force between the tibia and femur is referred to as the tibiofemoral joint reaction force.

Figure 10.25a shows the foot, shank and distal end of the thigh while in a sitting position with the shank and foot held off the floor at an angle of $42°$ with respect to the horizontal and the foot at a right angle to the shank. In this position, the weight W of the shank and foot will exert an anticlockwise moment about the mediolateral axis through the knee that tends to flex the knee, but the shank and foot will be held in equilibrium by a clockwise moment exerted by the force L in the patellar ligament. The magnitude of the moment of L will depend upon

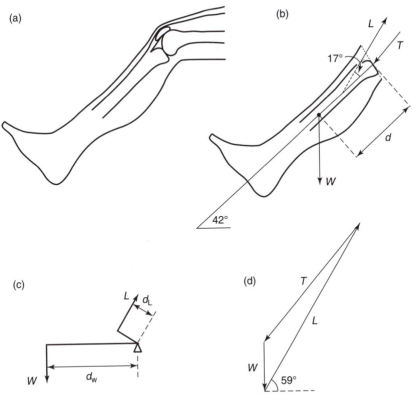

Figure 10.25 Patellar ligament force and tibiofemoral joint reaction force while holding shank and foot off of ground in sitting position. (a) Sitting with shank and foot held at an angle of 42° to the horizontal. (b) Free body diagram of shank and foot segment. (c) Force–moment arm diagram with respect to mediolateral axis through point of application of tibiofemoral joint reaction force. (d) Vector chain determination of tibiofemoral joint reaction force.

the moment exerted by the hamstrings, which will tend to flex the knee. In this example, it will be assumed that the force in the hamstrings is zero and, therefore, the moment exerted by the hamstrings is zero. Consequently, the moment of L will be equal and opposite to that of W. Figure 10.25b shows the corresponding free body diagram of the combined shank and foot. Figure 10.25c shows the corresponding force–moment arm diagram. Force T is the tibiofemoral joint reaction force. When the shank and foot segment is in equilibrium, the resultant of W, L and T will be zero.

In women, the length of the shank (the distance between the knee joint centre and the ankle joint centre) is approximately 25% of height (Plagenhoef *et al.* 1983). Consequently, for a woman of height 170 cm, the length of the shank will be approximately 42.5 cm and the corresponding distance d between the point of application of T and the location of the centre of gravity of the combined shank and foot will be approximately 21 cm (assuming that the distance between the knee joint centre and the point of application of T is approximately 3 cm and that the knee joint centre, point of application of T and centre of gravity of the shank and foot all lie on the same line with respect to Figure 10.25b). Consequently, with the shank and foot held at an angle of 42°, the moment arm d_W of W about the mediolateral axis through

377

the point of application of T will be approximately 15.6 cm. The line of action of L will be approximately $17°$ with respect to the line joining the point of application of T and the centre of gravity of the shank and foot, i.e. approximately $59°$ with respect to the horizontal and the length of the moment arm d_L of L will be approximately 4 cm through the $0°–90°$ range of knee flexion (Chow 1999). For a woman of weight 62 kgf, W will be approximately 4.14 kgf (Table 10.2). By taking moments about the mediolateral axis through the point of application of T,

$$W \cdot d_W - L \cdot d_L = 0$$

where: $W = 4.14$ kgf,
$d_W = d \cdot \cos 42° = 15.6$ cm,
$d_L = 4$ cm,

i.e. $L = \dfrac{W \cdot d_W}{d_L} = \dfrac{4.14 \text{ kgf} \times 15.6 \text{ cm}}{4 \text{ cm}} = 16.5$ kgf.

The vector chain determination of T is shown in Figure 10.25d; $T = 12.8$ kgf at an angle of $49°$ to the horizontal. The determination of T by trigonometry is shown in Figure 10.26; $J = 12.78$ kgf at an angle of $49.4°$ to the horizontal.

Figure 10.27a shows a free body diagram of the patella corresponding to the position of the shank and foot in Figure 10.25a. In this position, the patella is held in equilibrium under

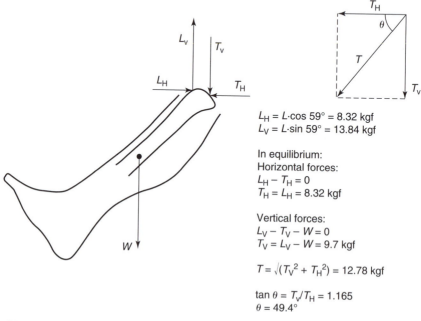

$L_H = L \cdot \cos 59° = 8.32$ kgf
$L_V = L \cdot \sin 59° = 13.84$ kgf

In equilibrium:
Horizontal forces:
$L_H - T_H = 0$
$T_H = L_H = 8.32$ kgf

Vertical forces:
$L_V - T_V - W = 0$
$T_V = L_V - W = 9.7$ kgf

$T = \sqrt{(T_V^2 + T_H^2)} = 12.78$ kgf

$\tan \theta = T_V / T_H = 1.165$
$\theta = 49.4°$

Figure 10.26 Determination of tibiofemoral joint reaction force by trigonometry (where forces are in equilibrium)

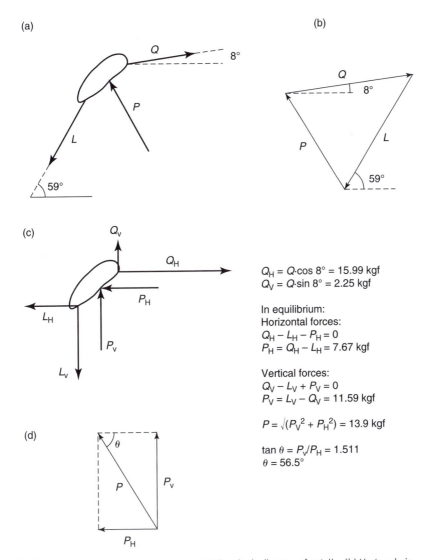

(a)

(b)

(c)

$Q_H = Q \cdot \cos 8° = 15.99$ kgf
$Q_V = Q \cdot \sin 8° = 2.25$ kgf

In equilibrium:
Horizontal forces:
$Q_H - L_H - P_H = 0$
$P_H = Q_H - L_H = 7.67$ kgf

Vertical forces:
$Q_V - L_V + P_V = 0$
$P_V = L_V - Q_V = 11.59$ kgf

$P = \sqrt{(P_V^2 + P_H^2)} = 13.9$ kgf

$\tan \theta = P_V/P_H = 1.511$
$\theta = 56.5°$

(d)

Figure 10.27 Patellofemoral joint reaction force. (a) Free body diagram of patella. (b) Vector chain determination of patellofemoral joint reaction force. (c,d) Determination of patellofemoral joint reaction force by trigonometry (where forces are in equilibrium)

the action of the force L in the patellar ligament (equal in magnitude, but opposite in direction to L in Figure 10.25b), the force Q in the quadriceps tendon (which can be assumed to be equal in magnitude to L) acting at an angle of 8° to the horizontal and the patellofemoral joint reaction force P. The vector chain determination of P is shown in Figure 10.27b; $P = 13.9$ kgf at an angle of 56° to the horizontal. The determination of P by trigonometry is shown in Figure 10.27c and d; $P = 13.9$ kgf at an angle of 56.5° to the horizontal.

The results show that to hold the shank and foot, weight approximately 4 kgf, at an angle of 42° to the horizontal requires a quadriceps muscle force of approximately 16 kgf, which, in turn, results in a patellar ligament force of approximately 16 kgf, a tibiofemoral joint reaction force of approximately 13 kgf and a patellofemoral joint reaction force of approximately 14 kgf. This illustrates the price that the body pays for the open-chain arrangement of the bones of the skeleton. The arms and legs form four peripheral chains, free at their extremities, which attach onto a central chain (the vertebral column). This open-chain arrangement allows any part of the body to move more-or-less independently of the rest and, as such, allows the body to adopt a very wide range of postures. However, this movement capability is only pos-sible because the muscles are attached to the skeleton close to the joints that they control, i.e. the muscles have very low mechanical advantages and, as such, generally have to exert much larger forces than the weights of the body segments that they control. Furthermore, the larger the muscle forces, the larger the associated joint reaction forces.

Forces at the knee in knee extension from a standing position

Knee extension exercises from a sitting position, with and without additional load (such as resistance training equipment), are widely used in rehabilitation programmes following knee injury. As illustrated in the previous section, the quadriceps muscle force and the tibiofemoral and patellofemoral forces are relatively small when there is no additional load (in the form of resistance training equipment) on the shank and foot segment. In a rehabilitation strength training programme, the load on the quadriceps muscles can be progressively increased by increasing the load on the shank and foot. Figure 10.28a shows a man performing a knee flexion and extension exercise from a standing position. In this situation, the load on each leg tending to flex the knee is half of body weight, i.e. if the exercise is performed slowly, avoiding high acceleration and deceleration at the start and end of each downward (knee flexion) and upward (knee extension) phase, the ground reaction force on each leg during the exercise will be approximately half of body weight. Figure 10.28b shows a free body diagram of one shank and foot corresponding to the position in Figure 10.28a.

In men, the length of the shank (the distance between the knee joint centre and the ankle joint centre) is approximately 25% of height (Plagenhoef et al. 1983). Consequently, for a man of height 180 cm, the length of the shank will be approximately 45 cm and the corresponding distance d_1 between the point of application of the tibiofemoral joint reaction force T and the location of the centre of gravity of the combined shank and foot will be about 24 cm (assum-ing that the distance between the knee joint centre and the point of application of T is about 3.2 cm and that the knee joint centre, point of application of T and centre of gravity of the shank and foot all lie on the same line with respect to Figure 10.28b). In the position shown in Figure 10.28a, the long axis of the shank (line joining the point application of the T and the ankle joint centre) is approximately 70° to the horizontal and the line of action of the patellar ligament will be approximately 68° to the horizontal (based on Van Eijden et al. 1985). The moment arm d_L of the patellar ligament force L about the mediolateral axis through the point of application of T will be approximately 4.5 cm (based on Chow 1999). The moment arm of the ground reaction force R will be approximately 9 cm (based on Wallace et al. 2002). For a man of weight 80 kgf, the weight of the shank and foot W will be approximately 4.94 kgf (see Table 10.1, Plagenhoef et al. data). In this example, it must be assumed that the hamstrings are active, as they normally work with the quadriceps to stabilise the knee joint. In the posi-tion shown in Figure 10.28a, the moment arm d_S of the force S exerted by hamstring muscles

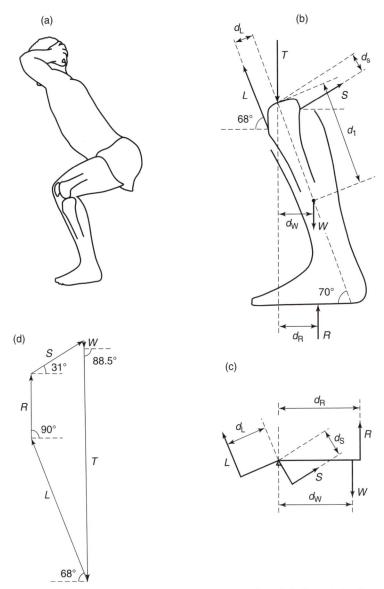

Figure 10.28 Patellar ligament force and tibiofemoral joint reaction force in half-squat standing position. (a) Half-squat standing position. (b) Free body diagram of shank and foot segment of one leg. (c) Force–moment arm diagram with respect to mediolateral axis through point of application of tibiofemoral joint reaction force. (d) Vector chain determination of tibiofemoral joint reaction force.

about the mediolateral axis through the point of application of T will be about 3 cm (based on Lieber 1992). It will be assumed that S is 40% of L (based on the ratio of the cross-sectional areas of the quadriceps and hamstring muscle groups; Lieber 1992). When the shank and foot segment is in equilibrium, the resultant of W, R, L, S and T will be zero. Figure 10.28c shows the corresponding force–moment arm diagram. By taking moments about the mediolateral axis through the point of application of T,

381

$$L \cdot d_L + W \cdot d_W - S \cdot d_S - R \cdot d_R = 0,$$

where: d_L = 4.5 cm,
W = 4.94 kgf,
$d_W = d_1 \cdot \cos 70° = 8.21$ cm,
S = 0.4L,
d_S = 3 cm,
R = 40 kgf,
d_R = 9.0 cm,

i.e. $L(d_L - 0.4d_S) = R \cdot d_R - W \cdot d_W$

$$L = \frac{R \cdot d_R - W \cdot d_W}{d_L - 0.4d_S} = \frac{(40 \text{ kgf} \times 9 \text{ cm}) - (4.94 \text{ kgf} \times 8.21 \text{ cm})}{4.5 \text{ cm} - 1.2 \text{ cm}} = 96.8 \text{ kgf.}$$

As L = 96.8 kgf, S = 38.72 kgf.

The vector chain determination of T is shown in Figure 10.28d; T = 145 kgf at an angle of 88.5° to the horizontal. The determination of T by trigonometry is shown in Figure 10.29; T = 144.78 kgf at an angle of 88.5° to the horizontal.

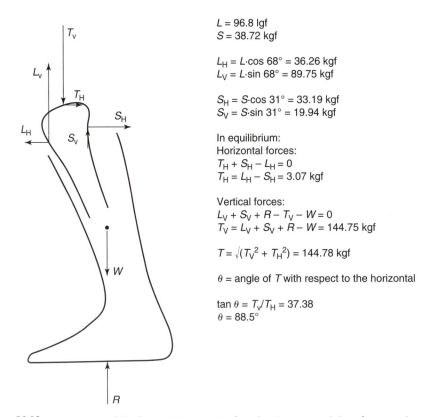

L = 96.8 lgf
S = 38.72 kgf

$L_H = L \cdot \cos 68° = 36.26$ kgf
$L_V = L \cdot \sin 68° = 89.75$ kgf

$S_H = S \cdot \cos 31° = 33.19$ kgf
$S_V = S \cdot \sin 31° = 19.94$ kgf

In equilibrium:
Horizontal forces:
$T_H + S_H - L_H = 0$
$T_H = L_H - S_H = 3.07$ kgf

Vertical forces:
$L_V + S_V + R - T_V - W = 0$
$T_V = L_V + S_V + R - W = 144.75$ kgf

$T = \sqrt{(T_V^2 + T_H^2)} = 144.78$ kgf

θ = angle of T with respect to the horizontal

$\tan \theta = T_V / T_H = 37.38$
$\theta = 88.5°$

Figure 10.29 Determination of tibiofemoral joint reaction force by trigonometry (where forces are in equilibrium)

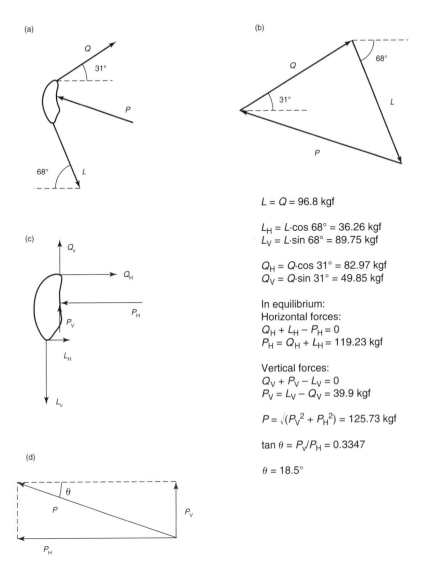

$$L = Q = 96.8 \text{ kgf}$$

$$L_H = L{\cdot}\cos 68° = 36.26 \text{ kgf}$$
$$L_V = L{\cdot}\sin 68° = 89.75 \text{ kgf}$$

$$Q_H = Q{\cdot}\cos 31° = 82.97 \text{ kgf}$$
$$Q_V = Q{\cdot}\sin 31° = 49.85 \text{ kgf}$$

In equilibrium:
Horizontal forces:
$$Q_H + L_H - P_H = 0$$
$$P_H = Q_H + L_H = 119.23 \text{ kgf}$$

Vertical forces:
$$Q_V + P_V - L_V = 0$$
$$P_V = L_V - Q_V = 39.9 \text{ kgf}$$

$$P = \sqrt{(P_V{}^2 + P_H{}^2)} = 125.73 \text{ kgf}$$

$$\tan \theta = P_V/P_H = 0.3347$$

$$\theta = 18.5°$$

Figure 10.30 Patellofemoral joint reaction force. (a) Free body diagram of patella. (b) Vector chain determination of patellofemoral joint reaction force. (c,d) Determination of patellofemoral joint reaction force by trigonometry (where forces are in equilibrium).

Figure 10.30a shows a free body diagram of the patella corresponding to the position of the shank and foot in Figure 10.28a. In this position, the patella is held in equilibrium by the action of the force L in the patellar ligament (equal in magnitude, but opposite in direction to L in Figure 10.28b), the force Q in the quadriceps tendon (which can be assumed to be equal in magnitude to L) acting at an angle of 31° to the horizontal and the patellofemoral joint reaction force P. The vector chain determination of P is shown in Figure 10.30b; P = 126 kgf at an angle of 18.5° to the horizontal. The determination of P by trigonometry is shown in Figure 10.30c and d; P = 125.73 kgf at an angle of 18.5° to the horizontal.

In the half-squat position shown in Figure 10.28a, the external forces acting on the shank and foot segment of each leg are the weight of the shank and foot, approximately 0.062 body weight (BW), and the ground reaction force, approximately 0.5 BW. Force analysis demonstrates that to maintain the equilibrium of the shank and foot in this position, five internal forces are required at the knee: quadriceps muscle force (approximately 1.2 BW), patellar ligament force (approximately 1.2 BW), hamstrings muscle force (approximately 0.5 BW), tibiofemoral joint reaction force (approximately 1.8 BW), patellofemoral joint reaction force (approximately 1.6 BW).

The use of body segments as levers in strength and endurance training

In any training exercise, such as a pull-up, sit-up or press-up, the muscles involved must overcome the moment of resistance exerted by the resistance force. The moment of resistance and, therefore, the load on the muscles can be varied by changing the resistance force or the moment arm of the resistance force. This is the basis of progressive strength and local (muscular) endurance training. Whereas strength training for sport is likely to involve the use of resistance equipment to increase the load and, therefore, the training effect on the muscles, subtle changes in body posture can provide adequate resistance for the development of strength and endurance that is consistent with good health without the need for additional load.

Trunk curl and sit-up

Consider a man lying on his back with his arms straight and hands, palms down, on the front of his thighs (Figure 10.31a). To sit up, the abdominal muscles and hip flexor muscles must overcome the moment of upper body weight about the mediolateral axis a_H through the hip joints. The first stage in the sit-up exercise usually involves what is called a trunk curl, i.e. flexion of the neck and thoracic region by the neck and abdominal flexor muscles. This movement results in a decrease in the moment arm of upper body weight about a_H (Figure 10.31b). The sit-up is completed by the action of the hip flexors, which rotate the upper body about the hips. As the upper body moves from the lying to the sit-up position, the moment arm of upper body weight about a_H gradually decreases (Figure 10.31b,c). Therefore, the moment of force required to raise the upper body into the sitting position also gradually decreases. As the moment arm of the hip flexor muscles gradually increases throughout the range of hip movement from lying to sitting up, the force exerted by the hip flexors gradually decreases as the upper body assumes the sit-up position. It follows that the most strenuous part of the whole sit-up movement occurs just after the start of hip flexion as the upper body is raised clear of the floor. The sit-up exercise can be made more strenuous by starting with the hands behind the head as shown in Figure 10.31d. The movement of the arms redistributes the upper body weight such that the moment arm of upper body weight about a_H is increased (Figure 10.31a,d; $d_2 > d_1$). Consequently, in raising the upper body into the sitting position, the hip flexors would need to exert a greater force than would be necessary from the starting position shown in Figure 10.31a. The exercise could be made even more strenuous by starting with the arms extended by the side of the head (Figure 10.31d,e; $d_3 > d_2$).

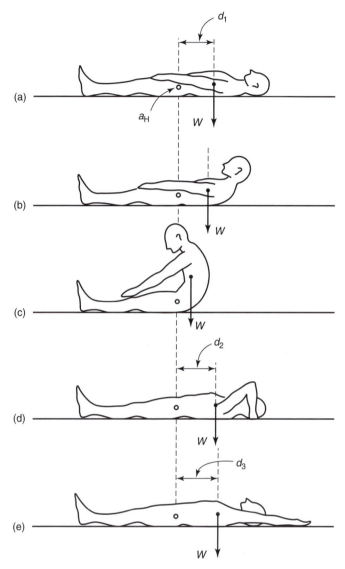

Figure 10.31 (a,b) Trunk curl. (a–c) Sit-up. (d) Effect of putting hands behind head on moment arm of upper body weight. (e) Effect of putting the arms by side of head on moment arm of upper body weight. *W*, weight of trunk, head, neck and arms.

Bent-leg sit-up

If the abdominal and hip flexor muscles are not strong enough for the person to perform a sit-up from the straight-leg starting position (Figure 10.31a), it may be possible for the person to perform a bent-leg sit-up (Figure 10.32). With the hips flexed at 45° to the horizontal in the starting position (Figure 10.32a), the moment arm of the hip flexors will be greater than in the straight-leg starting position. Consequently, the hip flexors will be able to raise the upper body into the sitting position with less force than that required in the straight-leg

385

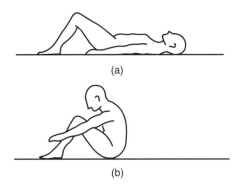

Figure 10.32 Bent-leg sit-up.

starting position. The moment arm of the abdominal muscles will be about the same in both starting positions.

Leg raise

When the hip flexor and abdominal muscles are very weak, such that the person cannot perform a bent-leg sit-up, a suitable exercise to start training these muscles is alternate single-leg raises (Figure 10.33a,b). The moment arm of the weight of each leg is about the same as that of the upper body, about a_H, after the trunk curl stage of the sit-up (Figures 10.31b and 10.33a). However, as the upper body (trunk, head, neck and arms) and each leg constitute about 68% and 16%, respectively, of total body weight (Table 10.1), the moment of resistance that the hip flexors of each leg are required to overcome when performing a single-leg raise is much less than that required to perform a bent-leg sit-up. Furthermore, the load on the abdominal muscles is much less in a single-leg raise than in a bent-leg sit-up. It might be assumed that a reasonable progression from alternate single-leg raises is to raise both legs together (Figure 10.33c). However, in order to perform this exercise correctly, i.e. without risk of injury to the low back, the abdominal muscles must exert considerable force, to prevent the pelvis from rotating forward (anticlockwise with respect to Figure 10.33c). The sacrum forms the lower end of the vertebral column and the rear part of the pelvis. Forward rotation of the pelvis increases the curvature of the lumbar region of the vertebral column (continuous with the sacrum), which may result in low back pain due to strain of the lumbosacral plexuses, i.e. the peripheral nerves of the lumbar region.

The single-leg raise can be made less strenuous by flexing the knee before raising the leg (Figure 10.33d,e). Flexing the knee reduces the moment arm of the weight of the leg about a_H, thereby reducing the moment of resistance that the hip flexors need to overcome. A suitable progression of exercises for increasing the strength and endurance of the hip flexors and abdominal muscles would be:

1. Trunk curls;
2. Alternate single bent-leg raises;
3. Double bent-leg raises;
4. Single straight-leg raises;

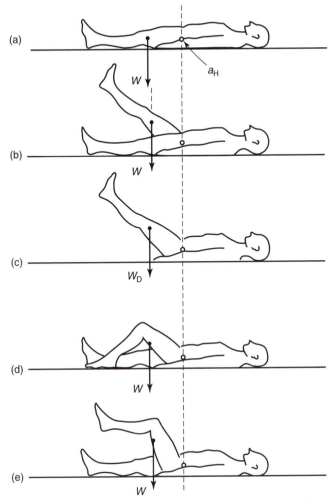

Figure 10.33 (a,b) Single straight-leg raise. (c) Double straight-leg raise. (d,e) Single bent-leg raise. W, weight of one leg; W_D, weight of both legs.

5. Bent-leg sit-ups;
6. Straight-leg sit-ups.

Press-up

During a press-up from the floor, as shown in Figure 10.34a and b, the body segment consisting of head, neck, trunk and legs is held in line and rotated about the balls of the feet by the action of the arms. To complete a press-up, the elbow extensors and shoulder flexors must overcome the moment of body weight about the mediolateral axis a_F through the points of contact between the feet and the floor. Provided that the head, neck, trunk and legs are held in line, the moment arm d_A of the force A exerted by the arms about a_F will be more-or-less the same, irrespective of the inclination of the head, neck, trunk and legs (Figure 10.34f).

387

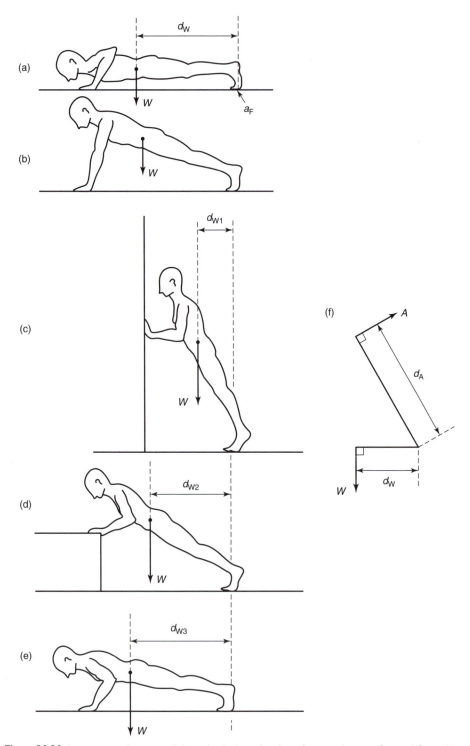

Figure 10.34 Press-up exercise: a_F, mediolateral axis through points of contact between feet and floor; W, body weight; A, force exerted by arms; d_W, moment arm of W about a_F; d_A, moment arm of A about a_F.

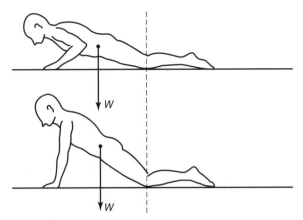

Figure 10.35 Modified press-up using knees rather than feet as fulcrum.

However, the greater the inclination of the head, neck, trunk and legs to the vertical, the greater the moment arm d_W of body weight W about a_F and, therefore, the greater the force A required to extend the arms. Therefore, in order to gradually increase the training effect of the exercise, it is necessary to gradually increase d_W. This can be achieved by gradually lowering the position of the hand support with respect to the feet. For example, a reasonable progression would be to start with a press-up against a wall followed by the edge of a table, then a low box or bench and finally the floor (Figure 10.34c–e; $d_{W1} < d_{W2} < d_{W3}$).

Press-ups against the floor can be made less strenuous by using the knees as a fulcrum (with suitable cushioning) rather than the feet, as shown in Figure 10.35. In this form of press-up, the moment of resistance about the mediolateral axis through the knees–floor fulcrum is considerably less than the moment of resistance about the feet–floor fulcrum in Figure 10.34a.

Squat

The half-squat with a barbell weight across the shoulders, as shown in Figure 10.36, is one of the most frequently used weight training exercises for increasing the strength of the leg extensor muscles, i.e. hip extensors, knee extensors and ankle plantar flexors. The effect that the exercise has on these three groups of muscles depends upon the moment of resistance about each corresponding joint. The resistance W is the combined weight of the body and the barbell. As W is the same in positions 1 and 2, the effect on each muscle group depends upon the moment arm of W about each joint. In position 1, the trunk is inclined forward at about $45°$ to the horizontal, such that the moment arm d_{K1} of W about the mediolateral axis a_K through the knee joint is less than the moment arm d_{H1} of W about the mediolateral axis a_H through the hip joint. In position 2, the trunk is more upright (an inclination of about $63°$ to the horizontal), such that the moment arm d_{K2} of W about a_K is greater than the moment arm d_{H2} of W about a_H. Consequently, the training effect on the hip extensors will be greater in position 1 than in position 2 and the training effect on the knee extensors will be greater in position 2 than in position 1. Similarly, as the moment arm of W about the mediolateral axis a_A through the ankle joint is greater in position 1 than in position 2, the training effect on the ankle plantar flexors will be greater in position 1 than in position 2.

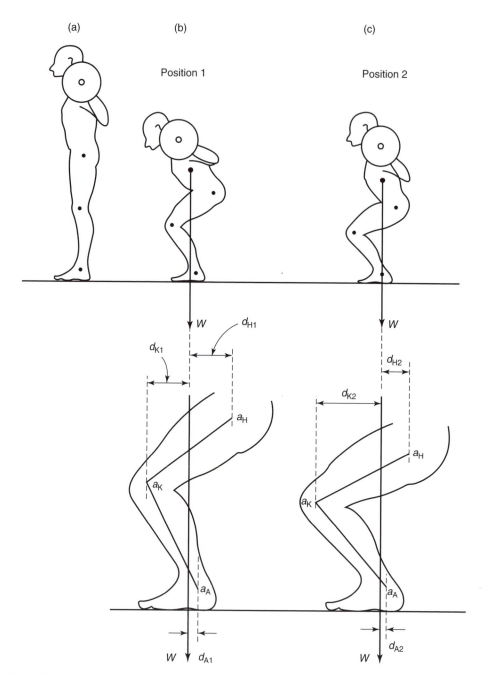

Figure 10.36 Half-squat with a barbell.

Leg press

The leg press, like the half-squat, is also a popular weight training exercise for strengthening the leg extensors. One form of leg press is shown in Figure 10.37. In this exercise, the trainer lies on his back and lifts and lowers a weight vertically by extending and flexing his legs. In position 1, the line of action of the weight W passes through the mediolateral axis through the hip joint, a_H. Consequently, the moment of W about a_H is zero and there will be little training effect on the hip extensors. However, the moment arm of W about the mediolateral axis through the knee joint, a_K, and the mediolateral axis through the ankle joint, a_A, is relatively large, such that the training effect on the knee extensors and ankle plantar flexors is likely to be significant. In position 2, W exerts a moment of resistance about all three joints, with the largest moment about the hip joint. The half-squat and leg press show that slight changes in body posture can significantly alter the way in which the musculoskeletal system responds to a particular external load on the body.

> Appropriate changes in body posture in training exercises can provide adequate resistance for the development of strength and endurance consistent with good health without the need for resistance equipment.

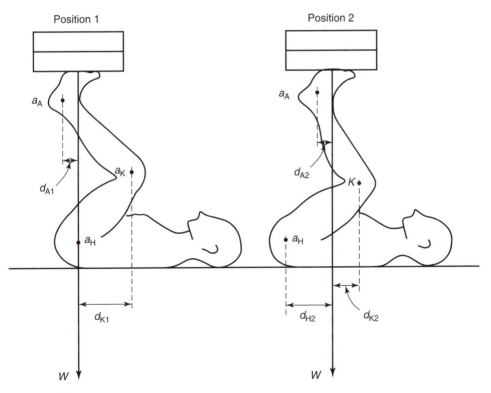

Figure 10.37 Leg press.

ANGULAR DISPLACEMENT, ANGULAR VELOCITY AND ANGULAR ACCELERATION

Figure 10.38 shows a man performing a single-leg raise from a lying position. In raising his left leg from position 1 to position 2, the centre of gravity of his leg moves a linear distance s, i.e. the arc of the circle of radius r about the mediolateral axis a_H through the left hip joint. Simultaneously, his leg rotates an angular distance θ (Greek lower case letter theta) about a_H.

In trigonometry, angular distance is usually measured in degrees. There are $360°$ in one complete revolution. Figure 10.39a shows a gymnast performing a giant circle on a horizontal bar. By rotating about the bar, i.e. about the axis a_B, from position A to position D, the gymnast will rotate an angular distance of $180°$ and an angular displacement (angular distance in a clockwise direction) of $180°$. By rotating from position A back to position A, the gymnast will have travelled an angular distance of $360°$, i.e. one revolution. Angular displacement must reflect the number of revolutions between the initial and final positions of the object following a period of rotation.

In mechanics, angular distance is usually measured in radians (rad). One radian is the angle subtended at the centre of a circle by an arc of the circle that is the same length as the radius of the circle (Figure 10.40). The circumference of a circle $= 2\pi \cdot r$, where r is the radius of the circle, i.e.

$$360° = 2\pi \cdot r/r \text{ rad}$$
$$= 2\pi \text{ rad}$$
$$= 6.2832 \text{ rad } (\text{as } \pi = 3.1416).$$

$$\text{Therefore, } 1° = 0.01745 \text{ rad } (6.2832/360)$$
$$1 \text{ rad} = 57.3°(360/6.2832).$$

Angular speed is the rate of change of angular distance. In mechanics, angular speed is usually measured in rad/s (radians per second). When the direction of rotation is specified, the term angular velocity is used rather than angular speed. The symbol for angular velocity is ω (Greek lower case letter omega). Figure 10.39b shows the movement of the gymnast between positions B and C. The average angular velocity of the gymnast between positions B and C is given by

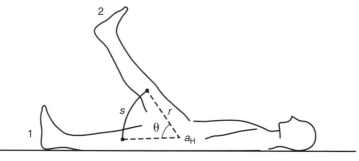

Figure 10.38 Linear movement (s) of centre of gravity of leg and angular movement (θ) of leg in single-leg raise: a_H, mediolateral axis through the hip joint, r, distance between a_H and centre of gravity of leg.

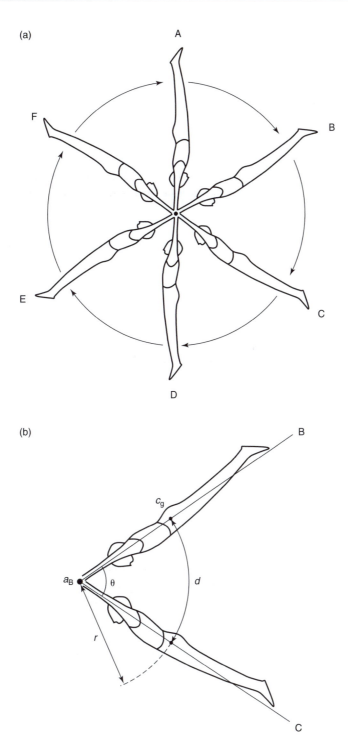

(a)

A

F

B

E

C

D

(b)

B

c_g

a_B

θ

d

r

C

Figure 10.39 Gymnast performing a giant circle on a horizontal bar: cg, centre of gravity; a_B, horizontal axis along centre of bar; r, distance between a_B and cg = radius of the circle followed by cg; d, linear distance travelled by cg; θ = angular distance travelled by body.

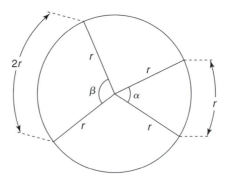

Figure 10.40 A radian is the angle subtended at the centre of a circle by an arc on the circumference of the circle that is the same length as the radius of the circle: r, radius of circle; $\alpha = 1$ radian; $\beta = 2$ radians.

$$\omega = \frac{\theta_C - \theta_B}{t_C - t_B},$$ (10.6)

where: θ_B = angular displacement of position B relative to position A,
          θ_C = angular displacement of position C relative to position A,
          t_B = time at position B with respect to position A,
          t_C = time at position C with respect to position A.

If $\theta_B = 60°$,
         $\theta_C = 125°$,
         $t_B = 1.43$ s,
         $t_C = 1.69$ s,

then: $\omega = \dfrac{125° - 60°}{1.69\,\text{s} - 1.43\,\text{s}} = 250°/\text{s}$ (degrees per second) $= 4.36$ rad/s.

Angular acceleration is the rate of change of angular velocity. In mechanics, angular acceleration is usually measured in rad/s² (radians per second per second). The symbol for angular acceleration is α (Greek lower case letter alpha). The average angular acceleration of the gymnast between positions B and C is given by

$$\alpha = \frac{\omega_C - \omega_B}{t_C - t_B},$$ (10.7)

where: ω_B = angular velocity at position B,
          ω_C = angular velocity at position C,
          t_B = time at position B with respect to position A,
          t_C = time at position C with respect to position A.

If $\omega_B = 3.13$ rad/s,
         $\omega_C = 5.55$ rad/s,
         $t_B = 1.43$ s,
         $t_C = 1.69$ s,

then $\alpha = \dfrac{5.55\,\text{rad/s} - 3.13\,\text{rad/s}}{1.69\,\text{s} - 1.43\text{s}} = 9.31\,\text{rad/s}^2.$

394

Relationship between linear velocity and angular velocity

In Figure 10.39b, if the orientation of the gymnast's body segments to each other remains the same between positions B and C, i.e. if the centre of gravity moves along the arc d of a circle of radius r in a time t, then the average linear velocity v of the centre of gravity during this period is given by

$$v = \frac{d}{t}. \tag{10.8}$$

If the body rotates through an angle θ during the same period, then the average angular velocity of the body is given by

$$\omega = \frac{\theta}{t}. \tag{10.9}$$

As θ degrees $= d/r$ radians, then

$$d = r \cdot \theta. \tag{10.10}$$

By substitution of d from Equation 10.10 into Equation 10.8,

$$v = \frac{r \cdot \theta}{t}. \tag{10.11}$$

By substitution of θ/t from Equation 10.9 into Equation 10.11,

$$v = r \cdot \omega, \tag{10.12}$$

i.e. the linear velocity of the centre of gravity is equal to the product of the radius of the circle (distance from the axis of rotation to the centre of gravity) and the angular velocity of the body. The radian is a dimensionless variable, i.e. it has no unit because it is the ratio of two distances (the arc of the circle and the radius of the circle). Consequently, the product $r \cdot \omega$ is in m/s (where r is in metres and ω is in rad/s). For example, in Figure 10.39b, if $r = 1$ m and $\omega = 3.13$ rad/s at position B, then v at B $= 3.13$ m/s.

Relationship between linear acceleration and angular acceleration

From Equation 10.12, it follows that $v_B = r \cdot \omega_B$ and $v_C = r \cdot \omega_C$ where v_B, v_C and ω_B, ω_C are the linear and angular velocities of the centre of gravity of the gymnast at positions B and C in Figure 10.39b. Consequently, the average linear acceleration a (Roman lower case letter a) of the centre of gravity between positions B and C is given by

$$a = \frac{v_C - v_B}{t} = \frac{r(\omega_C - \omega_B)}{t}.$$

As $\dfrac{\omega_C - \omega_B}{t} = \alpha = $ angular acceleration (Eq. 10.7),

395

it follows that,

$$a = r \cdot \alpha, \tag{10.13}$$

i.e. the linear acceleration of the centre of gravity in the direction of v is equal to the product of the radius of the circle (distance from the axis of rotation to the centre of gravity) and the angular acceleration of the body. As the direction of a is perpendicular to r, i.e. tangent to the circle, a is referred to as tangential acceleration and sometimes denoted a_T. In Figure 10.39b, if $r = 1$ m and $\alpha = 9.31$ rad/s^2 at position C, then a_T at C $= 9.31$ m/s^2.

CENTRIPETAL AND CENTRIFUGAL FORCE

It is clear from Figure 10.39b that the direction of the centre of gravity is continuously changing in order to maintain its circular path. In accordance with Newton's first law of motion, there must be a force acting on the centre of gravity that is responsible for its continuous change of direction. This force cannot be the weight of the body because weight acts vertically downward. Consequently, there must be another force acting on the centre of gravity that is responsible for its continuous change of direction. Intuitively, this force is the force exerted by the bar on the body, i.e. the equal and opposite reaction to the force exerted by the gymnast on the bar. To derive the magnitude and direction of this force, it is better to use an example, unlike a giant circle, where the force is not influenced by the weight of the moving body. Consider, for example, the movement of a small weight, such as a plumb bob, attached to a piece of string, which is being swung around with constant linear velocity v in a horizontal plane (Figure 10.41a) (Ninio 1993). If the object is rotating anticlockwise with respect to Figure 10.41a, the components of velocity v_X and v_Y at the point A in the directions of X (positive to the right) and Y (positive upward) respectively, are given by

$$v_X = -v \cdot \sin\theta = -\frac{v \cdot y}{r} \quad (\sin\theta = y/r); \tag{10.14}$$

$$v_Y = v \cdot \cos\theta = \frac{v \cdot x}{r} \quad (\cos\theta = x/r). \tag{10.15}$$

As v/r is constant, it follows from Equation 10.14 that the rate of change of v_X is the product of v/r and the rate of change of y. As the rate of change of v_X is a_X, the linear acceleration of the object in the X direction and the rate of change of y is v_Y, the linear velocity of the object in the Y direction, then

$$a_X = (-v/r) \cdot v_Y = (-v/r) \cdot (v \cdot x/r) = -(v^2/r) \cdot \cos\theta.$$

Similarly, it follows from Equation 10.15 that the rate of change of v_Y is the product of v/r and the rate of change of x. As the rate of change of v_Y is a_Y, the linear acceleration of the object in the Y direction and the rate of change of x is v_X, the linear velocity of the object in the X direction, then

$$a_Y = (v/r) \cdot v_X = (v/r) \cdot (-v \cdot y/r) = -(v^2/r) \cdot \sin\theta.$$

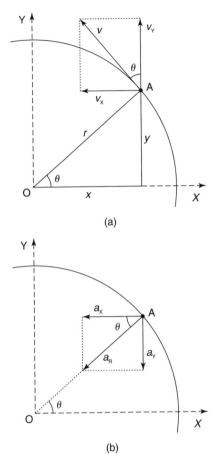

Figure 10.41 (a) Velocity components v_x and v_y of object moving in circle with constant velocity v. (b) Components a_x and a_y of centripetal acceleration a_R. O, centre of circle.

The resultant linear acceleration a of the object is given by Pythagoras' theorem:

$$a^2 = a_X^2 + a_Y^2 = (v^4/r^2 \cdot \cos^2\theta) + (v^4/r^2 \cdot \sin^2\theta)$$

$$a^2 = (v^4/r^2) \cdot (\cos^2\theta + \sin^2\theta).$$

As $\quad \cos^2\theta + \sin^2\theta = 1$,

then $\quad a^2 = v^4/r^2$

$$a = v^2/r.$$

The direction of a with respect to the horizontal is given by the angle β where,

$$\tan\beta = \frac{a_Y}{a_X} = \frac{-(v^2/r) \cdot \sin\theta}{-(v^2/r) \cdot \cos\theta}.$$

As $\sin \theta / \cos \theta = \tan \theta$,

then $\tan \beta = \tan \theta$,

i.e. $\beta = \theta$.

Therefore, the magnitude of a is v^2/r and its direction is toward the centre of the circle. As a is directed along the radius of the circle, it is referred to as radial acceleration and sometimes denoted a_R to distinguish it from the tangential acceleration a_T. Figure 10.41b shows a_R, a_X and a_Y. From Newton's second law of motion, a_R is due to a force of magnitude $m \cdot v^2/r$, where m is the mass of the object. This force is called the centripetal (centre-seeking) force, as it is directed toward the centre of the circle. Any object that moves on a curve (a circle is a regular curve) will do so due to the centripetal force F_C acting on it. As $F_C = m \cdot v^2/r$ and $v = r \cdot \omega$ (Equation 10.12), it follows that

$$F_C = m \cdot v^2/r = m \cdot r \cdot \omega^2 \tag{10.16}$$

In this example, the centripetal force is applied to the plumb-bob by the string. In accordance with Newton's third law of motion, the plumb-bob will exert an equal and opposite force on the string. This force is called the centrifugal (centre-fleeing) force.

The centrifugal force is due to the inertia of the plumb-bob resisting the change in its direction of motion by the centripetal force. As soon as the centripetal force disappears, so does the centrifugal force. Consequently, if the string attached to the plumb-bob breaks, the plumb-bob will continue to move (with respect to the plane of rotation) in the direction it had at the instant that the string broke, i.e. in a straight line, tangent to the circle (Figure 10.41a).

Centripetal force in throwing the hammer

In the hammer event in track and field athletics, the hammer consists of a metal ball (mass = 4 kg and diameter = 10 cm for women; mass = 7.26 kg and diameter = 12 cm for men) attached to a handle by a flexible wire (the total length of the handle and wire is approximately 1.13 m for women and men). The aim of the athlete is to maximise the range of the hammer, i.e. the horizontal distance travelled by the hammer following release.

As in the shot put, the main influences on the range of the hammer are release speed, release angle, release height and air resistance. Air resistance will have a greater effect on the range of a hammer throw (about 1.5% reduction in range) than on the range of a shot put (about 0.5% reduction in range), largely because of the greater release velocity of the hammer. Most elite male athletes release the hammer at about shoulder height, with a release angle of about 45° to the horizontal (Dapena 1984). Consequently, the main determinant of range is release speed. The angular and linear velocity of the hammer is built up over a period of about 4 seconds by a swinging-turning action performed within a circle 2.135 m (7 ft) in diameter. With the thrower standing in the back of the circle, facing the opposite direction to that of the throw, the action is usually initiated by two or three swings (lasting about 2.5 s) in which the hammer is swung overhead around the body. This is followed by three or four increasingly rapid whole body turns (each turn lasting about 0.5 s) in which the hammer is swung around the body as the body rotates about a vertical axis and simultaneously moves to the front of the

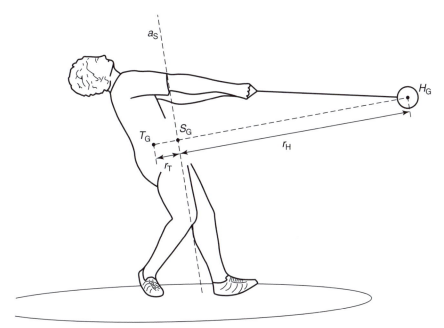

Figure 10.42 Position of thrower and hammer just before release: T_G, centre of gravity of thrower; H_G, centre of gravity of hammer; S_G, centre of gravity of combined thrower and hammer; a_S, axis passing through centre of gravity of combined thrower and hammer and perpendicular to plane of rotation; r_H, radius of curvature of hammer; r_T, radius of curvature of thrower.

circle. During the turns, the plane of motion of the hammer progressively increases so that the release angle is about 45°. The hammer is launched, ideally with maximum linear velocity, at the end of the final turn.

The current men's world record is 86.74 m (Yuriy Sedykh, Russia, mass = 110 kg, height = 1.85 m). Assuming a release height of 1.65 m and release angle of 45°, a release speed of approximately 29 m/s would be required for a throw of 86.74 m. The radius of curvature of the hammer (the distance from the instantaneous axis of rotation to the centre of gravity of the metal ball) at release for a male athlete of mass 110 kg and height 1.85 m will be approximately 1.80 m (Dyson 1977) (Figure 10.42). Consequently, from Equation 10.16, the centripetal force F_C acting on the hammer immediately before release will be approximately 3392 N, which is equivalent to 3.14 times the body weight (BW) of the athlete:

$$F_C = \frac{m \cdot v^2}{r} = \frac{7.26 \text{ kg} \times (29 \text{ m/s})^2}{1.80 \text{ m}} = 3392 \text{ N} = 345.8 \text{ kgf} = 3.14 \text{ BW}.$$

As the thrower pulls on the hammer with a force of 3.14 BW, the hammer will exert an equal and opposite force on the thrower, tending to pull him off balance. To maintain the centripetal force on the hammer and, therefore, the linear velocity (magnitude and direction) of the hammer, the thrower must counteract this force. The only way that this can be achieved is for the thrower to rotate his body in the same direction as the hammer about the same axis of rotation and thereby create a centripetal force on his centre of gravity that is equal and opposite to

399

the centripetal force on the hammer, i.e. the thrower and hammer rotate at the same angular velocity on opposite sides of the axis that passes through the centre of gravity of the combined thrower and hammer and is perpendicular to the plane of rotation (Figure 10.42). In this situation, the centrifugal force on the thrower will be equal and opposite to the centrifugal force on the hammer, so that the thrower can maintain his balance. It should be clear that the technique of throwing the hammer (usually referred to as throwing, but it is really a slinging action) not only requires great strength to produce and maintain such a large centripetal force on the hammer, especially in the final turn when the linear velocity of the hammer rapidly increases, but also a very high level of coordination and timing.

As the mass of the thrower is much greater than the mass of the hammer, the radius of curvature of the centre of mass of the thrower will be much smaller than the radius of curvature of the centre of mass of the hammer. A reasonable estimate of the radius of curvature of the centre of mass of the thrower can be made by considering the components of the centripetal forces on the hammer and thrower. Immediately prior to release, the centripetal force on the hammer will be more-or-less equal and opposite to the centripetal force on thrower. Consequently, from Equation 10.16,

$$m_H \cdot r_H \cdot \omega^2 = m_T \cdot r_T \cdot \omega^2, \qquad (10.17)$$

where: m_H = mass of the hammer,
r_H = radius of curvature of the hammer,
m_T = mass of the thrower,
r_T = radius of curvature of the thrower,
ω = angular velocity of the hammer and the thrower.

It follows from Equation 10.17 that

$$m_H \cdot r_H = m_T \cdot r_T \qquad (10.18)$$

If m_H = 7.26 kg, r_H = 1.8 m and m_T = 110 kg, then it follows from Equation 10.18 that

$$r_T = \frac{m_H \cdot r_H}{m_T} = \frac{7.26 \text{ kg} \times 1.8 \text{ m}}{110 \text{ kg}} = 0.119 \text{ m},$$

i.e. the radius of curvature of the centre of mass of the thrower is approximately 12 cm (Figure 10.42).

Centripetal force in cycling around a curved track

To cycle around a curve, the cyclist must create centripetal force between the wheels of the bike and the road. This is achieved by leaning toward the centre of curvature so that the horizontal component of the ground reaction force (in the plane of the radius of curvature) creates the required centripetal force. Figure 10.43a shows a rear-view free body diagram of a cyclist moving around a left-hand bend. As the cyclist and bike will be in rotational equilibrium with

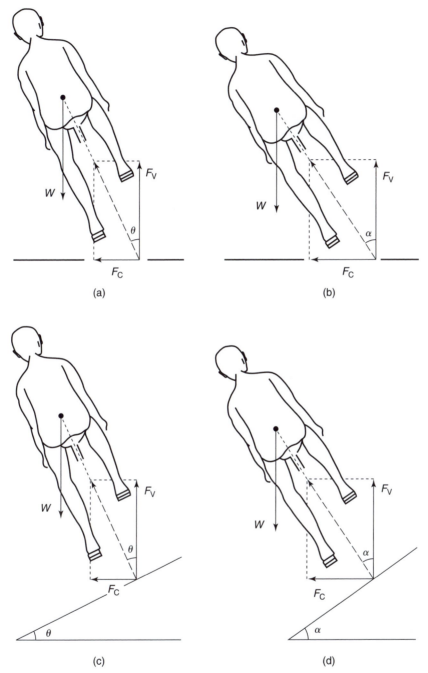

Figure 10.43 Rear-view free body diagram of cyclist riding around left-hand bend with linear velocity 13.41 m/s (30 mph). (a) Horizontal surface, radius of curvature, 37 m. (b) Horizontal surface, radius of curvature, 27 m. (c) Banked curve of slope θ, radius of curvature, 37 m. (d) Banked curve of slope α, radius of curvature, 27 m. θ, 26.3°; α, 34.2°; W, weight of rider and bike; F_c, horizontal component of ground reaction force = centripetal force; F_v, vertical component of ground reaction force = W.

respect to the plane of the radius of curvature (as in Figure 10.43a), the ground reaction force F (resultant of F_V and F_C) will act through the combined centre of gravity of the cyclist and bike. To maintain this situation, the cyclist and bike must lean at an angle θ, which is given by

$$\tan \theta = \frac{F_C}{F_V}. \tag{10.19}$$

If the combined mass of the cyclist and bike is 72 kg, and they are moving with a linear velocity of 13.41 m/s (30 mph) around a curve with radius of curvature 37 m (similar to a bend on a standard 400 m running track), the centripetal force F_C on the cyclist and bike will be

$$F_C = \frac{m \cdot v^2}{r} = \frac{72 \text{ kg} \times (13.41 \text{ m/s})^2}{37 \text{ m}} = 349.9 \text{ N}.$$

As $F_V = 72 \text{ kgf} = 706.3 \text{ N}$, then

$$\tan \theta = \frac{F_C}{F_V} = \frac{349.9 \text{ N}}{706.3 \text{ N}} = 0.4953$$

$$\theta = 26.3°.$$

If the cyclist wanted to cycle at the same speed around a tighter curve, i.e. a smaller radius of curvature, the centripetal force and lean angle would both increase. For example, for a radius of curvature of 27 m, $F_C = 479.5$ N and $\alpha = 34.2°$ (Figure 10.43b).

In these examples, it is assumed that the road is horizontal and, therefore, the centripetal force is the result of friction between the wheels and the road. In this situation, the maximum speed that can be achieved (for a given radius of curvature) is limited by the maximum friction that can be created (maximum friction $= \mu \cdot W$, where μ is the coefficient of friction and W is the normal reaction force, which is the weight of the cyclist and the bike; Equation 9.1). However, when riding on a banked curve, the need for friction can be significantly reduced or even eliminated. For example, Figure 10.43c shows the cyclist in Figure 10.43a riding at the same speed with the same radius of curvature on a banked curve with a slope that corresponds to the lean angle. Figure 10.43d shows the corresponding situation to that in Figure 10.43b. In these situations, centripetal force is provided by the horizontal component of the ground reaction without the need for friction. Consequently, if the angle of the slope is appropriate for the maximum speed likely to be achieved, friction is not a limiting factor. Velodromes (indoor cycling tracks) and indoor running tracks are banked for this reason. The slopes of velodromes range from approximately 15° on the straights to approximately 45° on the bends. The slopes of indoor running tracks range from 0° on the straights to approximately 15° on the bends (Wikipedia 2005).

Centripetal force in running around a curved track

As in cycling around a bend, a runner running around a bend leans toward the centre of curvature so that the horizontal component of the ground reaction force creates centripetal force. In cycling, the wheels are continuously in contact with the track so that the change of direction is fairly continuous. Furthermore, there is very little vertical motion of the combined centre of gravity of the cyclist and bike. However, in running, contact with the track is intermittent (each step consists of a ground contact phase and a flight phase), such that change of direction of the runner (in the transverse plane) only occurs during the ground contact phases. During the flight phase of each step, the centre of gravity of the runner moves in a straight line in the transverse plane and up and down in the median plane.

In a standard 400 m running track, each straight is 85 m and each bend is 115 m on the kerb. Consequently, the radius of each bend on the kerb is 36.6 m. The current men's world record for 200 m is 19.19 s (Usain Bolt, Jamaica, mass = 93 kg, height = 1.96 m), which represents an average velocity of 10.42 m/s. To maintain this average speed around the bend in lane 1 (radius of curvature approximately 36.6 m), a male sprinter of mass 93 kg would need to maintain an average centripetal force F_C of 275.9 N, equivalent to 0.3 times his body weight (BW), i.e.

$$F_C = \frac{m \cdot v^2}{r} = \frac{93 \text{ kg} \times (10.42 \text{ m/s})^2}{36.6 \text{ m}} = 275.9 \text{ N} = 28.12 \text{ kgf} = 0.30 \text{ BW}.$$

As the average magnitude of the vertical component of the ground reaction force F_V (over the total race time, i.e. the sum of ground contact time and flight time) is body weight, it follows from Equation 10.19 that the sprinter would need to lean toward the centre of curvature at an angle θ of 16.7° (Figure 10.44a).

$$\tan \theta = \frac{F_C}{F_V} = \frac{0.3 \text{ BW}}{1.0 \text{ BW}} = 0.3$$

$$\theta = 16.7°.$$

The lane width in outdoor tracks is approximately 1.22 m. Consequently, the radius of curvature in lane 8 is approximately 45.1 m (36.6 m in lane1 plus 7 × 1.22 m). To maintain an average speed of 10.42 m/s in lane 8, the sprinter would need to maintain an average centripetal force of 0.245 BW, which would require a lean angle of 13.8° (Figure 10.44b).

In these examples, the average values for F_V and F_C are based on continuous contact with the track. However, in maximum speed sprinting, approximately 55% of the time is spent in flight, i.e. only about 45% of the time is spent in contact with the track (Weyand et al. 2000). Consequently, the average magnitude of F_V would be approximately 2.2 BW (100/45 = 2.2) and the corresponding average magnitude of F_C in the lane 1 example would be 0.66 BW (2.2 × 0.3 BW = 0.66 BW). Therefore, the average magnitude of the resultant ground reaction force during each period of ground contact would be approximately 2.3 BW rather than 1.04 BW with continuous contact. As the ratio F_C/F_V would remain same, so would the lean angle (16.7°).

> Centripetal force is the force acting on a body that causes it to move on a curved path. Centrifugal force is the reaction exerted by a rotating object to the centripetal force; it is due to the inertia of the object, which resists a change in direction.

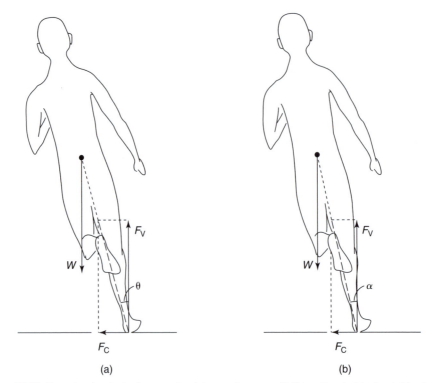

Figure 10.44 Rear-view free body diagram of sprinter running around left-hand bend of horizontal track with linear velocity 10.42 m/s (23.31 mph). (a) Radius of curvature, 36.6 m (lane 1); θ, 16.7°. (b) Radius of curvature, 45.1 m (lane 8), α, 13.6°. W, weight of sprinter; F_C, horizontal component of ground reaction force = centripetal force; F_V, vertical component of ground reaction force = W.

CONCENTRIC FORCE, ECCENTRIC FORCE AND COUPLE

In the earlier sections on moments of force and levers, most of the examples involved rotation or the tendency to rotate about a fixed axis. For example, a see-saw can only rotate about a horizontal axis through its fulcrum and a door can only rotate about a vertical axis through its hinges. When an object is free to rotate within a particular plane, i.e. it is not constrained to rotate about any particular axis, and a force acts on the object that causes or tends to cause the object to rotate, the rotation will occur about an axis that passes through the centre of gravity of the object. For example, Figure 10.45a shows an overhead view of a curling stone resting on a perfectly flat horizontal ice rink. The stone is acted on by a horizontal force F, which is concentric, i.e. the line of action of F passes through the centre of gravity of the stone. A concentric force produces or tends to produce rectilinear translation. Assuming that the friction between the stone and the ice is negligible, the only horizontal force acting on the stone is the concentric force F. Consequently, the stone will experience or tend to experience rectilinear translation, i.e. move in a straight line in the direction of F (Figure 10.45a,b). In a vertical jump, i.e. when the purpose of the movement is simply to raise the centre of gravity as high as possible off the ground without rotation or horizontal movement, the ground reaction force will be concentric (Figure 10.46).

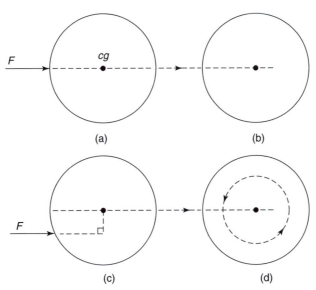

Figure 10.45 Overhead view of curling stone. (a) Concentric force. (c) Eccentric force. cg, centre of gravity of stone.

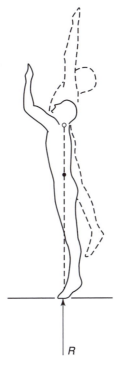

Figure 10.46 Concentric ground reaction force R in vertical jump without rotation or horizontal movement.

405

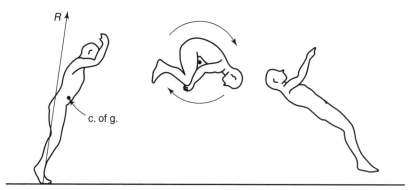

Figure 10.47 Eccentric ground reaction force R during take-off in forward somersault.

In Figure 10.45c, the horizontal force *F* is eccentric, i.e. its line of action does not pass through the centre of gravity of the stone. An eccentric force produces or tends to produce simultaneous rectilinear translation and rotation of an object about an axis that passes through the centre of gravity of the object and is perpendicular to the eccentric force. Consequently, in response to the eccentric force *F*, the stone will experience or tend to experience simultaneous rectilinear translation and rotation about the vertical axis passing through its centre of gravity (Figure 10.45c,d).

Most movements in sport that involve rotation of the whole body during flight are preceded by a ground contact phase prior to take-off, in which the ground reaction force is eccentric to the performer's centre of gravity. For example, Figure 10.47 shows a gymnast performing a front somersault following a run-up. Prior to take-off, the line of action of the ground reaction force *R* passes behind the gymnast's centre of gravity. The effect of the eccentric ground reaction force will be to move the centre of gravity in the direction of *R* (mainly upward, but also slightly forward, as in Figure 10.47) and simultaneously to help to generate forward rotation of the body about the mediolateral axis through the centre of gravity.

Similarly, in the final stages of a headspring, the line of action of the ground reaction force (the thrust resulting from arm extension) passes behind the centre of gravity of the body, resulting in translation of the centre of gravity (upward and forward) and the generation of forward rotation of the body (Figure 10.48).

Another example of the effect of an eccentric force can be seen in the flight of a rugby ball (Figure 10.49). If the ball is kicked such that the line of action of the kicking force passes

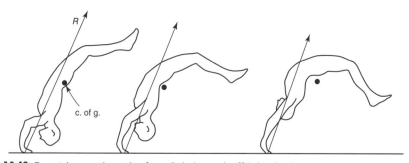

Figure 10.48 Eccentric ground reaction force R during push-off in headspring.

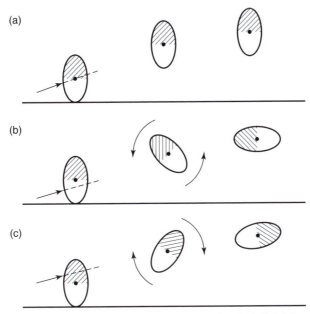

Figure 10.49 Effect of line of action of kicking force on movement of rugby ball. (a) Concentric force. (b) Eccentric force resulting in backward rotation. (c) Eccentric force resulting in forward rotation.

through the centre of gravity of the ball, i.e. it is a concentric force, then the ball will move through the air without rotation (Figure 10.49a). However, if the line of action of the kicking force passes directly below the centre of gravity of the ball, i.e. it is an eccentric force, the ball will rotate backward about the mediolateral axis through the centre of gravity of the ball as it moves through the air (Figure 10.49b). Similarly, if the line of action of the kicking force passes directly above the centre of gravity of the ball, the ball will rotate forward about the mediolateral axis through the centre of gravity of the ball as it moves through the air (Figure 10.49c).

Figure 10.50 shows an overhead view of a child's roundabout, which is designed to

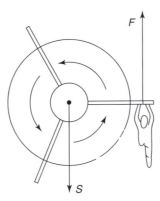

Figure 10.50 Overhead view of child's roundabout: F, eccentric force exerted on a handrail; S, horizontal force, equal and opposite to F, exerted by vertical support of roundabout; F and S form a couple resulting in rotation with no translation.

407

rotate about a fixed vertical axis through its point of support. In response to an eccentric horizontal force F applied to one of the handrails of the roundabout, the vertical support exerts an equal and opposite force S on the roundabout. The tendencies of F and S to translate the roundabout (F upward and S downward with respect to Figure 10.50) cancel each other out, but the turning effect of F rotates the roundabout, i.e. the roundabout rotates but does not translate. The force system produced by F and S is called a couple, i.e. a system of two parallel, equal and opposite forces, one concentric and one eccentric (as in Figure 10.50) or both eccentric, that tend to rotate an object in the same direction about a particular axis. A couple produces or tends to produce rotation without translation. Rotation of any object about a fixed axis is the result of a couple. The magnitude of a couple is the product of one of the forces and the perpendicular distance between the two forces. The larger the couple, the greater the angular acceleration and, therefore, the greater the angular velocity.

The systems of forces that result in translation, rotation or simultaneous translation and rotation may be summarised as follows. Consider an object that is free to translate and rotate within a particular plane, i.e. it is not constrained to translate in any particular direction or to rotate about any particular axis:

Concentric force system: If the line of action of the resultant force acting on the object is parallel to the plane of movement and acts through the centre of gravity of the object, the object will experience or tend to experience rectilinear translation, but will not rotate. This is a concentric force system.

Eccentric force system: If the line of action of the resultant force acting on the object is parallel to the plane of movement, but does not act through the centre of gravity of the object, the object will experience or tend to experience simultaneous rectilinear translation and rotation about an axis perpendicular to the plane of movement that passes through the centre of gravity of the object. This is an eccentric force system.

Couple: If the resultant of the forces acting on the object rotate or tend to rotate the object about an axis which does not move (translate) in the plane of movement, the force system is a couple.

ROTATION AND NEWTON'S FIRST LAW OF MOTION

From the previous section, an object at rest will only begin to rotate about a particular axis when the resultant force acting on the object is an eccentric force or couple. Newton's laws of motion apply to linear motion and angular motion. With regard to angular motion, the first law of motion may be expressed as follows:

> The resultant moment acting on a body at rest or rotating about a particular axis with constant angular velocity (assuming no change in the shape of the object while rotating) is zero and the body will remain at rest or continue to rotate with constant angular velocity unless acted upon by an unbalanced eccentric force or couple.

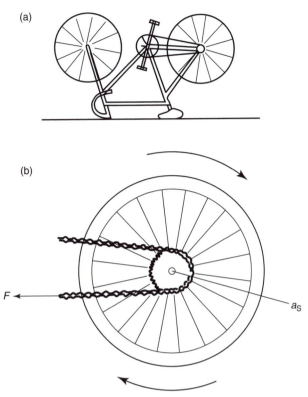

Figure 10.51 Application of unbalanced eccentric force to rear wheel of bicycle by chain through rotation of pedals: F, force exerted by chain; a_S, axis through wheel spindle.

For example, consider a bicycle turned upside down so that it rests on its handle bars and saddle (Figure 10.51a). Each wheel will remain at rest until an eccentric force or couple is applied to it with respect to the horizontal axis a_S through the spindle of the wheel. When the pedals are turned clockwise with respect to Figure 10.51a, the chain will exert an eccentric force on the rear wheel such that the wheel will start to rotate in a clockwise direction about a_S (Figure 10.51b). When the pedals are brought to rest (provided that the wheel is not a fixed wheel that rotates clockwise and anticlockwise in direct response to corresponding rotation of the pedals), the wheel will continue to rotate even though there is no couple or eccentric force acting on it. Furthermore, the wheel is likely to rotate for some considerable time unless a counter-rotation eccentric force, in the form of a brake, is applied to the wheel. If a brake is not applied to the wheel, the duration of rotation of the wheel will depend entirely on the amount of friction between the wheel and its spindle. The friction exerts a counter-rotation couple on the wheel and eventually brings it to rest; the greater the friction, the sooner the wheel is brought to rest. If the friction could be eliminated, the wheel would continue to rotate for ever with constant angular velocity.

In such movements as somersaults (Figure 10.47), in which the human body rotates freely in space during the flight phase of the movement, the rotation of the body will take place about an axis that passes through the centre of gravity of the body. Furthermore, the angular velocity of the body about the axis of rotation will remain constant, provided that the orientation of

409

the body segments to each other does not change. The rotation of the body in such movements is ultimately reduced to zero by the action of the ground reaction force on landing (which exerts an unbalanced counter-rotation eccentric force).

MOMENT OF INERTIA

The resistance of an object to an attempt to change its linear motion (resistance to start moving if it is at rest and resistance to change its speed or direction if it is moving) is referred to as its inertia. The inertia of an object is directly proportional to its mass; the larger the mass, the greater the inertia. The resistance of an object to an attempt to change its angular motion (resistance to start rotating about a particular axis if it is at rest and resistance to change its angular speed or direction if it is rotating) is referred to as its moment of inertia. The moment of inertia of an object about a particular axis depends not only on the mass of the object, but also on the distribution of the mass of the object about the axis of rotation. The closer the mass of the object to the axis of rotation or the more concentrated the mass of the object around the axis of rotation, the smaller will be the moment of inertia of the object and the easier it will be (the smaller the moment of force) to start the object rotating or to keep it rotating if is already rotating.

Figure 10.52 shows a gymnast swinging about the axis a_B of a horizontal bar. The human body can be considered to consist of any number of separate masses joined together. Consider the motion of a tiny particle of mass m of the gymnast's body. From Equation 10.13, it follows that the linear acceleration a of the mass m is equal to $r \cdot \alpha$, where r = radius of curvature of m about a_B and α = angular acceleration of m about a_B. From Newton's second law of motion, the force F responsible for a is given by

$$F = m \cdot r \cdot \alpha.$$

The moment of F about a_B is $F \cdot r$, i.e.

$$F \cdot r = m \cdot r^2 \cdot \alpha. \tag{10.20}$$

The total or resultant moment M of all the forces acting on all the particles that comprise the body is given by

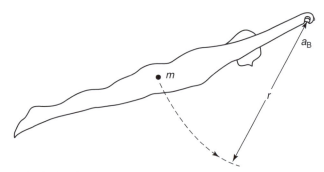

Figure 10.52 Gymnast swinging about horizontal bar: r, radius of curvature of particle of mass m.

$$M = F_1 \cdot r_1 + F_2 \cdot r_2 + F_3 \cdot r_3 + \ldots + F_n \cdot r_n, \qquad (10.21)$$

where n is the number of particles that comprise the body. It follows from Equations 10.20 and 10.21 that

$$M = m_1 \cdot r_1^2 \cdot \alpha + m_2 \cdot r_2^2 \, \alpha + m_3 \cdot r_3^2 \cdot \alpha + \ldots m_n \cdot r_n^2 \cdot \alpha \qquad (10.22)$$

$$M = I \cdot \alpha, \qquad (10.23)$$

where $\quad I = \left(\displaystyle\sum_{n=1}^{n=n} m_n \cdot r_n^2 \right) = $ moment of inertia of the body about the axis of rotation.

In this example, as the axis of rotation is fixed, the resultant moment is a couple.

Equations 10.22 and 10.23 show that the moment of inertia of an object about a particular axis of rotation is obtained by multiplying the mass of each particle of the object by the square of its distance from the axis of rotation and summing for the whole object. In the SI system, the unit of moment of inertia is kilogram metres squared ($kg \cdot m^2$). As the distribution of the mass of an object about a particular axis changes, so will the distance of some or all of the particles of mass from the axis of rotation. Consequently, the moment of inertia of the object about the axis of rotation will also change. Figure 10.53 and Table 10.5 show the effect of changing body position on the moment of inertia of the human body about the principal X, Y and Z axes (Figure 9.1) (Santschi et al. 1963).

> The moment of inertia of an object about a particular axis of rotation is the resistance of the object to an attempt to change its angular motion.

Measurement of moment of inertia

It is relatively easy to calculate the moment of inertia about a particular axis of a regular-shaped object of uniform density. For example, Figure 10.54a shows a side view of an object of uniform density of length 1 m, square cross section 0.05 m × 0.05 m and mass 2 kg. For the purpose of the illustration, the object is considered to consist of ten pieces of length 0.1 m joined end to end. As the object is of uniform density, each piece will have the same mass $m = 0.2$ kg and the centre of gravity of each piece will be at its geometric centre. The moment of inertia I_O of the object about an axis (perpendicular to the page) through the end O is given by

$$I_O = \left(\displaystyle\sum_{n=1}^{n=10} m_n \cdot r_n^2 \right) = m_1 \cdot r_1^2 + m_2 \cdot r_2^2 + m_3 \cdot r_3^2 + \ldots + m_{10} \cdot r_{10}^2,$$

where $m_1, m_2, \ldots, m_{10}$ are the masses and $r_1, r_2, \ldots, r_{10}$ are the distances of the centres of gravity of the masses from the axis through O. As all of the masses are the same, i.e. 0.2 kg,

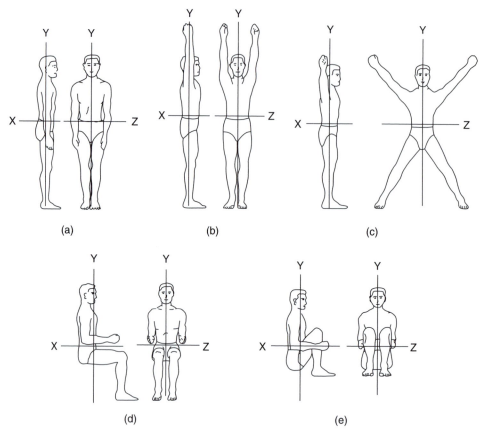

Figure 10.53 Effect of change in body position on moment of inertia of human body about X, Y and Z axes. (a) Standing. (b) Standing, arms overhead. (c) Star shape. (d) Sitting. (e) Tucked. Moments of inertia for each position are given in Table 10.5.

Table 10.5 Effect of change in body position on moment of inertia of human body about X, Y and Z axes.

	Moment of inertia (kg·m²)			Moment of inertia relative to standing		
	X	Y	Z	X	Y	Z
Standing	13.01	1.28	11.64	1	1	1
Standing, arms overhead	17.20	1.25	15.50	1.32	0.97	1.33
Star shape	17.07	4.14	12.89	1.31	3.23	1.11
Sitting	6.96	3.79	7.53	0.53	2.96	0.65
Tucked	4.42	2.97	4.30	0.34	2.32	0.37

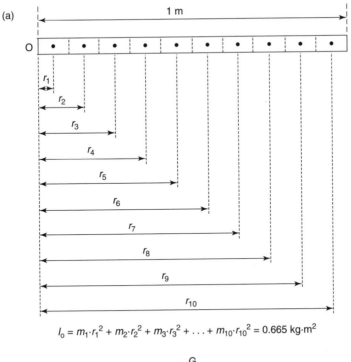

$$I_o = m_1 \cdot r_1^2 + m_2 \cdot r_2^2 + m_3 \cdot r_3^2 + \ldots + m_{10} \cdot r_{10}^2 = 0.665 \text{ kg·m}^2$$

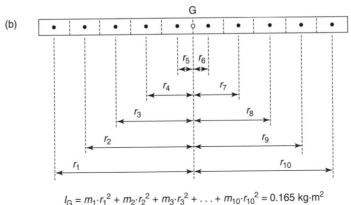

$$I_G = m_1 \cdot r_1^2 + m_2 \cdot r_2^2 + m_3 \cdot r_3^2 + \ldots + m_{10} \cdot r_{10}^2 = 0.165 \text{ kg·m}^2$$

Figure 10.54 Side view of an object of uniform density of length 1 m, square cross section 0.05 m × 0.05 m, mass 2 kg. (a) Determination of moment of inertia of object about axis (perpendicular to the page) through end 0. (b) Determination of moment of inertia of object about parallel axis through centre of gravity of object.

and $r_1 = 0.05$ m, $r_2 = 0.15$ m, $r_3 = 0.25$ m, $r_4 = 0.35$ m, $r_5 = 0.45$ m, $r_6 = 0.55$ m, $r_7 = 0.65$ m, $r_8 = 0.75$ m, $r_9 = 0.85$ m and $r_{10} = 0.95$ m, then

$$I_o = m\left((0.05 \text{ m})^2 + (0.15 \text{ m})^2 + (0.25 \text{ m})^2 + (0.35 \text{ m})^2 + (0.45 \text{ m})^2 + (0.55 \text{ m})^2 + \right.$$

$$\left. (0.65 \text{ m})^2 + (0.75 \text{ m})^2 + (0.85 \text{ m})^2 + (0.95 \text{ m})^2 \right)$$

$$I_o = 0.2 \text{ kg} \times 3.625 \text{ m}^2 = 0.665 \text{ kg·m}^2.$$

Parallel axis theorem

In this example, the axis of rotation was through the end O of the object. For any object, as the axis of rotation (perpendicular to a given plane) moves closer to the centre of gravity of the object, the sum of r^2 where $r_1, r_2, r_3, \ldots, r_n$ are the distances from the axis of rotation of the particles of equal mass that comprise the object, becomes smaller. Consequently, the sum of r^2 and, therefore, the moment of inertia of the object are least when the axis of rotation passes through the centre of gravity of the object. Conversely, the moment of inertia progressively increases with increased distance of the axis of rotation (perpendicular to a given plane) from the centre of gravity of the object. For parallel axes (within a given plane), the moment of inertia I_A of an object about an axis A that does not pass through the centre of gravity of the object is given by

$$I_A = I_G + m_t \cdot d^2, \tag{10.24}$$

where: I_A = moment of inertia of the object about axis A,
I_G = moment of inertia of the object about an axis passing through the centre of gravity of the object that is parallel to axis A,
m_t = total mass of the object.
d = distance from A to the centre of gravity of the object.

Equation 10.24 is referred to as the parallel axis theorem. Figure 10.54b shows the same piece of material as in Figure 10.54a. The moment of inertia I_G of the object about the axis passing through its centre of gravity (G), parallel to the axis through O, is given by

$$I_G = \left(\sum_{n=1}^{n=10} m_n \cdot r_n^2 \right) = m_1 \cdot r_1^2 + m_2 \cdot r_2^2 + m_3 \cdot r_3^2 + \ldots + m_{10} \cdot r_{10}^2,$$

where $m_1, m_2, \ldots, m_{10}$ are the masses and $r_1, r_2, \ldots, r_{10}$ are the distances of the centres of gravity of the masses from the axis through G. Since all of the masses are the same, i.e. 0.2 kg, and $r_1 = 0.45$ m, $r_2 = 0.35$ m, $r_3 = 0.25$ m, $r_4 = 0.15$ m, $r_5 = 0.05$ m, $r_6 = 0.05$ m, $r_7 = 0.15$ m, $r_8 = 0.25$ m, $r_9 = 0.35$ m and $r_{10} = 0.45$ m, then

$$I_G = m((0.45 \ m)^2 + (0.35 \ m)^2 + (0.25 \ m)^2 + (0.15 \ m)^2 + (0.05 \ m)^2 + (0.05 \ m)^2$$
$$+ (0.15 \ m)^2 + (0.25 \ m)^2 + (0.35 \ m)^2 + (0.45 \ m)^2)$$
$$I_O = 0.2 \ kg \times 0.825 \ m^2 = 0.165 \ kg \cdot m^2.$$

According to the parallel axis theorem,

$$I_O = I_G + m_t \cdot d^2,$$

where: m_t = total mass of the object = 2 kg,
d = distance between the parallel axes through O and G = 0.5 m,

i.e. $I_O = 0.165 \text{ kg·m}^2 + (2 \text{ kg} \times (0.5 \text{ m})^2) = 0.165 \text{ kg·m}^2 + 0.5 \text{ kg·m}^2 = 0.665 \text{ kg·m}^2.$

As expected, this is the same result for I_O as that obtained by the summation method ($\Sigma m_n \cdot r_n^2$).

Radius of gyration

When the density of an object is not uniform, like the human body, the summation method cannot be used to determine the moment of inertia of the object. Even if the object could be considered to consist of a number of exactly similar volumes (as in the example in Figure 10.54), it would not be possible to determine the mass of each volume and it cannot be assumed that the centre of gravity of each volume is at its geometric centre.

Various methods, summarised by Hay (1974), have been devised to measure the moment of inertia of the human body and body segments. These methods involve complex equipment and are, in general, fairly impractical. Consequently, in most biomechanical analyses of human movement, moments of inertia are estimated from average data on the mass distribution of body segments obtained from cadaver studies.

The mass distribution of an object (of uniform or non-uniform density) about a particular axis is reflected in the radius of gyration of the object about the axis. The moment of inertia I of an object about a particular axis is equivalent to that of a mass m_t, equal to the mass of the object, rotating about the axis at a distance k from the axis, where k is the radius of gyration, i.e.

$$I = m_t \cdot k^2. \tag{10.25}$$

For comparative purposes, the moment of inertia of an object about a particular axis is often expressed in terms of $m_t \cdot k^2$. For a given object, m_t is constant, but k and, therefore, the moment of inertia of the object, depend upon the distribution of the mass of the object about the axis of rotation. For example, in Figure 10.54a, $I_O = 0.665 \text{ kg·m}^2$ and $m_t = 2 \text{ kg}$. Therefore, from Equation 10.25,

$$k_O = \sqrt{(I_O/m_t)} = 0.5766 \text{ m},$$

where k_O is the radius of gyration of m_t about the axis through O. Similarly, in Figure 10.54b, $I_G = 0.165 \text{ kg·m}^2$ and $m_t = 2 \text{ kg}$. Therefore, from Equation 10.25,

$$k_G = \sqrt{(I_G/m_t)} = 0.2872 \text{ m},$$

where k_G is the radius of gyration of m_t about the axis through G. k_O and k_G are illustrated in Figure 10.55. k_O is approximately twice the size of k_G ($0.5766/0.2872 = 2.01$). However, as moment of inertia is proportional to the square of the radius of gyration, I_O is approximately four times the size of I_G ($0.665 \text{ kg·m}^2/0.165 \text{ kg·m}^2 = 4.03$).

For objects with the same shape and the same distribution of mass (even if the density is not uniform), but different size, the radius of gyration (with respect to any axis through or

415

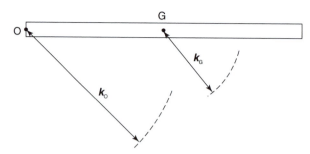

Figure 10.55 Radius of gyration of object of Figure 10.54 about axis through O (k_O) and parallel axis through G (k_G).

Table 10.6 Radii of gyration of human body segments about the mediolateral axis through the centre of gravity of the segments, as a proportion of segment length (adapted from Winter 1990).

Segment	Segment endpoints	Radius of gyration
Upper arm	shoulder joint, elbow joint	0.322
Forearm	elbow joint, wrist	0.303
Forearm and hand	elbow joint, wrist	0.468
Hand	wrist, knuckle of 2nd finger	0.297
Whole upper limb	shoulder joint, wrist	0.368
Thigh	hip joint, knee joint	0.323
Shank	knee joint, ankle joint	0.302
Shank and foot	knee joint, ankle joint	0.416
Foot	lateral malleolus, head of 2nd metatarsal	0.475
Whole lower limb	hip joint, ankle joint	0.326
Trunk, head and neck	shoulder joint, hip joint	0.503

on the surface of the object), as a proportion of the length of the segment, is the same. This also applies to the segments of the human body, i.e. corresponding segments of different individuals are very similar in shape and distribution of mass and, therefore, the radii of gyration of corresponding segments, as a proportion of the length of the segments, are very similar. Table 10.6 shows average data, obtained mainly from cadaver studies, for the radii of gyration of body segments as a proportion of segment length about the mediolateral axis through the centre of gravity of the segments (Winter 1990).

Determination of the moment of inertia of a gymnast about the axis of a horizontal bar

Figure 10.56 shows three positions of a gymnast rotating about a horizontal bar. In position 1, the mass of the gymnast is distributed as far away as possible from the axis of rotation. Consequently, the moment of inertia of the gymnast about the axis of rotation will be highest in this position. In position 2, the legs are much closer to the bar than in position 1, such that the moment of inertia of the gymnast about the bar will be smaller in position 2 than in posi-

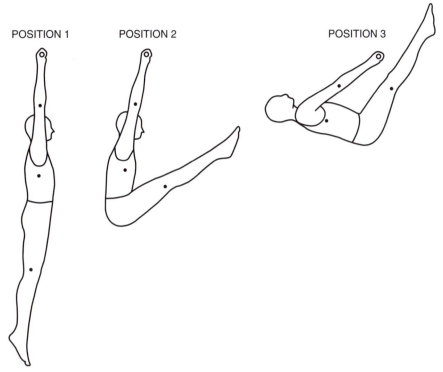

POSITION 1   POSITION 2   POSITION 3

Figure 10.56 Three positions of gymnast rotating about horizontal bar: dots indicate centres of gravity of arm, leg and combined trunk, head and neck (see Table 10.7).

tion 1. In position 3, the trunk and legs are much closer to the bar than in positions 1 and 2, and the moment of inertia of the gymnast about the bar will be smaller in position 3 than in positions 1 and 2.

Table 10.7 shows the stages in the calculation of the moment of inertia of the gymnast about the long axis of the bar in the three positions. The calculations are based on a five-segment model consisting of trunk, head and neck (one segment), right arm, left arm, right leg and left leg. It is assumed that the movement of the gymnast is symmetrical about the median plane, such that the movement of the right arm is the same as that of the left arm and the movement of the right leg is the same as that of the left leg. The data on segment mass as a proportion of whole body mass are taken from Plagenhoef *et al.* (1983) (Table 10.1). The data on segment length were taken from a video of the gymnast. The data on radius of gyration as a proportion of segment length are taken from Winter (1990) (Table 10.6) and the data on the distance of the centre of gravity of each segment from the axis of the bar were obtained by applying the centre of gravity locus data of Plagenhoef *et al.* (1983) (Table 10.1) to the segment length data.

Columns 1 to 6 of Table 10.7 show the calculation of I_G for each segment, i.e. the moment of inertia of the segment about an axis parallel with the bar through the centre of gravity of the segment. For example, in position 1, I_G for the arm is given by

$$I_G = m \cdot k_G^2 = 4.04 \text{ kg} \times (0.22 \text{ m})^2 = 0.1955 \text{ kg} \cdot \text{m}^2,$$

417

Table 10.7 Determination of the moment of inertia of a gymnast about the axis of a horizontal bar in three positions (see Figure 10.56).

		Mass of segment as percentage of whole body mass (%)	Mass (kg)	Length of segment (m)	k_G (as proportion of length)	k_G (m)	I_G (kg·m²)	d (m)	$m·d^2$ (kg·m²)	I_O (kg·m²)	I_O (kg·m²)
Position 1	Upper arm, forearm and hand	5.77	4.04	0.60	0.368	0.22	0.1955	0.37	0.5531	0.7486	1.4972
	Trunk, head and neck	55.1	38.6	0.53	0.503	0.27	2.8118	0.87	29.194	32.005	32.005
	Thigh, shank and foot	16.7	11.7	0.81	0.326	0.26	0.7896	1.55	28.061	28.851	57.702
	Total										91.204
Position 2	Upper arm, forearm and hand	5.77	4.04	0.60	0.368	0.22	0.1955	0.37	0.5531	0.7486	1.4972
	Trunk, head and neck	55.1	38.6	0.53	0.503	0.27	2.8118	0.85	27.888	30.699	30.699
	Thigh, shank and foot	16.7	11.7	0.81	0.326	0.26	0.7896	0.97	11.008	11.798	23.596
	Total										55.792
Position 3	Upper arm, forearm and hand	5.77	4.04	0.60	0.368	0.22	0.1955	0.37	0.5531	0.7486	1.4972
	Trunk, head and neck	55.1	38.6	0.53	0.503	0.27	2.8118	0.60	13.896	16.708	16.708
	Thigh, shank and foot	16.7	11.7	0.81	0.326	0.26	0.7896	0.26	0.7896	1.5792	3.1584
	Total										21.364

Whole body mass, 70 kg; k_G, radius of gyration of the segment about mediolateral axis a_G through its centre of gravity, first as proportion of segment length and then in metres; I_G, moment of inertia of the segment about a_G and the axis of the bar; d, distance between a_G and the axis of the bar; I_O (column 9), moment of inertia of the segment about the axis of the bar; I_O (column 10) = moment of inertia of both arms, both legs and the trunk head and neck about the axis of the bar and the total moment of inertia.

where m is the mass of the arm (upper arm, forearm and hand), 4.04 kg and k_G is the radius of gyration of the arm about the mediolateral axis through the centre of gravity of the arm,

$$\text{segment length} \times k_G \text{ (as a proportion of segment length)} = 0.6 \text{ m} \times 0.368 = 0.22 \text{ m}.$$

Columns 7 and 8 show the calculation of $m \cdot d^2$ for the arm in position 1, i.e.

$$m \cdot d^2 = 4.04 \text{ kg} \times (0.37 \text{ m})^2 = 0.5531 \text{ kg·m}^2,$$

where m is the mass of the arm, 4.04 kg, and d is the distance of the centre of gravity of the arm from the axis of the bar, 0.37 m.

Column 9 shows the parallel axis theorem calculation of I_O for the arm in position 1, i.e. the moment of inertia of the arm about the axis of the bar

$$I_O = I_G + m \cdot d^2 = 0.1955 \text{ kg·m}^2 + 0.5531 \text{ kg·m}^2 = 0.7486 \text{ kg·m}^2.$$

Column 10 shows the sum of the moments of inertia of both arms about the axis of the bar in position 1, i.e. 1.4972 kg·m².

Table 10.7 shows that the moment of inertia of the body about the axis of the bar in positions 1, 2 and 3 is approximately 91.2 kg·m², 55.8 kg·m², and 21.4 kg·m², respectively.

ANGULAR MOMENTUM

Just as an object of mass m (kg) moving with linear velocity v (m/s) has linear momentum $m \cdot v$ (kg·m/s), an object rotating about a particular axis has angular momentum $I \cdot \omega$ (kg·m²/s), where I (kg·m²) is the moment of inertia of the object about the axis and ω (rad/s) is the angular velocity of the object about the axis. Whereas the mass of an object is constant (unless part of the mass is removed or more mass is added), the moment of inertia of a rotating object can be changed by simply redistributing the mass about the axis of rotation. From Newton's first law of motion, the angular momentum of an object about a particular axis of rotation will remain constant until the object is acted upon by an unbalanced eccentric force or couple. Therefore, if the moment of inertia of an object rotating freely about a particular axis is changed, there will be a simultaneous change in the angular velocity of the object so that the angular momentum of the object remains unchanged. This principle is referred to as the conservation of angular momentum and it has great significance in movements of the human body that involve rotation during flight.

Figure 10.57 shows the successive positions of a gymnast during the performance of a front somersault following a run-up. During the flight phase (positions 2 to 9), the gymnast rotates in the median plane about the mediolateral axis a_Z through his centre of gravity. Since there are no unbalanced turning moments acting on the gymnast during flight, the angular momentum of the gymnast about a_Z will be conserved, i.e. remain constant. To land on his feet, the gymnast must complete the forward somersault very quickly. By tucking his body (positions 2 to 5), the gymnast reduces the moment of inertia of his body about a_Z; this simultaneously results in an increase in his angular velocity about a_Z. Suppose that the moment of inertia of

419

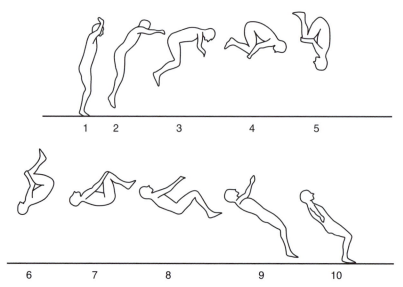

Figure 10.57 Successive positions of gymnast performing front somersault following run-up.

his body about a_Z in position 5 is half that in position 2. Since his angular momentum about a_Z is the same in both positions, it follows that

$$I_2 \cdot \omega_2 = I_5 \cdot \omega_5,$$

where I_2, I_5 and ω_2, ω_5 are the moments of inertia and angular velocities of the gymnast about a_Z in positions 2 and 5, respectively. As $I_5 = I_2/2$, then

$$I_2 \cdot \omega_2 = \frac{I_2}{2}\omega_5,$$

i.e. $\omega_5 = 2\omega_2.$

By halving the moment of inertia, the angular velocity is doubled. The increased angular velocity will enable the gymnast to complete the forward somersault in half the time that it would have taken if he had not tucked his body. In the second part of the flight phase (positions 6 to 9) the gymnast extends his body, which increases his moment of inertia and decreases his angular velocity about a_Z, in preparation for landing. Figure 10.58 shows the change in I and ω about a_Z during the flight phase.

> The angular momentum of an object about a particular axis is the product of its moment of inertia and angular velocity about the axis.

Figure 10.59 shows a skater rotating about the vertical axis a_Y through his centre of gravity. If the skater goes into a spin with his arms outstretched at his sides (Figure 10.59a) and then suddenly brings in his arms close to his sides (Figure 10.59b), his moment of inertia about a_Y

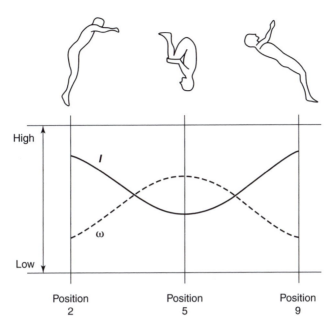

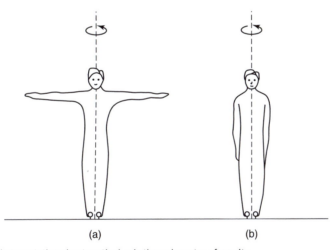

Figure 10.58 Relationship between moment of inertia I and angular velocity ω of gymnast about mediolateral axis through centre of gravity during flight phase of front somersault following run-up (see Figure 10.57).

Figure 10.59 Skater rotating about vertical axis through centre of gravity.

will decrease and his angular velocity about a_Y will simultaneously increase. In this movement, the skater's angular momentum about a_Y will not be entirely conserved, since the friction between his skates and the ice will exert a small counter-rotation moment, such that if the skater could rotate for long enough, his angular momentum would eventually be reduced to zero and he would stop spinning.

The change in angular velocity that accompanies a change in moment of inertia of an object in situations where angular momentum is conserved can be experienced by using a chair, stool

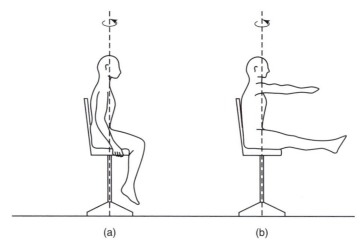

(a)   (b)

Figure 10.60 Use of freely rotating chair to experience change in angular velocity accompanying change in moment of inertia in situations where angular momentum is conserved.

or turntable that is free to rotate about a vertical axis. With the subject and chair rotating, as in Figure 10.60a, extending the arms or the legs (or both) away from the axis of rotation (Figure 10.66) will increase the moment of inertia and decrease angular velocity, and vice versa. The effect is more marked if the subject holds a weight in each hand or wears weighted shoes, since the movement of the limbs will result in more marked changes in the moment of inertia of the body about the axis of rotation and, consequently, more marked changes in angular velocity. The angular momentum of subject and chair is not entirely conserved, as there will be a certain amount of friction between the chair and its spindle.

ROTATION AND NEWTON'S SECOND LAW OF MOTION

From Equation 10.23 ($M = I \cdot \alpha$), when a resultant moment M acts on an object about a particular axis of rotation, the angular acceleration α experienced by the object about the axis of rotation will be directly proportional to the magnitude of M and inversely proportional to the moment of inertia I of the object about the axis of rotation, i.e. $\alpha = M/I$. This equation (directly analogous to $a = F/m$; see Equation 9.14) represents Newton's second law of motion in relation to rotation and may be expressed as follows:

> When a moment (i.e. a resultant moment greater than zero) acts on an object about a particular axis of rotation, the angular acceleration experienced by the object takes place in the direction of the moment and is directly proportional to the magnitude of the moment and inversely proportional to the moment of inertia of the object about the axis of rotation.

As $M = I \cdot \alpha$, then $M = I(\omega_2 - \omega_1)/t$ (from Equation 10.7) and

$$M \cdot t = I\omega_2 - I \cdot \omega_1,$$
(10.26)

422

where t is the duration of the moment M and ω_1 and ω_2 are the angular velocities of the object at t_1 and t_2, where $t = t_2 - t_1$.

Newton's second law of motion in relation to rotation is often expressed in terms of Equation 10.26 (directly analogous to $F \cdot t = m \cdot v - m \cdot u$; see Equation 9.15) as follows:

> When a moment (resultant moment greater than zero) acts on an object about a particular axis of rotation, the change in angular momentum experienced by the object takes place in the direction of the moment and is directly proportional to the magnitude of the moment and the duration of the moment.

When the amount of force and size of the moment arm that comprise a particular moment are not specified, for example, in describing the turning effect on part of a machine, the term torque is used rather than moment.

From Equation 10.26, it is clear that to maximise the angular momentum of an object about a particular axis, it is necessary to apply as much moment as possible for as long as possible. The product $M \cdot t$ of the moment M and duration t of the moment is called the impulse of the moment, i.e. the angular impulse. The angular impulse–angular momentum principle is widely used in sports, especially those involving rotation of the whole body, such as gymnastics and diving.

Figure 10.61 shows four successive positions of a gymnast prior to take-off during the performance of a standing back somersault. Prior to take-off, the gymnast needs to generate sufficient upward linear momentum and sufficient backward angular momentum about the mediolateral axis a_z through his centre of gravity to perform the somersault and land on his feet. These requirements are met by a vertical eccentric ground reaction force, which passes in front of a_z (Figure 10.61). Assuming that the gymnast starts the movement from a resting

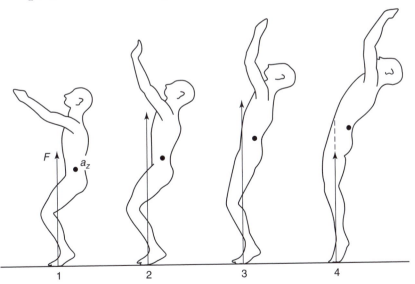

Figure 10.61 Eccentric ground reaction force F prior to take-off in standing back somersault: the linear impulse of F generates linear momentum of the whole body centre of gravity in the direction of F; the angular impulse of F about a_z generates backward angular momentum of the body about a_z.

position, then the vertical velocity at take-off, v (which will determine flight time), and the angular momentum at take-off, $I \cdot \omega$ (which, together with changes in the moment of inertia about a_z, will determine the time required to complete the somersault), are given by,

$$v = \frac{F \cdot t}{m} \text{ (from Equation 9.15, where } u = 0),$$

$I \cdot \omega = M \cdot t$ (from Equation 10.26, where $\omega_1 = 0$),

where: $\quad t \quad$ = time from the start of movement to take-off,

$\quad F \quad$ = average resultant vertical force acting on the gymnast during t,

$\quad d \quad$ = average moment arm of F,

$\quad M \quad = F \cdot d$ = average moment about a_z during t (clockwise with respect to Figure 10.61),

$\quad m \quad$ = mass of the gymnast,

$\quad I \quad$ = moment of inertia of the gymnast about a_z at take-off,

$\quad \omega \quad$ = angular velocity of the gymnast about a_z at take-off.

F will be largely determined by the strength of the gymnast's leg extensor muscles, t will be determined by the range of motion in the gymnast's hips, knees and ankles and the extent to which this range of motion is utilised and d will be determined by the ability of the gymnast to push vertically downward eccentrically, i.e. with a_z behind the line of action of F. The line of action of F will determine the extent to which the centre of gravity of the gymnast moves horizontally during the movement. In a standing back somersault, F would ideally be vertical prior to take-off, resulting in vertical displacement but no horizontal displacement of the centre of gravity.

Figure 10.62 shows four successive positions of a gymnast prior to take-off during the performance of a headspring. To land on his feet, the gymnast needs to generate sufficient upward linear momentum and sufficient forward angular momentum about the mediolateral axis a_z through his centre of gravity during the push-off. These requirements are met by an eccentric

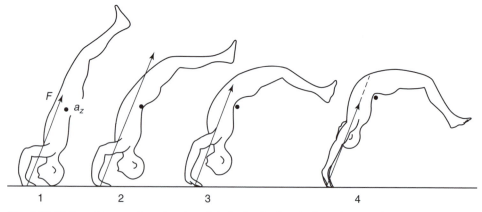

Figure 10.62 Eccentric ground reaction force F during headspring: the linear impulse of F generates linear momentum of the whole body centre of gravity in the direction of F; the angular impulse of F about a_z generates forward angular momentum of the body about a_z.

ground reaction force F, which passes in front of a_z. The linear impulse of F generates upward linear momentum and the angular impulse of F about a_z generates forward angular momentum about a_z. As in the standing back somersault, the line of action of F will determine the extent of horizontal movement of the centre of gravity.

In Practical Worksheet 8, students use a turntable to determine the moment of inertia and radius of gyration of the human body about a vertical axis while in a seated position.

> To maximise the change in angular momentum of an object about a particular axis of rotation, it is necessary to maximise the angular impulse applied to the object.

TRANSFER OF ANGULAR MOMENTUM

From Equations 10.22 and 10.23,

$$I \cdot \alpha = m_1 \cdot r_1^2 \cdot \alpha + m_2 \cdot r_2^2 \cdot \alpha + m_3 \cdot r_3^2 \cdot \alpha + \ldots + m_n \cdot r_n^2, \tag{10.27}$$

where: I = moment of inertia of an object about a particular axis of rotation,
  α = angular acceleration of the object about the axis of rotation,
  $m_1, m_2, m_3, \ldots, m_n$ = mass of parts of the object,
  $r_1, r_2, r_3, \ldots, r_n$ = distances of the parts of the object from the axis of rotation.

As $\alpha = \omega/t$ (Equation 10.7), it follows from Equation 10.27 that

$$I \cdot \frac{\omega}{t} = m_1 \cdot r_1^2 \cdot \frac{\omega}{t} + m_2 \cdot r_2^2 \cdot \frac{\omega}{t} + m_3 \cdot r_3^2 \cdot \frac{\omega}{t} + \ldots + m_n \cdot r_n^2 \cdot \frac{\omega}{t}$$

$$I \cdot \omega = m_1 \cdot r_1^2 \cdot \omega + m_2 \cdot r_2^2 \cdot \omega + m_3 \cdot r_3^2 \cdot \omega + \ldots + m_n \cdot r_n^2 \cdot \omega$$

$$I \cdot \omega = I_1 \cdot \omega + I_2 \cdot \omega + I_3 \cdot \omega + \ldots + I_n \cdot \omega, \tag{10.28}$$

where $I_1, I_2, I_3, \ldots I_n$ are the respective moments of inertia of the parts about the axis of rotation. It follows, therefore, that the angular momentum of the object about the axis of rotation is equal to the sum of the angular momenta of all the individual parts that comprise the object. Consequently, when an object is rotating with constant angular momentum about a particular axis, any change in the angular momentum of one or more parts of the object as a result of internal forces will simultaneously result in a change in the angular momentum of one or more of the other parts of the body, so that the angular momentum of the object remains the same.

Demonstration of transfer of angular momentum using a rotating turntable

Figure 10.63 shows a man standing with his arms outstretched at his sides on a turntable, which is free to rotate about a vertical axis a_Y. If the turntable is rotated by an external

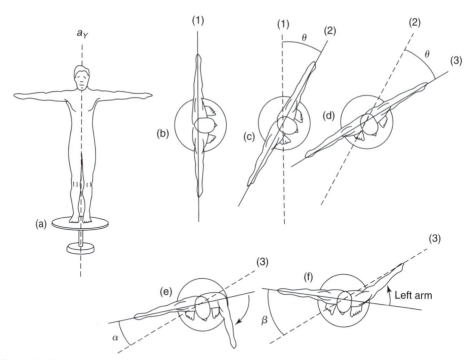

Figure 10.63 Man standing on turntable and rotating about vertical axis a_Y through centre of gravity with constant angular momentum (subject to friction around spindle): images are at equal time intervals.

moment, which is then removed, the system consisting of man and turntable will continue to rotate with constant angular momentum about a_Y (Figure 10.63b–d). If the man suddenly rotates his left arm relative to the rest of the system, in a horizontal plane and in the direction of rotation of the whole system, the angular velocity of the rest of the system about a_Y will be seen to decrease for the same period of time that the left arm is rotating relative to the rest of the system, i.e. in the same time that it takes the left arm to rotate through 90° about a vertical axis through the left shoulder, the rest of the system rotates through a smaller angle about a_Y than it would have done if the left arm had not rotated relative to the rest of the system (Figure 10.63d,e, where $\alpha < \theta$). The angular momentum of the whole system about a_Y is equal to the sum of the angular momentum of the left arm about a_Y and the angular momentum of the rest of the system about a_Y. As rotation of the left arm relative to the rest of the system results in a decrease in the angular momentum of the rest of the system about a_Y, it follows that there must be a simultaneous increase in the angular momentum of the left arm about a_Y, so that the angular momentum of the whole system about a_Y is conserved. In effect, rotation of the left arm relative to the rest of the system results in a transfer of angular momentum from the rest of the system to the left arm for as long as the left arm is moving relative to the rest of the system.

If the left arm is rotated relative to the rest of the system in the direction of rotation of the whole system, then angular momentum will be transferred from the rest of the system to the left arm. However, if the left arm is rotated in the opposite direction to that of the whole system, angular momentum will be transferred from the left arm to the rest of the system;

426

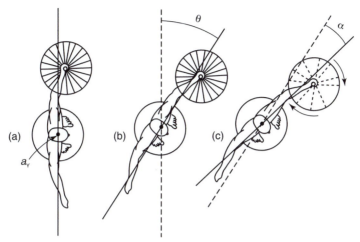

Figure 10.64 Man standing on turntable, holding a wheel that is free to rotate about its spindle, with the whole system of turntable, man and wheel rotating about a vertical axis a_Y with constant angular momentum (subject to friction around spindle): images are at equal time intervals.

the angular velocity of the rest of the system about a_Y will be seen to increase during the same period that the left arm is rotating relative to the rest of the system (Figure 10.63d,f, where $\beta > \theta$).

It is evident that for a body, such as the human body, that is comprised of a number of segments that can move relative to each other, angular momentum can be transferred from one segment to another by the action of internal forces exerted between the segments. The angular momentum of any particular segment can be increased or decreased by increasing or decreasing the angular velocity of the segment relative to the axis of rotation of the whole system. This phenomenon is referred to as the principle of transfer of angular momentum. The principle may be demonstrated by using a turntable that is free to rotate about a vertical axis a_Y and a bicycle wheel that has a handle attached to each end of its spindle, in line with the spindle, so that the wheel can rotate independently of the handles. A person stands on the turntable and holds the wheel, with its spindle vertical, in one hand, as shown in Figure 10.64. If the turntable is then rotated by an external moment, which is subsequently removed, the whole system (turntable, person and wheel) will continue to rotate about a_Y with constant angular momentum (Figure 10.64a,b). If the person then rotates the wheel about its spindle in the direction of rotation of the whole system, the angular velocity and, therefore, the angular momentum of the rest of the system, i.e. the turntable and person, will decrease (Figure 10.64b,c, where $\alpha < \theta$). As the angular momentum of the whole system about a_Y is conserved, the angular momentum lost by the turntable and person is gained by the wheel; by rotating the wheel in the direction of rotation of whole system, angular momentum is transferred from the turntable and person to the wheel. If the person then stops the wheel rotating by touching the wheel against his chest and holds the wheel in its original position, the whole system will rotate about a_Y with the same angular velocity as at the start of the experiment, i.e. after removal of the external moment. Therefore, by stopping the wheel rotating, angular momentum is transferred back from the wheel to the rest of the system. The angular momentum of the system about a_Y will not be entirely conserved because of friction around the turntable spindle.

427

Transfer of angular momentum in a forward pike dive

The principle of transfer of angular momentum is of great significance in many sports. Figure 10.65 shows four successive positions of a diver performing a forward pike dive. The diver leaves the board with a certain amount of linear momentum (upward and forward) and forward angular momentum about the mediolateral axis a_z through his centre of gravity. The linear momentum and angular momentum of the diver are the result of the impulse (linear and angular) of the ground reaction force prior to take-off. Just after take-off, the diver flexes his hips and achieves the pike position shown in Figure 10.65b. The piking action increases the angular velocity and, therefore, the angular momentum of the upper body (trunk, head and arms) about a_z; this results in a simultaneous decrease in the angular velocity and angular momentum of the legs about a_z, as the angular momentum of the whole body about a_z is conserved. If the piking action is carried out very quickly, i.e. the angular velocity of the upper body is rapidly increased, the angular velocity of the legs may be reduced to zero or the direction of rotation of the legs may even be reversed, as shown in Figure 10.65b (compare the position of the legs in Figure 10.65a and b). In the last part of the pike dive, the diver needs to straighten out his body in preparation for entry into the water. This is achieved by extension of the hips, which increases the angular velocity and angular momentum of the legs about a_z and simultaneously decreases the angular velocity and angular momentum of the upper body about a_z as the angular momentum of the whole body about a_z is conserved (Figure 10.65b–d). In the time that it takes for the position of the body to change from that in Figure 10.65b to that in Figure 10.65d, the legs rotate approximately 145° about a_z and the upper body rotates approximately 20°.

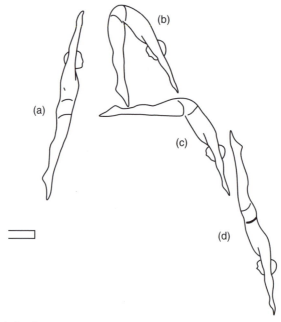

Figure 10.65 Forward pike dive.

Transfer of angular momentum in the long jump

The hitch-kick technique of long jumping involves transfer of angular momentum, in order to control forward rotation during flight. At take-off, the jumper would like to maximise vertical velocity v_V (to maximise flight time t) and horizontal velocity v_H (to maximise jump distance d where $d = v_H \cdot t$). However, v_V and v_H are not independent of each other, i.e. it is not possible to maximise both at the same time (see the section on the trajectory of a long jumper in Chapter 9). Maximal performance (jump distance) involves a compromise between v_V and v_H.

v_H is almost entirely due to the run-up, but v_V is entirely due to the impulse of the vertical component of the ground reaction force acting on the jumper during the thrust from the board. Consequently, to generate vertical velocity at take-off, the jumper pushes down on the board, which results in the ground reaction force passing behind the jumper's centre of gravity prior to take-off (Figure 10.66a). The near-vertical eccentric ground reaction force generates not only upward linear momentum, but also forward angular momentum of the body, which is conserved about the mediolateral axis a_z through the jumper's centre of gravity during the flight phase of the jump. If the forward angular momentum is not controlled during flight, the jumper is likely to rotate forward and land face down (Figure 10.67). To control the forward angular momentum, i.e. prevent forward rotation of the body as a whole, the angular momentum of the trunk, head and neck can be transferred to the arms and legs by increasing

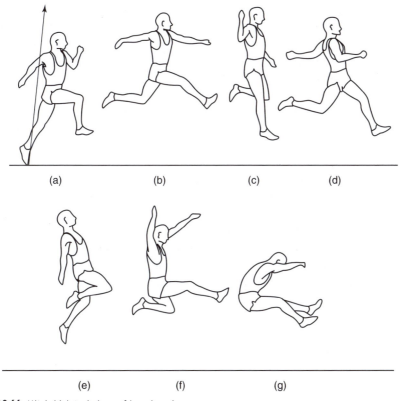

(a)   (b)   (c)   (d)

(e)   (f)   (g)

Figure 10.66 Hitch-kick technique of long jumping.

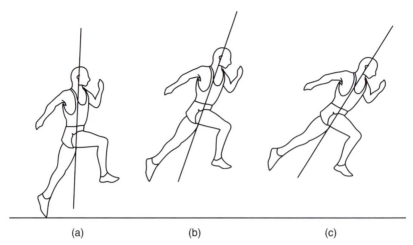

(a)   (b)   (c)

Figure 10.67 Forward rotation in long jumping: if the forward angular momentum is not controlled during flight, the jumper is likely to rotate forward and land face down.

the angular velocity of the arms and legs relative to a_z. This is achieved by forward rotation of the arms about the shoulders and similar rotation of the legs about the hips (Figure 10.66b–f). These actions, referred to as hitch-kick, enable the jumper to keep the trunk upright during flight or even reverse the direction of rotation of the trunk, if the action of the arms and legs is sufficiently vigorous (Figure 10.66d,e). In preparation for landing, the arms and legs are brought to rest in front of the trunk; this transfers angular momentum back from the arms and legs to the trunk, head and neck. Consequently, the trunk, head and neck rotate forward prior to landing, thus increasing the chance of rotating over the feet rather than falling back in the sand (Figure 10.66g). The hitch-kick technique enables the jumper to make full use of the ground reaction force in generating vertical velocity at take-off and also facilitates an effective landing.

Transfer of angular momentum in a standing back somersault

Figure 10.68 shows a gymnast performing a standing back somersault. The movement is initiated by hip flexion and shoulder extension into a position from which a powerful upward thrust can be made (position 1 in Figure 10.68). The arms are then swung rapidly forward (shoulder flexion; clockwise rotation of the arms with respect to Figure 10.68) such that much of the backward angular momentum of the body at take-off is contained in the arms (position 11). After take-off, rotation of the body takes place about the mediolateral axis through the gymnast's centre of gravity. Just after take-off, the angular velocity and, therefore, the angular momentum of the arms, is rapidly reduced to zero which is maintained for most of the flight phase (positions 13–22). Therefore, during this period, the angular momentum of the arms is transferred to the rest of the body, as the angular momentum of the whole body is conserved during flight.

In a study of platform diving, Hamill *et al.* (1986) showed that in a backward single somersault dive, which is similar to a standing back somersault, about half of the backward

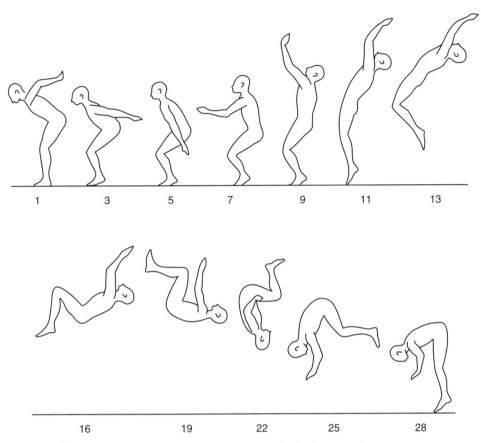

Figure 10.68 Successive positions of gymnast performing standing back somersault.

angular momentum of the body at take-off is contained in the arms. In both movements, the magnitude and direction of the ground reaction force will vary prior to take-off, but the end result, in terms of linear and angular momentum of the body at take-off, will depend upon the impulse of the resultant force and impulse of the resultant moment acting on the body.

Figure 10.69 shows four possible positions of a gymnast at take-off in a standing back somersault, together with the line of action of the ground reaction force F in relation to the mediolateral axis a_z through the centre of gravity of the gymnast in each position. If it is assumed that the line of action of F in each position is typical of the whole of the upward thrust, it will be interesting to consider the effects of F in the different types of actions. In Figure 10.69a, the line of action of F is vertical and passes through a_z. This action will produce upward linear momentum but no backward angular momentum, i.e. the gymnast would jump upward without backward rotation. In Figure 10.69b, the line of action of F is vertical and passes in front of a_z. This action will produce upward linear momentum and backward angular momentum, i.e. the gymnast would jump upward and rotate backward during flight. In both situations (Figure 10.69a,b) the ground reaction force is vertical and therefore the centre of gravity will move vertically (up and down) throughout the whole movement, i.e. the centre of gravity will not move horizontally. If the orientation of the body is the same at take-off and

431

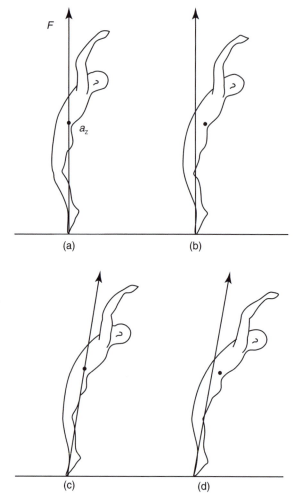

F

a_z

(a)   (b)

(c)   (d)

Figure 10.69 Four variations in the line of action of the ground reaction force at take-off in a standing back somersault: a_z, mediolateral axis through gymnast's centre of gravity.

landing, the feet will land in the same place from which they left the ground. In Figure 10.69c the line of action of F passes through a_z and is inclined with respect to the vertical. This action will produce linear momentum in the direction of F, but no backward angular momentum, i.e. the gymnast's centre of gravity will move up and down (vertically) and backward (horizontally) during flight. In Figure 10.69d, the line of action of F passes in front of a_z and is inclined with respect to the vertical. This action will produce linear momentum in the direction of F, similar to that in Figure 10.69c, and backward angular momentum.

> The angular momentum of a body is conserved during flight, but angular momentum can be transferred between body segments by internal (muscle) forces.

ROTATION AND NEWTON'S THIRD LAW OF MOTION

From Newton's first law of motion, when an object is rotating about a particular axis with constant angular momentum, the resultant moment acting on the object is zero. Internal forces may alter the moment of inertia of the object about the axis of rotation, but angular momentum will be conserved. When internal forces change the moment of inertia of an object about a particular axis, there is a simultaneous change in the angular momentum of each part of the object. For example, in the pike dive shown in Figure 10.65, the pike is achieved by flexion of the hips, simultaneously increasing the angular momentum of the upper body and decreasing the angular momentum of the legs about the mediolateral axis a_Z through the centre of gravity so that angular momentum is conserved. When the hip flexors contract to produce the pike position, they pull equally on both of their attachments, the upper body and the legs. Therefore, the angular impulse of the hip flexors on the upper body is exactly the same in magnitude but opposite in direction to that exerted on the legs, so that the angular momentum of the body about the mediolateral axis a_H through the hip joints is unchanged, i.e. it remains zero. To straighten his body in preparation for entry into the water, the diver extends his hips. The hip extensor muscles pull equally on both of their attachments, the upper body and the legs. Therefore, the angular impulse of the hip extensors on the upper body is equal in magnitude but opposite in direction to that exerted on the legs, so that the angular momentum of the body about a_H is unchanged, i.e. it remains zero. The action of the hip extensors also results in an increase in the angular momentum of the legs about a_Z and a simultaneous decrease in the angular momentum of the upper body about a_Z, so that angular momentum about a_Z is conserved. This example illustrates that when an object is rotating about a particular axis with constant angular momentum, such as in the flight phase of a jump, dive or somersault, the angular momentum of the body about any joint axis will be zero.

In a pike dive, the actions of the hip flexors in piking the body and the hip extensors in straightening the body by rotating the upper body and legs in opposite directions are examples of the operation of Newton's third law of motion in relation to rotation. The law may be expressed as follows:

> When an object A exerts a moment on another object B, there will be an equal and opposite moment exerted by object B on object A.

The law may be demonstrated by using a turntable, which is free to rotate about a vertical axis through its point of support. A man stands on the turntable, perfectly still, with his arms outstretched at his sides (Figure 10.70a). If the man flexes his left shoulder, such that his left arm is rotated with respect to the rest of the system of man and turntable through an angle β in a horizontal plane about the local vertical axis a_S through his left shoulder joint, the rest of the system will be seen to rotate about a_S in the opposite direction through an angle θ (Figure 10.70b). As the angular impulse exerted by the shoulder flexors on the left arm is equal and opposite to that exerted on the rest of the system, the angular momentum of the system about a_S remains unchanged, i.e. zero. In Figure 10.70b,

$$I_A \cdot \omega_A = I_R \cdot \omega_R,$$

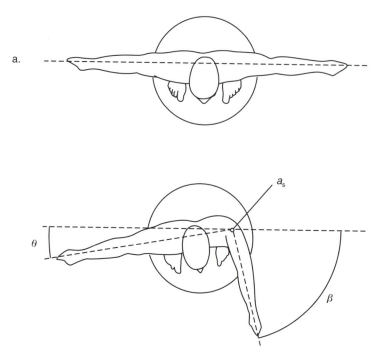

Figure 10.70 Overhead view of man standing on turntable that is free to rotate about vertical axis through its spindle: a_S, vertical axis through left shoulder joint.

where: I_A = moment of inertia of the left arm about a_S,
ω_A = angular velocity of the left arm about a_S,
I_R = moment of inertia of the rest of the system about a_S,
ω_R = angular velocity of the rest of the system about a_S.

As $\omega_A = \dfrac{\beta}{t}$ and $\omega_R = \dfrac{\theta}{t}$,

where t is the duration of the angular impulse of the shoulder flexors, it follows that

$$I_A \cdot \beta = I_R \cdot \theta.$$

Therefore, $\theta = \dfrac{I_A \cdot \beta}{I_R}.$

If, for example, $I_A/I_R = \frac{1}{3}$ and $\beta = 90°$, then $\theta = 30°$. The reaction of the rest of the body to rotation of one part of the body is not always discernible, especially when the larger part is in contact with the ground. In such cases, the reaction of the larger part may be prevented from occurring by friction between the larger part and the ground. The effect of Newton's third law is most clearly seen in movements that occur during flight when the body has little, if any, angular momentum as, for example, in a pike jump (Figure 10.71a,b) and spiking a volleyball (Figure 10.71c,d).

434

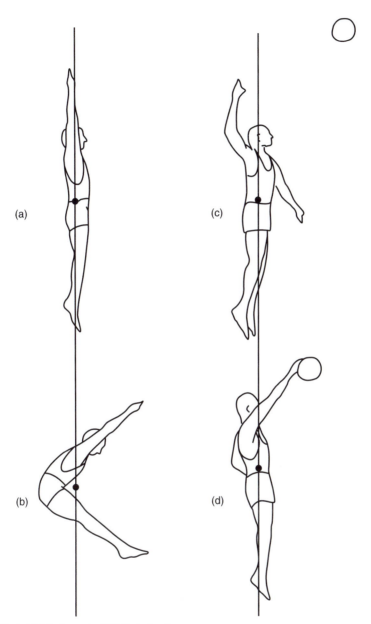

Figure 10.71 (a,b) Pike jump. (c,d) Volleyball spike.

SOMERSAULTING AND TWISTING

In a number of sports, including gymnastics, diving, trampolining and freestyle skiing, the main features of the movements are twisting somersaults during flight, i.e. movements that involve simultaneous rotation of the body about the mediolateral axis a_Z and vertical axis a_Y through the centre of gravity of the body (Figure 9.4). Rotation about a_Z is referred to as somersaulting and rotation about a_Y is referred to as twisting. Twisting can be produced in

435

three ways: contact twist, counter-rotation twist and tilt twist (Frohlich 1979, 1980; Yeadon 1993a–d). Contact twist generates angular momentum about a_Y prior to take-off; this angular momentum is conserved during flight and, consequently, results in constant rotation about a_Y during flight. Counter-rotation twist and tilt twist only occur during flight and, by contrast with contact twist, can be initiated and stopped by the performer. Counter-rotation twist is produced as a reaction to rotation of the body or part of the body about a_Y in a manner that facilitates twist but does not change the angular momentum of the body about a_Y. Tilt twist is produced by partitioning existing somersault angular momentum into somersault and twist components by tilting the a_Y axis of the body away from the vertical by asymmetric movements of the arms, chest or legs.

Contact twist

Contact twist is generated prior to take-off by a pushing or pulling action with the feet or hands against the floor or apparatus in such a way that the forces acting on the feet or hands exert a turning moment (in the form of a couple or two eccentric forces) on the body in the required direction of rotation around a_Y. For example, most people of average physical fitness will be able to demonstrate contact twist by jumping vertically and rotating a certain amount about a_Y before landing. This is achieved by a jumping action involving simultaneous whole body extension along a_Y and torsion of the body around a_Y, i.e. as the body extends upward, the body is forcibly rotated, involving a vigorous upward and lateral swing of both arms, around a_Y in the required direction (Figure 10.72). If torsion about a_Y occurs during flight, with no angular momentum about a_Y, rotation of the upper body in one direction about a_Y will result in the lower body rotating in the opposite direction, in order to conserve zero angular momentum (similar to the situations in Figures 10.70 and 10.71a and b). However, friction between the feet and the support surface (the horizontal components of the ground reaction forces acting on the feet) normally prevents movement of the feet and simultaneously exerts a turning moment on the body about a_Y. Consequently, the body takes off with an angular momentum about a_Y that is conserved during flight. Contact twist is a source of angular momentum about a_Y in all sports that involve twisting somersaults (Frohlich 1979, 1980; Yeadon 1997).

Counter-rotation twist

There are two forms of counter-rotation twist, the two-axes twist and the hula twist. Both forms are based on the ability of the body to twist about a_Y even though the body has no angular momentum about a_Y.

Two-axes twist

The most frequently cited example of the two-axes twist or 'cat-twist' form of counter-rotation twist is that of the falling cat (McDonald 1960). If a cat is held upside down by it legs about 0.5 m above the floor and then released, it will rotate 180° about its head-to-toe axis a_j in about 0.12 s to land safely on its feet after its 0.3 s fall (Frohlich 1979). This is achieved

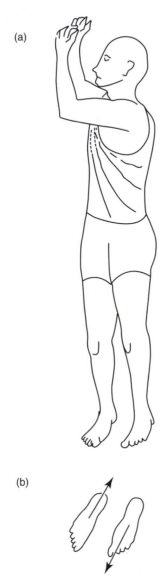

(a)

(b)

Figure 10.72 Contact twist during take-off from the floor. (a) Contact twist to the gymnast's right, involving vigorous upward and lateral swing of the arms. (b) Horizontal components of ground reaction forces acting on feet.

by a combination of flexion and extension of the trunk with alternate rotation of the upper part of the body (head, neck, upper part of the trunk and front legs) and lower part of the body (lower part of the trunk and back legs). Flexion and extension of the trunk results in the upper body portion a_U of a_j being at an angle to that of the lower part a_L. Consequently, in flexion and extension, the moment of inertia of the upper body about a_U is less than the moment of inertia of the lower body about a_U and the moment of inertia of the lower body about a_L is less than the moment of inertia of the upper body about a_L; the greater the angle between a_U and a_L, the greater the difference in moment of inertia of the upper and lower

437

(a)   (b)   (c)   (d)   (e)

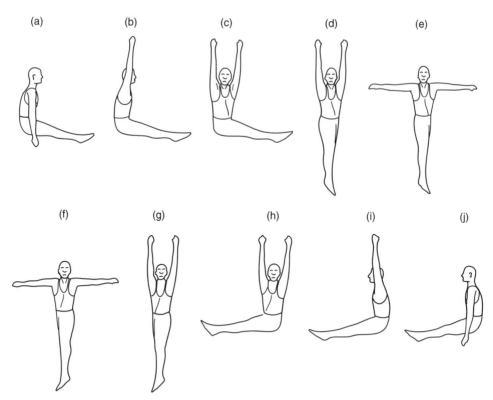

(f)   (g)   (h)   (i)   (j)

Figure 10.73 Swivel hips move on trampoline. (a,b) As body moves upward, arms rotate upward in frontal plane to overhead position. (b) The moment of inertia of the upper body (trunk, head, neck and arms) about the vertical axis a_Y through the whole body centre of gravity is much smaller than the moment of inertia of the legs about a_Y. (b,c) Upper body rotates about a_Y (shoulders about 90°). The legs hardly move in the opposite direction because of their much larger moment of inertia about a_Y in the pike position. (c,d) Body straightens, as upper body and legs rotate in opposite directions about mediolateral axis a_Z through whole body centre of gravity; the movement of the upper body is much smaller than that of the legs because of its much greater moment of inertia about a_Z. (d,e) Arms rotate in frontal plane to horizontal position; moment of inertia of the upper body about a_Y is considerably increased. (e,f) Legs rotate (swivel) approximately 180° about $a_{Y'}$ with hardly any reaction from the upper body because of its much larger moment of inertia about a_Y. (f,g) Arms rotate in frontal plane to overhead position. (g,h) Body pikes as upper body and legs rotate in opposite directions about a_Z; movement of the upper body is much less than that of legs because of its much greater moment of inertia about a_Z. (h,i) Upper body rotates about a_Y to complete the 180° turn with very little reaction from the legs because of their much larger moment of inertia about a_Y in pike position. (i,j) Arms rotate downward in the frontal plane in preparation for landing.

body about a_U and a_L. Consequently, when the upper body rotates about a_U, the simultaneous rotation of the lower body in the opposite direction is relatively small, owing to its larger moment of inertia. Similarly, when the lower body rotates about a_L, the simultaneous rotation of the upper body in the opposite direction is relatively small, owing to its larger moment of inertia. Coordinated flexion and extension of the trunk and rotation about a_U and a_L enables the cat to complete the 180° twist. The action of 'swivel hips' on a trampoline (seat drop, half twist to seat drop) is an example of two-axes counter-rotation twist in human movement (Figure 10.73).

Hula twist

In the Hawaiian hula dance, and when keeping a hula hoop rotating around the body, the hips are moved in a continuous circular manner, effectively rotating the body about a_Y. If this circular movement of the hips occurs during flight, with no angular momentum about a_Y, the body as a whole will rotate in the opposite direction to that of the hips, in order to conserve zero angular momentum about a_Y. This can be demonstrated by a gymnast hanging from a ring that is free to rotate about a_Y. If the gymnast starts to rotate his hips clockwise in a hula manner, he will simultaneously twist anticlockwise (Figure 10.74). Similarly, if the gymnast starts to rotate his hips anticlockwise in a hula manner, he will simultaneously twist clockwise.

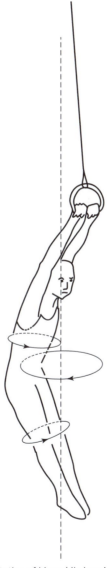

Figure 10.74 Hula twist in response to rotation of hips while hanging from ring.

Tilt twist

Like linear velocity and linear momentum, angular velocity and angular momentum are vector quantities. At any particular point in time, the angular velocity of an object is the sum of the component angular velocities. For example, when a gymnast is performing a twisting somersault, the angular velocity of the gymnast at any point in time is the resultant of his angular velocities about a_Y (twisting speed) and a_Z (somersaulting speed). Similarly, the angular momentum of the gymnast is the resultant of his angular momentum about a_Y and a_Z. During flight, the total amount of angular momentum of the gymnast will be conserved, but asymmetric movements of the body can vary the amounts of angular momentum and, therefore, angular velocity about a_Y and a_Z. This is the basis of tilt twist.

Figure 10.75 shows a gymnast during the flight phase of a vertical jump in which he has no angular momentum about any axis. If the gymnast rotates his left arm about the anteroposterior axis a_S through his left shoulder from an overhead position (Figure 10.75a) to a side position (Figure 10.75b), the rest of his body will simultaneously rotate in the opposite direction about a_S so that zero angular momentum about a_S is conserved. The moment of inertia of the

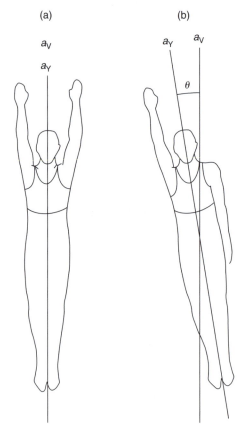

(a)   (b)

Figure 10.75 Effect of asymmetric arm action on rotation of rest of body during the flight phase of vertical jump without angular momentum: a_V, longitudinal axis through centre of gravity of gymnast, a_V; vertical axis through centre of gravity of gymnast; θ, tilt angle.

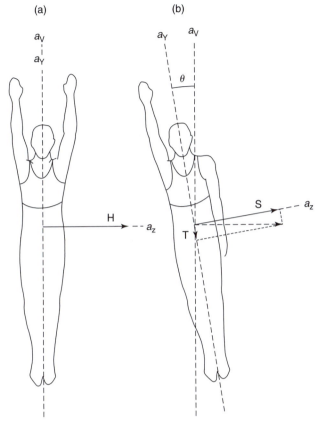

Figure 10.76 Development of tilt twist by asymmetric arm action during somersaulting: a_y, longitudinal axis through centre of gravity of gymnast; a_z, mediolateral axis through centre of gravity of gymnast; a_v, vertical axis through centre of gravity of gymnast; H, angular momentum of gymnast; S, component of H about a_z. T, component of H about a_y.

left arm about a_s will be approximately one-twentieth of the moment of inertia of the rest of the body about a_s, thus, as the arm rotates about 180°, the rest of the body will rotate about 9°. Consequently, the effect of the arm action is to tilt the body with respect to the vertical. In the absence of any further movement of body segments, this tilted posture will be maintained until landing. If the same arm action is made while the gymnast somersaults forward, he will immediately start twisting to his right while continuing to somersault forward, as described next.

Figure 10.76a shows the front view of a gymnast just after take-off from the floor following a run-up. It is assumed that the gymnast has considerable forward angular momentum about the mediolateral axis a_z through his centre of gravity, but no angular momentum about the anteroposterior axis a_X or vertical axis a_Y. When showing angular momentum vectors, it is convention that the direction of the arrow indicates clockwise rotation. Consequently, in Figure 10.76a, the angular momentum H of the gymnast is shown as a vector pointing to his left because he is rotating forward about a_z. If he had been rotating backward about a_z, the vector would have pointed to his right.

In the absence of a change in posture, the direction of H will be aligned with a_Z of the gymnast such that he will somersault forward about a_Z with constant angular velocity. However, if the gymnast rotates his left arm in the frontal plane (Figure 10.76b), his body will tilt with respect to the vertical such that the direction of H will no longer be aligned with a_Z. The tilt will effectively partition H into two components, one along a_Y and one along a_Z, so that the gymnast will immediately start twisting to his right about a_Y as well as somersault forward about a_Z, with the total amount of angular momentum being conserved. Furthermore, the gymnast will continue twisting to his right even though there may be no further change in body posture. This source of twist is referred to as tilt twist. Tilt twist can be stopped by the reverse action to that which caused it, i.e. in the above example, reversing the left arm movement. The direction of twist depends upon the direction and amount of tilt. In this example, anticlockwise rotation of the right arm instead of clockwise rotation of the left arm (with respect to Figure 10.76) would tilt the body in the opposite direction, resulting in tilt twist to the left. Here, tilt twist was caused by asymmetric arm action, but any movements that result in left–right asymmetry will result in tilt twist when somersaulting (Yeadon 1993c).

Twist speed depends upon the resultant angular momentum H, the tilt angle and the moments of inertia of the gymnast about a_Y and a_Z while twisting. For example, from Figure 10.76b,

$$T = H \cdot \sin \theta$$

where:
$$
\begin{aligned}
S &= H \cdot \cos \theta \\
\theta &= \text{tilt angle,} \\
T &= \text{component of angular momentum about } a_Y, \\
S &= \text{component of angular momentum about } a_Z.
\end{aligned}
$$

Therefore,
$$
\begin{aligned}
I_T \cdot \omega_T &= H \cdot \sin \theta \\
I_S \cdot \omega_S &= H \cdot \cos \theta,
\end{aligned}
$$

where:
$$
\begin{aligned}
I_T &= \text{moment of inertia of the gymnast about } a_Y, \\
\omega_T &= \text{angular velocity (twist velocity) of the gymnast about } a_Y, \\
I_S &= \text{moment of inertia of the gymnast about } a_Z, \\
\omega_S &= \text{angular velocity (somersault velocity) of the gymnast about } a_Z.
\end{aligned}
$$

It follows that,

$$\frac{I_T \cdot \omega_T}{I_S \cdot \omega_S} = \tan \theta \ (\text{as } \sin \theta / \cos \theta = \tan \theta)$$

and
$$\omega_T = \frac{I_S \cdot \omega_S \cdot \tan \theta}{I_T}.$$

If I_S is 15 times larger than I_T, i.e. $I_S / I_T = 15$ and $\theta = 9°$ ($\tan 9° = 0.158$), then,

$$\omega_T = 2.37 \omega_S,$$

i.e. the body will make 2.37 twists for every somersault.

Elite trampolinists, divers and gymnasts achieve twist speeds of 4 to 6 twists per somersault (Frohlich 1979; Yeadon 1993c). To maintain counter-rotation twist, the performer needs to continuously change his body shape, and this tends to restrict the twist speed that can be achieved. High twisting speeds can only be achieved by tilt twisting.

The contribution of contact twist, counter-rotation twist and tilt twist varies between different performers for the same action, but tilt twist appears to be the most important source of twist in multiple twisting somersaults (Yeadon 1993c).

> Twisting can be produced in three ways: contact twist, counter-rotation twist and tilt twist.

REVIEW QUESTIONS

Moment of a force and levers

1. Define the following terms: moment of a force, resultant moment, equilibrium, lever, centripetal force, eccentric force, moment of inertia, angular momentum.

2. In Figure 10.3, the see-saw is horizontal and at rest with both boys off the floor. If the centre of gravity of the see-saw coincides with the fulcrum, determine W_B, the weight of boy B, if: W_A = weight of boy A = 45 kgf, d_A = moment arm of W_A about the fulcrum = 3 m and d_B = moment arm of W_B about the fulcrum = 3.75 m.

3. In Figure 10.10, if S_1 = 10 kgf, S_2 = 42 kgf, W_S = 80 kgf, l = 2.5 m and the height h of the man = 1.8 m, determine:

   i. the distance d between the vertical plane containing the centre of gravity of the man lying on the board and the parallel plane through knife-edge support A;
   ii. d as a percentage of h.

4. In Figure 10.14, if E = 20 kgf, d_E = 25 cm and d_R = 7 cm, calculate R if the nail does not move.

5. In Figure 10.15, calculate the minimum force required to lift the lid further if R = 40 kgf, d_R = 7 cm and d_E = 25 cm.

6. In Figure 10.34c–e, calculate the forces (A_1, A_2, A_3, respectively) that the arms have to exert against the floor in order to raise the body if d_A = 1.45 m, d_{W1} = 0.35 m, d_{W2} = 0.79 m, d_{W3} = 0.99 m and W = 70 kgf.

7. In Figure 10.19, if W = 5 kgf, d_W = 2.5 cm, d_F = 7.5 cm and F, J and W are all vertical forces, calculate F and J.

8. In Figure 10.20, if W = 5 kgf, d_w = 4.5 cm, d_F = 7.5 cm and the line of action of F is 45° with respect to the horizontal, calculate the magnitude of F and the magnitude and direction of J.

9. In Figure 10.23, if W = 60 kgf, d_w = 12 cm, d_A = 7 cm and the line of action of A is 80° with respect to the horizontal, calculate the magnitude of A and the magnitude and direction of J.

10. In Figure 10.25, if W = 4.5 kgf, d_L = 4 cm, d = 20 cm, the line of action of L is 17° with respect to the long axis of the shank (as shown in Figure 10.25b) and the long axis of the shank is at an angle of 30° with respect to the horizontal, calculate the magnitude of L and the magnitude and direction of T.

11. Figure 10Q.1a shows a gymnast performing an iron cross manoeuvre on the rings. Figure 10Q.1b shows a free body diagram of the right upper limb of the gymnast. Calculate the magnitude and direction of the shoulder joint reaction force S if:

   R = force exerted by the ring on the right hand = 35.54 kgf, and its line of action with respect to the horizontal = 80°,

   A = weight of the right upper limb = 3.5 kgf (total body weight = 70 kgf),

   P = force exerted by the pectoralis major muscle, and its line of action with respect to the horizontal = 20°,

   L = force exerted by the latissimus dorsi muscle = 2P (force exerted by L is twice that of P), and its line of action with respect to the horizontal = 55°,

   H = point of application of R,

   G = point of application of A,

   I = point of application of P and L,

   J = point of application of S,

   where H, G, I and J all lie on the same horizontal line,

   d_1 = distance between I and J = 10 cm,

   d_2 = distance between G and J = 29 cm,

   d_3 = distance between H and J = 60 cm.

Segmental analysis

12. Figure 10Q.2 shows the outline of a male pole vaulter clearing the bar, superimposed onto a centimetre grid. X and Y axes are shown on the grid with origin O. The following points are marked on the vaulter's body: top of the head, shoulder joint, wrist joint, hip joint, ankle joint. Assume that the position of the right arm is the same as that of the left arm with respect to the X–Y plane and that the position of the right leg is the same as that of the left leg with respect to the X–Y plane. Use a five-segment model (combined trunk, head and neck, right upper limb, left upper limb, right lower limb and left lower limb) and the segmental data from Plagenhoef et al. (1983) in Table 10.1 to determine the x and y coordinates of the centre of gravity of the vaulter with respect to O. It is not necessary to use the vaulter's mass in the calculations (the masses of the segments can

444

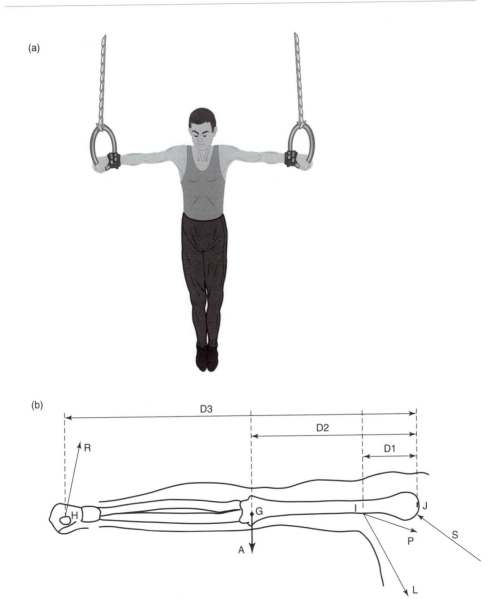

(a)

(b)

Figure 10Q.1 (a) Gymnast performing iron cross manoeuvre on rings. (b) Free body diagram of right upper limb of gymnast.

be incorporated as proportions of the total mass), but in order to calculate moments in N·cm, a nominal body mass of 70 kg should be used.

Angular displacement, angular velocity and angular acceleration

13. Define angular displacement, angular velocity, angular acceleration, tangential acceleration, radial acceleration, centripetal force and centrifugal force.

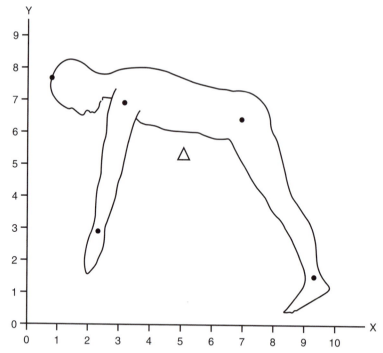

Figure 10Q.2 Pole vaulter clearing bar, superimposed onto centimetre grid. The x, y coordinates of the points on the vaulter's body are as follows: top of head (0.7, 7.7), left shoulder joint (3.1, 6.9), left wrist (2.3, 2.9), left hip joint (6.9, 6.4), left ankle (9.3, 1.5).

14. In Figure 10.39a, if position A is the reference position, i.e. 0°, and positions B, C, D, E and F are 60°, 125°, 180°, 240° and 305° clockwise from A, calculate:

   i.   The angular displacement θ_C of the gymnast at position C with respect to A and the angular displacement θ_E of the gymnast at position E with respect to A, in degrees and radians.
   ii. The average angular velocity ω in °/s and rad/s of the gymnast between positions B and D, if the time between positions B and D is 0.3 s.
   iii. The average angular acceleration α in °/s² and rad/s² between positions B and D, if the time between positions B and D is 0.3 s and ω_B and ω_D are 3.1 rad/s and 5.5 rad/s, respectively.
   iv. The linear velocity of the centre of gravity of the gymnast at positions B and D, if the distance between the bar and the gymnast's centre of gravity is 1 m in both positions and ω_B and ω_D are 3.1 rad/s and 5.5 rad/s, respectively.
   v.   The linear acceleration of the centre of gravity of the gymnast at positions B and D, if the distance between the bar and the gymnast's centre of gravity is 1 m in both positions and α_B and α_D are 7.1 rad/s² and 9.3 rad/s², respectively.

15. In Figure 10.42, if the mass of the thrower = 100 kg, the mass of the hammer = 7.26 kg, the linear velocity of the hammer = 27.5 m/s and the radius of curvature of the

hammer $= 1.78$ m, calculate the centripetal force F_C on the hammer and the radius of curvature of the thrower r_T.

16. In Figure 10.43, if the mass of the cyclist and bike $m_C = 70$ kg and the radius of curvature of the cyclist and bike $r_C = 35$ m, calculate the centripetal force F_C on the cyclist and bike and the lean angle θ with respect to the vertical required to ride at a speed of 13.5 m/s.

Angular impulse and angular momentum

17. In Table 10Q.1, list the metric units and their abbreviations for each variable.

18. Use the data from the solution to question 12 to calculate the moment of inertia of the pole vaulter about the mediolateral axis a_G through his centre of gravity. Use the same five-segment model, the segmental data from Plagenhoef *et al.* (1983) in Table 10.1 and the radius of gyration data from Winter (1990) in Table 10.6. Total mass of vaulter $= 70$ kg; 1 cm on the figure ~ 0.132 m.

19. In Figure 10.57, if the angular momentum of the gymnast about the mediolateral axis a_z through his centre of gravity just after take-off is 65 kg·m²/s and his moment of inertia I_z about a_z in positions 2 and 5 is 15 kg·m² and 5 kg·m², respectively, calculate the angular velocity of the gymnast about a_z in positions 2 and 5.

Table 10Q.1

Variable	Unit	Unit abbreviation
Moment of a force		
Time		
Angular impulse		
Moment of inertia		
Angular velocity		
Angular momentum		

Chapter 11

Work, energy and power

There are a number of different forms of energy, including heat, light, sound, electricity, chemical energy and various forms of mechanical energy. The total amount of energy in the universe is constant; it cannot be created or destroyed, it can only be transformed from one form to another. All interactions in nature are the result of transformation of energy from one form to another. For example, the combustion of oil, gas or coal produces heat that can be used to produce electricity that can be used to produce heat in a toaster, heat and light in a light bulb, heat, light and sound in a television or mechanical energy in the form of movement in a model train. Living organisms consume nutrients in order to produce chemical energy to maintain all of the life processes. The majority of the energy produced from nutrients is used to produce mechanical energy in the form of movement of the body segments. Transformation of energy into mechanical energy is referred to as work. All forms of energy are equivalent in their capacity to do work, i.e. to bring about the transfer of energy from one body to another through the action of a force or forces that deform or change the position or speed of movement of the bodies. Power is the rate of transformation of energy from one form to another. Mechanical power is the rate at which energy is transformed in the form of work. The purpose of this chapter is to describe the relationships between work, mechanical energy and mechanical power in human movement. Before reading this chapter, the reader should read the sections in Chapter 6 concerning energy and the different forms of mechanical energy.

OBJECTIVES

After reading this chapter, you should be able to do the following:

1. Differentiate the work of a force and the work of the moment of a force.
2. Differentiate average power and instantaneous power.
3. Describe the principle of conservation of energy.
4. State the first and second laws of thermodynamics.
5. Describe the components of mechanical energy.
6. Describe the conservation of mechanical energy.
7. With respect to human movement, differentiate internal work and external work.

WORK OF A FORCE

Newton's second law of motion expresses the relationship between impulse and momentum. With regard to linear motion,

$$F \cdot t = m \cdot v - m \cdot u, \qquad (9.15)$$

where: F = resultant force (greater than zero) acting on an object of mass m,
  t = duration of the resultant force,
  u = velocity of the object at the start of force application,
  v = velocity of the object at the end of force application.

If F is a constant force, resulting in constant acceleration, the average velocity v_a of the object during the period t is given by

$$v_a = \frac{u + v}{2}. \qquad (9.21)$$

If $u = 0$, then

$$F \cdot t = m \cdot v \qquad (11.1)$$

and

$$v_a = \frac{v}{2}. \qquad (11.2)$$

If d is the distance moved by the object during the period t, then

$$v_a = \frac{d}{t}. \qquad (11.3)$$

It follows from Equations 11.2 and 11.3 that

$$t = \frac{2d}{v}. \qquad (11.4)$$

By substitution of t from Equation 11.4 into Equation 11.1,

$$F \cdot d = \frac{m \cdot v^2}{2}. \qquad (11.5)$$

The quantity $F \cdot d$ is the work done by the force on the mass m. A force does work when it moves its point of application in the direction of the force; the amount of work done is defined as the product of the force and the distance moved by the point of application of the force. The quantity $m \cdot v^2/2$ is the change in translational (linear) kinetic energy of the mass m resulting from the work done on it. The translational kinetic energy of an object is the energy possessed by the object due to its linear motion. An object of mass m moving with linear velocity v has translational kinetic energy equal to $m \cdot v^2/2$. A stationary object has no translational kinetic energy, as $v = 0$. Energy is the capacity to do work. A body can do work if it has energy. There are a number of different forms of energy, including heat, light, sound, electricity, chemical energy and various forms of mechanical energy. Translational kinetic energy is a form of mechanical energy, and work is the transformation of any form of energy into mechanical energy. Equation 11.5 is referred to as the

449

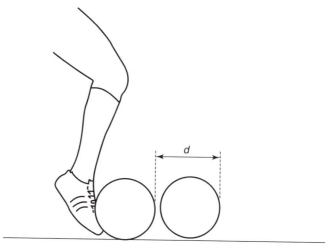

Figure 11.1 Distance *d* moved by soccer ball while in contact with kicker's foot when kicked from rest.

work–energy equation in relation to the work of a force; it expresses the relationship between the work done on an object by a force and the resulting change in the translational kinetic energy of the object. As will be described shortly, the moment of a force can also do work.

When a body A does work on another body B, energy is transferred from A to B. In this process, body B is moved or its type of movement is changed, i.e. it experiences acceleration or deceleration, usually combined with deformation. Figure 11.1 shows the movement of a soccer ball from the instant of contact with the kicker's foot to the instant of separation of foot and ball. If the ball is at rest before the kick, the velocity of the ball after the kick can be determined by applying Equation 11.5. For example, if

$F = 607.5 \text{ N}$ = the average force exerted on the ball during the kick,

$d = 0.27 \text{ m}$ = contact distance (distance moved by the ball in the direction of F while in contact with the kicker's foot)

$m = 0.45 \text{ kg}$ = the mass of the ball,

then the work done on the ball by the kicker, W, is given by

$$W = F \cdot d = 607.5 \text{ N} \times 0.27 \text{ m} = 164 \text{ J}.$$

In the SI system, the unit of work is the joule (J) (after James Prescott Joule 1818–1889). One joule is the work done by a force of 1 newton (N) when it moves its point of application a distance of 1 metre (m) in the direction of the force. The units of work, energy and moment of a force consist of the same combination of base units, $\text{kg} \cdot \text{m}^2/\text{s}^2$. To distinguish these quantities, the unit for work and energy is the joule (J) and the unit for moment of a force is the newton metre (N·m). From Equation 11.5, the velocity v of the ball after the kick is given by

$$v = \sqrt{\frac{2F \cdot d}{m}} = 27.0 \, \text{m/s} \, (60.4 \, \text{mph}).$$

> All interactions in nature are the result of a transformation of energy from one form to another. The transformation of energy into mechanical energy is referred to as work. In the SI system, the unit of work is the joule.

POWER

Power is work rate, i.e. the rate of doing work. In the SI system, the unit of power is the watt (W). One watt (after James Watt, 1736–1819) is a work rate of 1 J/s. Power can be measured over a period of time, in which case the average power can be calculated, or instantaneously, in which case it is referred to as the instantaneous power.

Average power

In the example of kicking a soccer ball, the contact time t between the kicker's foot and the ball can be determined by applying Newton's second law of motion, i.e.

$$F \cdot t = m \cdot v \tag{11.1}$$

$$t = \frac{m \cdot v}{F} = \frac{0.45 \, \text{kg} \times 27.0 \, \text{m/s}}{607.5 \, \text{N}} = 0.02 \, \text{s}.$$

As the kicker does 164 J of work on the ball in 0.02 s, the average power P_a of the kick, i.e. the average rate at which the kicker transfers energy to the ball in the form of work, is given by

$$P_a = \frac{W}{t} = \frac{164 \, \text{J}}{0.02 \, \text{s}} = 8200 \, \text{W} = 8.2 \, \text{kW} \, (1 \, \text{kW} = 1 \, \text{kilowatt} = 1000 \, \text{W}).$$

A soccer player kicking a stationary ball is similar, in terms of energy transfer, to a hammer hitting nail (Figure 11.2). As the hammer contacts the nail, the hammer has a certain amount of translational kinetic energy due to the work done on it by the person swinging it. As the hammer is rapidly brought to rest, its translational kinetic energy is equally rapidly transferred to the nail in the form of work, which drives the nail a distance d into the wood. Some of the energy of the hammer may be dissipated as heat and sound. If it is assumed that all of the translational kinetic energy of the hammer is transferred to the nail in the form of work, and if

$$m = 0.45 \, \text{kg} = \text{the mass of the hammer},$$

$$v = 1.8 \, \text{m/s} = \text{the velocity of the hammer on impact with the nail},$$
$$d = 0.01 \, \text{m},$$

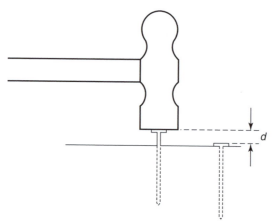

Figure 11.2 Impact of hammer on nail: d, distance that nail is driven into wood by impact.

then, from Equation 11.5, the average force F exerted by the hammer on the nail is given by

$$F = \frac{m \cdot v^2}{2d} = \frac{0.45 \text{ kg} \times (1.8 \text{ m/s})^2}{0.02 \text{ m}} = 72.9 \text{N} = 7.43 \text{ kgf}.$$

The duration of the impact t can be determined from Newton's second law of motion, i.e. $F \cdot t = m \cdot v - m \cdot u$, where $F = -72.9$ N, $u = 1.8$ m/s and $v = 0$.

$$t = \frac{-(0.45 \text{ kg} \times 1.8 \text{ m/s})}{-72.9 \text{ N}} = 0.011 \text{ s}.$$

The average power of the hammer strike on the nail is given by

$$P_a = \frac{W}{t} = \frac{F \cdot d}{t} = \frac{72.9 \text{ N} \times 0.01 \text{ m}}{0.011 \text{ s}} = 66.3 \text{W}.$$

Instantaneous power

Figure 11.3 shows the force–time graph and corresponding velocity–time graph and instantaneous power–time graph of the force exerted by the kicker on the soccer ball in the example. The corresponding data are shown in Table 11.1. The area between the force–time graph and the time axis represents the impulse of the force; the velocity of the ball increases as the impulse increases. The instantaneous power P_i of the kick, i.e. the instantaneous rate at which the kicker transfers energy to the ball in the form of work, is given by

$$P_i = F_i \cdot v_i,$$

where F_i and v_i are the force and velocity of the ball at the instant of time t_i. For example, when $t_i = 0.01$ s, $F_i = 1130$ N and $v_i = 14.79$ m/s. Consequently, P_i is given by

$$P_i = 1130 \text{ N} \times 14.79 \text{ m/s} = 1671.4 \text{ W} = 16.714 \text{ kW}.$$

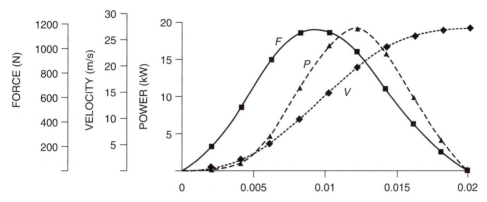

Figure 11.3 Force–time, velocity–time and instantaneous power–time graphs pertaining to soccer ball that is kicked from rest (see data in Table 11.1): F, force; v, velocity; P, power.

Table 11.1 Force–time, velocity–time and instantaneous power–time data pertaining to a soccer ball that is kicked from a resting position (see Figure 11.3).

Time (s)	Force (N)	Velocity (m/s)	Instantaneous power (W)
0	0	0	0
0.002	200	0.41	0.081
0.004	520	1.99	1.035
0.006	910	5.15	4.683
0.008	1130	9.77	11.039
0.010	1130	14.79	16.714
0.012	970	19.59	19.004
0.014	670	23.24	15.568
0.016	380	25.55	9.708
0.018	150	26.68	4.003
0.020	0	26.99	0

Peak instantaneous power, in the region of 19 kW, occurs at approximately $t_i = 0.012$ s (see Table 11.1 and Figure 11.3).

The transformation of relatively small amounts of energy can have a considerable effect when sufficient power is involved. For example, exposure of a piece of steel to a beam of light for ten seconds has no visible effect on the steel. However, if the same amount of light is discharged in one picosecond (one millionth of one millionth of a second, 10^{-12} s) it will burn a hole in the steel (Frost 1967). This is the basis of laser technology.

> Power is the rate of transformation of energy from one form to another. Mechanical power is the rate at which energy is transformed in the form of work. In the SI system, the unit of power is the watt.

CONSERVATION OF ENERGY

In the example of a hammer striking a nail, the work done by the hammer is clearly evident in the distance that the nail is driven into the wood. Similarly, in the example of kicking a soccer ball, the work done by the kicker on the ball is clearly apparent in the velocity of the ball as it flies away from the kicker's foot. However, most energy transfers are less dramatic and involve relatively small amounts of energy in relation to the masses of the objects upon which the work is done. Figure 11.4a shows a free body diagram of a box resting on the floor. Figure 11.4b shows a free body diagram of the box when a man pushes on the box with a horizontal force S. To slide the box across the floor, it is necessary to overcome the friction between the box and the floor. If the weight of the box $B = 30$ kgf and the coefficient of sliding friction between the box and the floor $= 0.45$, then the friction F that resists sliding is given by

$$F = \mu \cdot R = 0.45 \times 294.3 \text{ N} = 132.4 \text{ N},$$

where $R =$ the normal reaction force $= B = 294.3$ N (30 kg $\times$ 9.81 N).

Consequently, to slide the box across the floor, it is necessary to do work on the box equivalent to the work done by friction on the box in the opposite direction. For example, to slide the box a distance $d = 3.5$ m, work W must be done on the box equivalent to $F \cdot d$, i.e.

$$W = F \cdot d = 132.4 \text{ N} \times 3.5 \text{ m} = 463.5 \text{ J.}$$

The speed attained by the box will depend upon the work rate. A relatively low work rate will produce a relatively low speed, resulting in steady movement. A high work rate (a powerful thrust) is likely to generate sufficient translational kinetic energy in the box for it to slide, albeit briefly, in the absence of S. Whether the work rate is low or high, the work done on the box will be quickly dissipated as heat due to the friction, i.e. as energy is transferred to the box in the form of work, the box immediately transfers the energy to itself and the floor in the form of heat; this is reflected in an increase in the temperature of the bottom of the box and the floor. The transfer of energy from work to translational kinetic energy to heat is an

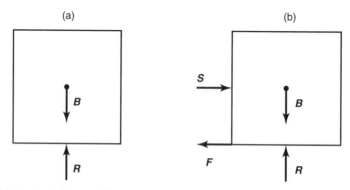

Figure 11.4 (a) Free body diagram of box resting on level floor. (b) Free body diagram of box when it is pushed from one side by horizontal force S: B, weight of box; R, ground reaction force exerted on box; F, friction between box and floor.

illustration of the conservation of energy, i.e. the continual transfer of energy from one form to another while the total amount of energy remains the same.

The principle of conservation of energy was established in the mid-nineteenth century, largely through the work of James Joule and Hermann von Helmholtz (1821–1894) (Brancazio 1984). Its formulation originated from observations that friction produces heat and heat can be used to do work, as in, for example, a steam engine (heat boils water, which produces steam, which drives the engine). Joule carried out experiments in which he measured the amount of heat generated by electricity, chemical reactions, work in various forms and friction. He discovered that work and heat are equivalent, i.e. a specific amount of work produces an equivalent amount of heat in terms of the amount of energy transformed. It was later discovered that all forms of energy are equivalent. Helmholtz is generally credited with the formulation of the principle of conservation of energy in its most general form, i.e. the principle that the total amount of energy (all forms) in a closed system is constant. A closed system is a system that is completely isolated from its surroundings. The earth is not a closed system, since it receives most of its energy from the sun, but the universe as a whole is considered a closed system (Brancazio 1984).

Thermodynamics

Thermodynamics is the branch of physics concerning the nature of heat and its association with other forms of energy. The first law of thermodynamics incorporates the principle of conservation of energy, i.e. the principle that the total amount of energy in a closed system is constant; energy cannot be created or destroyed, it can only be converted from one form to another. In the example of sliding a box across the floor, the work done on the box was transformed to translational kinetic energy of the box and then to heat almost immediately. The heat gained by the floor and the box would then be dissipated in the form of an increase in the temperature of the surrounding air. Consequently, the total amount of energy transformed in the action of pushing the box across the floor is still in the system, but it is present as heat rather than as chemical energy in the muscles of the man just prior to doing the work. The energy transformed to heat is no longer available to do work, even though it is still part of the total amount of energy in the system. This is the basis of the second law of thermodynamics, i.e. in any transformation of energy there is always an increase of entropy, or in other words, energy is transformed into forms that cannot be recovered to do work.

Heat energy

In the SI system, the base units are the metre, the kilogram and the second. In an older system of units, referred to as the c.g.s. system, the base units are the centimetre, the gram and the second. In the SI system, the unit of heat is the joule. In the c.g.s. system, the unit of heat is the calorie (cal), which is defined as the energy required to raise the temperature of 1 g (gram) of water by 1 °C. 1 cal = 4.186 J. One calorie is equivalent to the work done in lifting a weight of 4.186 N (0.43 kgf) vertically a distance of 1 m. It is also equivalent to pushing a mass of 1 kg a distance of 1 m across a level surface with coefficient of friction = 0.4267.

Work done in pushing a load up a slope

Figure 11.5a shows a free body diagram of a box resting on a slope of angle θ with respect to the horizontal. There are two forces acting on the box, the weight of the box B and the equal and opposite ground reaction force R. In Figure 11.5b, B and R have been replaced by their components perpendicular and parallel to the slope. The component of B perpendicular to the slope $B_N = B \cdot \cos\theta$ is equal and opposite to the normal reaction force N (component of R perpendicular to the slope). The component of B parallel to the slope $B_P = B \cdot \sin\theta$ is equal and opposite to the friction force F (component of R parallel to the slope). The box will remain at rest on the slope if $F > B_P$. As $F = \mu \cdot N = \mu \cdot B \cdot \cos\theta$, and $B_P = B \cdot \sin\theta$, the box will remain at rest provided that:

$$\mu \cdot B \cdot \cos\theta > B \cdot \sin\theta$$

$$\mu > \frac{B \sin\theta}{B \cos\theta}$$

$$\mu > \tan\theta \text{ (as } \tan\theta = \sin\theta / \cos\theta).$$

Since $\tan\theta$ increases as θ increases and μ is constant for any two surfaces, it follows that the box will start to slide down the slope when the slope reaches a critical angle. In Figure 11.5b, if $\mu = 0.45$ and $B = 30$ kgf, the box will be on the point of sliding down the slope when $\tan\theta = 0.45$, i.e. when $\theta = 24.23°$. In this situation, $F = B_P$:

$$F = \mu \cdot B \cdot \cos\theta = 0.45 \times 30 \text{ kgf} \times 0.9119 = 12.31 \text{ kgf}$$
$$B_P = B \cdot \sin\theta = 30 \text{ kgf} \times 0.4104 = 12.31 \text{ kgf}.$$

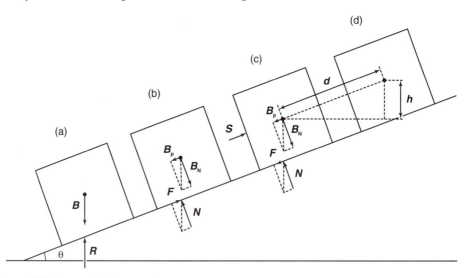

Figure 11.5 (a) Free body diagram of box resting on slope. (b) Free body diagram of box resting on slope with weight of box B and reaction force R resolved into their components perpendicular (B_N, N) and parallel (B_P, F) to the slope. (c) Free body diagram of box when it is being pushed up slope by force S parallel to slope. (d) Position of box after it has been pushed up slope a distance d.

In Figure 11.5, $\theta = 20°$, so the box will remain at rest if $\mu = 0.45$. If the angle of the slope is constant and the surface of the slope is even, N will be constant in magnitude and direction. Consequently, the magnitude of F will be constant ($= \mu \cdot N$). However, the direction of F will depend upon the movement of the box across the slope. F will always act on the box in the opposite direction to the movement of the box or opposite to the direction in which the box tends to move. In Figure 11.5b the box is at rest, but tending to slide down the slope due to B_p. Consequently, in this situation, F acts on the box up the slope and is equal in magnitude to B_p. However, if someone pushes the box up the slope, F will act on the box down the slope for the period of time that the box is moving up the slope or tending to move up the slope.

Figure 11.5c shows a free body diagram of the box when it is being pushed up the slope by someone applying a force S. To push the box up the slope, the person pushing the box must overcome F and B_p, which both oppose the movement of the box up the slope. The work done by S in pushing the box up the slope is the sum of the work done against F (the work done by F on the box) and the increase in the gravitational potential energy of the box as it moves up the slope. For example, if the box moves a distance d up the slope (Figure 11.5c,d), the work done W by S is given by

$$W = S \cdot d = F \cdot d + m \cdot g \cdot h,$$

where $m =$ mass of the box and $h =$ vertical displacement of the box, as it moves a distance d up the slope. If $m = 30$ kgf, $\mu = 0.45$, $\theta = 20°$, $d = 3.5$ m, then

$$N = B \cdot \cos 20° = 30 \text{ kgf} \times 9.81 \text{ m/s}^2 \times 0.9397 = 276.55 \text{ N}$$
$$F = \mu \cdot N = 0.45 \times 276.55 \text{ N} = 124.45 \text{ N}$$
$$h = d \cdot \sin 20° = 3.5 \text{ m} \times 0.3420 = 1.197 \text{ m}$$
$$W = (124.45 \text{ N} \times 3.5 \text{ m}) + (30 \text{ kg} \times 9.81 \text{ m/s}^2 \times 1.197 \text{ m})$$
$$= 435.5 \text{ J} + 352.28 \text{ J} = 787.85 \text{ J}.$$

As $W = S \cdot d$, then the average magnitude of S is given by

$$S = \frac{787.85 \text{ J}}{3.5 \text{ m}} = 225.1 \text{ N}.$$

The first law of thermodynamics incorporates the principle of conservation of energy, i.e. the total amount of energy in a closed system is constant; energy cannot be created or destroyed, it can only be converted from one form to another.

WORK OF THE MOMENT OF A FORCE

Newton's second law of motion in relation to angular motion expresses the relationship between angular impulse and angular momentum, i.e.

$$M \cdot t = I \cdot \omega_2 - I \cdot \omega_1 \tag{10.27}$$

457

where: M = resultant moment of force (greater than zero) acting on an object with moment of inertia I about a particular axis,

t = duration of the resultant moment,

ω_1 = angular velocity of the object at the start of the application of the resultant moment,

ω_2 = angular velocity of the object at the end of the application of the resultant moment.

If M is a constant moment, resulting in constant angular acceleration, the average angular velocity ω_a of the object during the period t is given by

$$\omega_a = \frac{\omega_1 + \omega_2}{2}.$$

If $\omega_1 = 0$, then

$$M \cdot t = I \cdot \omega \quad (\text{where } \omega = \omega_2) \tag{11.6}$$

and

$$\omega_a = \frac{\omega}{2} \tag{11.7}$$

If θ is the angular distance in radians moved by the object during the period t, then

$$\omega_a = \frac{\theta}{t}. \tag{11.8}$$

It follows from Equations 11.7 and 11.8 that

$$t = \frac{2\theta}{\omega}. \tag{11.9}$$

By substitution of t from Equation 11.9 into Equation 11.6,

$$\frac{2M \cdot \theta}{\omega} = I \cdot \omega$$

$$M \cdot \theta = \frac{I \cdot \omega^2}{2}. \tag{11.10}$$

The quantity $M \cdot \theta$ is the work done by the moment of force on the object. As the unit of M is newton metres and the unit of θ is radians, the unit of $M \cdot \theta$ is joules, the same as the unit of work done by a force. The work done by the moment of a force is the product of the moment and the angular distance in radians moved by the object during the impulse of the moment. The quantity $I \cdot \omega^2 / 2$ is the change in rotational (angular) kinetic energy of the object resulting from the work done on it by the moment of force. The rotational kinetic energy of an object is the energy possessed by the object due to its angular motion. An object with moment of inertia I and angular velocity ω about a particular axis has rotational kinetic energy equal

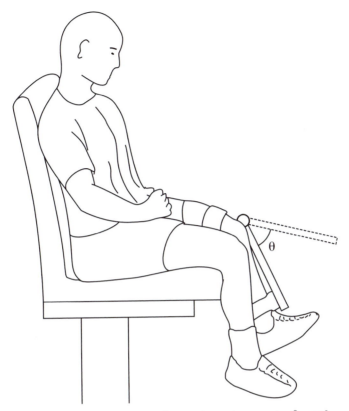

Figure 11.6 Football player performing knee extension exercise on dynamometer: $\theta = 50°$.

to $I{\cdot}\omega^2/2$. A stationary object has no rotational kinetic energy, as $\omega = 0$. Equation 11.10 is referred to as the work–energy equation in relation to the work of the moment of a force; it expresses the relationship between the work done on an object by the moment of a force and the resulting change in the rotational kinetic energy of the object.

Figure 11.6 shows a football player performing a knee extension training exercise on a dynamometer. In this type of dynamometer, the resistance exerted by the lever arm matches the force exerted by the trainer. If the player exerts a constant force of 140 N perpendicular to the lever arm of the dynamometer at a distance of 0.25 m from the axis of the lever arm and in extending the knee rotates the lever through 50°, the work done by the player on the dynamometer is given by

$$M \cdot \theta = (140 \text{ N} \times 0.25 \text{ m}) \times 0.8727 \text{ rad } (50° = 50 \times 0.017.45 \text{ rad} = 0.8727 \text{ rad})$$

$$= 35 \text{ N} \cdot \text{m} \times 0.8727 \text{ rad} = 30.5 \text{ J}.$$

In this exercise, the work done by the trainer on the dynamometer is equivalent to the work done by the friction (or electromagnetic brake) around the axis of the lever arm on the dynamometer in the opposite direction. Consequently, the work done by the trainer on the dynamometer is immediately dissipated as heat within the machine.

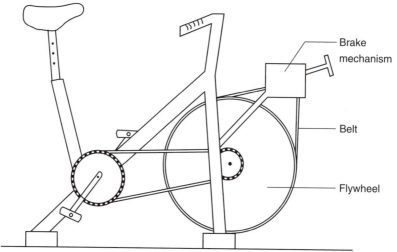

Figure 11.7 Friction-braked cycle ergometer: the friction between the belt and the flywheel can be adjusted by the brake mechanism.

Figure 11.7 shows an exercise cycle. Clockwise rotation of the pedals results in clockwise rotation of the flywheel. If the flywheel is a solid mass, the moment of inertia of the flywheel I about its spindle $= m \cdot r^2 / 2$, where m = mass of the flywheel and r = radius of the flywheel. If $m = 7$ kg and $r = 0.3$ m, then $I = 0.315$ kg·m². If a trainer exerts a constant moment of 0.75 N·m via the pedals for five revolutions of the pedals (with no friction between the belt and flywheel), the work done by the trainer on the flywheel is given by

$$M \cdot \theta = 0.75 \text{ N·m} \times (5 \text{ rev} \times 2\pi \text{ rad/rev}) \left(1 \text{ rev} = 2\pi \text{ rad} = 6.28 \text{ rad}\right)$$
$$= 0.75 \text{ N·m} \times 31.4 \text{ rad} = 23.55 \text{ J}.$$

The work done on the flywheel is equivalent to the increase in rotational kinetic energy of the flywheel, i.e. from Equation 11.10

$$\frac{I \cdot \omega^2}{2} = 23.55 \text{ J}$$
$$\omega = \sqrt{(47.1 \text{ J}/0.315 \text{ kg·m}^2)} = 12.2 \text{ rad/s}.$$

CONSERVATION OF MECHANICAL ENERGY

At any particular instant in time, the total mechanical energy of an object is the sum of its kinetic energy (translational and rotational) and its gravitational potential energy (Winter 1979). Transformation of mechanical energy from one form to another within an object is a common occurrence. For example, in a falling object, there will be a continuous transformation of gravitational potential energy to translational kinetic energy; as the height of the object and, therefore, its gravitational potential energy decreases, there will be a corresponding increase in its translational kinetic energy. Figure 11.8 shows the

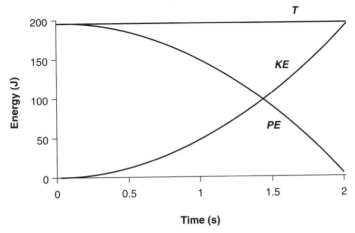

Figure 11.8 Transformation of gravitational potential energy *PE* to translational kinetic energy *KE* of 1 kg ball that is dropped from height of 20 m. In the absence of air resistance, the total mechanical energy *T* of the ball, i.e. the sum of *PE* and *KE*, would remain constant during the fall.

transformation of gravitational potential energy to translational kinetic energy of a 1 kg ball after being dropped from a height of 20 m in the absence of air resistance. In this situation, the loss in gravitational potential energy would be equal to the gain in translational kinetic energy so that the total amount of mechanical energy of the ball would be conserved, i.e. remain constant. This concept is referred to as the conservation of mechanical energy.

When an object is acted on by a resultant force that changes the proportions of the different forms of mechanical energy of the object, but does not change the total amount of mechanical energy of the object, the resultant force acting on the object is referred to as a conservative force. There are no conservative force systems in nature, as the movement of objects is always resisted to a certain extent by friction or fluid (air, water) resistance. However, a number of situations approximate to the action of a conservative force system, such as the effect of weight on a falling object. Whereas weight is constant, air resistance will increase as the velocity of the falling object increases (Equation 9.24). Air resistance will dissipate the energy of a falling object by transforming some of its energy into an increase in the kinetic energy of the layer of air in contact with the falling object.

Another situation that closely approximates a conservative force system is the movement of a pendulum. If a pendulum is stopped from swinging, it will hang vertically; this is the equilibrium position of the pendulum (Figure 11.9a). If the equilibrium position is the reference position for the measurement of gravitational potential energy ($h = 0$), then the pendulum will possess no mechanical energy in the equilibrium position. If the pendulum is rotated through an angle θ with respect to the vertical and held at rest, the work done on the pendulum will be equivalent to the gain in gravitational potential energy, i.e. $m·g·h$. If the pendulum is then released, it will oscillate about the equilibrium position for some considerable time and display a continuous transformation of mechanical energy from gravitational potential energy to translational kinetic energy in the downswings and from translational kinetic energy to gravitational potential energy in the upswings (Figure 11.9b). In the absence of friction

461

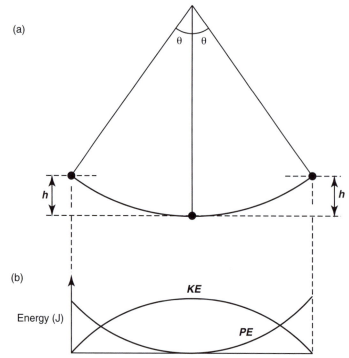

(a)

(b)

Energy (J)

KE

PE

h

h

θ θ

Figure 11.9 Movement of pendulum. (a) In the absence of friction around the axis of rotation and air resistance, the total mechanical energy of the pendulum would be conserved. (b) Transformation of gravitational potential energy *PE* and translational kinetic energy *KE* of the pendulum during each swing.

around its axis of rotation and air resistance, the pendulum would oscillate for ever and the total mechanical energy would be conserved. However, there will always be a certain amount of friction around its axis and air resistance. The friction around the axis will dissipate the energy of the pendulum in the form of heat, and air resistance will dissipate the energy of the pendulum in the form of an increase in the kinetic energy of the layer of air in contact with the pendulum.

Conservation of mechanical energy in a gymnast rotating about a horizontal bar

The rotation of a gymnast around a horizontal bar is similar to that of a pendulum in terms of transformation of mechanical energy. Figure 11.10 shows a gymnast swinging from rest in a clockwise direction from A through B. If B is the reference position for the measurement of gravitational potential energy ($h = 0$), then the mechanical energy of the gymnast at A and B is given by

Gravitational potential energy at $A = 2m \cdot g \cdot h$,
Translational kinetic energy at $A = 0$,
Rotational kinetic energy at $A = 0$,
Total mechanical energy at $A = 2m \cdot g \cdot h$, (11.11)

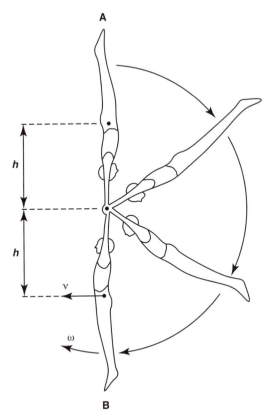

A

h

h

v

ω

B

Figure 11.10 Gymnast swinging around horizontal bar from position of rest directly above bar: h, distance between bar and centre of gravity of gymnast; v, linear velocity of the gymnast at B; ω, angular velocity of gymnast about bar at B.

Gravitational potential energy at $B = 0$,
Linear kinetic energy at $B = m{\cdot}v^2/2$,
Rotational kinetic energy at $B = I{\cdot}\omega^2/2$,
Total mechanical energy at $B = m{\cdot}v^2/2 + I{\cdot}\omega^2/2$, (11.12)

where: m = mass of the gymnast,
   h = distance between the bar and the centre of gravity of the gymnast,
   v = linear velocity of the gymnast at B,
   ω = angular velocity of the gymnast about the bar at B,
   I = moment of inertia of the gymnast about the bar.

From Equations 11.11 and 11.12,

$$2m{\cdot}g{\cdot}h = m{\cdot}v^2/2 + I{\cdot}\omega^2/2.$$ (11.13)

As $v = h{\cdot}\omega$ (Equation 10.12), substitution for v in Equation 11.13 gives

463

$$2m \cdot g \cdot h = \frac{m \cdot (h \cdot \omega)^2}{2} + \frac{I \cdot \omega^2}{2}$$

$$4m \cdot g \cdot h = \omega^2 (m \cdot h^2 + I)$$

$$\omega^2 = \frac{4m \cdot g \cdot h}{m \cdot h^2 + I}. \tag{11.14}$$

If $m = 70$ kg, $h = 0.9$ m and $I = 90$ kg·m^2, then from Equation 11.14

$$\omega^2 = \frac{4 \times 70 \text{ kg} \times 9.81 \text{ m/s} \times 0.9 \text{ m}}{(70 \text{ kg} \times 0.81 \text{ m}^2) + 90 \text{ kg} \cdot \text{m}^2} = 16.85 \text{ rad}^2/\text{s}^2$$

$$\omega = 4.105 \text{ rad/s}.$$

As $v = h \cdot \omega$, then $v = 0.9$ m $\times$ 4.105 rad/s $= 3.694$ m/s.

The total mechanical energy of the gymnast at $A = 2m \cdot g \cdot h = 1236$ J. The total mechanical energy of the gymnast at B is

$$m \cdot v^2/2 + I \cdot \omega^2/2 = 477.59 \text{ J} + 758.25 \text{ J} = 1236 \text{ J}.$$

Consequently, in rotating about the bar from A to B the composition of the mechanical energy of the gymnast changes from 100% gravitational potential energy at A (1236 J) to 38.6% translational kinetic energy (477.59 J) and 61.4% rotational kinetic energy (758.25 J) at B. The mechanical energy of the gymnast would not be completely conserved, owing to friction between the gymnast's hands and the bar.

Conservation of mechanical energy in pole vaulting

In the pole vault, the vaulter produces translational kinetic energy in the run-up. During the period between take-off and maximum pole bend, much of this translational kinetic energy is transformed into gravitational potential energy (as the centre of gravity of the vaulter rises), rotational kinetic energy (as the body swings about the hand grip) and strain energy in the pole (Figure 11.11a–c). Some of the strain energy in the pole will be dissipated as heat, but most of it will be available to do work in lifting the vaulter during the period between maximum pole bend and maximum height (Figure 11.11c–d). During the same period (while the pole is straightening), the vaulter normally pushes down on the pole in order to lift his body. Consequently, whereas some mechanical energy is lost as heat, a certain amount of new mechanical energy is added to the system of pole and vaulter in the form of work done by the vaulter in pushing down on the pole. It is difficult to measure the mechanical energy dissipated as heat and gained by muscular effort, but some insight into the loss and gain can be made by considering the mechanical energy of the vaulter at take-off and maximum height.

At take-off, the total mechanical energy E_T of the system of vaulter and pole is equal to the

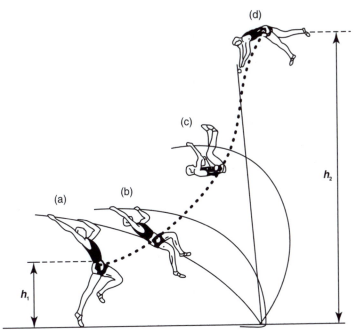

Figure 11.11 Movement of pole vaulter. (a) Take-off. (b) Forward swing between take-off and maximum pole bend. (c) Maximum pole bend. (d) Maximum height. h_1, height of vaulter's centre of gravity at take-off; h_2, height of vaulter's centre of gravity at maximum height.

sum of the gravitational potential energy and translational kinetic energy of the vaulter (assuming negligible energy in the pole and negligible rotational kinetic energy of the vaulter), i.e.

$$E_T = m{\cdot}g{\cdot}h_1 + m{\cdot}v_1^2/2, \tag{11.15}$$

where h_1 is the height of the vaulter's centre of gravity above the ground at take-off and v_1 is the linear velocity of the vaulter at take-off (Figure 11.11). At maximum height, the total mechanical energy E_M of the vaulter is equal to the sum of his gravitational potential energy and translational kinetic energy (assuming negligible rotational kinetic energy), i.e.

$$E_M = m{\cdot}g{\cdot}h_2 + m{\cdot}v_2^2/2, \tag{11.16}$$

where h_2, is the height of the vaulter's centre of gravity above the ground and v_2 is the linear velocity of the vaulter, which is the small amount of forward horizontal velocity required to ensure that the vaulter continues to move forward instead of coming to rest over the bar. Consequently, if all of the mechanical energy available at take-off is transformed into mechanical energy at maximum height (assuming no losses due to heat and no gains due to muscular effort), then from Equations 11.15 and 11.16

$$m{\cdot}g{\cdot}h_1 + m{\cdot}v_1^2/2 = m{\cdot}g{\cdot}h_2 + m{\cdot}v_2^2/2$$
$$h_2 - h_1 = (v_1^2 - v_2^2)/2g.$$

465

The term $(v_1{}^2 - v_2{}^2)/2g$ represents the theoretical gain in height between take-off and maximum height for given values of v_1 and v_2. When the theoretical gain is less than the actual gain, this indicates that the work done by the vaulter during the period when the pole is straightening (Figure 11.11c–d) is greater than the energy losses during the vault; this would be regarded by the coach as good technique. For example, if $h_1 = 1.18$ m, $h_2 = 5.58$ m, $v_1 = 9.3$ m/s and $v_2 = 1.5$ m/s (data from Bogdanis and Yeadon 1994), then the theoretical gain in height is $(v_1{}^2 - v_2{}^2)/2g = 4.29$ m. However, the actual gain in height is $h_2 - h_1 = 4.4$ m.

> There are no conservative force systems in nature as the movement of objects is always resisted to a certain extent by friction or fluid resistance.

INTERNAL AND EXTERNAL WORK

All voluntary human movement is the result of work done by the skeletal muscles, i.e. muscle contractions transform chemical energy stored in the muscles into mechanical energy in the form of internal work W_I and external work W_E (Winter 1979). W_I is the work done on the body itself, i.e. changes in the mechanical energy of the body segments. W_E is the work done by the body in moving objects in the environment. Over a period of time t, W_I is given by

$$W_I = W_{GI} + W_{TI} + W_{RI},$$
(11.17)

where W_{GI} is the work done in changing the gravitational potential energy of the body, W_{TI} is the work done in changing the translational kinetic energy of the body and W_{RI} is the work done in changing the rotational kinetic energy of the body. Over the same period of time t, W_E is given by

$$W_E = W_{GE} + W_{TE} + W_{RE},$$
(11.18)

where W_{GE} is the work done in changing the gravitational potential energy of objects in the environment, W_{TE} is the work done in changing the translational kinetic energy of the objects and W_{RE} is the work done in changing the rotational kinetic energy of the objects. W_E includes, for example,

- Changes in the gravitational potential energy of other objects, e.g. lifting and lowering a box;
- Changes in the kinetic energy of other objects, e.g. throwing and catching a ball or accelerating the flywheel of a cycle ergometer;
- Work done against friction, e.g. pushing a box across a floor, pedalling a cycle ergometer against the friction brake mechanism or turning a screw.

Consequently, the total work done W_T by the human body and the corresponding average power output P_a during any particular period of time t are given by

$$W_T = W_I + W_E \tag{11.19}$$

$$P_a = W_T/t \tag{11.20}$$

Equation 11.20 should be used to determine the average power output of the human body over a particular period of time. To do so, it is necessary to measure W_{GI}, W_{TI}, W_{RI}, W_{GE}, W_{TE} and W_{RE}. However, all six work components are rarely, if ever, measured.

Measurement of internal work

At any instant in time, the mechanical energy E of a body segment is the sum of the gravitational potential energy (GPE), translational kinetic energy (TKE), and rotational kinetic energy (RKE) of the segment, i.e.

$$E = GPE + TKE + RKE. \tag{11.21}$$

The mechanical energy of the whole body E_b at any particular instant in time is the sum of the energies of all the body segments, i.e.

$$E_b = \sum_{i=1}^{i=N} GPE_i + \sum_{i=1}^{i=N} TKE_i + \sum_{i=1}^{i=N} RKE_i, \tag{11.22}$$

where N is the number of body segments.

The change in E_b during an infinitely small period of time t is the internal work done by the body over the time period t. Net concentric muscular activity, referred to as positive work, increases E_b and net eccentric work, referred to as negative work, decreases E_b. However, both positive and negative work contribute to the metabolic cost of the activity. Consequently, the internal work W_I done by the body over a period of time T consisting of k consecutive time periods of t (i.e. $T = k \cdot t$) is given by

$$W_I = \sum_{i=1}^{i=k} |\Delta E_{bi}|, \tag{11.23}$$

where ΔE_{bi} is the change (increase or decrease) in E_b in the ith change and k is the number of changes.

The shorter the time period t, the greater the accuracy of the measurement of internal work over the period of time T. However, because of the practical difficulty of determining the linear velocity of each segment, the angular velocity of each segment and the height of the centre of gravity of each segment relative to some zero reference level at each instance of time t, the total internal work over a period of time is rarely measured. Consequently, most published reports of internal work and power output of the human body do not provide accurate measures of internal work and power output (Winter 1979). For example, many published reports concerning internal work and power output of the human body are based on the movement of the whole body centre of gravity (CG) (considering the body as a single or point

467

mass) rather than the movement of the individual body segments (as in Equations 11.22 and 11.23). Using this approach, referred to as the point mass method, it is possible to measure the *GPE* and *TKE* components of internal work (the first two elements on the right side of Equation 11.22), but it is not possible to measure the *RKE* component (the third element on the right side of Equation 11.22). Winter (1979) compared the point mass and segmental methods of measuring internal work in eight adult subjects (5 men, 3 women) walking at different speeds and found that the point mass method underestimated internal work in the segmental method by an average ± SD of −16.2 ± 10.6% (range of −41.7% to + 5.4%).

The point mass method has been widely used to determine peak power output of the human body in a vertical jump on a force platform (Davies and Rennie 1968; Canavan and Vescovi 2004). In this approach, the *GPE* and *TKE* components of internal work are measured, but not the *RKE* component. As there are no published reports of power output in a vertical jump based on the segmental approach, it is not clear how much the point mass method underestimates actual peak power output in a vertical jump.

Stair climbing (Margaria *et al*. 1966) and running up a slope (Kyle and Caiozzo 1985) have been used for many years to measure average power output of the human body. However, the method only measures the gross change in *GPE* of the *CG*; the variations in the height of the *CG* during each stride and the *TKE* and *RKE* components of internal work are not measured.

In Practical Worksheet 9, students determine average power output in stair climbing and running up a slope. In Practical Worksheet 10, students use a force platform to determine average and peak power output in a vertical jump.

Internal work and average power output in walking

Figure 11.12a–e shows one stride of a man walking at 1.3 m/s (2.9 mph). The time interval between the pictures is approximately 0.25 s. Figures 11.12f and g show the thigh, shank and foot segments of the right leg in Figure 11.12d (just after toe-off) and Figure 11.12e (just before heel-strike) and the corresponding linear velocity *v* of the centre of gravity of each segment, the angular velocity ω of each segment about the mediolateral axis through its centre of gravity and the height *h* of the centre of gravity of each segment above the level floor. The mechanical energy of each segment in each position is the sum of its gravitational potential energy, translational kinetic energy and rotational kinetic energy. For example, the mechanical energy of the thigh segment in Figure 11.12d = 49.68 J (Table 11.2), i.e.

$$E_{\text{thigh}} = m \cdot g \cdot h + \frac{m \cdot v^2}{2} + \frac{I \cdot \omega^2}{2}$$

$$= 38.23\,\text{J} + 10.97\,\text{J} + 0.48\,\text{J}$$

$$= 49.68\,\text{J}.$$

The mechanical energy of each leg in each position is the sum of the mechanical energy of the thigh, shank and foot segments. For example, the mechanical energy of the leg in Figure 11.12d is 75.51 J (Table 11.2), i.e.

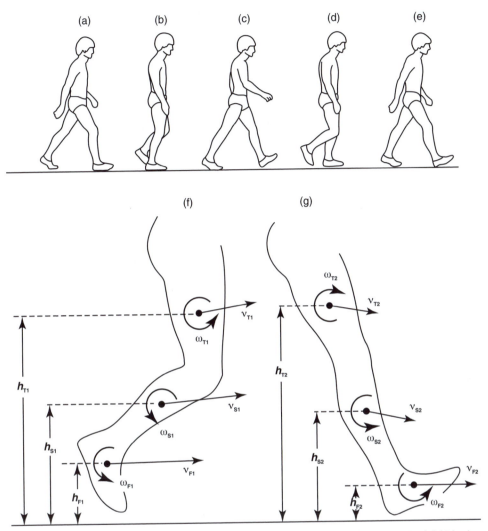

Figure 11.12 (a–e) One stride of man walking at 1.3 m/s. (f,g) Thigh, shank and foot segments of right leg in (d,e), showing height h of centre of gravity of each segment above floor, linear velocity v of centre of gravity of each segment and angular velocity ω of each segment about mediolateral axis through its centre of gravity (see data in Table 11.2).

$$E_{\text{leg}} = E_{\text{thigh}} + E_{\text{shank}} + E_{\text{foot}}$$

$$= 49.68\,\text{J} + 20.26\,\text{J} + 5.57\,\text{J}$$

$$= 75.51\,\text{J}.$$

Figure 11.13 shows the mechanical energy–time graphs of the arms, legs, combined trunk, head and neck and whole body (E_b) during one stride (right heel-strike to right heel-strike) of a man of approximate mass 72 kg walking at approximately 1.5 m/s (3.3 mph) (based on Pierrynowski *et al.* 1980). The time interval between the data points is 0.062 s

Table 11.2 Determination of the components of mechanical energy of the right leg of a man just after toe-off (Figure 11.12d) and just before heel-strike (Figure 11.12e) while walking at 1.3 m/s.

	Mass of segment (kg)	Length of segment (m)	k_G (as a percentage of segment length)	k_G (m)	I_G (kg·m²)	h (m)	v (m/s)	ω (rad/s)	Gravitational potential energy (J)	Translational kinetic energy (J)	Rotational kinetic energy (J)	Total energy (J)	Segment energy (%)
Just after TO													
Thigh	5.95	0.314	0.323	0.1014	0.0612	0.655	1.92	3.98	38.23	10.97	0.48	49.68	65.79
Shank	2.69	0.425	0.302	0.1283	0.0443	0.370	2.79	1.24	9.76	10.47	0.03	20.26	26.83
Foot	0.81	0.122	0.475	0.0579	0.0027	0.180	3.19	2.75	1.43	4.13	0.01	5.57	7.38
Total									49.42	25.57	0.52	75.51	
Energy component %									65.45	33.86	0.69		
Just before HS													
Thigh	5.95	0.314	0.323	0.1014	0.0612	0.675	1.54	-0.79	39.40	7.06	0.02	46.48	75.03
Shank	2.69	0.425	0.302	0.1283	0.0443	0.340	1.69	1.75	8.97	3.84	0.07	12.88	20.79
Foot	0.81	0.122	0.475	0.0579	0.0027	0.105	2.07	1.94	0.84	1.74	0.01	2.59	4.18
Total									49.21	12.64	0.10	61.95	
Energy component %									79.44	20.40	0.16		

Whole body mass, 56.7 kg; masses of segments are based on segmental percentage data of Plagenhoef et al. (1983); k_G, radius of gyration of the segment about a mediolateral axis a_G through its centre of gravity, as a percentage of segment length (from Winter 1990) and in metres; I_G, moment of inertia of the segment about a_G; h, height of the centre of gravity of the segment above the floor; v, linear velocity of centre of gravity of the segment; ω, angular velocity of the segment about a_G; segment energy and energy component are given as a percentage of the total energy of the leg.

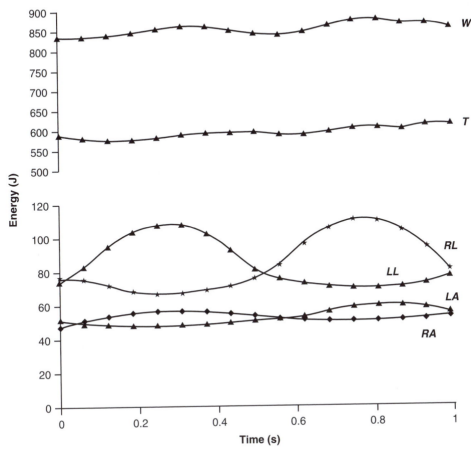

Figure 11.13 Mechanical energy–time graphs of arms, legs, combined trunk, head and neck and whole body during one stride (heel-strike to heel-strike of same leg) of man walking at approximately 1.5 m/s (adapted from Pierrynowski *et al.* 1980) (see data in Table 11.3): *LA*, left arm; *RA*, right arm; *LL*, left leg; *RL*, right leg; *T*, trunk, head and neck; *W*, whole body.

and the data corresponding to Figure 11.13 are shown in Table 11.3. The average of E_b is 845.31 J. The range of E_b is 33.87 J, (829.10 J–862.87 J) which is only 4.0% of the average. The arms, legs and combined trunk, head and neck contribute an average of approximately 12%, 19% and 69%, respectively to E_b (S% in Table 11.3). The change in E_b per time interval is shown in the eighth column of Table 11.3. The absolute changes are shown in the ninth column of Table 11.3. The sum of the absolute changes in E_b corresponds to the internal work during the single stride (Equation 11.23), i.e. $W = 106.72$ J. As the stride time is 0.99 s, the average power output (work rate) is 107.8 W (106.72 W / 0.99 s).

Table 11.3 Determination of the total mechanical energy of the human body and work done during a single stride of a man walking at 1.5 m/s on a treadmill (adapted from Pierrynowski et al. 1980) (see Figure 11.13).

Time (s)	Right arm (J)	Left arm (J)	Right leg (J)	Left leg (J)	Trunk, head and neck (J)	E_b (J)[1]	ΔE (J)[2]	Abs ΔE (J)[3]
0	47.57	50.37	75.56	73.69	586.57	833.77	0	0
0.062	49.81	48.51	74.63	82.09	579.10	834.14	0.373	0.373
0.124	52.24	47.57	70.89	94.22	573.51	838.43	4.291	4.291
0.186	54.10	46.64	67.16	102.61	572.57	843.10	4.664	4.664
0.248	55.04	46.27	65.67	106.34	578.17	851.49	8.395	8.395
0.310	55.04	46.27	65.67	106.34	582.84	856.16	4.664	4.664
0.372	53.73	46.64	67.16	100.75	585.63	853.92	−2.239	2.239
0.434	52.24	47.20	69.03	90.48	584.70	843.66	−10.261	10.261
0.496	50.37	48.13	73.13	78.17	584.70	834.51	−9.142	9.142
0.557	48.51	48.51	81.16	72.76	578.17	829.10	−5.410	5.410
0.620	47.57	49.81	93.28	69.22	575.37	835.26	6.157	6.157
0.681	46.64	52.24	102.05	67.16	581.90	850.00	14.739	14.739
0.743	46.27	54.48	106.34	65.86	588.43	861.38	11.381	11.381
0.805	46.08	55.22	106.34	65.86	589.36	862.87	1.492	1.492
0.867	46.08	54.85	99.81	66.23	584.70	851.68	−11.194	11.194
0.929	46.64	53.17	89.55	68.10	594.03	851.49	−0.186	0.186
0.991	47.57	50.37	76.49	71.83	593.10	839.37	−12.127	12.127
Mean	49.74	49.78	81.41	81.28	583.11	845.31		
S%	5.88	5.89	9.93	9.61	68.98			
ΣAbs ΔE								106.72

[1] E_b, total energy at time t; [2] ΔE, change in E_b; [3] Abs ΔE, absolute value of ΔE.

Mechanical efficiency of the human body in walking

Metabolic rate refers to the rate at which the human body consumes energy (measured as oxygen consumption) to maintain all of the involuntary bodily functions that are necessary to sustain life (e.g. breathing and circulation of blood) and all of the voluntary activities, such as movement. The energy expenditure of involuntary processes varies throughout the day; for example, the energy expenditure of the digestive system increases following a meal. However, changes in metabolic rate that occur as a result of changes in the energy expenditure of involuntary functions are small compared with the effect of physical activity. For example, during maximal effort, the energy expenditure of skeletal muscles may increase over one hundred times compared with that spent at rest (McArdle et al. 1991). The increase in metabolic rate that accompanies an increase in the level of physical activity is mainly due to the large amount of heat that is generated by skeletal muscle contractions. Consequently, when the skeletal muscles do work (external or internal), the total energy expenditure of the muscles E_T is the sum of the energy expended by the muscles in doing the work E_W and the energy expended as heat E_H while doing the work, i.e. $E_T = E_W + E_H$. E_H is usually much higher than E_W, such that the metabolic rate is usually much higher than the work rate. Mechanical efficiency is a measure of the effectiveness with which metabolic energy expenditure is transformed into work, i.e.

$$\eta = \frac{W}{C} \times 100\%,$$

where η (lower case Greek letter eta) is mechanical efficiency, W is work done, and C is metabolic energy expenditure. For a given amount of work done by the body, the lower the corresponding metabolic energy expenditure, the higher the mechanical efficiency of the body and vice versa.

In the preceding section, the work rate of the man of mass 72 kg walking at approximately 1.5 m/s was 107.8 W. The oxygen consumption (metabolic rate) of a man walking at 1.5 m/s is approximately 13.4 ml/kg·min (McArdle *et al.* 1991). Consequently, the oxygen consumption of a man of mass 72 kg walking at 1.5 m/s is approximately 965 ml/min. As 1 l oxygen is approximately equivalent to 4.825 kcal and 1 kcal is approximately equivalent to 4.183 kJ, then an oxygen consumption of 0.965 l/min is approximately equivalent to 324.6 W:

$$1 \, l \, O_2 \approx 4.825 \text{ kcal},$$
$$1 \text{ kcal} \approx 4.183 \text{ kJ},$$

i.e. $1 \, l \, O_2 \approx 20.183 \text{ kJ}$

and $0.965 \, l \, O_2/\text{min} \approx 19.476 \text{ kJ/min} = 324.6 \text{ W}.$

The mechanical efficiency of walking at a work rate of 107.8 W with a metabolic rate of 324.6 W is 33.2%:

$$\eta = \frac{107.8 \text{ W}}{324.6 \text{ W}} \times 100\% = 33.2\%.$$

In general, the mechanical efficiency of human locomotion in walking and running ranges between 20% and 30% (McArdle *et al.* 1991).

In any given situation, work done W by the body is the result of muscular activity (active work) and the utilisation of strain energy in the musculoskeletal system (passive work, which has no energy cost). Consequently, W = active work + passive work, and

$$\eta = \frac{\text{active work} + \text{passive work}}{C} \times 100.$$

As C reflects only active work, a decrease in C indicates a decrease in active work. Consequently, an increase in mechanical efficiency is likely to reflect greater utilisation of strain energy.

REVIEW QUESTIONS

1. Define the following terms: work of a force, work of the moment of a force, energy, joule, power, watt, conservation of energy, potential energy, strain energy, entropy, conservative force, conservation of mechanical work, internal work, external work, positive work, negative work.

2. If a soccer ball of mass 0.45 kg is kicked from rest and leaves the kicker's foot with a linear velocity of 25 m/s, calculate:
   i.   The average force exerted on the ball;
   ii. The power of the kick if the ball and the kicker's foot were in contact for 0.3 m.

3. If a sledge hammer of mass 2.25 kg has a translational kinetic energy of 7 J at impact with a wall, calculate:
   i.   The average force exerted on the wall if the hammer is brought to rest in 0.03 m;
   ii. The power of the impact.

4. If a box of mass 20 kg is at rest on a level floor that has a coefficient of friction with the bottom of the box of 0.4, calculate the work required to push the box a distance of 3 m across the floor.

5. If a box of mass 20 kg is resting on an even 15° slope, calculate the friction between the bottom of the box and the slope.

6. If a box of mass 20 kg is being pushed steadily up an even 15° slope by a force S that is parallel to the slope, calculate:
   i.   The friction between the bottom of the box and the slope if the coefficient of friction between the box and the slope is 0.4;
   ii. The work required to push the box up the slope a distance of 5 m;
   iii. The average magnitude of force S.

7. An iron ball of mass 7.26 kg is dropped from a height of 1.5 m onto the ground. Calculate the average force exerted on the ball by the ground if the ball is brought to rest in:
   i.   0.04 m;
   ii. 0.01 m.

8. If a ball of mass 0.25 kg is dropped from a height of 1.2 m and bounces up 0.8 m, calculate:
   i.   The amount of mechanical energy dissipated during the impact with the ground;
   ii. The resilience of the ball.

9. If an arrow of mass 0.015 kg separates from a bowstring with a linear velocity of 60 m/s, calculate:
   i.   The average force exerted on the arrow by the bowstring after release by the archer if the arrow and bowstring are in contact for 0.70 m;

ii.   The average force exerted by the target on the arrow if the arrow is brought to rest in 0.04 m (assume no loss of energy during flight).

10. In the most common form of friction-braked cycle ergometer, one revolution of the pedals moves a point on the rim of the flywheel a distance of 6 m. If the friction between the belt and flywheel rim is 2 kgf, calculate the work rate of the cyclist if she pedals at a constant rate of 50 pedal revolutions per minute.

11. At take-off, a pole vaulter of mass 70 kg has a linear velocity of 9.1 m/s and his centre of gravity is 1.1 m above the ground. If the linear velocity of the vaulter at maximum height is 1.0 m/s and all of the remaining mechanical energy available at take-off was transformed into gravitational potential energy at maximum height, calculate:
   i.   The theoretical gain in height;
   ii. The theoretical maximum height of the vaulter's centre of gravity.

Assume that the mechanical energy in the pole and the rotational kinetic energy of the vaulter at take-off and maximum height is negligible.

Chapter 12

Fluid mechanics

Mass exists in three forms, solids, liquids and gases. Structurally, the main difference between solids, liquids and gases is in the strength of their intermolecular bonds. Most substances become less stable (the intermolecular bonds become progressively weaker) with increase in temperature and vice versa, such that a substance may change its state from one form to another. For example, water can exist as a solid (ice), liquid or gas (steam). In general, the stronger the intermolecular bonds, the more stable the structure, and the less likely it is to deform in response to load. Whereas the strength of the intermolecular bonds is different in different solids, i.e. some solids deform more easily than others in response to load, a solid is characterised by a fixed volume and a fixed shape when subjected to no external force other than its own weight. In contrast, a liquid will tend to deform under its own weight and is characterised by a fixed volume and variable shape. In comparison with solids and liquids, the intermolecular bonds in gases are very weak, such that in response to external pressure, a gas is likely to change not only its shape, but also its volume, i.e. gases are characterised by variable volume and variable shape.

Liquids and gases share the characteristic of variable shape; this is reflected in their natural tendency to flow or change shape. A substance that has a natural tendency to flow is called a fluid (Fuchs 1985). Liquids and gases are both fluids. Whenever an object moves through a fluid or a fluid flows over a stationary object, the fluid exerts pressure on the object; thereby tending to move the object or change the way the object is moving. Fluid mechanics is the study of the forces that act on bodies in fluids and the effects of those forces on the movement of the bodies. Human movement is affected by two fluids, air and water, often simultaneously, as in swimming and sailing. The purpose of this chapter is to describe the fluid mechanics of air and water in relation to the movement of the human body and projectiles.

OBJECTIVES

After reading this chapter, you should be able to do the following:

1. Differentiate atmospheric pressure and hydrostatic pressure.
2. Differentiate centre of gravity and centre of buoyancy.
3. Differentiate viscous drag, pressure drag and wave drag.
4. Describe the ways in which hydrodynamic lift can be produced.
5. Differentiate paddle propulsion and screw propulsion.
6. Describe the effects of lift and drag on ball flight.

ATMOSPHERIC PRESSURE

The atmosphere is the layer of gas surrounding any planet or star (Clugston 1998). The earth's atmosphere consists of air, which is a mixture of gases, largely comprising nitrogen (about 78%), oxygen (about 21%) and argon (about 1%) with small amounts of other gases, including carbon dioxide. The earth's atmosphere extends upward from the surface of the earth for a distance of approximately 1000 km (620 miles). Like all gases, air has mass. The downward pressure exerted by the atmosphere, referred to as atmospheric pressure, increases with decrease in altitude, owing to the progressive increase in the weight of air above. Consequently, atmospheric pressure is greatest at sea level (zero altitude), i.e. 101 325 Pa (101 325 N/m² = 10 328.7 kgf/m² = 14.69 lbf/in²). Atmospheric pressure at sea level is frequently used as a unit of pressure in meteorology and oceanography, where 1 atm (1 atmosphere) is defined as a pressure of 101 325 Pa. The progressive increase in atmospheric pressure with decrease in altitude results in a progressive increase in the density of air, which is greatest at sea level (1.25 kg/m³); over half the total mass of the atmosphere is contained within the lowest 5.5 km of the atmosphere. Atmospheric pressure at sea level is equivalent to the pressure exerted by a vertical column of air of height 8263 m, horizontal cross-sectional area 1 m² and uniform density 1.25 kg/m³ (Figure 12.1). Density is generally reported in terms of mass per unit volume rather than weight per unit volume, i.e. the mass density of air = 1.25 kg/m³ and the weight density of air = 1.25 kgf/m³ = 12.262 N/m³. When density is used to determine pressure, density is usually given as weight density because pressure is derived from force.

Weight of the column of air $W = V \cdot \rho$ 1
where
V = volume of air
ρ = weight density of the air
   = 1.25 kgf/m³
   = 12.2625 N/m³

$V = h \cdot A$ 2
where
h = height of the column
A = horizontal square cross-sectional area = 1 m²

From equations 1 and 2,
$W = h \cdot A \cdot \rho$ 3

If the pressure on A = 101 325 Pa then W = 101 325 N

From equation 3,
101 325 N = $h \times 1$ m² $\times$ 12.2625 N/m³
h = 8263 m

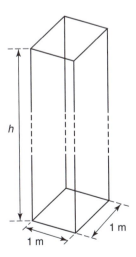

Figure 12.1 The dimensions of a column of air of uniform density exerting a pressure equivalent to atmospheric pressure at sea level

477

Archimedes' principle

The atmospheric pressure at any particular altitude is exerted in all directions. Figure 12.2 shows a side view of the volume of air V (shaded region) of uniform horizontal cross-sectional area A between altitude L_1 and a higher altitude L_2. If P_1 is the upward atmospheric pressure on V at L_1 and P_2 is the downward atmospheric pressure on V at L_2, it follows that

$$P_1 = P_2 + W/A,$$ (12.1)

where W is the weight of V and W/A is the downward pressure exerted by W at L_1. From Equation 12.1,

$$F_1 = F_2 + W,$$ (12.2)

where $F_1 = P_1 \cdot A$ is the upward force exerted on V at L_1 and $F_2 = P_2 \cdot A$ is the downward force exerted on V at L_2. From Equation 12.2, $F_1 - F_2 = W$, i.e. V will experience a resultant upward force $B = F_1 - F_2$ that is equal in magnitude to its own weight. If V is replaced by an object of mass m with the same dimensions and, therefore, the same volume as V, the surrounding air will be exactly the same as that previously surrounding the volume of air V. Consequently, the atmospheric pressure at L_1 and L_2 will be the same as that previously acting on the volume of air V and the mass m will experience an upward force that is equal in magnitude to the weight of the displaced air. The force B is referred to as the buoyancy force and buoyancy is a characteristic of all fluids that are within the earth's gravitational field. The equivalence between the magnitude of the buoyancy force and the weight of fluid displaced was discovered by the Greek mathematician Archimedes (c 287–212 BC) and is expressed in Archimedes' principle,

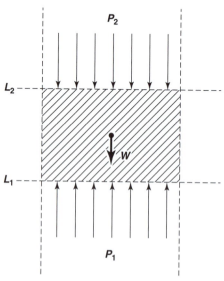

Figure 12.2 Atmospheric pressure increases with decrease in altitude: P_1, atmospheric pressure at altitude L_1; P_2, atmospheric pressure at altitude L_2; W, weight of air between L_1 and L_2.

i.e. an object that is partially or completely immersed in a fluid will experience a buoyancy force that is equal to the weight of the fluid displaced.

Floating in air

Figure 12.3 shows a child's party balloon floating in the air. The balloon will experience atmospheric pressure over the whole of its surface; this effectively results in four forces, a downward force F_1, an upward force F_2, where $F_1 < F_2$ due to the difference in altitude, and a pair of forces, one at each side, of equal magnitude F_3. Consequently, the resultant upward force R on the balloon (using the convention of positive upward) is given by

$$R = F_2 - F_1 - W, \tag{12.3}$$

where W is the weight of the balloon envelope W_E and the weight of air in the balloon W_A. As the buoyancy force $B = F_2 - F_1$ and $W = W_E + W_A$, then from Equation 12.3,

$$R = B - W_E - W_A. \tag{12.4}$$

Consequently, the balloon will float (not move up or down) when $R = 0$, i.e. when $B = W_E + W_A$. If the density of the air inside the balloon is equal to the density of the air

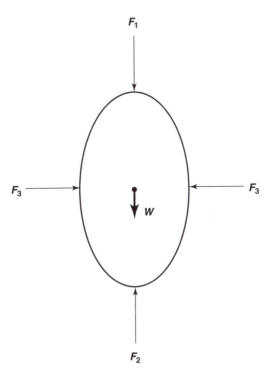

Figure 12.3 Forces acting on child's party balloon surrounded by air: F_1, F_2 and F_3 are forces due to atmospheric pressure; W is the weight of the balloon.

outside the balloon, $W_A = B$, i.e. $B < W_E + W_A$ and the balloon will fall to the ground, owing to the resultant downward force W_E. However, as the density of air decreases with increase in temperature, it should be possible to make the balloon float by filling it with hot air, such that $B = W_E + W_A$. For example, if

> V = the volume of the inflated balloon = 0.007 24 m³ (the volume of a sphere of
> radius 0.12 m),
> ρ_1 = weight density of the air outside the balloon = 1.25 kgf/m³,
> B = $V \cdot \rho_1$ = 0.007 24 m³ × 1.25 kgf/m³ = 0.009 05 kgf,

and W_E = 0.5 gf (grams force) = 0.0005 kgf,

then the balloon will float if

$$W_A = B - W_E = 0.009\ 05\ \text{kgf} - 0.000\ 5\ \text{kgf} = 0.008\ 55\ \text{kgf},$$

i.e. if $W_A = V \cdot \rho_2 = 0.008\ 55\ \text{kgf}$,

where ρ_2 is the weight density of the air inside the balloon. Consequently, the balloon will float if

$$\rho_2 = \frac{W_A}{V} = \frac{0.008\ 55\ \text{kgf}}{0.007\ 24\ \text{m}^3} = 1.18\ \text{kgf/m}^3.$$

If the density of the air inside the balloon is less than 1.18 kgf/m³, the balloon will move upward as B will then be greater than $W_E + W_A$. In competitions to see how far a balloon will travel before falling to earth, balloons (like permanent large advertisement balloons) are usually filled with a gas such as helium, which has a much lower density than air. If the balloon in this example is filled with helium (weight density $\rho_H = 0.1787$ kgf/m³) instead of hot air, then, from Equation 12.4, the resultant upward force on the balloon will be given by

$$R = B - W_E - W_H = m \cdot a \tag{12.5}$$

where: $W_H = V \cdot \rho_H$ = 0.007 24 m³ × 0.1787 kgf/m³ = 0.001 29 kgf = the weight of
helium in the balloon,

$m = m_E + m_H$ = 0.000 5 kg + 0.001 29 kg = 0.001 79 kg = the mass of the
balloon envelope and helium in the balloon,

a = acceleration of the balloon.

As B and W_E remain the same as before, it follows from Equation 12.5 that

$$R = 0.009\ 05\ \text{kgf} - 0.000\ 5\ \text{kgf} - 0.001\ 29\ \text{kgf} = 0.007\ 26\ \text{kgf} = 0.071\ 2\ \text{N},$$

i.e. $a = \dfrac{R}{m} = \dfrac{0.071\ 2\ \text{N}}{0.001\ 79\ \text{kg}} = 39.8\ \text{m/s}^2.$

Consequently, the balloon would initially accelerate upward at 39.8 m/s².

> An object that is partially or completely immersed in a fluid will experience a buoyancy force that is equal to the weight of the fluid displaced.

HYDROSTATIC PRESSURE

The density of air (1.25 kg/m³) is very much lower than that of water (1000 kg/m³) and atmospheric pressure is normally imperceptible. In contrast, the pressure exerted by water on the body, referred to as hydrostatic pressure, is normally clearly noticeable. For example, walking from a beach into the sea will result in a noticeable progressive increase in buoyancy; the greater the degree of immersion, the greater the buoyancy force. Just as atmospheric pressure increases with decrease in altitude, hydrostatic pressure increases with increase in depth. As the density of water is much greater than that of air, hydrostatic pressure increases much more rapidly than atmospheric pressure. For example, 1 atm is equivalent to the pressure exerted by an 8263 m high column of air of horizontal cross-sectional area 1 m² (Figure 12.1); the same amount of pressure is produced by a 10.3 m high column of water, i.e.

$$W = h \cdot A \cdot \rho$$

where: W = weight of the column of water = 101 325 N,
h = height of the column of water,
A = horizontal cross-sectional area of the column = 1 m²,
ρ = weight density of water = 1000 kgf/m³ = 9810 N/m³,

i.e. $h = \dfrac{W}{A \cdot \rho} = \dfrac{101\ 325\ N}{1\ m^2 \times 9810\ N/m^3} = 10.33\ m.$

Consequently, the pressure on a scuba diver at a depth of 10.33 m = 2 atm, i.e. the combined pressure of the atmosphere and the water.

Floating in water

From Archimedes' principle, an object will float at the surface of water if the weight of the object W_O is less than the weight of an equal volume of water W_W. The ratio of these two weights is referred to as the specific gravity of the object (a dimensionless number), i.e.

$$\text{Specific gravity of an object} = \frac{W_O}{W_W}. \tag{12.6}$$

Consequently, an object will float in water if its specific gravity is less than or equal to 1.0. An object with a specific gravity less than 1.0 will be able to float by displacing a volume of water that is less than its own volume, i.e. it will float with part of its mass above the surface of the water (Figure 12.4a,b). An object with a specific gravity of 1.0 will just float with all of its volume immersed (Figure 12.4c). In Figure 12.4a, the object floats with half of its volume below the surface of the water, i.e.

481

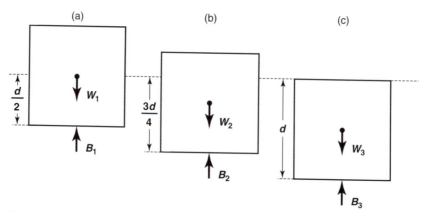

Figure 12.4 Three cubic objects with the same volume, but different weights (W_1, W_2, W_3) and, therefore, different specific gravities ($SG_1 = 0.5$, $SG_2 = 0.75$, $SG_3 = 1.0$): B_1, B_2 and B_3 are the buoyancy forces corresponding to W_1, W_2 and W_3.

$$W_1 = V_1 \cdot \rho = \frac{V_1 \cdot \rho_W}{2} = \frac{W_W}{2},$$

where W_1, V_1 and ρ_1 are the weight, volume and density of the object and ρ_W and W_W are the density and weight of the displaced water. As $W_1 = W_W/2$, then

$$\frac{W_1}{W_W} = 0.5,$$

i.e. the specific gravity of the object is 0.5. Similarly, as the object in Figure 12.4b floats with three-quarters of its volume below the surface of the water, its specific gravity is 0.75.

From Equation 12.6, the specific gravity of an object can be expressed as

$$\frac{W_O}{W_W} = \frac{V_O \cdot \rho_O}{V_O \cdot \rho_W} = \frac{\rho_O}{\rho_W}, \tag{12.7}$$

where W_O, V_O and ρ_O are the weight, volume and density of the object, respectively, W_W is the weight of an equal volume of water and ρ_W is the density of water. Consequently, an object will float in water if its density is less than or equal to that of water and it will sink if its density is greater than that of water. The ratio of the density of the object to the density of water, ρ_O/ρ_W (dimensionless number), is referred to as its relative density. An object will float in water if its relative density is less than or equal to 1.0 and it will sink if its relative density is greater than 1.0. The specific gravity and relative density of an object have the same value.

The density of water varies depending upon the type and amount of substances that are dissolved in it. The density of fresh water is 1000 kg/m³. The density of seawater is higher than that of fresh water due to its relatively high concentration of salt; the density of seawater ranges between 1020 kg/m³ and 1030 kg/m³ with an average value of 1026 kg/m³ (Pickard and Emery 1990). As the specific gravity of the human body is normally close to 1.0, most people who cannot float in fresh water will be able to float in seawater, owing to its

Table 12.1 Specific gravity of human body tissues and other materials (average values).

Adult man	0.98
Adult woman	0.97
Fat (adipose tissue)	0.94
Muscle	1.05
Bone	1.80
Rubber	0.92
Ice	0.87
Cork	0.21
Expanded polystyrene	0.02

slightly higher density. Corlett (1980) provides a good illustration of the effect on buoyancy of increasing the salinity of water. A shelled boiled egg will sink if it is placed in a glass of tap water. If salt is gradually dissolved in the water, the density of the water will gradually increase and the egg will soon rise to the surface.

The human body comprises a number of different tissues, including bone, muscle and fat, which have different specific gravities (Table 12.1). The specific gravity of the whole body depends upon the proportions of the different tissues. These proportions change with age, so the specific gravity and, therefore, the floating ability of the body also change with age (Whiting 1963, 1965). In general, non-obese children have a lower specific gravity than non-obese adults, owing to a relatively higher proportion of fat (specific gravity = 0.94) and relatively lower proportions of bone (specific gravity = 1.8) and muscle (specific gravity = 1.05) (Malina and Bouchard 1991). Consequently, children tend to float more easily than adults; for this reason, childhood is a good time to learn to swim (Corlett 1980). Women tend to be more buoyant than men at all ages; this is also due to a greater proportion of fat (McArdle *et al.* 1994).

Fully inflating the lungs by maximal inspiration increases the volume of the body as a whole and, therefore, increases the buoyancy force when floating in water. The increase in buoyancy force is greater than the increase in body weight resulting from the increased volume of air in the lungs. Consequently, the specific gravity of the body will be lower following maximal inspiration and the body will float more easily. Following maximal inspiration, most people will float with at least the face above the surface of the water (Figure 12.5). However, it is unlikely that two people will be able to float in the same position, owing to differences in body composition (distribution and proportions of body tissues). The position in which a person can float motionless in water depends upon the points of application of body weight and the buoyancy force. Body weight W acts downward at the whole body centre of gravity C_G. The buoyancy force B acts upward at the centre of buoyancy C_B, i.e. the centre of gravity of the displaced water. As the density of the water is uniform and the density of the body is non-uniform, it is unlikely that C_G and C_B will coincide. For the person to float motionless, W and B must be equal in magnitude and opposite in direction and act along the same vertical line. C_B is usually closer to the head than C_G, such that when the body is in a horizontal position, as in Figure 12.5a, W and B form a couple that rotates the body, so that the legs sink until an equilibrium position is reached where C_B is directly above C_G (Figure 12.5b). The

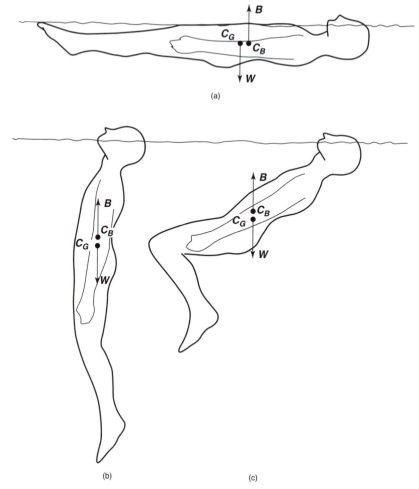

(a)

(b)   (c)

Figure 12.5 Effect of position of centre gravity C_G and centre of buoyancy C_B on equilibrium position when floating in water: W, body weight, B, buoyancy force.

distance between C_G and C_B in the position shown in Figure 12.5a is approximately 0.5 cm in adult men and 0.8 cm in adult women (Gagnon and Montpetit 1981). Consequently, a fairly small change in posture is likely to have a significant effect on the magnitude of the $W–B$ couple (by changing the positions of C_G and C_B) and on the orientation of the body in the equilibrium position. For example, most people who normally float in a fairly upright position (Figure 12.5b) will be able to float in a more horizontal position by flexing the hips and knees (Figure 12.5c).

The specific gravity of the whole body depends upon the proportions of the different tissues. These proportions change with age, resulting in a change in specific gravity and, therefore, the floating ability of the body.

DRAG

When an object moves through a fluid, i.e. when the velocity of the object relative to that of the fluid (referred to as the relative velocity of the object) is greater than zero, the pressure of the fluid on the object exerts a retarding force on the object, which tends to decelerate the object. This retarding force is referred to as drag. Drag has three components; viscous drag, pressure drag and wave drag.

Viscous drag

A fluid flowing over an object can be considered to consist of layers of fluid called streamlines (Daish 1972). When the relative velocity of the object is low, the streamlines tend to flow fairly smoothly over the object, as in Figure 12.6a. This type of flow is called laminar flow or

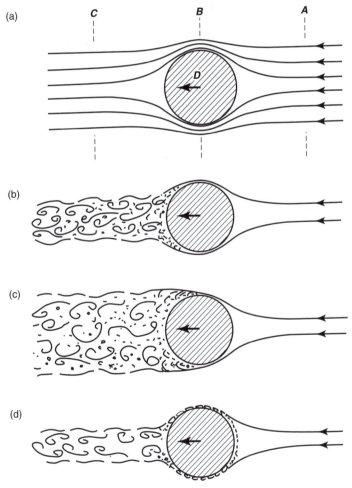

Figure 12.6 Types of fluid flow over a cylinder. (a) Laminar or streamlined flow. (b) Partially turbulent flow at moderate relative velocity. (c) Partially turbulent flow at high relative velocity. (d) Fully turbulent flow. D, drag force on cylinder.

streamlined flow. Whereas the flow is fairly smooth, the layer of fluid adjacent to the surface of the object, referred to as the boundary layer, sticks to the surface of the object and is dragged along with the object. As the layer of fluid next to the boundary layer flows over the boundary layer, a certain amount of friction is created between the two layers, which resists the movement of both layers and, consequently, resists the movement of the object. Similarly, friction is exerted between all of the layers of fluid within a certain distance of the surface of the object, but the amount of friction between the layers decreases with distance from the surface of the object. The cumulative effect of the friction between the layers of fluid is a force called viscous drag (also referred to as friction drag and surface drag) that retards the movement of the object. The magnitude of viscous drag depends upon the viscosity of the fluid, the surface area of the object in contact with the fluid, the relative velocity of the object and the volume of fluid surrounding the object.

The viscosity of a fluid is a measure of the fluid's resistance to flow (how quickly it changes shape in response to external forces) and its stickiness (how strongly it adheres to the surface of the object moving through it). Specifically, it is the resistance of the fluid to shear strain in response to a shear load. Shear stress = viscosity × shear strain rate, i.e. for a given amount of shear stress, the lower the viscosity, the greater the shear strain rate. Figure 12.7a shows a flat piece of card separated from a larger flat fixed surface by a layer of fluid. If the area of the card in contact with the fluid is A and a horizontal force F is applied to the card, then the shear stress experienced by the fluid is F/A. The movement of the card is resisted by the viscosity of the fluid; the greater the viscosity, the greater the resistance and the more slowly the card will move. Figure 12.7b shows the displacement of the card in time t. The shear strain experienced by the fluid is d/h, where d is the horizontal distance moved by the card in time t in the direction of F and h is the thickness of the layer of fluid between the card and the fixed support surface. The shear strain rate experienced by the fluid is $d/(h \cdot t) = v/h$ where $v = d/t$ is the average velocity of the card in the direction of F in time t. The term v/h is referred to as the velocity gradient. Shear strain rate and velocity gradient are equivalent. As shear stress = viscosity × shear strain rate, it follows that

$$\frac{F}{A} = \frac{\eta \cdot v}{h}$$

$$F = \frac{\eta \cdot A \cdot v}{h},$$

(12.8)

where η is the viscosity of the fluid. Equation 12.8 is the general expression for the viscous drag acting on an object moving through a fluid, where F is the viscous drag, η is the viscos-

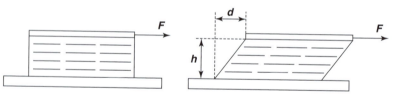

Figure 12.7 Response of fluid to shear stress. (a) Start of application of shear stress. (b) Strain on fluid after time t. F, force exerted on card; d, horizontal displacement of card in time t; h, thickness of fluid layer.

ity of the fluid, A is the surface area in contact with the fluid, v is the relative velocity of the object and h is the radius of the tube of fluid around the object in which the layers of fluid experience friction. From Equation 12.8, it is clear that viscous drag is directly proportional to η, A and v and inversely proportional to h. The SI unit of viscosity is the pascal second (Pa·s). (1 Pa·s = 1 kg/(m·s) = 1 kg·m^{-1}·s^{-1}), but the poise (P), which is named after Jean Louis Poiseuille (1799–1869), is also sometimes used (1 P = 1 g/(cm·s) = 1 g·cm^{-1}·s^{-1}). 1 P = 0.1 Pa·s. The viscosity of fluids decreases with increase in temperature, but the viscosity of liquids is always much greater than that of gases (Brancazio 1984). For example, at 20 °C the viscosity of water (0.01002 Pa·s) is approximately 55 times higher than that of air (0.00018 Pa·s). It is difficult to measure viscous drag on the human body during movement, as it is difficult to measure the velocity gradient and to separate viscous drag from pressure drag.

Pressure drag

At low relative velocities, the viscosity of a fluid may be sufficient to overcome the inertia of the boundary layer, i.e. the layer adhering to the surface of the object resulting in laminar flow. However, as relative velocity increases, there comes a point where the viscosity of the fluid is no longer able to overcome the inertia of the boundary layer, which becomes detached from the surface of the object, initially toward the rear of the object. The separation of the boundary layer results in a drop in pressure in the region of separation and, in turn, a turbulent wake, which is characterised by disorganised whirls of fluid or eddies (Figure 12.6b). As the pressure in the turbulent wake is less than the pressure at the front of the object, a pressure gradient is created, referred to as pressure drag, which retards the movement of the object.

As relative velocity increases, boundary layer separation occurs earlier, i.e. the region around the object where the boundary layer separates from the surface of the object moves progressively forward toward the front of the object. This increases the width of the turbulent wake and, consequently, increases the pressure drag (Figure 12.6c). At this stage, the flow around the object is described as partially turbulent, as there is still a region at the front of the object where the flow is laminar. However, as relative velocity increases further, there comes a point where the whole of the boundary layer becomes turbulent. This results in a decrease in the pressure differential between the front and back of the object and, consequently, a decrease in drag. The decrease in drag is associated with delayed boundary layer separation, which moves back toward the rear of the object, and a reduction in the width of the turbulent wake (Figure 12.6d). When the whole of the boundary layer becomes turbulent, the flow around the object is described as fully turbulent.

The magnitude of the pressure drag depends upon the shape, surface texture, relative velocity and profile area of the object and the density of the fluid. The profile area is the cross-sectional area of the object perpendicular to the direction of movement. Pressure drag is also referred to as profile drag and form drag. Figure 12.8 shows a rod of cross-sectional area A moving in the direction of its long axis through a fluid. If the rod moves a distance d it will displace a mass of fluid $m = A{\cdot}d{\cdot}\rho$ where ρ is the density of the fluid. The work done by the rod is $F{\cdot}d$, where F is the average force exerted by the rod on m. The work done by the rod is equal to the change in translational kinetic energy of the mass m, i.e. $F{\cdot}d = m{\cdot}v^2/2$, where v is the change in velocity of m. As $m = A{\cdot}d{\cdot}\rho$ then $F{\cdot}d = A{\cdot}d{\cdot}\rho{\cdot}v^2/2$, i.e. $F = A{\cdot}\rho{\cdot}v^2/2$. From

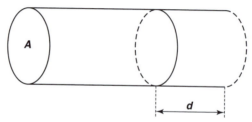

Figure 12.8 Displacement of mass of fluid $m = A \cdot d \cdot \rho$ by a rod of cross-sectional area A moving a distance d in the direction of its long axis, where ρ is the density of the fluid.

Newton's third law, the rod will experience an equal and opposite force F, i.e. pressure drag, which will retard its movement. Depending upon the shape and surface texture of the rod, the movement of the rod will affect the fluid around it as well as in front of it which, in turn, will affect the magnitude of the pressure drag experienced by the rod. Consequently, pressure drag F is usually expressed as

$$F = \frac{C_D \cdot A \cdot \rho \cdot v^2}{2},$$ (12.9)

where C_D = the coefficient of drag, a dimensionless number that reflects the surface texture and shape of the object.

Effect of surface texture and shape on drag

At low to moderate relative velocity, boundary layer separation and, therefore, a marked increase in drag occurs earlier on rough surfaces than on smooth surfaces. However, pressure drag on objects with smooth surfaces still increases with an increase in relative velocity when the flow is partially turbulent. For a given object, pressure drag is lower when the flow is fully turbulent than when it is partially turbulent. Consequently, in some situations, it may be appropriate to roughen the surface of an object so that fully turbulent flow and, therefore, reduced pressure drag occurs at a lower relative velocity. This explains the fuzzy surface of a tennis ball and the dimples on a golf ball (Brancazio 1984); the roughened surfaces reduce drag, enabling these balls to travel farther.

Table 12.2 lists the range of drag coefficients for a number of shapes. Streamlined objects tend to have lower drag coefficients than non-streamlined objects. A streamlined object, like an aerofoil, aircraft fuselage or torpedo (Figure 12.9), is rounded at the front and tapers to a point at the rear. In comparison with non-streamlined shapes, streamlined shapes reduce the disruption of fluid flow by reducing the rate of change of direction of the layers of fluid closest to the surface of the object. This delays boundary layer separation (boundary layer separation occurs at a higher relative velocity) and, therefore, reduces pressure drag. The degree of streamlining of an object is reflected in the fineness ratio, i.e. the ratio of the length of the object to the diameter of the object with respect to the direction of fluid flow. In general, the higher the fineness ratio, the lower the drag coefficient. For objects of equal volume, total drag is least (other variables held constant) when the fineness ratio is about 4.5 (Alexander 1968). Not surprisingly, the fineness ratio of the fuselages of passenger aircraft tends to be

Table 12.2 Drag coefficients for various shapes: adapted from Wright (2005) and Filippone (2004).

Aerofoil, torpedo, aircraft fuselage[1]	0.006–0.12
Airship[1]	0.02–0.025
Sphere: smooth	0.07–0.1
Bullet[1]	0.15–295
Sphere: rough	0.4–0.5
Sports car[1]	0.3–0.4
Economy car[1]	0.4–0.5
Flat plate[2]	1.28–2.0
Freestyle swimmer	0.4–0.5
Bobsleigh[3]	0.4–0.45
Racing cyclist[3]	0.8–0.97
Adult man or woman[4]	1.0–1.3
Downhill skier in crouch position[3]	1.0–1.1
Parachutist[3]	1.0–1.4
Ski jumper in flight[3]	1.2–1.3
Motor cyclist[3]	1.4–1.8

[1], Flow parallel to the long axis of the structure; [2], flow perpendicular to the plane of the plate; [3], flow parallel to direction of movement; [4], flow perpendicular to the front of the body when standing upright.

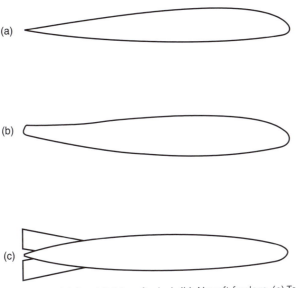

Figure 12.9 Streamlined shapes. (a) Aerofoil (aircraft wing). (b) Aircraft fuselage. (c) Torpedo.

about 4.5, as this is the best compromise between drag, which determines fuel consumption, and volume, which determines the number of passengers.

Drag on a rugby ball

The total drag on an object that is completely immersed in a fluid is the sum of the viscous drag and the pressure drag. Whereas it is relatively easy to measure the total drag, for example, in a wind tunnel, it is difficult to measure the viscous drag and pressure drag components. Equation 12.8 shows that viscous drag is proportional to v and Equation 12.9 shows that pressure drag is proportional to v^2. Consequently, pressure drag tends to increase much more rapidly than viscous drag as relative velocity increases. At the high speeds of movement generated in most sports (of participants and implements, such as bats and balls), viscous drag is very small relative to pressure drag, such that pressure drag provides a reasonable estimate of total drag.

The fineness ratio of a rugby ball in flight depends upon the orientation of the ball to the air flow. Changing the orientation of the ball changes the fineness ratio and, consequently, changes the drag coefficient and the profile area. When the long axis of the ball is parallel to the air flow (nose-on), its fineness ratio, drag coefficient and profile area are approximately 1.47, 0.1 and 0.0287 m², respectively (Figure 12.10a). When the short axis of the ball is parallel to the air flow (broadside), its fineness ratio, drag coefficient and profile area are approximately 0.68, 0.6 and 0.0435 m² respectively (Figure 12.10b). Consequently, if $v = 22.35$ m/s (50 mph) and $\rho = 1.25$ kg/m³, then (from Equation 12.9) the pressure drag on the ball in the nose-on and broadside orientations is approximately 0.9 N and 8.15 N, respectively. Clearly, changing the orientation of the ball has a marked effect on pressure drag.

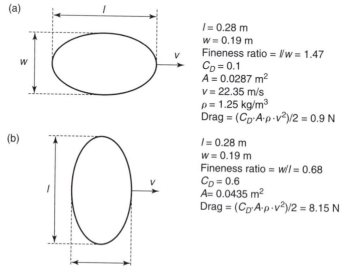

(a)

$l = 0.28$ m
$w = 0.19$ m
Fineness ratio $= l/w = 1.47$
$C_D = 0.1$
$A = 0.0287$ m²
$v = 22.35$ m/s
$\rho = 1.25$ kg/m³
Drag $= (C_D \cdot A \cdot \rho \cdot v^2)/2 = 0.9$ N

(b)

$l = 0.28$ m
$w = 0.19$ m
Fineness ratio $= w/l = 0.68$
$C_D = 0.6$
$A = 0.0435$ m²
Drag $= (C_D \cdot A \cdot \rho \cdot v^2)/2 = 8.15$ N

Figure 12.10 (a) Long axis of the ball in the same direction as the velocity of the ball (b) Long axis of the ball at right angles to the direction of the velocity of the ball

Drag on a skier in a wind tunnel

At the elite level, the time between the medal winners in bobsleigh, luge, skeleton and ski races is usually a fraction of a second. In such events, the difference between the times of the competitors is largely dependent upon differences in drag, which is a combination of air resistance and friction with the slope. Not surprisingly, considerable effort is made to reduce drag as much as possible. Friction drag is largely dependent upon the quality of the turns; the smoother the turns, the lower the friction drag. Air resistance is largely dependent on shape and surface texture. With regard to skiing, smooth, skin-tight clothing tends to reduce drag, but changes in shape and profile area are likely to be more important sources of drag. Changes in body shape are necessary to negotiate turns and sudden changes in slope, but downhill skiers try to maintain a compact crouch position, referred to as the egg position, as much as possible, since this position has been shown to minimise drag. Figure 12.11 shows the drag on a skier in four different positions while standing in a wind tunnel with a wind velocity of 22.2 m/s (50 mph). It is clear that the compact crouch position produces the least drag

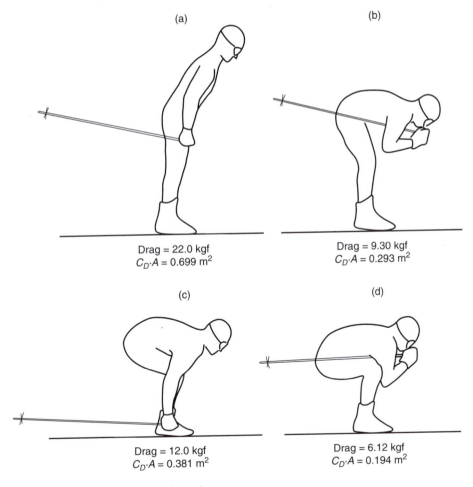

(a)

Drag = 22.0 kgf
$C_D{\cdot}A = 0.699$ m²

(b)

Drag = 9.30 kgf
$C_D{\cdot}A = 0.293$ m²

(c)

Drag = 12.0 kgf
$C_D{\cdot}A = 0.381$ m²

(d)

Drag = 6.12 kgf
$C_D{\cdot}A = 0.194$ m²

Figure 12.11 Drag on a skier in a wind tunnel.

(Figure 12.11d). It is, perhaps, surprising that dropping the arms outside the lower legs from the compact crouch increases the drag more than extending the legs from the crouch position (Figure 12.11b, c).

Terminal velocity of a downhill skier

Even though downhill skiers experience both air resistance and friction with the slope, very high speeds can be produced when conditions are favourable, i.e. minimal turns, dry snow and a steep slope (Armenti 1984). The maximum velocity that a downhill skier may achieve can be estimated through consideration of the pressure drag on the skier. There are three forces acting on a downhill skier, body weight W, the ground reaction force S and the drag force D (Figure 12.12a). D is parallel to the slope. In Figure 12.12b, W and S have been replaced by their components parallel and perpendicular to the slope. W_P is the component of W parallel to the slope. The component of W perpendicular to the slope W_N is equal and opposite to the normal reaction force N, which is the component of S perpendicular to the slope. F is the frictional force, which is the component of S parallel to the slope. The resultant force R acting on the skier down the slope (positive down) is given by

$$R = W_P - F - D = m \cdot a,$$ (12.10)

where m is the mass of skier and skis and a is the linear acceleration of the skier. When $R > 0$, the skier will accelerate down the slope. Whereas W_P and F will remain fairly constant, D is proportional to relative velocity, i.e. it increases as relative velocity increases, such that terminal (maximal) velocity will occur when $R = 0$ and, therefore, $a = 0$. Consequently, from Equation 12.10, terminal velocity v will occur when $W_P - F - D = 0$, i.e. when

$$W \cdot \sin \theta - \mu \cdot W \cdot \cos \theta - C_D \cdot A \cdot \rho \cdot v^2 / 2 = 0,$$ (12.11)

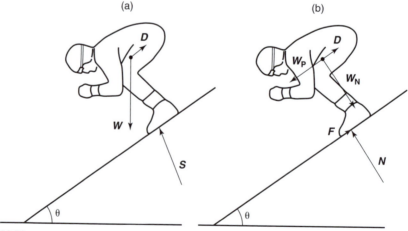

Figure 12.12 Free body diagram of downhill skier: W, weight of skier, clothing and skis; D, drag force; S, ground reaction force; W_P, component of W parallel to slope; W_N, component of W perpendicular to slope; F, component of S parallel to slope; N, component of S perpendicular to slope.

where: μ = coefficient of friction between the skis and the slope,
         C_D = coefficient of drag,
         A = profile area,
         ρ = density of air.

From Equation 12.11

$$v = \sqrt{\frac{2(W \cdot \sin\theta - \mu \cdot W \cdot \cos\theta)}{(C_D \cdot A \cdot \rho)}}. \qquad (12.12)$$

Determinations of drag on particular objects are usually made in wind tunnels so that the density of air (ρ) and velocity of air (v) can be held constant. Under these circumstances, drag varies directly with change in shape, which simultaneously changes C_D and A. As it is difficult to measure A, it is usual to report the product $C_D \cdot A$ rather than C_D and A separately. For a downhill skier, $C_D \cdot A$ is approximately 0.25 m^2 (Wagner and Wood 1996). Consequently, if $W = 80$ kgf, $\theta = 35°$, $\mu = 0.04$ (dry snow), $C_D \cdot A = 0.25$ m^2 and $\rho = 1.2$ kg/m^3, then

$$W \cdot \sin\theta = 80 \text{ kg} \times 9.81 \text{ m/s}^2 \times 0.5736 = 450.1 \text{ N}$$

$$\mu \cdot W \cdot \cos\theta = 0.04 \times 80 \text{ kg} \times 9.81 \text{ m/s}^2 \times 0.8191 = 25.7 \text{ N}$$

$$C_D \cdot A \cdot \rho = 0.25 \text{ m}^2 \times 1.2 \text{ kg/m}^3 = 0.3 \text{ kg/m}.$$

From Equation 12.12,

$$v = \sqrt{\frac{2(450.1 \text{ N} - 25.7 \text{ N})}{0.3 \text{ kg/m}}} = \sqrt{2829.3 \text{ m}^2/\text{s}^2} = 53.19 \text{ m/s} = 119 \text{ mph}.$$

The world record speed for a downhill skier is reported to be 124.23 mph (Armenti 1984).

Terminal velocity of a skydiver

By contrast with a downhill skier, the only source of drag on a skydiver is air resistance. There are two forces acting on a skydiver, body weight W and air resistance D (Figure 12.13). The resultant force R acting on the skydiver (positive down) is given by

$$R = W - D = m \cdot a, \qquad (12.13)$$

where m is the mass of skydiver, clothing and parachute and a is the linear acceleration of the skydiver. Terminal velocity v will occur when $R = 0$. Consequently, from Equation 12.13, terminal velocity v will occur when $W - D = 0$, i.e. when

$$W - C_D \cdot A \cdot \rho \cdot v^2 / 2 = 0, \qquad (12.14)$$

where C_D is the coefficient of drag, A is the profile area and ρ is the density of air. From Equation 12.14,

493

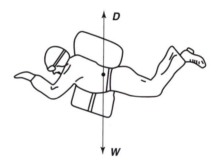

Figure 12.13 Free body diagram of skydiver: W, weight of skydiver, clothing and parachute; D, drag force.

$$v = \sqrt{\frac{2W}{C_D \cdot A \cdot \rho}}. \tag{12.15}$$

For a skydiver, $C_D \cdot A$ is approximately $0.56 \ m^2$ before the parachute opens (Wagner and Wood 1996). Consequently, if $W = 80 \ kgf$, $C_D \cdot A = 0.56 \ m^2$ and $\rho = 1.2 \ kg/m^3$, then from Equation 12.15

$$v = \sqrt{\frac{2 \times 80 \ kg \times 9.81 \ m/s^2}{0.56 \ m^2 \times 1.2 \ kg/m^3}}$$

$$v = \sqrt{2335.7 \ m^2/s^2} = 48.33 \ m/s = 108.1 \ mph.$$

Consequently, it is possible for the terminal velocity of a downhill skier to be greater than that of a skydiver. Terminal velocity in the two activities depends largely on the profile area A, which, in turn, determines C_D. In these examples, $C_D \cdot A$ is $0.25 \ m^2$ for the skier and $0.56 \ m^2$ for the skydiver.

After the skydiver opens his parachute, C_D and A change considerably. A typical parachute has a diameter of approximately $8.5 \ m$ when fully opened. Consequently, A is approximately $57 \ m^2$. In this situation, C_D is approximately 1.42 (Wagner and Wood 1996). Therefore, from Equation 12.15, if W is $80 \ kgf$, C_D is 1.42 and ρ is $1.2 \ kg/m^3$, the terminal velocity v of the skydiver with parachute fully open is given by

$$v = \sqrt{\frac{2 \times 80 \ kg \times 9.81 \ m/s^2}{1.42 \times 57 \ m^2 \times 1.2 \ kg/m^3}}$$

$$v = \sqrt{16.2 \ m^2/s^2} = 4.02 \ m/s = 9.0 \ mph.$$

Consequently, the terminal velocity of the skydiver with parachute fully open is the same as free-falling a distance of just $0.82 \ m$.

Slipstreaming

As the pressure drag on a runner increases with an increase in relative velocity, so does the metabolic cost of overcoming the drag. In sprint events, where the runners run in lanes, the drag experienced by each runner is largely dependent upon his speed. Similarly, the drag on the leading runner in a middle-distance to long-distance event is largely dependent upon his speed. However, the drag on the other runners is significantly affected by their positions with respect to each other. As the air pressure on the front of each runner is higher than the pressure in the turbulent wake at his back, a runner can reduce the drag on his body by running in the turbulent wake or 'slipstream' of the runner in front. Whereas the second to last runners all benefit from the slipstream effect between the leading and second runner by a reduction in drag of approximately 4% (assuming that the runners are in single file, one behind the other), their place in the line appears to confer no additional benefit (Pugh 1971).

The beneficial effect of slipstreaming increases with increase in relative velocity. For example, the reduction in drag due to streamlining in cycling is approximately 40%, which results in a 33% decrease in energy expenditure (Kyle 1979). Not surprisingly, the members of cyclist teams usually take turns at leading, as this is likely to maximise team performance.

Wave drag

In addition to viscous drag and pressure drag, an object moving through the boundary between two different fluids experiences wave drag. For example, swimming, with part of the body in the water and part of the body out of the water, creates a wave in front of the body. The wave is the result of work done on the water by the body; the amount of work done is directly proportional to the size and speed of the wave. As the body pushes against the wave, the body experiences a force, wave drag, that is equal and opposite to that exerted by the body on the wave. Barthels (1977) likens wave drag to the force exerted by the water against a bridge support in a fast flowing river. As flow velocity increases, so does the size of the wave and the force exerted by the wave against the support. In flood conditions, the support may collapse under the strain.

> Drag has three components; viscous drag, pressure drag and wave drag.

BERNOULLI'S PRINCIPLE

Figure 12.6a shows the streamlines of a fluid flowing smoothly over a cylindrical object. The closer the streamlines are to the object, the more they are disrupted as they flow over the object. The greater the disruption, the greater the distance that the particles of fluid in these streamlines have to travel as they pass over the object. As the particles of fluid in these streamlines have to travel a greater distance in the same time as particles of fluid in the undisrupted streamlines, it follows that the speed of the particles of fluid in the disrupted streamlines must be greater than the speed of the particles in the undisrupted streamlines as they flow between the regions of undisrupted flow upstream and downstream of the object, i.e. between regions

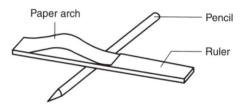

Figure 12.14 Demonstration of Bernoulli's principle.

A and *C* in Figure 12.6a. In Figure 12.6a, the speed of the particles in the disrupted stream-lines increases between regions *A* and *B* and decreases between regions *B* and *C*. The changes in the speed of the particles of fluid in the disrupted streamlines are due to differences in pressure, i.e. pressure decreases between regions *A* and *B* resulting in an increase in speed and pressure increases between regions *B* and *C* resulting in a decrease in speed. The inverse relationship between the pressure in a fluid and its speed is a well-established phenomenon, referred to as Bernoulli's principle, after Daniel Bernoulli (1700–1782), i.e. when a fluid flows over a surface, the pressure exerted by the fluid on the surface is inversely proportional to the speed of flow, or the higher the speed the lower the pressure and vice versa.

Gardner (1993) describes a good demonstration of Bernoulli's principle. One end of a strip of paper about 20 cm long and 3.5 cm wide (the width of a ruler) is attached to one end of a 30 cm ruler and the other end of the strip of paper is attached to the ruler about 18 cm along the ruler so that the piece of paper forms an arch (Figure 12.14). The ruler is placed on a round-stemmed pencil lying on a table. The pencil is rotated until the end of the ruler with the paper arch just overbalances the other end. If air is then blown along the ruler from the end that is elevated, the speed of the air flow decreases the pressure above the paper arch so that the ruler tips the other way.

HYDRODYNAMIC LIFT

In accordance with Bernoulli's principle, differences in the speed of flow of fluid over the opposite sides of an object will result in differences in pressure and, therefore, a pressure gradient, which will tend to move the object in the direction of the pressure gradient, i.e. from the region of higher pressure to the region of lower pressure. Consequently, whereas all objects moving through fluids experience drag, an object may also simultaneously experience a force at right angles to the drag force if the speeds of fluid flow over the opposite sides of the object are different. This force is referred to as a hydrodynamic lift force and its effect is referred to as hydrodynamic lift, where lift is a general term indicating movement or tendency to move in a direction at right angles to the drag force. Hydrodynamic lift can be produced in four ways: asymmetric shape, asymmetric orientation of a regular shape, asymmetric surface texture and spin.

Lift due to asymmetric shape

Objects that are specifically designed to produce hydrodynamic lift by asymmetric shape are referred to as aerofoils. An aircraft wing is an aerofoil. Figure 12.15a shows the cross

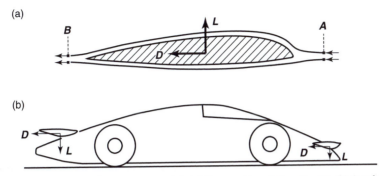

Figure 12.15 Drag D and lift L forces on an aerofoil. (a) Cross section of aircraft wing. (b) Aerofoils on front and rear of sports car.

section of an aircraft wing. The distance from the front edge of the wing to the back edge is greater over the upper surface than over the lower surface. Consequently, as each particle of air must move between A and B in Figure 12.15a in the same time, the speed of air flowing over the upper surface must be greater than the speed over the lower surface, which, in accordance with Bernoulli's principle, results in a pressure gradient (the pressure on the lower surface is greater than the pressure on the upper surface) tending to lift the wing.

Like pressure drag (Equation 12.9), the magnitude of the hydrodynamic lift force F_L on an aerofoil depends upon the density of the fluid ρ, the relative velocity v of the aerofoil through the fluid, the profile area A perpendicular to v and a dimensionless coefficient, referred to as the coefficient of lift C_L, reflecting the surface texture and shape of the aerofoil, i.e.

$$F_L = C_L \cdot A \cdot \rho \cdot v^2 / 2. \tag{12.16}$$

For example, consider the lift force required for a fighter aircraft to take off. The aircraft will take off if the lift force F_L is greater than the weight of the aircraft W, i.e. if

$$\frac{C_L \cdot A \cdot \rho \cdot v^2}{2} > W$$

$$v > \sqrt{\frac{2W}{C_L \cdot A \cdot \rho}}. \tag{12.17}$$

If $C_L = 0.8$, A = wing area = 55.74 m^2, ρ = density of air = 1.25 kg/m^3 and m = mass of the aircraft = 11800 kg (NASA 1999), then the aircraft will take off when

$$v > \sqrt{\frac{2 \times 11\,800 \text{ kg} \times 9.81 \text{ m/s}^2}{0.8 \times 55.74 \text{ m}^2 \times 1.25 \text{ kg/m}^3}}$$

$v > 64.44$ m/s $= 144.15$ mph.

497

Whereas aerofoils in the form of wings are used to produce upward force in aircraft, aerofoils are fitted to the front and rear of racing cars to produce downward force, in order to increase the grip between the tyres and the track. In this situation, the downward pressure differential is created by an aerofoil in which the lower surface is larger than the upper surface, i.e. the reverse of an aircraft wing (Figure 12.15b).

Lift due to asymmetric orientation

The lift force produced by an aerofoil can be increased to a certain extent by increasing the angle of attack of the aerofoil, i.e. the angle that the axis of the aerofoil makes with respect to the linear velocity of the aerofoil (Figure 12.16a). As the angle of attack increases from zero, there is an increase in both hydrodynamic lift and drag with hydrodynamic lift increasing at a faster rate than drag. However, as the angle of attack increases, there comes a point where the increase in drag decreases the linear velocity of the aerofoil so much that hydrodynamic lift cannot be maintained and the aerofoil stalls, i.e. the aerofoil experiences a dramatic decrease in hydrodynamic lift and forward movement (Figure 12.16b). A typical aerofoil will stall when the angle of attack is approximately 15° to 20°. In an aircraft, stalling results in an almost vertical, often uncontrollable, fall (Brancazio 1984).

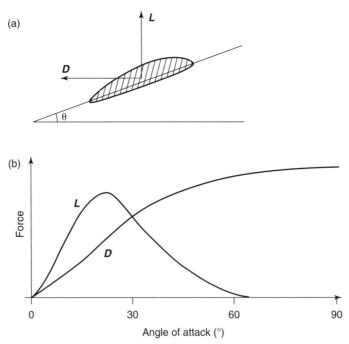

Figure 12.16 Effect of angle of attack on the magnitude of the lift L and drag D forces on a typical aerofoil for a given relative velocity. (a) Angle of attack θ. (b) Change in drag and lift forces with increase in angle of attack.

Paddle propulsion

In contrast with lift force, which decreases rapidly after the stall point, drag continues to increase over the 0° to 90° range, if the relative velocity of the object is maintained (Figure 12.16b). In terms of the type of force created, the action of an oar or paddle in producing propulsion in water is similar to an aerofoil with an angle of attack of 90° (Figure 12.17a). Figure 12.17b shows a person rowing a boat with two oars. As the oar blades sweep downstream through the water, turbulence is created on the upstream side of each blade, such that the pressure on the upstream side of each blade is less than the pressure on the downstream side. Consequently, the pressure differential on each blade results in drag, which resists its movement. If the resultant drag force on the oar blades is greater than the drag force on the boat, the boat will be accelerated upstream as the oar blades move downstream. This form of propulsion is called paddle propulsion or drag propulsion (Brown and Counsilman 1971).

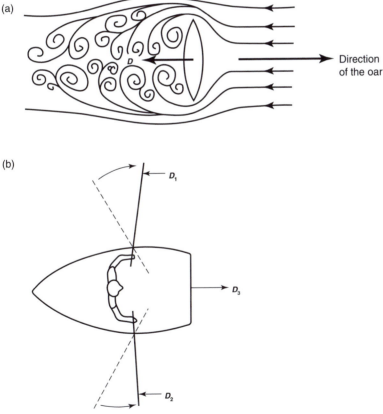

Figure 12.17 Paddle propulsion in water. (a) Drag D on oar blade. (b) Drag forces D_1 and D_2 on oars and D_3 on boat.

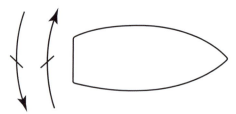

Figure 12.18 Screw propulsion using single oar operated from rowlock in stern of rowing boat.

Screw propulsion

Even fairly flat symmetrical objects can experience lift force if orientated asymmetrically to the linear velocity of the object. For example, Figure 12.18 shows a boat being propelled forward by one oar operated from a rowlock in the stern. If the oar is moved sideways alternately left and right, i.e. in a direction at right angles to the intended direction of travel, and the oar blade is angled in order to create an angle of attack with respect to the water flow, the movement of the blade will produce hydrodynamic lift force on the blade and the boat will move forward. The movement of the oar blade, referred to as sculling, will also produce drag such that the boat will zigzag as it moves forward. The form of propulsion produced by sculling is similar to that produced by a propeller and is referred to as screw propulsion (Barthels 1977).

The blades of a propeller in a ship cut through the water in a plane at right angles to the intended direction of the ship. As the propeller blades are angled on the propeller shaft, the angle of attack with respect to the water creates hydrodynamic lift force on the blades; this force pushes the propeller and, therefore, the ship forward. The rotation of the propeller also produces drag on the blades, but as the drag force is evenly distributed around the propeller and acts at right angles to the lift force, it has no effect on the movement of the ship. Consequently, propulsion in a propeller-driven ship is entirely due to hydrodynamic lift force. In a propeller-driven aircraft, both the forward movement (resulting from the rotation of the propellers) and the upward movement (resulting from air flow over the wings) are due to hydrodynamic lift force.

Propulsion in swimming

Prior to the advent of the equipment (notably, slow-motion cameras) and facilities (notably, observation windows) necessary for the detailed analysis of underwater movements, it was assumed that swimmers propelled themselves through the water by pulling the arm or arms straight back through the water, i.e. paddle propulsion. However, slow-motion underwater filming showed that elite swimmers do not pull straight back in any of the swimming strokes, but move the hands in a three-dimensional path involving considerable mediolateral movement. This is illustrated in Figure 12.19a, which shows a typical bottom-view right-hand–body plot of an elite freestyle swimmer, i.e. the path of the right hand in relation to the body as seen from underneath the swimmer. Of even greater significance in terms of coaching was the discovery of how the hand moved in relation to the water, as it is the flow of water over

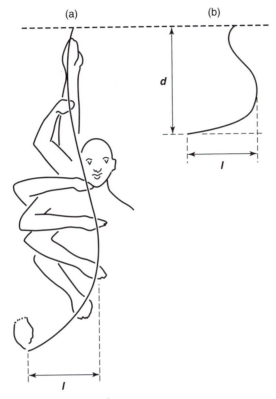

(a)   (b)

d

l

l

Figure 12.19 (a) Hand–body plot of movement of right hand of elite freestyle swimmer during propulsion phase of stroke as seen from underneath. (b) Corresponding hand–water plot. *d*, backward displacement of hand during propulsion phase of stroke; *l*, range of mediolateral movement of hand during propulsion phase of stroke.

the hands that produces most of the propulsion. Figure 12.19b shows a hand–water plot corresponding to the hand–body plot shown in Figure 12.19a. The analysis of three-dimensional hand–water plots led some coaches to suggest that elite swimmers derived some propulsion from hydrodynamic lift force by asymmetric orientation of their hands to the flow of water over them (Brown and Counsilman, 1971). It is now generally accepted that elite swimmers use a combination of paddle and screw propulsion (Costill *et al.* 1992; Counsilman and Counsilman 1994).

Figure 12.20a shows a typical bottom-view right-hand–water plot of an elite breaststroke swimmer during the propulsion phase of the stroke. The hand–water plot can be described as an elongated loop at right angles to the direction of body movement. Throughout the stroke, the plane of the hand maintains an angle of attack with respect to the flow of water; this results in a lift force as well as drag on the hand. The hand position is shown at two points, *A* and *B*, in the stroke and the flow of water over the hand in position *B* and the associated lift force and drag is shown in Figure 12.20b.

When a swimmer's hand produces lift and drag forces, it is the resultant of the two forces that determine the effect of the hand movement on body movement. Ideally, the resultant force acting on each hand in the alternate arm action events (freestyle and backstroke) and the

501

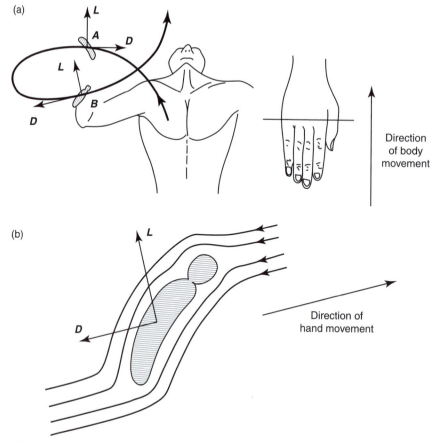

Figure 12.20 (a) Hand–water plot of right hand of elite breaststroke swimmer during propulsion phase of stroke as seen from underneath. (b) Angle of attack of hand at point B. D, drag; L, lift force.

resultant of the resultant forces acting on both hands in the dual arm action events (butterfly and breaststroke) would act in the intended direction of body movement. It is reasonable to assume that swimmers differ in their ability to produce the most effective combination of paddle and screw propulsion and also to direct the resultant propulsion force in the intended direction of body movement. However, it would appear that elite swimmers naturally adopt a sculling–pulling (or screw–paddle) action. The main advantage of a sculling–pulling action over a pulling action is reduced backward displacement of the hand relative to the water during the propulsion phase (d in Figure 12.19b). Consequently, stroke length (the distance moved forward by the body per stroke) is increased; this, in turn, increases the speed of body movement (assuming the same stroke frequency).

Propulsion from a sail

Depending on the number and distribution of sails, sailing boats utilise both drag and screw propulsion. Drag propulsion is used when running with the wind, i.e. sailing with the wind

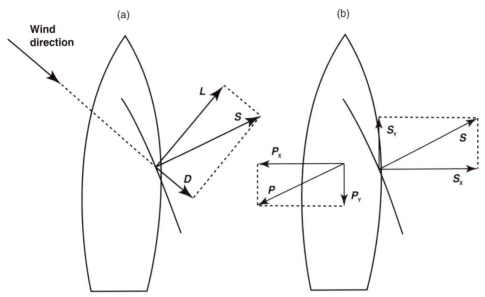

Figure 12.21 Lift and drag forces on sail. *L*, lift force on sail; *D*, drag force on sail; *S*, resultant of *L* and *D*; *P*, force exerted by water on hull in reaction to *S*; P_X and S_X, transverse components of *P* and *S*; P_Y and S_Y, anteroposterior components of *P* and *S*.

blowing directly from behind. In this situation, the wind creates a drag force on the sails, pushing the boat forward (similar to the drag on an oar in Figure 12.17a). Screw propulsion is used when tacking, i.e. moving obliquely into the wind. In this situation, the sails act as aerofoils and experience both drag and lift forces. Figure 12.21a shows a sailing dinghy with a single sail. The wind produces lift force *L* and drag *D* on the sail with resultant *S*. The tendency of *S* to move the boat in the direction of *S* is resisted by the reaction force *P* exerted by the water on the hull (Figure 12.21b). The tendency of S_X, the transverse component of *S*, to move the boat sideways is resisted by P_X, the transverse component of *P*. P_Y, the posterior component of *P* is the drag force exerted by the water on the hull. The boat will move forward if S_Y, the anterior component of *S*, is greater than P_Y.

Lift due to asymmetric surface texture

When shape, orientation, relative velocity and fluid density are constant, surface texture will determine the timing of transitions between the different types of fluid flow (laminar, partially turbulent, fully turbulent) and, therefore, the pressure on different parts of the surface of an object. Consequently, differences in surface texture on opposite sides of an object are likely to result in differences in pressure and, therefore, create a hydrodynamic lift force, which will tend to move the object sideways as it moves forward. This is the principle underlying the swing of a cricket ball in flight. The surface of a cricket ball consists of two leather hemispheres that are bound together around a solid core by several parallel rows of stitches that constitute the seam. In a new ball, the leather is highly polished and the seam is slightly proud of the rest of the surface. At fast bowling speeds, 40 m/s–45 m/s (90 mph–100 mph), the ball can

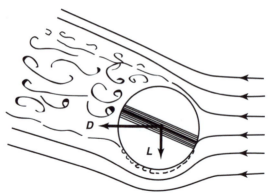

Figure 12.22 Drag D and lift force L on cricket ball released without spin.

be made to swing by releasing the ball with the seam asymmetric to the linear velocity of the ball. Figure 12.22 shows an overhead view of a cricket ball projected left to right with respect to the figure. On the left side of the ball (upper part of the figure), the air flows over the uninterrupted highly polished surface. At fast bowling speeds, this tends to produce partially turbulent flow with boundary layer separation close to the front of the ball and, consequently, considerable turbulence. On the right side of the ball (lower part of the figure), the seam presents a region of roughness to the air flow, which tends to produce fully turbulent flow, delayed boundary layer separation and, consequently, reduced turbulence. The different types of flow on the left and right sides of the ball are associated with differences in pressure (the pressure on the left side is higher than that on the right side), resulting in a hydrodynamic lift force that tends to move the ball sideways from left to right. The combination of simultaneous sideways and forward movement is referred to as swing. The amount and direction of the swing will be influenced by any change in the surface of the ball. Cricketers frequently polish one side of the ball and roughen the other side with moisture or grease, in order to affect swing.

Lift due to spin

Figure 12.23 shows an overhead view of a ball with uniform surface texture projected left to right with respect to the figure and spinning clockwise about a vertical axis. The left side of the ball (the upper part of the figure) is moving in the opposite direction to that of the adjacent streamlines. This results in a significant increase in the friction (relative to when the ball is not spinning) between the boundary layer and the adjacent streamlines. The increased friction results in early boundary layer separation, which is associated with an increase in pressure and a decrease in the speed of flow of air. The right side of the ball (the lower part of the figure) is moving in the same direction as the adjacent streamlines. This results in a significant decrease in the friction (relative to when the ball is not spinning) between the boundary layer and the adjacent streamlines. The decreased friction delays boundary layer separation and is associated with a decrease in pressure and an increase in the speed of flow of air. The pressure differential results in a hydrodynamic lift force that tends to move the ball sideways from left to right. The production of hydrodynamic lift as a result of spin is referred to as the Magnus effect after Heinrich Gustav Magnus (1802–1870).

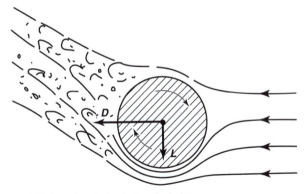

Figure 12.23 Drag D and lift force L on ball spinning clockwise.

Swing due to the Magnus effect is an important feature of many ball games, especially at the elite level. The Magnus effect can be used to produce swing in any direction, but topspin and backspin (about a horizontal axis perpendicular to the linear velocity of the ball) and sidespin (about a vertical axis perpendicular to the linear velocity of the ball) are the most common forms. Topspin produces a downward lift force (as in Figure 12.23, if the plane of the figure is assumed to be vertical) and is used in situations where the player wants to hit the ball hard, but also keep the ball in court, as in tennis, or on the table, as in table tennis. Backspin produces an upward lift force and is the key feature of drop shots in tennis and table tennis. Backspin is also the major feature of golf shots. The angled face of golf clubs produces considerable backspin on the ball, which, due to lift force, significantly increases the range through the air. Sidespin (as in Figure 12.23) is also an important feature of golf shots. A shot that is intended to swing left to right (for a right hander) is referred to as a fade. Similarly, a shot that is intended to swing right to left is referred to as a draw. Recreational golfers are more familiar with unintended shots in these directions; these shots are referred to as a slice and a hook, respectively.

All objects moving through fluids experience drag; they may simultaneously experience hydrodynamic lift force due to asymmetric shape, asymmetric orientation, asymmetric surface texture, spin or a combination of these influences.

Effect of drag and lift force on ball flight

In the absence of air resistance (no drag or lift force), the trajectory of a ball when projected into the air would be a parabola, i.e. the second half of the trajectory (from maximum height to landing) would be a mirror image of the first part of the trajectory (from release to maximum height) and the only force acting on the ball would be its weight (Figure 12.24a). If projected at the same velocity in air, without spin (and uniform surface texture), the ball would experience two forces, drag and weight, and the drag force would result in reduced range (Figure 12.24b). If projected at the same velocity with topspin, the ball would

505

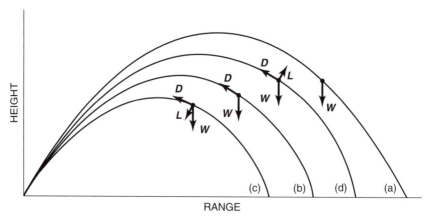

Figure 12.24 Effect of drag and lift force on trajectory of ball flight. (a) No air resistance. (b) Air resistance, no spin. (c) Air resistance and topspin. (d) Air resistance and backspin. W, weight of ball; D, drag; L, lift force.

experience three forces; drag, lift force and weight. The net effect of the three forces would be a shorter range than when the ball is projected without spin (Figure 12.24c). If it is projected at the same velocity with backspin, the ball would experience three forces, drag, lift force and weight, but the lift force would be in the opposite direction to that of topspin. The net effect of the three forces would be a longer range than when projected without spin (Figure 12.24d).

REVIEW QUESTIONS

1. Define the following terms: atmospheric pressure, hydrostatic pressure, fluid, Archimedes' principle, buoyancy force, centre of buoyancy, specific gravity, viscosity, boundary layer, drag, viscous drag, pressure drag, slipstreaming, paddle propulsion, Bernoulli's principle, hydrodynamic lift force, screw propulsion and the Magnus effect.

2. When fully inflated, a balloon used to provide overhead views at televised golf tournaments has a volume of 1000 m³. Calculate the maximum load that the balloon can carry in order to be able to float if the weight of the balloon envelope W_E is 50 kgf, the weight density of air outside the balloon ρ_o is 1.25 kgf/m³ and the weight density of hot air inside the balloon ρ_i is 1.10 kgf/m³.

3. If the density of seawater ρ_w is 1025 kg/m³, what is the weight of a boat that floats with 1.5 m³ of its hull submerged.

4. In freestyle swimming events, each swimmer dives into the water and then glides underwater for a short distance before rising to the surface and starting to swim. During the glide, each swimmer tries to adopt a streamlined position (fully extended body in line with the linear velocity of the swimmer), in order to minimise drag.

   i. Calculate the viscous drag and pressure drag on a swimmer during the glide (assume no change in body position) if:

linear velocity of the swimmer $v = 3.5$ m/s,

viscosity of water $\eta = 0.010\ 02$ Pa·s,

density of water $\rho = 1000$ kg/m³,

body surface area $A_s = 1.8$ m²,

velocity gradient $v/h = 1.75$ /s,

coefficient of drag $C_D = 0.2$,

profile area $A_p = 0.06$ m².

    ii.   Calculate the instantaneous deceleration of the swimmer if the mass of the swimmer m is 70 kg.

5.   i.   Calculate the viscous drag and pressure drag on a soccer ball moving through the air if:

linear velocity of ball $v = 22.35$ m/s (50 mph);

viscosity of air $\eta = 0.000\ 18$ Pa·s,

density of air $\rho = 1.25$ kg/m³,

surface area of the ball $A_s = 0.152$ m²,

velocity gradient $v/h = 2.2$ /s,

coefficient of drag $C_D = 0.2$,

profile area $A_p = 0.04$ m².

    ii.   Calculate the instantaneous deceleration of the ball if the mass of the ball m is 0.45 kg.

6.   Calculate the theoretical terminal velocity of a two-man team in a bobsleigh sliding down a consistent slope of 5° with no turns if:

combined mass of bobsleigh and two-man team $m = 390$ kg,

coefficient of sliding friction between the sleigh and the slope $\mu = 0.03$,

coefficient of drag of the sleigh $C_D = 0.45$,

profile area of the sleigh $A = 0.413$ m²,

density of air $\rho = 1.25$ kg/m³.

7.   Following a free kick in soccer, if the ball moves through the air with a sidespin that results in a 0.1% difference in atmospheric pressure on opposite sides of the ball, calculate the distance that the ball swings sideways during a flight of one second if the mass of the ball m is 0.45 kg and the radius of the ball r is 0.11 m.

Origins, insertions, and actions of the major muscles of the human body

Table A.1 Major muscles of the trunk (Figures A.1 and A.2).

Muscles	Origin	Insertion	Action
External oblique	Borders of lower eight ribs at sides of chest	Anterior half of iliac crest	Flexion (together) and lateral flexion (single) of trunk
Internal oblique	Lateral half of inguinal ligament (links the pubic tubercle and anterior-superior iliac spine)	Eighth, ninth and tenth costal cartilages and linea alba (narrow aponeurosis between left and right parts of rectus abdominis)	Flexion (together) and lateral flexion (single) of trunk
Transversus abdominis	Lateral third of inguinal ligament Inner aspect of iliac crest Costal cartilages of lower six ribs Lumbar fascia (merges with origin of latissimus dorsi)	Pubic crest and linea alba	Compression of abdomen
Rectus abdominis	Pubic crest	Fifth, sixth, and seventh costal cartilages and xiphoid process	Flexion of trunk
Erector spinae	Posterior aspect of sacrum and crest of ilium Angles of lower seven ribs Spines of L1 to L5 and T9 to T12 Transverse processes of T1 to T12.	Transverse processes of all vertebrae Between superior and inferior nuchal lines on occipital bone	Extension of trunk

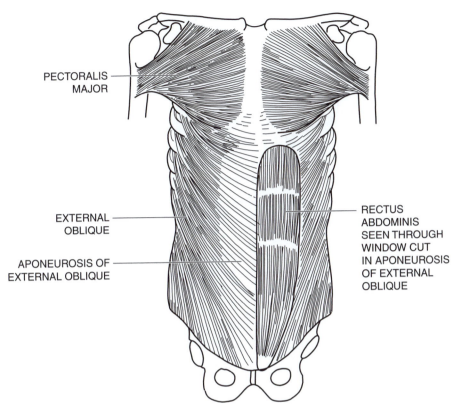

PECTORALIS
MAJOR

EXTERNAL
OBLIQUE

APONEUROSIS OF
EXTERNAL OBLIQUE

RECTUS
ABDOMINIS
SEEN THROUGH
WINDOW CUT
IN APONEUROSIS
OF EXTERNAL
OBLIQUE

Figure A1 Superficial muscles of the anterior aspect of the trunk.

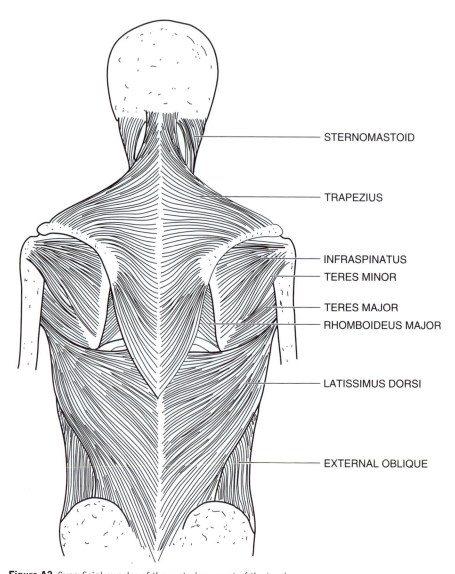

Figure A2 Superficial muscles of the posterior aspect of the trunk.

Table A.2 Major muscles of the upper limb (Figure A.3)

Muscles	Origin	Insertion	Action
Trapezius	Between superior and inferior nuchal lines either side of occipital protuberance Ligamentum nuchae Spines of C7 and T1 to T12 and adjacent supraspinous ligament	Lateral third of superior aspect of clavicle Superior aspect of acromion process and spine of scapula	Elevation and rotation of scapulae
Deltoid	Lateral third of anterior aspect of clavicle Lateral aspect of acromion process Inferior aspect of border of spine of scapula	Deltoid tuberosity of humerus	Flexion, abduction, and extension of shoulder joint
Pectoralis major	Medial third of anterior aspect of clavicle Lateral border of sternum and adjoining costal cartilages	Lateral aspect of bicipital groove of humerus	Flexion, adduction, and medial rotation of shoulder joint
Latissimus dorsi	Posterior aspect of sacrum Posterior third of iliac crest Spines of T8 to T12 and L1 to L5	Medial aspect of bicipital groove of humerus	Extension, adduction, and medial rotation of shoulder joint
Supraspinatus	Supraspinous fossa of scapula	Superior aspect of greater tuberosity of humerus	Abduction of shoulder joint
Infraspinatus	Infraspinous fossa of scapula	Posterior aspect of greater tuberosity of humerus	Lateral rotation of shoulder joint
Teres minor	Posterior-lateral aspect of scapula	Posterior aspect of greater tuberosity of humerus	Lateral rotation of shoulder joint
Subscapularis	Subscapular fossa of scapula	Anterior aspect of lesser tuberosity of humerus	Medial rotation of shoulder joint
Teres major	Inferior lateral-posterior aspect of scapula below origin of teres minor	Medial aspect of bicipital groove of humerus	Extension, medial rotation, and adduction of shoulder joint
Biceps brachii	Superior aspect of glenoid fossa (long head) Tip of coracoid process (short head)	Radial tuberosity of humerus	Flexion of shoulder and elbow joints
Triceps brachii	Superior third of lateral border of scapula below glenoid fossa (long head)	Olecranon process of ulna	Extension of elbow Adduction of shoulder joint

Table A.2 (continued)

Muscles	Origin	Insertion	Action
	Medial line on superior-posterior half of humerus (lateral head) Lower two-thirds of posterior-medial aspect of humerus (medial head)		
Brachioradialis	Lateral supracondylar ridge of humerus	Styloid process of radius	Flexion of elbow
Brachialis	Anterior-inferior half of humerus	Coronoid process of ulna	Flexion of elbow
Pronator teres	Medial supracondylar ridge of humerus Medial aspect of coronoid process	Middle third of lateral aspect of radius	Flexion of elbow Pronation of forearm
Supinator	Lateral epicondyle of humerus Lateral aspect of coronoid process of ulna	Proximal lateral third of radius	Supination of forearm
Flexor carpi radialis	Medial aspect of humerus above trochlea	Anterior aspect of bases of second and third metacarpals	Flexion of wrist and elbow
Flexor carpi ulnaris	Medial aspect of humerus above trochlea	Anterior aspect of base of fifth metacarpal	Flexion of wrist and elbow
Extensor carpi radialis	Posterior aspect of lateral epicondyle of humerus	Posterior aspect of base of third metacarpal	Extension of wrist and elbow
Extensor carpi ulnaris	Posterior aspect of the lateral epicondyle of humerus	Posterior aspect of base of fifth metacarpal	Extension of wrist and elbow
Flexor digitorum sublimis	Medial epicondyle of humerus Anterior aspect of ulna distal to coronoid process Lateral third of radius	Four tendons to sides of bases of middle phalanges of fingers	Flexion of wrist and fingers
Extensor digitorum communis	Lateral epicondyle of humerus	Four tendons to bases of middle and distal phalanges of fingers (dorsal surface)	Extension of wrist and fingers

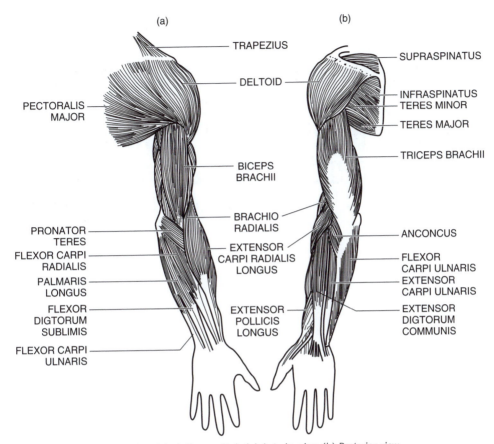

Figure A3 Superficial muscles of the left upper limb. (a) Anterior view. (b) Posterior view.

Table A.3 Major muscles of the lower limb (Figure A.4)

Muscles	Origin	Insertion	Action
Iliopsoas (psoas and iliacus)	Transverse processes and sides of bodies of T12 and L1 to L5 Anterior aspect of ilium	Lesser trochanter	Flexion of hip joint
Gluteus medius	Superior half of lateral aspect of ilium	Superior and lateral aspects of greater trochanter	Abduction of hip joint
Gluteus maximus	Posterior-lateral aspect of iliac crest and sacrum	Gluteal ridge on posterior aspect of the femur, and iliotibial tract*	Extension, abduction and lateral rotation of hip joint
Tensor fasciae latae	Anterior-lateral aspect of anterior-superior iliac spine	Iliotibial tract*	Flexion and abduction of hip joint
Sartorius	Anterior aspect of ilium between anterior-superior and anterior-inferior iliac spines	Medial aspect of tibia below medial condyle	Flexion of hip joint
Gracilis	Inferior aspect of pubic symphysis Inferior aspect of inferior ramus of pubis	Posterior aspect of medial condyle of tibia	Adduction of hip joint
Adductor longus	Pubic crest	Middle third of linea aspera	Adduction and lateral rotation of hip
Pectineus	Anterior-medial aspect of pubis	Proximal medial third of femur	Flexion and adduction of femur
Rectus femoris	Anterior aspect of ilium between anterior-superior and anterior-inferior iliac spines	Patella tendon, which is continuous with patellar ligament, which attaches onto tibial tuberosity	Flexion of hip; Extension of knee
Vastus lateralis	Lateral aspect of linea aspera Gluteal ridge on femur	Patellar tendon	Extension of knee
Vastus medialis	Medial aspect of linea aspera Spiral line on femur	Patellar tendon	Extension of knee
Vastus intermedius	Superior two-thirds of anterior aspect of femur	Patellar tendon	Extension of knee

Table A.3 (continued)

Muscles	Origin	Insertion	Action
Biceps femoris	Ischial tuberosity Distal half of linea aspera Lateral supracondylar ridge of femur	Posterior-lateral aspect of lateral condyle of tibia Head of fibula	Extension of hip Flexion of knee
Semitendinosus	Ischial tuberosity	Anterior-medial aspect of tibia below medial condyle	Extension of hip Flexion of knee
Semimembranosus	Ischial tuberosity	Posterior aspect of medial condyle of tibia	Extension of hip Flexion of knee
Flexor digitorum longus	Lower two-thirds of posterior aspect of tibia	Under medial malleolus. The tendon splits into four branches, one to each of the lateral four toes. The tendons attach onto the bases of distal phalanges of the lateral four toes.	Plantar flexion of lateral four toes Plantar flexion and inversion of ankle
Tibialis posterior	Posterior aspect of upper half of interosseus membrane and adjoining borders of tibia and fibula	Under medial malleolus. The tendon splits into six branches that attach onto the plantar aspects of the navicular, the first cuneiform and the bases of the second to fifth metatarsals.	Plantar flexion and inversion of ankle
Peroneus longus	Head and upper two-thirds of lateral aspect of fibula	Under lateral malleolus. The tendon splits into two branches that attach onto the plantar aspects of the first cuneiform and the base of the first metatarsal.	Plantar flexion and eversion of the ankle
Peroneus brevis	Lower two-thirds of lateral aspect of fibula	Under the lateral malleolus to attach onto the tuberosity of the fifth metatarsal	Plantar flexion and eversion of the ankle
Tibialis anterior	Upper two-thirds of lateral aspect of tibia	Anterior to the ankle joint via the medial aspect of the foot to attach onto the plantar aspects of the first cuneiform and the base of the first metatarsal	Dorsiflexion and inversion of ankle

Table A.3 (continued)

Muscles	Origin	Insertion	Action
Extensor hallucis longus	Middle two-thirds of anteromedial aspect of fibula	Anterior to ankle joint to attach onto superior aspect of base of distal phalanx of hallux	Dorsiflexion of hallux Dorsiflexion of ankle
Extensor digitorum longus	Anterolateral aspect of lateral condyle of tibia and upper two-thirds of anterior aspect of fibula	Anterior to ankle joint. The tendon splits into four branches that attach onto the superior aspects of the bases of the middle and distal phalanges of the lateral four toes.	Dorsiflexion of lateral four toes Dorsiflexion of ankle
Gastrocnemius	Medial head: superior aspect of medial condyle of femur Lateral head: superior aspect of lateral condyle of femur	The two heads attach onto the upper Achilles tendon, which is inserted onto the upper half of the posterior aspect of the calcaneus.	Plantar flexion of ankle Flexion of knee
Soleus	Upper third of fibula and adjoining soleal line on upper third of tibia	Anterosuperior half of Achilles tendon, which is inserted onto upper half of posterior aspect of calcaneus	Plantar flexion of ankle

* The iliotibial tract is the thickened lateral region of the *fascia lata* (the connective tissue that encloses all of the muscles of the thigh). It extends from the iliac crest to the lateral aspect of the knee, where it blends with the fascia around the knee and inserts onto the anterolateral aspect of the tibia below the lateral condyle

(a)   (b)

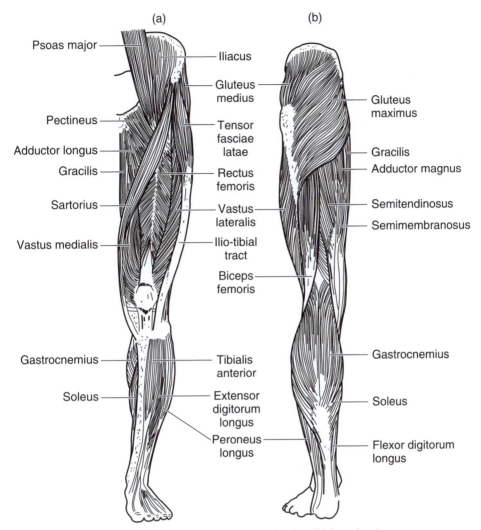

Psoas major
Iliacus
Gluteus medius
Gluteus maximus
Pectineus
Tensor fasciae latae
Adductor longus
Gracilis
Gracilis
Adductor magnus
Sartorius
Rectus femoris
Vastus lateralis
Semitendinosus
Semimembranosus
Vastus medialis
Ilio-tibial tract
Biceps femoris
Gastrocnemius
Tibialis anterior
Gastrocnemius
Soleus
Extensor digitorum longus
Soleus
Peroneus longus
Flexor digitorum longus

Figure A4 Superficial muscles of the left lower limb. (a) Anterior view. (b) Posterior view.

Linear kinematic analysis of a 15 m sprint

OBJECTIVE

To record 5 m split times during a 15 m sprint and use the distance–time data to produce the distance–time, speed–time and acceleration–time graphs of the sprint

LOCATION

Indoor or outdoor area with minimum length of 30 m

APPARATUS AND EQUIPMENT

Four sets of photocells linked to a timer

METHOD

Subject's clothing and footwear

Sports clothing and trainers

Layout of equipment

The four sets of photocells are arranged as in Figure PW1.1. Each set of photocells is arranged so that the photocells are placed approximately 3 m apart on either side of the running track. The photocells are mounted on tripods at a height of about 1 m. One set of photocells is located at the start, with the other sets located 5 m, 10 m and 15 m from the start line.

Data collection and analysis

1. Using a standing start from 1 m behind the start line (so that the first set of photocells will start the timer as you run between them), perform three maximum-effort trials and record the 5 m, 10 m and 15 m times for each trial in Table PW1.1 of the data collection sheet.
2. Plot the distance–time data (distance on the vertical axis and time on the horizontal axis) of your fastest trial on centimetre squared graph paper and draw a smooth curve through the origin and the three data points to produce the distance–time graph. If necessary,

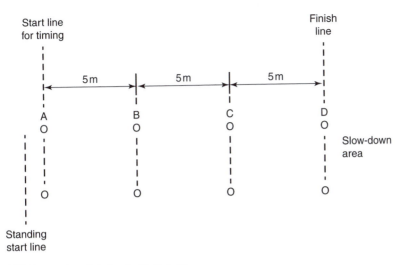

Figure PW1.1 Location of photocells (A, B, C, D).

extend the graph beyond the 3 second point on the time axis. A suitable scale to use would be 1 cm on the graph paper for 1 m for the distance axis and 5 cm on the graph paper for 1 s for the time axis.

3. From the distance–time graph, read the distance at 1, 2 and 3 seconds after the start and record these data in the second column of Table PW1.2 of the data collection sheet.

4. Calculate and record in the third column of Table PW1.2 the change in distance during each of the three one-second intervals.

5. Record the average speed in each of the three one-second intervals in the fourth column of Table PW1.2. (These will be the same numbers as in column 3.)

6. Plot the average speed–time data (column 4 of Table PW1.2) on the same sheet of graph paper, choosing an appropriate scale for speed (vertical axis). A suitable scale would be 2 cm on the graph paper for 1 m/s for the speed axis. As the data represent average speeds, plot the data at the midpoints of the corresponding time intervals.

7. Draw a smooth curve through the origin and the three data points to produce the speed–time graph. Extend the graph beyond the 3 second point on the time axis.

8. From the speed–time graph, read the speed at 1, 2 and 3 seconds after the start and record these data in the second column of Table PW1.3 of the data collection sheet.

9. Calculate and record in the third column of Table PW1.3 the change in speed during each of the three one-second intervals.

10. Record the average acceleration in each of the three one-second intervals in the fourth column of Table PW1.3. (These will be the same numbers as in column 3.)

11. Using the same axis and scale for acceleration as that used for speed, plot the average acceleration–time data (column 4 of Table PW1.3) on the same sheet of graph paper. As the data represent average acceleration, plot the data at the midpoints of the corresponding time intervals.

12. Draw a smooth curve through the origin and the three data points to produce the acceleration–time graph.

Table PW1.1 5 m, 10 m and 15 m times (s) in three maximum-effort trials.

Distance (m)	Trial 1	Trial 2	Trial3
5			
10			
15			

Table PW1.2 Average speed.

Time interval (s)	Distance (m)	Change in distance (m)	Average speed (m/s)
1			
2			
3			

Table PW1.3 Average acceleration.

Time interval (s)	Speed (m/s)	Change in speed (m/s)	Average acceleration (m/s^2)
1			
2			
3			

EXAMPLE RESULTS

Example data are shown in Tables PW1.4 to PW1.6. The distance–time, speed–time and acceleration–time graphs based on the data in Tables PW1.4 to PW1.6 are shown in Figure PW1.2. The speed–time graph indicates that speed continued to increase throughout the trial. This is clearly reflected in the progressive increase in the slope of the distance–time graph over the corresponding period. Whereas speed continued to increase throughout the trial, the slope of the speed–time graph progressively decreased, i.e. acceleration was always positive, but decreasing. This is clearly reflected in the acceleration–time graph.

Table PW1.4 5 m, 10 m and 15 m times (s) in three maximum-effort trials.

Distance (m)	Trial 1	Trial 2	Trial 3
5	1.33	1.35	1.32
10	2.22	2.11	2.12
15	3.25	3.01	2.83

Table PW1.5 Average speed.

Time interval (s)	Distance (m)	Change in distance (m)	Average speed (m/s)
1	3.45	3.45	3.45
2	9.25	5.80	5.80
3	16.25	7.00	7.00

Table PW1.6 Average acceleration.

Time interval (s)	Speed (m/s)	Change in speed (m/s)	Average acceleration (m/s^2)
1	4.875	4.875	4.875
2	6.45	1.575	1.575
3	7.50	1.05	1.05

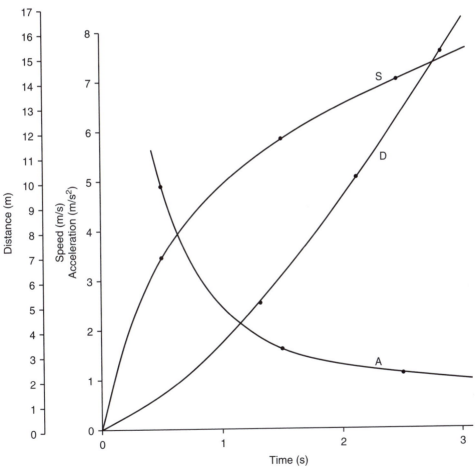

Figure PW1.2 Distance–time (D), speed–time (S), and acceleration–time (A) graphs based on the data in Tables PW1.4 to PW1.6.

Title: The effect of increase in speed on stride length, stride rate and relative stride length in running

OBJECTIVE

To obtain stride length, stride rate and relative stride length data for subjects running on a treadmill over a speed range of 1.5 m/s–3.5 m/s and to produce the corresponding stride length–speed, stride rate–speed and relative stride length–speed graphs

LOCATION

Motion analysis laboratory

APPARATUS AND EQUIPMENT

Variable speed treadmill with handrails, stopwatches, steel tape

METHOD

Subject's clothing and footwear

Sports clothing and trainers

Data collection and analysis

Height of subject

The subject's height is measured (m) with the subject standing upright without shoes and looking straight ahead. The height is recorded in Table PW2.1.

Leg length

1   The subject lies supine with legs straight and together.
2.   The subject relaxes legs so that legs rest naturally with feet turned out.
3.   The length of each leg is measured with a steel tape; this is the distance between the anterior-superior iliac spine and the medial malleolus.
4.   The subject's average leg length is recorded in Table PW2.1.

Time measurements

1. For each subject, in a single trial, the time for ten complete stride cycles at speeds of 1.5 m/s, 2.5 m/s and 3.5 m/s is measured and recorded in the results sheet.

2. At the start of each trial, the subject stands on the treadmill with hands on the handrails. The speed of the treadmill is gradually increased to 1.5 m/s (moderate walking pace) as the subject accommodates to the increase in speed.

3. After the subject has settled into a natural rhythm at a speed of 1.5 m/s, the time (s) for 10 complete stride cycles is measured using a stopwatch (heel-strike to heel-strike of the same foot). The time for ten complete stride cycles can be measured by any number of timers with the average time being recorded in Table PW2.1. For example, the class can be divided into groups of six people with each member of a group taking turns as subject, treadmill operator and timer.

4. After the time for ten complete stride cycles at a speed of 1.5 m/s has been measured, the speed of the treadmill is gradually increased to 2.5 m/s (slow jog). After the subject has settled into a natural rhythm at a speed of 2.5 m/s, the time (s) for ten complete stride cycles is measured and recorded in Table PW2.1.

5. The speed of the treadmill is then gradually increased to 3.5 m/s (moderate running pace) and the time for ten complete stride cycles is measured as before and recorded in Table PW2.1. The speed of the treadmill is then gradually reduced to zero.

6. After the times for ten complete stride cycles at all three speeds have been recorded, the stride rate, stride length, relative stride length with respect to height (RSL_H) and relative stride length with respect to leg length (RSL_L) are calculated for each speed, as follows:

$$\text{Stride rate (SR)} = \frac{10 \text{ cycles}}{t},$$

where: t = time for ten complete stride cycles.

Example:

If $t = 9.56$ s at a speed of 1.5 m/s, then $SR = \dfrac{10 \text{ cycles}}{9.56 \text{ s}} = 1.046$ Hz.

Stride length (SL) = Speed/SR.

Example:

If SR = 1.046 Hz at a speed of 1.5 m/s, then SL = 1.5 m/s/1.046 Hz = 1.434 m/str.

$$\text{Relative stride length with respect to height} = \frac{SL}{L}$$

Example:

If SL = 1.434 m/str and H = 1.694 m, then RSL_H = 0.846.

$$\text{Relative stride length with respect to leg length (}RSL_L\text{)} = \frac{SL}{L}.$$

Example:

If SL = 1.434 m/str and L = 0.90 m, then RSL_L = 1.593.

7. Record stride rate, stride length, and relative stride length with respect to height and leg length in Table PW2.1.

523

Table PW2.1 Individual and group mean results for height, leg length, stride rate, stride length, and relative stride length

Subject	H (m)	L (m)	1.5 m/s Time (s)	SR (Hz)	SL (m/str)	RSL$_H$ (H/str)	RSL$_L$ (L/str)	2.5 m/s Time (s)	SR (Hz)	SL (m/str)	RSL$_H$ (H/str)	RSL$_L$ (L/str)	3.5 m/s Time (s)	SR (Hz)	SL (m/str)	RSL$_H$ (H/str)	RSL$_L$ (L/str)
Females																	
1.																	
2.																	
3.																	
4.																	
5.																	
6.																	
Mean																	
SD																	
Females																	
1.																	
2.																	
3.																	
4.																	
5.																	
6.																	
Mean																	
SD																	

H = height; L = average leg length; SR = stride rate; SL = stride length

RSL$_H$ = relative stride length in relation to height; RSL$_L$ = relative stride length in relation to height

PRESENTATION OF RESULTS

1. Present a results table showing individual and group (mean and standard deviation) results for the subjects in your group. Show the results for women and men separately, i.e. list the subjects as two groups.
2. Present two sets of graphs of the results:
    i. Group mean results for stride rate and stride length (women and men separately). Plot speed (m/s) on the horizontal axis and stride rate (Hz) and stride length (m/str) on the vertical axis.
    ii. Group mean results for relative stride length (women and men separately). Plot speed (m/s) on the horizontal axis and relative stride length on the vertical axis.

n.b.: The unit of relative stride length for RSL_H is 'heights per stride' (length of stride relative to the subject's height) and that for RSL_L is 'leg lengths per stride' (length of stride relative to the subject's average leg length).

EXAMPLE RESULTS

Example data (obtained in an actual practical session with students) are shown in Table PW2.2. The corresponding group mean graphs for stride length–speed, stride rate–speed and relative stride length–speed are shown in Figure PW2.1. Figure PW2.1 shows that:

i. The women had a shorter average stride length and a higher average stride rate than the men at each of the three speeds.
ii. The average relative stride length (with respect to height and leg length) at each speed was very similar for both groups.

Table PW2.2 Individual and group mean results for height, leg length, stride rate, stride length, and relative stride length

Subject	H (m)	L (m)	1.5 m/s					2.5 m/s					3.5 m/s				
			Time (s)	SR (Hz)	SL (m/str)	RSL_H (H/str)	RSL_L (L/str)	Time (s)	SR (Hz)	SL (m/str)	RSL_H (H/str)	RSL_L (L/str)	Time (s)	SR (Hz)	SL (m/str)	RSL_H (H/str)	RSL_L (L/str)
Females																	
1.	1.65	0.89	10.35	0.97	1.55	0.94	1.74	7.8	1.28	1.95	1.18	2.19	7.1	1.41	2.49	1.51	2.80
2.	1.69	0.90	9.56	1.05	1.43	0.84	1.59	7.66	1.31	1.91	1.13	1.12	7.09	1.41	2.48	1.46	2.76
3.	1.61	0.81	10.4	0.96	1.56	0.97	1.93	7.6	1.32	1.89	1.17	2.33	7.19	1.39	2.52	1.56	3.11
4.	1.65	0.87	9.46	1.06	1.42	0.86	1.62	6.97	1.43	1.75	1.06	2.0	6.47	1.55	2.26	1.37	2.58
5.	1.68	0.91	10.3	0.97	1.55	0.92	1.70	7.53	1.33	1.88	1.12	2.07	6.69	1.49	2.34	1.39	2.57
6.	1.65	0.87	9.50	1.05	1.43	0.87	1.64	7.0	1.43	1.75	1.06	2.01	6.0	1.67	2.1	1.27	2.41
Mean	1.66	0.88	9.93	1.01	1.49	0.9	1.70	7.43	1.35	1.86	1.12	2.12	6.76	1.49	2.37	1.43	2.71
SD	0.03	0.04	0.47	0.05	0.07	0.05	0.12	0.35	0.06	0.08	0.05	0.12	0.46	0.11	0.16	0.10	0.24
Males																	
1.	1.85	0.96	11.04	0.91	1.65	0.89	1.72	8.13	1.23	2.03	1.10	2.11	7.60	1.32	2.66	1.44	2.77
2.	1.83	0.95	11.0	0.91	1.65	0.90	1.73	8.0	1.18	2.12	1.16	2.22	8.09	1.24	2.83	1.55	2.96
3.	1.81	0.85	10.63	0.94	1.60	0.89	1.88	7.84	1.28	1.95	1.08	2.29	7.63	1.31	2.67	1.48	3.14
4.	1.69	0.89	10.94	0.91	1.65	0.98	1.86	8.16	1.23	2.03	1.20	2.29	7.47	1.34	2.61	1.55	2.94
5.	1.88	0.98	10.50	0.95	1.58	0.84	1.61	7.87	1.27	1.97	1.05	2.0	7.53	1.33	2.64	1.40	2.69
6.	1.81	0.96	10.15	0.99	1.52	0.84	1.58	7.62	1.31	1.91	1.06	1.98	7.15	1.40	2.50	1.38	2.59
Mean	1.81	0.93	10.71	0.94	1.61	0.89	1.73	8.02	1.25	2.0	1.11	2.15	7.58	1.32	2.65	1.47	2.85
SD	0.07	0.05	0.35	0.03	0.05	0.05	0.12	0.31	0.05	0.07	0.06	0.14	0.30	0.05	0.11	0.07	0.20

H = height; L = average leg length; SR = stride rate; SL = stride length

RSL_H = relative stride length in relation to height; RSL_L = relative stride length in relation to height

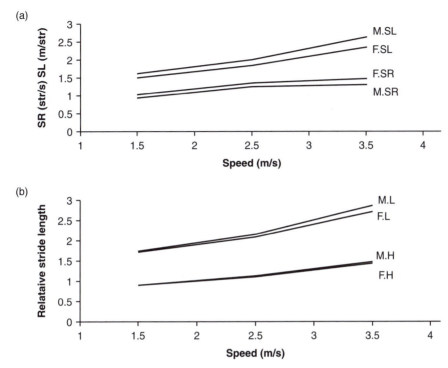

Figure PW2.1 (a) Group mean results for men (M) and women (F) for stride rate (SR) and stride length (SL) at speeds of 1.5 m/s, 2.5 m/s and 3.5 m/s. (b) Group mean results for men (M) and women (F) for relative stride length with respect to height (H) and average leg length (L) at speeds of 1.5 m/s, 3.5 m/s and 3.5 m/s.

Force–time analysis of the ground reaction force in walking

OBJECTIVE

To record the anteroposterior (F_X) and vertical (F_Y) components of the ground reaction force acting on a person during the ground contact phase of a single step when walking at a normal pace, and to perform a force–time analysis of the two recordings

LOCATION

Motion analysis laboratory

APPARATUS AND EQUIPMENT

Force platform system

METHOD
Subject's clothing and footwear

Everyday clothing and shoes

Data collection and analysis
Mass and weight of the subject

1. Measure the subject's mass (kg), with subject standing upright without shoes.
2. Record the mass of the subject in Table PW3.1.
3. Calculate and record the weight (N) of the subject in Table PW3.1.

Ground reaction force–time components

Record the anteroposterior (F_X) and vertical (F_Y) ground reaction force–time components during contact time of the right foot.

Table PW3.1 Analysis of the anteroposterior (F_X) and vertical (F_Y) ground reaction force components acting on the right foot of a person when walking at a normal steady pace.

Name of subject:			
		Mass (kg)	Weight (N)

Mass of subject			
	Time (s)	Force (N)	Force (BW)
1. Heel contact (t_1, F_{Y1})		0	0
2. Peak F_Y impact force peak (t_2, F_{Y2})			
3. Peak F_Y in the absorption phase (t_3, F_{Y3})			
4. End of the absorption phase (when $F_X = 0$) (t_4, F_{Y4})			
5. Peak F_Y in the propulsion phase (t_5, F_{Y5})			
6. Toe-off (t_6, F_{Y6})		0	0
7. Peak F_X in absorption phase (t_7, F_{Y7})			
8. Peak F_X in propulsion phase (t_8, F_{Y8})			

	Time (s)	Proportion of contact time (%)
9. Contact time $(t_6 - t_1)$		100
10. Duration of absorption phase $(t_4 - t_1)$		
11. Duration of propulsion phase $(t_6 - t_4)$		
12. Time to F_Y impact force peak $(t_2 - t_1)$		
13. Time to peak F_Y in the absorption phase $(t_3 - t_1)$		
14. Time to peak F_Y in the propulsion phase $(t_5 - t_1)$		
15. Time to peak F_X in the absorption phase $(t_7 - t_1)$		
16. Time to peak F_X in the propulsion phase $(t_8 - t_1)$		

	L_{RY} (N/s)	L_{RY} (BW/s)
17. Rate of F_Y loading (L_{RY}) during impact $(F_{Y2}/(t_2 - t_1))$		

1. On a signal from the system operator, the subject walks at a normal steady pace (approximately 1.2 m/s) across the force plate, making sure that only the right foot contacts the force plate.
2. The operator prints the anteroposterior (F_X) and vertical (F_Y) force–time components of the ground reaction force acting on the right foot during contact with the force plate. Figure PW3.1 shows typical F_X–time and F_Y–time records.

Analysis of the F_X–time and F_Y–time records

1. From the F_X–time and F_Y–time records, estimate the forces (N) and times (s) corresponding to the variables listed 1 to 8 in Table PW3.1. Record these forces and times in Table PW3.1.

529 ▪

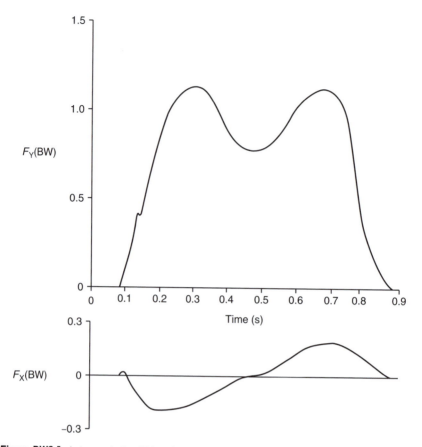

Figure PW3.1 Anteroposterior (F_X) and vertical (F_Y) ground reaction force–time components acting on the right foot of a person when walking at a normal steady pace.

2. Calculate the forces in units of body weight and record the forces in Table PW3.1.
3. Using the time data in Table PW3.1 for points 1 to 8, calculate and record the time variables 9 to 16 in Table PW3.1.
4. Calculate and record in Table PW3.1 the rate of F_Y loading (L_{RY}) during impact (the period t_1 to t_2) in N/s and BW/s.

PRESENTATION OF RESULTS

Your submission should consist of:

1. A figure of the F_X and F_Y force–time records showing the time points 1 to 8.
2. A table of results showing the force and time analysis of the F_X and F_Y force–time records.

EXAMPLE RESULTS

Figure PW3.2 shows the time points 1 to 8 on the F_X and F_Y force–time records of Figure PW3.1.

Table PW3.2 shows the force and time analysis of the F_X and F_Y force–time records of Figure PW3.2.

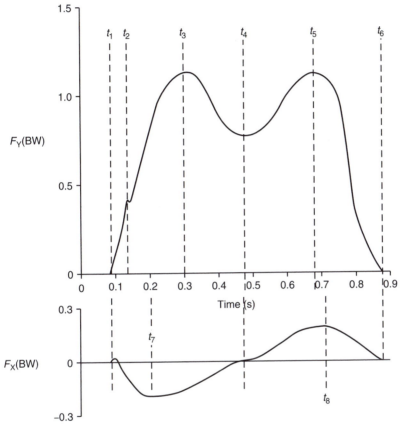

Figure PW3.2 Anteroposterior (F_X) and vertical (F_Y) ground reaction force–time components acting on the right foot of a person when walking at a normal steady pace. t_1, heel contact; t_2, peak F_Y (impact force peak); t_3, peak F_Y in the absorption phase; t_4, end of the absorption phase; t_5, peak F_Y in the absorption phase; t_6, toe-off; t_7, peak F_X in the absorption phase; t_8, peak F_X in the propulsion phase.

Table PW3.2 Analysis of the anteroposterior (F_X) and vertical (F_Y) ground reaction force components acting on the right foot of a person when walking at a normal steady pace.

Name of subject:

	Mass (kg)	Weight (N)	
Mass of subject	71.0	695.5	

	Time (s)	Force (N)	Force (BW)
1. Heel contact (t_1, F_{Y1})	0.084	0	0
2. Peak F_Y impact force peak (t_2, F_{Y2})	0.134	288.1	0.41
3. Peak F_Y in the absorption phase (t_3, F_{Y3})	0.297	779.9	1.12
4. End of the absorption phase (when $F_X = 0$) (t_4, F_{Y4})	0.469	531.6	0.76
5. Peak F_Y in the propulsion phase (t_5, F_{Y5})	0.672	775.0	1.11
6. Toe-off (t_6, F_{Y6})	0.870	0	0
7. Peak F_X in absorption phase (t_7, F_{Y7})	0.208	−132.1	0.18
8. Peak F_X in propulsion phase (t_8, F_{Y8})	0.701	136.1	0.19

	Time (s)	Proportion of contact time (%)
9. Contact time ($t_6 - t_1$)	0.786	100
10. Duration of absorption phase ($t_4 - t_1$)	0.385	49.0
11. Duration of propulsion phase ($t_6 - t_4$)	0.401	51.0
12. Time to F_Y impact force peak ($t_2 - t_1$)	0.050	6.4
13. Time to peak F_Y in the absorption phase ($t_3 - t_1$)	0.213	27.1
14. Time to peak F_Y in the propulsion phase ($t_5 - t_1$)	0.588	74.8
15. Time to peak F_X in the absorption phase ($t_7 - t_1$)	0.124	15.8
16. Time to peak F_X in the propulsion phase ($t_8 - t_1$)	0.617	78.4

	L_{RY} (N/s)	L_{RY} (BW/s)
17. Rate of F_Y loading (L_{RY}) during impact ($F_{Y2}/(t_2 - t_1)$)	5762.0	8.28

Force–time analysis of ground reaction force in running

OBJECTIVE

To record the anteroposterior (F_X) and vertical (F_Y) components of the ground reaction force acting on a runner during the ground contact phase of a single step when running at a moderate pace and to perform a force–time analysis of the two recordings

LOCATION

Motion analysis laboratory

APPARATUS AND EQUIPMENT

Force platform system

METHOD

Subject's clothing and footwear

Sports clothing and trainers

Data collection and analysis

Mass and weight of the subject

1. Measure the subject's mass (kg), with subject standing upright without shoes.
2. Record the mass of the subject in Table PW4.1.
3. Calculate and record the weight (N) of the subject in Table PW4.1.

Ground reaction force–time components

Record the anteroposterior (F_X) and vertical (F_Y) ground reaction force–time components during contact time of the right foot.

Table PW4.1 Analysis of the anteroposterior (F_X) and vertical (F_Y) ground reaction force components acting on the right foot of a runner when running at a moderate pace.

Name of subject:				
		Mass (kg)	**Weight (N)**	
Mass of subject				
	Time (s)	**Force (N)**	**Force (BW)**	
1. Heel contact (t_1, F_{Y1})		0	0	
2. Peak F_Y impact force peak (t_2, F_{Y2})				
3. End of the passive phase (t_3, F_{Y3})				
4. End of the absorption phase (when $F_X = 0$) (t_4, F_{Y4})				
5. Toe-off (t_5, F_{Y5})		0	0	
6. Peak F_X in absorption phase (t_6, F_{Y6})				
7. Peak F_X in propulsion phase (t_7, F_{Y7})				
	Time (s)	**Proportion of contact time (%)**		
8. Contact time ($t_5 - t_1$)		100		
9. Time to impact force peak ($t_2 - t_1$)				
10. Duration of passive phase ($t_3 - t_1$)				
11. Duration of active phase ($t_5 - t_3$)				
12. Duration of absorption phase ($t_4 - t_1$)				
13. Duration of propulsion phase ($t_5 - t_4$)				
	L_{RY} (N/s)	L_{RY} (BW/s)		
14. Rate of F_Y loading (L_{RY}) during impact ($F_{Y2}/(t_2 - t_1)$)				

1. On a signal from the system operator, the subject runs across the force plate at a moderate speed (approximately 3.5 m/s), making sure that only the right foot contacts the force plate.

2. The operator prints the anteroposterior (F_X) and vertical (F_Y) force–time components of the ground reaction force acting on the right foot during contact with the force plate. Figure PW4.1 shows typical F_X–time and F_Y–time records.

Analysis of the F_X–time and F_Y–time records

1. From the F_X–time and F_Y–time records, estimate the forces (N) and times (s) corresponding to the time points listed 1 to 7 in Table PW4.1. Record these forces and times in Table PW4.1.

2. Calculate the forces in units of body weight and record the forces in Table PW4.1.

3. Using the time data in Table PW4.1 for points 1 to 7, calculate and record the time variables 8 to 13 in Table PW4.1.

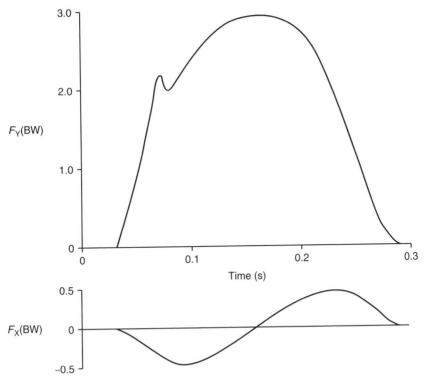

Figure PW4.1 Anteroposterior (F_X) and vertical (F_Y) ground reaction force–time components acting on the right foot of a runner when running at a moderate pace.

4. Calculate and record in Table PW4.1 the rate of F_Y loading (L_{RY}) during impact (the period t_1 to t_2) in N/s and BW/s.

PRESENTATION OF RESULTS

Your submission should consist of:

1. A figure of the F_X and F_Y force–time records showing the time points 1 to 7.
2. A table of results showing the force and time analysis of the F_X and F_Y force–time records.

EXAMPLE RESULTS

Figure PW4.2 shows the time points 1 to 7 on the F_X and F_Y force–time records of Figure PW4.1.

Table PW4.2 shows the force and time analysis of the F_X and F_Y force–time records of Figure PW4.2.

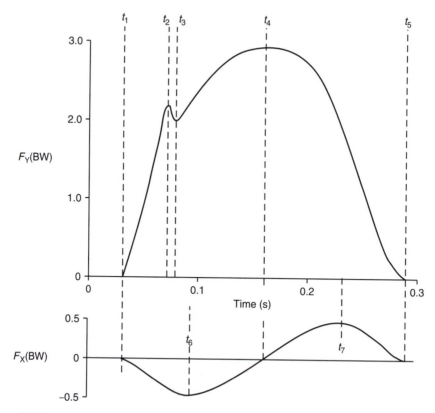

Figure PW4.2 Anteroposterior (F_X) and vertical (F_Y) ground reaction force–time components acting on the right foot of a runner when running at a moderate pace: t_1, heel contact; t_2, peak F_Y (impact force peak); t_3, end of passive phase; t_4, end of absorption phase; t_5, toe-off, t_6, peak F_X in absorption phase; t_7, peak F_X in propulsion phase.

Table PW4.2 Analysis of the anteroposterior (F_X) and vertical (F_Y) ground reaction force components acting on the right foot of a runner when running at a moderate pace.

Name of subject:			
	Mass (kg)	Weight (N)	
Mass of subject	75.2	737.7	
	Time (s)	Force (N)	Force (BW)
1. Heel contact (t_1, F_{Y1})	0.030	0	0
2. Peak F_Y impact force peak (IFP) (t_2, F_{Y2})	0.071	1615.6	2.19
3. End of the passive phase (t_3, F_{Y3})	0.078	1475.4	2.00
4. End of the absorption phase (when $F_X = 0$) (t_4, F_{Y4})	0.159	2161.4	2.93
5. Toe-off (t_5, F_{Y5})	0.288	0	0
6. Peak F_X in absorption phase (t_6, F_{Y6})	0.095	339.3	0.46
7. Peak F_X in propulsion phase (t_7, F_{Y7})	0.232	346.7	0.47
	Time (s)	Proportion of contact time (%)	
8. Contact time ($t_5 - t_1$)	0.258	100	
9. Time to IFP ($t_2 - t_1$)	0.041	15.9	
10. Duration of passive phase ($t_3 - t_1$)	0.048	18.6	
11. Duration of active phase ($t_5 - t_3$)	0.210	81.4	
12. Duration of absorption phase ($t_4 - t_1$)	0.129	50.0	
13. Duration of propulsion phase ($t_5 - t_4$)	0.129	50.0	
	L_{RY} (N/s)	L_{RY} (BW/s)	
14. Rate of F_Y loading (L_{RY}) during impact ($F_{Y2}/(t_2 - t_1)$)	39 404.9	53.4	

Determination of the position of the whole body centre of gravity by the direct method using a one-dimension reaction board

OBJECTIVES

1. To determine the position of the whole body centre of gravity in the anatomical position.
2. To examine the effect of changes in body shape on the position of the whole body centre of gravity relative to the anatomical position.

LOCATION

Motion analysis laboratory

APPARATUS AND EQUIPMENT

One-dimension reaction board (approximately 2.5 m × 0.5 m) with a centimetre scale running left to right on one side, one set of weighing scales

METHOD

Subjects' clothing

Shorts and shirt

Data collection and analysis

1. Record in Table PW5.1 the height h (cm) and weight W (kgf) of the subject without shoes.
2. Record in Table PW5.1 the distance l between the knife-edge supports of the reaction board.
3. Support the reaction board in a horizontal position with knife-edge support B resting on the weighing scales (Figure PW5.1a).
4. Record in Table PW5.1 the vertical force S_1 (kgf) exerted on the scales, i.e. the vertical support force acting on knife-edge support B.

5. Position 1: anatomical reference position.

   i. Have subject lie on the board with arms by sides and soles of feet in the same plane as knife-edge support A (Figure PW5.1b).

   ii. Record in Table PW5.1 the force S_2 on the scales.

   iii. Calculate the horizontal distance d (cm) between knife-edge support A and the parallel vertical plane containing the whole body centre of gravity of the subject using Equation PW5.1,

$$d = \frac{l(S_2 - S_1)}{W}. \qquad\qquad (\text{PW5.1})$$

   iv. Record d in Table PW5.1.

   v. Calculate d as a percentage of h and record the result in Table PW5.1.

6. Position 2: from Position 1, fold arms across chest (Figure PW5.2a).

   i. Record S_2 in Table PW5.1.

   ii. Calculate d (cm) using Equation PW5.1 and record the result in Table PW5.1.

   iii. Calculate d as a percentage of h and record the result in Table PW5.1.

   iv. Calculate the change in d (Δd, cm) between Positions 1 and 2 and record the result in Table PW5.1.

   v. Calculate Δd as a percentage of h and record the result in Table PW5.1.

7. Position 3: from Position 1, fully abduct both arms (Figure PW5.2b).

   i. Record S_2 in Table PW5.1.

   ii. Calculate d (cm) using Equation PW5.1 and record the result in Table PW5.1.

   iii. Calculate d as a percentage of h and record the result in Table PW5.1.

   iv. Calculate Δd between Positions 1 and 3 and record the result in Table PW5.1.

   v. Calculate Δd as a percentage of h and record the result in Table PW5.1.

8. Position 4: from Position 1, fully flex hips and knees (Figure PW5.2c).

   i. Record S_2 in Table PW5.1.

   ii. Calculate d (cm) using Equation PW5.1 and record the result in Table 2.

   iii. Calculate d as a percentage of h and record the result in Table PW5.1.

   iv. Calculate Δd between Positions 1 and 4 and record the result in Table PW5.1.

   v. Calculate Δd as a percentage of h and record the result in Table PW5.1.

9. Position 5: from Position 1, fully abduct both arms and fully flex hips and knees (Figure PW5.2d).

   i. Record S_2 in Table PW5.1.

   ii. Calculate d (cm) using Equation PW5.1 and record the result in Table PW5.1.

   iii. Calculate d as a percentage of h and record the result in Table PW5.1.

   iv. Calculate Δd between Positions 1 and 5 and record the result in Table PW5.1.

   v. Calculate Δd as a percentage of h and record the result in Table PW5.1.

539

10. Position 6: from Position 1, sit up and touch toes (Figure PW5.2e).
   i.   Record S_2 in Table 2.
   ii. Calculate d (cm) using Equation PW5.1 and record the result in Table PW5.1.
   iii. Calculate d as a percentage of h and record the result in Table PW5.1.
   iv. Calculate Δd between Positions 1 and 6 and record the result in Table PW5.1.
   v.   Calculate Δd as a percentage of h and record the result in Table PW5.1.

Table PW5.1 Individual results.

Name of subject:
Weight of subject W (kgf):
Height of subject h (cm):
l (cm):
S_1 (kgf):

Body position	S_2 (kgf)	d (cm)	$d\%$	Δd (cm)	$\Delta d\%$
1				0	0
2					
3					
4					
5					
6					

S_2, vertical force on knife-edge support B with subject lying on board in corresponding position; d, distance between knife-edge support A and vertical plane containing whole body centre of gravity of subject; $d\%$, d as a percentage of height h; Δd, change in d with respect to position 1; $\Delta d\%$, Δd as a percentage of h.

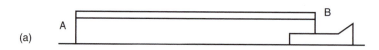

(a)

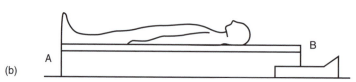

(b)

Figure PW5.1 (a) Reaction board resting horizontally with knife-edge support B resting on weighing scales. (b) Reaction board resting horizontally with knife-edge support B resting on weighing scales with subject lying on board in Position 1.

PRESENTATION OF RESULTS

1. Present your individual results in Table PW5.1.
2. Present the results for all of the subjects in your group and the group mean data in Table PW5.2.

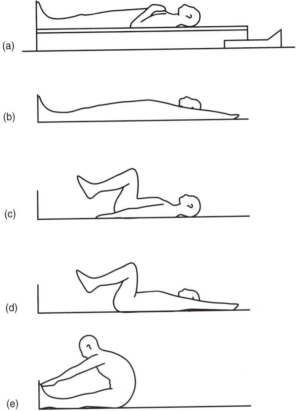

Figure PW5.2 Reaction board resting horizontally with knife-edge support B resting on weighing scales with subject lying on board. (a) Position 2: arms folded across chest. (b) Position 3: arms extended above head. (c) Position 4: hips and knees flexed. (d) Position 5: arms extended above head and hips and knees flexed. (e) Position 6: sitting up with fingers touching toes.

Table PW5.2 Individual and group results.

Subjects	h (cm)	W (kgf)	Position 1		Position 2		Positvion 3		Position 4		Position 5		Position 6	
			d%	Δd%	d%	Δd%	d%	Δd%	d%	Δd%	d%	Δd%	d%	Δd%
Women														
1				0										
2				0										
3				0										
4				0										
5				0										
Mean				0										
SD				0										
Men														
1				0										
2				0										
3				0										
4				0										
5				0										
Mean				0										
Standard deviation				0										

h, height of subject; W, weight of subject; $d\%$, d as a percentage of h; $\Delta d\%$; change in d with respect to Position 1 as a percentage of h.

EXAMPLE RESULTS

Example data (obtained from a practical session with students) are shown in Tables PW5.3 and PW5.4. Table PW5.4 shows group mean results for ten students (five women and five men). The group mean data show that the change in the position of the whole body centre of gravity is on average very similar for the men and women even though there is considerable variation in height and weight.

Table PW5.3 Individual results.

Name of subject: Anne
Weight of subject W (kgf): 67.0
Height of subject h (cm): 167.0
l (cm): 244.0
S_1 (kgf): 10.0

Body position	S_2 (kgf)	d (cm)	$d\%$	Δd (cm)	$\Delta d\%$
1	36.0	94.7	56.7	0	0
2	36.5	96.5	57.8	1.8	1.08
3	37.5	100.1	59.9	5.4	3.23
4	41.5	114.7	68.7	20.0	12.0
5	42.0	116.5	69.7	21.8	13.05
6	29.0	69.2	41.4	−25.5	−15.3

S_2, vertical force on knife-edge support B with subject lying on board in corresponding position; d, distance between knife-edge support A and vertical plane containing whole body centre of gravity of subject; $d\%$, d as a percentage of height h; Δd, change in d with respect to position 1; $\Delta d\%$, Δd as a percentage of h.

Table PW5.4 Individual and group results.

Subjects	h (cm)	W (kgf)	Position 1		Position 2		Position 3		Position 4		Position 5		Position 6	
			d%	Δd%	d%	Δd%	d%	Δd%	d%	Δd%	d%	Δd%	d%	Δd%
Women														
Anne	167	67	56.7	0	57.8	1.08	59.9	3.23	68.7	12.0	69.7	13.05	41.4	−15.3
Sarah	153.4	52	54.8	0	56.1	1.24	58.5	3.71	64.8	9.9	67.3	12.45	39.9	−14.9
Dawn	157	52.5	57.8	0	58.9	1.21	61	3.25	68.6	10.8	71	13.23	42.1	−15.6
Susan	172	68	53.2	0	54.2	1.04	56.3	3.13	64.7	11.5	66.7	13.56	41.7	−11.5
Kylie	167	61	55.6	0	56.6	0.96	59.5	3.89	65.4	9.75	67.3	11.7	41	−14.7
Mean	163.3	60.1	55.6	0	56.7	1.11	59.0	3.44	66.4	10.8	68.4	12.8	41.2	−14.4
SD	7.76	7.65	1.76	0	1.78	0.12	1.77	0.34	2.04	0.95	1.85	0.73	0.84	1.67
Men														
Paul	176.5	77	58.3	0	59.2	0.9	62.8	4.49	68.2	9.88	71.8	13.5	45.8	−12.6
Richard	181.3	76	61.9	0	62.9	0.88	65.5	3.54	69.1	7.08	72.6	10.6	46	−15.9
Bruce	189.4	80.5	59.8	0	60.4	0.63	63.1	3.27	68.9	9.13	72.8	13.0	44.8	−14.9
David	171	78	58.7	0	60.2	0.54	62.4	3.72	68.4	9.66	73.6	14.9	43.1	−15.6
John	169	68	59.6	0	60.5	0.89	62.2	2.66	68.6	8.99	70.4	10.8	43.3	−16.3
Mean	177.4	75.9	59.7	0	60.6	0.77	63.2	3.54	68.6	8.95	72.2	12.6	44.6	−15.1
Standard deviation	1.65	0.94	0.28	0	0.27	0.03	0.27	0.13	0.07	0.22	0.24	0.36	0.27	0.3

h, height of subject; W, weight of subject; $d\%$, d as a percentage of h; $\Delta d\%$; change in d with respect to Position 1 as a percentage of h.

Comparison of the direct and segmental analysis methods of determining the position of the whole body centre of gravity of the human body

OBJECTIVE

To compare the direct and segmental analysis methods of determining the transverse plane containing the centre of gravity (CG) of the human body in static equilibrium in the anatomical position using a one-dimension reaction board

LOCATION

Motion analysis laboratory

APPARATUS AND EQUIPMENT

One-dimension reaction board (approximately 2.5 m × 0.5 m) with a centimetre scale running left to right on one side, one set of weighing scales

METHOD

Subject's clothing

Shorts and a sleeveless top so that the following points on the skin on *left side of the body* can be easily identified:

- A point on the skin of the left arm at a distance of 3 cm below the tip of the acromion process, i.e. 3 cm to the left of the acromion process when the subject is lying horizontally in the anatomical position. This point will indicate the plane of the left shoulder joint centre when lying on the reaction board.
- The tip of the styloid process of the left ulna. This point will indicate the plane of the left wrist when lying on the reaction board.
- The tip of the left greater tuberosity. This point will indicate the plane of the left hip joint centre when lying on the reaction board.

■ The tip of the lateral malleolus of the left fibula. This point will indicate the plane of the left ankle joint centre when lying on the reaction board.

Data collection

1. Record in Table PW6.1 the weight W (kgf) of the subject (shorts, sleeveless top, no shoes).
2. Record in Table PW6.1 the height h (cm) of the subject (no shoes).
4. Record in Table PW6.1 the distance l (cm) between the two knife-edge supports of the reaction board.
3. Support the board in a horizontal position with knife-edge support B resting on the scales (Figure PW6.1a).
5. Record in Table PW6.1 the vertical force S_1 (kgf) exerted on the scales.
6. Have the subject lie on the board with arms by sides and soles of feet against the foot block, i.e. with the soles of the feet in the vertical plane containing knife-edge support A (Figure PW6.1b).
7. Record in Table PW6.1 the vertical force S_2 (kgf) exerted on end B.
8. Using the centimetre scale on the side of the board, record in Table PW6.1 the horizontal distances (cm) between the plane of the soles of the feet (reference zero) and the following points on the left side of the body (see Figure PW6.2): lateral malleolus (d_M), greater trochanter (d_H), styloid process of the ulna (d_U), shoulder joint (d_S), vertical plane through the top of the head (d_D).

Table PW6.1 Individual results.

Subject	
W (kgf)	
h (cm)	
l (cm)	
S_1 (kgf)	
S_2 (kgf)	
d_M (cm)	
d_H (cm)	
d_U (cm)	
d_S (cm)	
d_D (cm)	
W_A (kgf)	
W_L (kgf)	
W_{THN} (kgf)	
d_{GA} (cm)	
d_{GL} (cm)	
d_{GTHN} (cm)	
M_C (kgf·cm)	
d_W (cm)	
d (cm)	

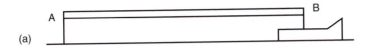

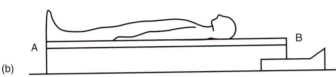

Figure PW6.1 (a) Reaction board resting horizontally with knife-edge support B resting on weighing scales. (b) Reaction board resting horizontally with knife-edge support B resting on weighing scales with subject lying on board.

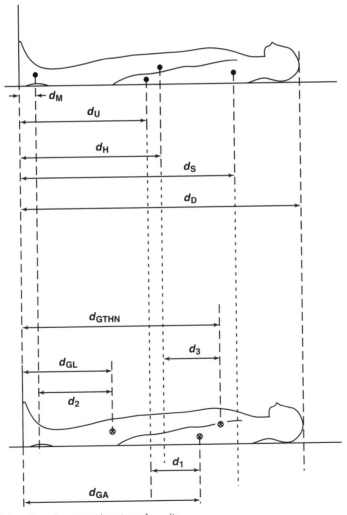

Figure PW6.2 Location of segmental centres of gravity.

Data analysis

1. Calculate the horizontal distance d between the plane of the soles of the feet and the plane containing the CG of the body by the direct method using Equation PW6.1 and record the result in Table PW6.1.

$$d \text{ (cm)} = \frac{1(S_2 - S_1)}{W}. \tag{PW6.1}$$

2. Calculate the horizontal distance dw between the plane of the soles of the feet and the plane containing the CG of the body by the indirect method (segmental analysis method):

   i. Calculate the weight (kgf) of each upper limb W_A, the weight of each lower limb W_L and the weight of the combined trunk, head and neck W_{THN}. Record the results in Table PW6.1. Use the Plagenhoef et al. (1983) data for segment weight percentages in Table 10.1 for men and Table 10.2 for women, i.e.

Men: W_A (kgf) = 0.0577 × W,
W_L (kgf) = 0.1668 × W,
W_{THN} (kgf) = 0.551 × W,

Women: W_A (kgf) = 0.0497 × W,
W_L (kgf) = 0.1843 × W,
W_{THN} (kgf) = 0.532 × W.

   ii. Calculate the moment arms, about end A of the board, of the centres of gravity of each upper limb (d_{GA}) (assume that the moment arms are the same for the left and right upper limbs), each lower limb (d_{GL}) (assume that the moment arms are the same for the left and right lower limbs) and the combined trunk, head and neck (d_{GTHN}). See Figure PW6.2. Record the results in Table PW6.1. Use the Plagenhoef et al. (1983) data for segment centre of gravity loci in Table 10.1 for men and Table 10.2 for women, i.e.

Men: d_{GA} (cm) = $d_U + d_1 = d_U + 0.50(d_S - d_U)$,
d_{GL} (cm) = $d_M + d_2 = d_M + 0.564(d_H - d_M)$,
d_{GTHN} (cm) = $d_H + d_3 = d_H + 0.434(d_D - d_H)$,

Women: d_{GA} (cm) = $d_U + d_1 = d_U + 0.514(d_S - d_U)$,
d_{GL} (cm) = $d_M + d_2 = d_M + 0.580(d_H - d_M)$,
d_{GTHN} (cm) = $d_H + d_3 = d_H + 0.397(d_D - d_H)$.

   iii. Calculate the combined moment (M_C) about end A of the board of the five segments of the body (two upper limbs, two lower limbs and combined trunk, head and neck). Record the result in Table PW6.1.

$$M_C \text{ (kgf} \cdot \text{cm)} = 2(W_A \times d_{GA}) + 2(W_L \times d_{GL}) + (W_{THN} \times d_{GTHN}).$$

iv. Calculate the moment arm of total body weight (d_W) about end A by the principle of moments. Record the result in Table PW6.1.

$$d_W \text{ (cm)} = M_C/W.$$

v. Compare d with d_W. If the anthropometric data (segmental masses and mass centre loci) used in the calculation of M_C were accurate, then d and d_W should be exactly the same. This is unlikely, since the anthropometric data were estimated from mean data obtained by volumetric analysis. Nevertheless, the anthropometric data are accurate enough for most analyses of human movement.

PRESENTATION OF RESULTS

1. Present your individual results in Table PW6.1.
2. Present the results for all of the subjects in your group and the group mean data in Table PW6.2

Table PW6.2 Individual and group results.

Subjects	h (cm)	W (kgf)	d (cm)	d as a percentage of h (%)	d_W (cm)	d_W as a percentage of h (%)	$d_W - d$ (cm)	$(d_W - d)$ as a percentage of h (%)
Women								
1.								
2.								
3.								
4.								
5.								
Mean								
SD								
Men								
1.								
2.								
3.								
4.								
5.								
Mean								
SD								

EXAMPLE RESULTS

Example data (obtained from a practical session with students) are shown in Tables PW6.3 and PW6.4. The group mean data show that the indirect result was greater than the direct result for both the women and the men by an average of 2.4 cm (1.5% of height) and 4.1 cm (2.3% of height), respectively.

Table PW6.3 Individual results.

Subject	Pamela
W (kgf)	57
h (cm)	165.8
l (cm)	198.8
S_1 (kgf)	13
S_2 (kgf)	40.5
d_M (cm)	8
d_H (cm)	86
d_U (cm)	91
d_S (cm)	139
d_D (cm)	168
W_A (kgf)	2.9
W_L (kgf)	9.2
W_{THN} (kgf)	32.8
d_{GA} (cm)	114.4
d_{GL} (cm)	52.1
d_{GTHN} (cm)	118.5
M_C (kgf·cm)	5509
d_W (cm)	96.6
d (cm)	95.9

Table PW6.4 Individual and group results.

Subjects	h (cm)	W (kgf)	d (cm)	d as a percentage of h (%)	d_w (cm)	d_w as a percentage of h (%)	$d_w - d$ (cm)	$(d_w - d)$ as a percentage of h (%)
Women								
1. Pamela	165.8	57	95.9	57.8	96.6	58.3	0.7	0.4
2. Jane	164.2	52	96.5	58.8	99	60.3	2.5	1.5
3. Susan	172	66	102.4	59.5	106.7	62	4.3	2.5
4. Sally	160.3	49	91.8	57.3	95.8	59.8	4.0	2.5
5. Fiona	155.5	55	90.4	58.1	91.1	58.6	0.7	0.5
Mean	163.6	55.8	95.4	58.3	97.8	59.8	2.4	1.5
SD	6.2	6.5	4.7	0.9	5.7	1.5	1.7	1.0
Men								
1. Stuart	169.3	68.5	91.7	54.2	96.3	56.9	4.6	2.7
2. Paul	176.5	77	103	58.4	108.9	61.7	5.9	3.3
3. John	170.2	71	99.6	58.5	100.4	59	0.8	0.5
4. Graeme	184.8	79.5	102.9	55.7	109.2	59.1	6.3	3.4
5. Richard	181.3	76	109.2	60.2	111.9	61.7	2.7	1.5
Mean	176.4	74.4	101.3	57.4	105.3	59.7	4.1	2.3
SD	6.8	4.5	6.4	2.4	6.6	2.0	2.3	1.2

Determination of take-off distance, flight distance and landing distance in a standing long jump

OBJECTIVE

1. To video a person performing a standing long jump
2. To determine the take-off distance, flight distance and landing distance components of the jump distance by analysing the video

LOCATION

Motion analysis laboratory

APPARATUS AND EQUIPMENT

Video camera and computer with appropriate video analysis software

METHOD
Subject's clothing and preparation of the subject

In the analysis of the video it is necessary to record the sagittal plane X (left to right) and Y (vertical) coordinates of the approximate positions of the following points and joints on the right side of the subject: shoulder joint, elbow joint, wrist joint, hip joint (greater trochanter), knee joint, heel and great toe. Consequently, the subject should wear tight-fitting shorts, a tight-fitting sleeveless top and shoes without socks so that the points can be easily identified and marked as shown in Figure PW7.1. The points should be marked with pieces of coloured tape of approximately 1.5 cm².

Mass and height of the subject

The mass (kg) and height (cm) of the subject are measured with the subject standing upright without shoes. The mass and height are recorded in Table PW3.1.

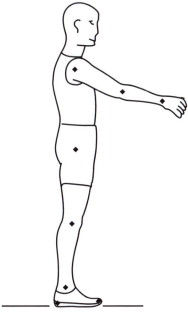

Figure PW7.1 Preparation of the subject.

Table PW7.1 Individual results.

Name of subject:
Mass of subject (kg):
Height of subject h (cm):

Coordinates of the segmental model

Segmental model	Take-off		Landing	
	X (cm)	Y (cm)	X (cm)	Y (cm)
Shoulder				
Elbow				
Wrist				
Hip				
Knee				
Ankle				
Toe, T_{TX} and T_{TY}				
Heel, H_{LX} and H_{LY}				

Table PW7.1 (continued)

Name of subject:

Mass of subject (kg):

Height of subject h (cm):

Coordinates of the whole body centre of gravity (CG)

	Take-off		Landing	
	CG_{TX} (cm)	CG_{TY} (cm)	CG_{LX} (cm)	CG_{LY} (cm)
		Distance (cm)	Distance as a proportion of D (%)	Distance as a percentage of h (%)

Jump distance $D = H_{LX} - T_{TX}$

Take-off distance $TD = CG_{TX} - T_{TX}$

Landing distance $LD = H_{LX} - CG_{LX}$

Flight distance $FD = D - TD - LD$

$CG_Y = CG_{TY} - CG_{LY}$

T_{TX}, X coordinate of toe at take-off; T_{TY}, Y coordinate of toe at take-off; H_{LX}, X coordinate of the heel on landing; H_{LY}, Y coordinate of the heel on landing; CG_{TX}, X coordinate of the whole body CG at take-off; CG_{TY}, Y coordinate of the whole body CG at take-off; CG_{LX}, X coordinate of the whole body CG on landing; CG_{LY}, Y coordinate of the whole body CG on landing.

Video recording of standing long jump

1. A white line approximately 2.5 m long is marked on the floor parallel to and approximately 1 m from a suitable vertical non-reflective background.
2. The camera is set up at a distance of approximately 10 m from the line with the optical axis of the camera perpendicular to the line and passing through the centre of the line.
3. With respect to the camera, the subject stands at the left end of the line with the line in the median plane of the subject.
4. The subject performs two or three practice trials of a standing long jump while attempting to jump along the line (left to right in relation to the camera view) and trying to maintain symmetrical movements of the arms and legs. As the subject performs the practice trials, the camera operator should observe where the subject lands and adjust the zoom of the camera to ensure that all of the movement will be visible in the recorded trials.
5. A metre stick is placed along the line with the centre of the stick over the centre of the line. The picture of the subject standing at the left end of the line ready to jump and the metre stick is recorded for 1–2 seconds. The metre stick is then removed.
6. On the command from the camera operator the subject then performs a maximal effort standing long jump, which is recorded. Two more trials are recorded with a recovery period of approximately 30 s between trials.

Video analysis

1. Using the playback facility of the motion analysis system in use, select one of the trials for analysis. The selected trial should be one in which the subject demonstrates a high level of symmetry in the movement of the arms and legs.

2. Use the origin function to set the origin for the measurement of the X and Y coordinates of points in the display to the left of and just below the feet of the subject in the stationary starting position. The location of the origin may be set automatically or manually, depending upon the motion analysis system in use.

3. Using the reference distance function, identify and record the coordinates of the left end of the metre stick followed by the right end of the metre stick. Input the reference distance, i.e. 1 m.

4. In the selected trial, identify the take-off frame, i.e. the last frame in which the right toe is still in contact with the floor before take-off. The accuracy with which this instant can be determined will depend upon the sampling frequency of the camera (the number of frames per second), but 50 Hz should be adequate.

5. In the take-off frame, digitise the following points on the subject, as in Figure PW7.2, and record the X and Y coordinates of the points in Table PW7.1.

   ■ Shoulder;
   ■ Elbow;
   ■ Wrist;
   ■ Hip;
   ■ Knee;
   ■ Ankle;
   ■ Toe.

6. In the selected trial, identify the landing frame, i.e. the frame in which the heels first make contact with the floor. The accuracy with which this instant can be determined will depend upon the sampling frequency of the camera, but 50 Hz should be adequate.

7. In the landing frame, digitise the following points on the subject, as in Figure PW7.2, and record the X and Y coordinates of the points in Table PW7.1.

   ■ Shoulder;
   ■ Elbow;
   ■ Wrist;
   ■ Hip;
   ■ Knee;
   ■ Ankle;
   ■ Heel.

555

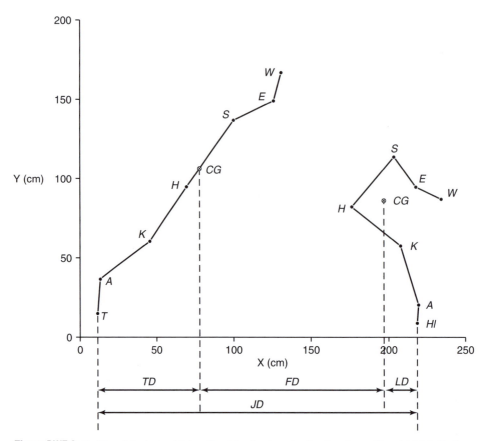

Figure PW7.2 Position of the body at take-off and landing in a standing long jump: *W*, wrist joint; *E*, elbow joint; *S*, shoulder joint; *H*, hip joint (greater trochanter); *K*, knee joint; *A*, ankle joint (lateral malleolus); *HI*, heel; *T*, great toe; *JD*, jump distance; *TD*, take-off distance; *FD*, flight distance; *LD*, landing distance; *CG*, whole body centre of gravity.

Determination of jump distance, take-off distance, flight distance, landing distance and vertical displacement of the centre of gravity in the jump

1. Use the Plagenhoef *et al.* (1993) data for segmental masses and mass centre loci (Tables 10.1 and 10.2) and the X–Y coordinate data in Table PW7.1 to determine the X–Y coordinates of the centre of gravity of the body in the take-off frame and the landing frame. Record the coordinates in Table PW7.1.
2. Use the segmental model coordinates and the centre of gravity coordinates in Table PW7.1 to determine the jump distance, take-off distance, landing distance, flight distance and vertical displacement of the centre of gravity in the jump. Record the data in Table PW7.1.

PRESENTATION OF RESULTS

1. Present your individual results in Table PW7.1.

Table PW7.2 Individual and group results.

Subjects	h (cm)	D (cm)	D_h (%)	TD (cm)	TD_D (%)	FD (cm)	FD_D (%)	LD (cm)	LD_D (%)	CGy (cm)	CGyh (%)
Women											
1.											
2.											
3.											
4.											
5.											
6.											
Mean											
SD											
Men											
1.											
2.											
3.											
4.											
5.											
6.											
Mean											
SD											

h, height; D, jump distance; D_h (%), jump distance as a percentage of h; TD, take-off distance; FD, flight distance; LD, landing distance; TD_D, take-off distance as a percentage of D; FD_D, flight distance as a percentage of D; LD_D, landing distance as a percentage of D; CGy, vertical displacement of CG at take-off relative to landing; CGyh, CGy as a percentage of h.

2. Draw a stick figure, as in Figure PW7.2, showing the position of the body and the centre of gravity of the body in the take-off and landing frames.
3. Present the results for all of the subjects in your group and the group mean data in Table PW7.2.

EXAMPLE RESULTS

Example data (obtained from a practical session with students) are shown in Tables PW7.3 and PW7.4. The stick figure corresponding to the data in Table PW7.3 is shown in Figure PW7.2. The group mean data show that the average jump distance of the men as a percentage of height (120.3%) was much greater than that of the women (96.9%). However, the average take-off, flight and landing distance components as a percentage of jump distance were similar for the men (32.6%, 54.8%, 12.6%) and women (30.2%, 56.3%, 13.6%).

Table PW7.3 Individual results.

Name of subject: Ross
Mass of subject (kg): 75.4
Height of subject h (cm): 171.5

Coordinates of the segmental model

Segmental model	Take-off		Landing	
	X (cm)	Y (cm)	X (cm)	Y (cm)
Shoulder	98.0	136.7	203.0	111.8
Elbow	123.8	148.8	216.7	93.7
Wrist	129.0	166.0	233.9	86.0
Hip	67.9	94.6	176.3	80.8
Knee	43.9	60.2	208.1	55.9
Ankle	12.0	36.1	219.3	19.8
Toe, T_{TX} and T_{TY}	11.2	14.6		
Heel, H_{LX} and H_{LY}			218.4	8.6

Coordinates of the whole body centre of gravity (CG)

	Take-off		Landing	
	CG_{TX} (cm)	CG_{TY} (cm)	CG_{LX} (cm)	CG_{LY} (cm)
	76.5	106.4	198.0	85.4

	Distance (cm)	Distance as a proportion of D (%)	Distance as a percentage of h (%)
Jump distance $D = H_{LX} - T_{TX}$	207.2	100	120.8
Take-off distance $TD = CG_{TX} - T_{TX}$	65.3	31.5	38.0
Landing distance $LD = H_{LX} - CG_{LX}$	20.4	9.8	11.9
Flight distance $FD = D - TD - LD$	121.5	58.6	70.8
$CG_Y = CG_{TY} - CG_{LY}$	21.0	10.1	12.2

T_{TX}, X coordinate of toe at take-off; T_{TY}, Y coordinate of toe at take-off; H_{LX}, X coordinate of the heel on landing; H_{LY}, Y coordinate of the heel on landing; CG_{TX}, X coordinate of the whole body CG at take-off; CG_{TY}, Y coordinate of the whole body CG at take-off; CG_{LX}, X coordinate of the whole body CG on landing; CG_{LY}, Y coordinate of the whole body CG on landing.

Table PW7.4 Individual and group results.

Subjects	h (cm)	D (cm)	D_h (%)	TD (cm)	TD_D (%)	FD (cm)	FD_D (%)	LD (cm)	LD_D (%)	CGy (cm)	$CGyh$ (%)
Women
Natalie	165.5	205.1	123.9	54.2	26.4	123.6	60.3	27.3	13.3	11.5	6.9
Pamela	165	169	102.4	54	32	94	55.6	21	12.4	11	6.7
Fiona	155.5	93.3	60	44.3	47.5	29.5	31.6	19.5	20.9	16.5	10.6
Janet	176	171	97.2	39.6	23.2	113	66.1	18.4	10.8	12.9	7.3
Hazel	172	173	100.6	50.3	29.1	99.3	57.4	23.4	13.5	21.1	12.3
Donna	176	171	97.2	39	22.8	114	66.7	18	10.5	12.9	7.3
Mean	168.3	163.7	96.9	46.9	30.2	95.6	56.3	21.3	13.6	14.3	8.5
SD	7.94	37.12	20.66	6.9	9.19	34.09	12.9	3.55	3.8	3.84	2.35
Men
Ross	171.5	207.2	120.8	65.3	31.5	121.5	58.6	20.4	9.8	21.0	12.2
Kevin	173.5	221	127.4	74	33.5	111	50.2	36	16.3	5.5	3.2
Robert	188	162	86.2	52	32.1	103	63.6	7	4.3	24	12.8
Carl	180.5	190.5	105.5	62.1	32.6	101	53	27.4	14.4	7.4	4.1
Michael	169	247	146.2	73.5	29.8	141	57.1	32.5	13.2	26.5	15.7
Nicholas	185	250.7	135.5	90.1	35.9	116.9	46.6	43.7	17.4	18.9	10.2
Mean	177.9	213.0	120.3	69.5	32.6	115.7	54.8	27.8	12.6	17.2	9.7
SD	7.73	34.01	21.61	12.96	2.05	14.66	6.14	12.88	4.84	8.75	5.01

h, height; D, jump distance; D_h (%), jump distance as a percentage of h; TD, take-off distance; FD, flight distance; LD, landing distance; TD_D, take-off distance as a percentage of D; FD_D, flight distance as a percentage of D; LD_D, landing distance as a percentage of D; CGy, vertical displacement of CG at take-off relative to landing; $CGyh$, CGy as a percentage of h

Measurement of the moment of inertia of the human body

OBJECTIVE

To measure the moment of inertia and radius of gyration of the human body about a vertical axis while in a seated position.

LOCATION

Motion analysis laboratory

APPARATUS AND EQUIPMENT

1. A turntable with a radial pointer extending from the turntable.
2. A stool that can be placed on the turntable with the vertical axis through the centre of the stool in line with the spindle of the turntable (see Figure PW8.1).
3. A pulley-based gravitational load system to apply an angular impulse to the turntable.
4. A timer linked to two sets of photocells to record the duration of the angular impulse (time for the load to descend from its starting point to the floor).
5. A timer linked to two sets of photocells defining an arc of one radian within the field of the pointer.
6. A set of weighing scales.

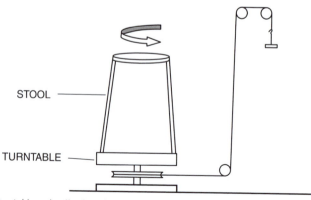

Figure PW8.1 Turntable and pulley-based gravitational load system.

METHOD

Subject's clothing

Shorts, shirt and trainers

Data collection

1. Record the mass (kg) of the subject in Table PW8.1.
2. With the stool resting on the turntable and the whole system at rest, a load is allowed to descend from its starting point to the floor. As the load descends, it applies, via the pulley system, an angular impulse to the turntable and stool about the vertical axis a_Y through the spindle of the turntable. The angular impulse generates a certain amount of angular momentum of the turntable and stool about a_Y, i.e.

$$M \cdot t = I \cdot \omega \quad \text{(Equation 10.26, where } \omega_1 = 0) \qquad \qquad \text{(PW8.1)}$$

where: F = load (N),
  d = moment arm (m) of F about a_Y,
  $M = F \cdot d$ = moment (N·m) exerted on turntable and stool about a_Y,
  t = duration (s) of angular impulse,
  I = moment of inertia (kg·m^2) of turntable and stool about a_Y,
  ω = angular velocity (rad/s) of turntable and stool about a_Y resulting from angular impulse.

3. The duration of the angular impulse t_1 is the time taken for the load to descend from rest to the floor (over a distance of about 1 m; see Figure PW8.1). After the load contacts the floor (at which point the string applying the load to the turntable disconnects from the turntable), the turntable and stool will continue to rotate about a_Y. If there is no friction around the spindle of the turntable, the turntable and stool will rotate with constant angular velocity, as angular momentum would be conserved. However, friction around the spindle will gradually reduce the speed of rotation. Consequently it is important to measure ω as soon as possible after the end of the angular impulse, i.e. after the load has contacted the floor. ω is calculated as $\omega = 1/t_2$, where t_2 is the time for the pointer to sweep through the arc of one radian after the string has disconnected from the turntable. Record F, d, t_1 and t_2 in Table PW8.1. In the example results in Table PW8.3, $F = 4.905$ N (0.5 kgf) and $d = 0.235$ m.
4. Repeat Steps 2 to 3 with the subject sitting on the stool.

Data analysis

1. Calculate the turning moment M and the impulse of the turning moment $M \cdot t_1$ for the turntable and stool and for the turntable, stool and subject. Record the results in Table PW8.1.

Table PW8.1 Individual results.

Name of subject:								
Mass of subject (kg):								
	F (N)	d (m)	M (N·m)	t_1 (s)	$M·t_1$ (N·m·s)	t_2 (s)	ω (rad/s)	I_1 (kg·m²)
Turntable and stool								
	F (N)	d (m)	M (N·m)	t_1 (s)	$M·t_1$ (N·m·s)	t_2 (s)	ω (rad/s)	I_2 (kg·m²)
Turntable, stool and subject								
		I_3 (kg·m²)				k (m)		
Subject								

2. Calculate $\omega = 1/t_2$ for the turntable and stool and for the turntable, stool and subject. Record the results in Table PW8.1.

3. Calculate the moment of inertia I_1 of the turntable and stool about a_Y and the moment of inertia I_2 of the turntable, stool and subject about a_Y from Equation PW8.1, i.e. $I = (M·t_1)/\omega$. Record the results in Table PW8.1.

4. Calculate the moment of inertia I_3 of the subject about a_Y from $I_3 = I_2 - I_1$. Record the result in Table PW8.1.

5. Calculate the radius of gyration k of the subject about a_Y from $k = \sqrt{(I_3/m)}$, where $m =$ mass of the subject. Record the result in Table PW8.1.

PRESENTATION OF RESULTS

1. Present your individual results in Table PW8.1.

2. Present the results for all of the subjects in your group and the group mean results in Table PW8.2.

EXAMPLE RESULTS

Example results are shown in Tables PW8.3 and PW8.4. The group mean results show that the average moment of inertia (I_3) and average radius of gyration (k) of the men (3.549 kg·m², 0.219 m) were very similar to those of the women (3.321 kg·m², 0.235 m), even though the average mass of the men (73.3 kg) was much greater than that of the women (60.6 kg).

Table PW8.2 Individual and group results.

Subjects	Mass (kg)	I_1 (kg·m²)	I_2 (kg·m²)	I_3 (kg·m²)	k (m)
Women					
1.					
2.					
3.					
4.					
5.					
Mean					
Standard deviation					
Men					
1.					
2.					
3.					
4.					
5.					
Mean					
Standard deviation					

Table PW8.3 Individual results.

Name of subject: Dan
Mass of subject (kg): 66.0

	F (N)	d (m)	M (N·m)	t_1 (s)	$M{\cdot}t_1$ (N·m·s)	t_2 (s)	ω (rad/s)	I_1 (kg·m²)
Turntable and stool	4.905	0.235	1.153	0.910	1.049	0.171	5.848	0.179

	F (N)	d (m)	M (N·m)	t_1 (s)	$M{\cdot}t_1$ (N·m·s)	t_2 (s)	ω (rad/s)	I_2 (kg·m²)
Turntable, stool and subject	4.905	0.235	1.153	3.751	4.325	0.826	1.210	3.571

	I_3 (kg·m²)	k (m)
Subject	3.392	0.227

Table PW8.4 Individual and group results.

Subjects	Mass (kg)	I_1 (kg·m²)	I_2 (kg·m²)	I_3 (kg·m²)	k (m)
Women					
1. Fiona	52.2	0.179	3.336	3.157	0.246
2. Jennifer	63.9	0.179	3.347	3.168	0.223
3. Natalie	59.7	0.179	3.843	3.664	0.248
4. Lynne	68.2	0.179	3.641	3.462	0.225
5. Sarah	59.1	0.179	3.333	3.154	0.231
Mean	60.6	0.179	3.500	3.321	0.235
Standard deviation	5.96	0	0.232	0.232	0.012
Men					
1. Dan	66.0	0.179	3.571	3.392	0.227
2. Stuart	69.6	0.179	3.131	2.952	0.206
3. Richard	78.2	0.179	3.650	3.471	0.211
4. Paul	74.8	0.179	4.016	3.837	0.226
5. Ross	77.9	0.179	4.270	4.091	0.229
Mean	73.3	0.179	3.728	3.549	0.219
Standard deviation	5.35	0	0.437	0.437	0.011

Determination of human power output in stair climbing and running up a slope

OBJECTIVES

To determine the power output of the human body (rate of increase in gravitational potential energy) in stair climbing and running up a slope

LOCATION, APPARATUS AND EQUIPMENT

Stair climbing

It is unlikely that a purpose-built stairway will be available, but any suitable stairway indoors or outdoors will suffice. In the test, the subject is required to run up a stairway or part of a stairway as fast as possible. The time to complete a particular number of steps, involving a certain vertical displacement of the body, is measured by a timer linked to pressure mats placed on specific steps or photocells placed at the sides of the stairway (Figure PW9.1). The average power output P_a of the body (rate of increase in gravitational potential energy) is given by

$$P_a = m \cdot g \cdot h / t, \tag{PW9.1}$$

where: m = mass of the subject (kg),
g = acceleration due to gravity = 9.81 m/s^2,
h = vertical displacement (m) of the whole body centre of gravity in time t.

For example, if m is 70 kg, the height of each step is 0.15 m, and the time to complete four steps is 0.5 s, P_a is given by

$$P_a = (70 \text{ kg} \times 9.81 \text{ m/s}^2 \times 4 \times 0.15 \text{ m})/0.5 \text{ s} = 824 \text{ W}.$$

Running up a slope

Any even slope of approximately 25 m in length that is not too steep should be suitable. In the test, the subject is required to run up the slope as fast as possible. The time to complete a particular distance up the slope, involving a certain vertical displacement of the body, is

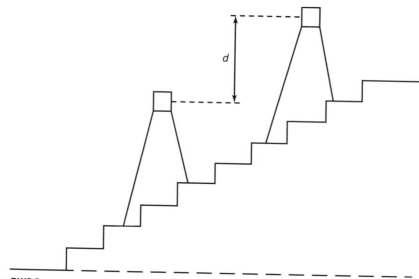

Figure PW9.1 Location of photocells in relation to stairway.

measured by a timer linked to photocells placed at the sides of the runway (Figure PW9.2). The subject begins her or his run about 5 m before the start of the test region and slows down after completing the test distance. The average power output P_a of the body (rate of increase in gravitational potential energy) is measured in the same way as in the stair climbing test. For example, if the angle of the slope is 5° and the test distance up the slope is 10 m, then the vertical displacement $h = 10 \text{ m} \times \sin 5° = 10 \text{ m} \times 0.0871 = 0.87 \text{ m}$. If the mass of the subject m is 60 kg and the time to complete the test distance is 1.8 s, then P_a is given by

$$P_a = (60 \text{ kg} \times 9.81 \text{ m/s}^2 \times 0.87 \text{ m})/1.8 \text{ s} = 284.5 \text{ W}.$$

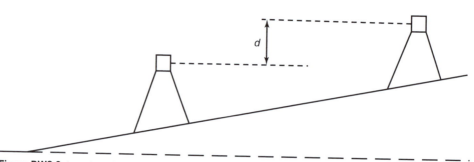

Figure PW9.2 Location of photocells in relation to slope.

METHOD

Subject's clothing

Shorts, shirt and trainers

Data collection and analysis: stair climbing

1. Ensure that each set of photocells is at the same height (approximately waist height) above the target steps.
2. Reset the timer.
3. Have the subject perform a trial, i.e. from a 5 m rolling start, the subject runs up the stairs between the sets of photocells (Figure PW9.1) as quickly as possible.
4. Record the time for the trial in Table PW9.1.
5. Repeat stages 2 to 4 for five 5 more trials.
6. Record the subject's mass (kg) in Table PW9.1.
7. Record the vertical displacement d between the photocells in Table PW9.1.
8. Calculate the average power P_a in each trial, using Equation PW9.1. Record P_a in Table PW9.1 in watts (W) and watts per kilogram of body mass (W/kg).
9. Calculate the mean and standard deviation of P_a and record the data in Table PW9.1.

Data collection and analysis: running up a slope

1. Ensure that each set of photocells is at the same height (approximately waist height) above the slope.
2. Reset the timer.
3. Have the subject perform a trial, i.e. from a 5 m rolling start, the subject runs up the slope between the sets of photocells (Figure PW9.2) as quickly as possible.
4. Record the time for the trial in Table PW9.2.

Table PW9.1 Stair climbing test.

Name of subject:
Mass (kg):
d (m):

Trial	time (s)	P_a (W)	P_a (W/kg)
1			
2			
3			
4			
5			
6			
Mean			
Standard deviation			

Table PW9.2 Running test.

Name of subject:			
Mass (kg):			
d (m):			

Trial	time (s)	P_a (W)	P_a (W/kg)
1			
2			
3			
4			
5			
6			
Mean			
Standard deviation			

5. Repeat stages 2 to 4 for five more trials.
6. Record the subject's mass (kg) in Table PW9.2.
7. Record the vertical displacement d between the photocells in Table PW9.2.
8. Calculate the average power P_a in each trial, using Equation PW9.1. Record P_a in Table PW9.2 in watts (W) and watts per kilogram of body mass (W/kg).
9. Calculate the mean and standard deviation of P_a and record the data in Table PW9.2.

Group results

1. Record the mean data for all of the subjects in your group in both tests in Table PW9.3.
2. Calculate the group mean and standard deviation for P_a for the subjects in your group in both tests and record the results in Table PW9.3.

Table PW9.3 Individual means and group mean results.

Name	Mass (kg)	Stair climbing test			Running test		
		Time (s)	Pa (W)	Pa (W/kg)	Time (s)	Pa (W)	Pa (W/kg)
1.							
2.							
3.							
4.							
5.							
Mean							
Standard deviation							

PRESENTATION OF RESULTS

1. Present your individual results for both tests, using Tables PW9.1 and PW9.2.
2. Present the group results for both tests, using Table PW9.3.

EXAMPLE RESULTS

Example results are shown in Tables PW9.4 to PW9.6. The group mean results in Table PW9.6 show that absolute average power output in the stair climbing test (846.0 W) was 2.55 times the absolute average power output in the running test (331.1 W). Even when normalised with respect to body mass, the average power output in the stair climbing test (12.03 W/kg) was 2.57 times the average power output in the running test (4.68 W/kg). In contrast, the average time in the stair climbing test (0.495 s) was 0.27 times the average time in the running test (1.824 s). These results are to be expected for two reasons:

1. When maximal effort is exerted for the duration of the exercise, the average power output of the human body is inversely proportional to the duration of the exercise, i.e. the shorter the duration of the exercise the higher the power output. These example results are consistent with the example results presented at the end of Practical Worksheet 10, which is concerned with the determination of peak power output and average power output in a vertical jump.
2. The change in gravitational potential energy in running up a slope is likely to be a much smaller proportion of the total work done by the body than when running up stairs. See the section on internal and external work in Chapter 11.

Table PW9.4 Stair climbing test*

Name of subject: John
Mass (kg): 61.7
d (m): 0.6 m

Trial	Time (s)	P_a (W)	P_a (W/kg)
1	0.528	687.8	11.14
2	0.491	739.3	11.98
3	0.453	801.3	12.98
4	0.471	770.7	12.49
5	0.484	750.0	12.15
6	0.469	774.0	12.54
Mean	0.483	753.8	12.21
Standard deviation	0.026	38.8	0.63

* Height of each step, 0.15 m: 4 steps × 0.15 m = 0.6 m. Depth of each step, 0.2 m

569

Table PW9.5 Running test*

Name of subject: John
Mass (kg): 61.7
d (m): 0.87

Trial	Time (s)	P_a (W)	P_a (W/kg)
1	1.890	278.6	4.51
2	1.864	282.5	4.58
3	1.870	281.6	4.56
4	1.902	276.9	4.49
5	1.879	280.2	4.54
6	1.877	280.5	4.55
Mean	1.880	280.0	4.54
Standard deviation	0.014	2.03	0.03

* 10 m test distance on a 5° slope: vertical displacement, 0.87 m.

Table PW9.6 Individual means and group mean results.

Name	Mass (kg)	Stair climbing test			Running test		
		Time (s)	Pa (W)	Pa (W/kg)	Time (s)	Pa (W)	Pa (W/kg)
1. John	61.7	0.483	753.8	12.21	1.880	280.0	4.54
2. James	82.1	0.565	854.9	10.42	1.901	368.5	4.49
3. Stephen	71.9	0.539	784.7	10.89	1.748	351.0	4.88
4. Callum	70.1	0.463	891.8	12.74	1.812	330.2	4.71
5. David	67.9	0.423	945.1	13.89	1.777	326.0	4.79
Mean	70.7	0.495	846.0	12.03	1.824	331.1	4.68
Standard deviation	7.43	0.06	77.9	1.40	0.07	33.3	0.16

Determination of human power output in a countermovement vertical jump

OBJECTIVES

To determine the peak power output and average power output of the human body during the upward propulsion phase of a countermovement vertical jump

LOCATION

Motion analysis laboratory

APPARATUS AND EQUIPMENT

Force platform system

METHOD

Subject's clothing

Shorts, shirt and trainers

Data collection

Record the vertical ground reaction force–time component of the subject performing a countermovement jump on a force platform.

1. Each subject should practice the jump a number of times before any trials are recorded. The jump is a countermovement jump without the use of the arms. The subject adopts a relaxed standing position on the force platform with hands on hips (to eliminate the use of the arms) and feet a shoulder width apart. The subject stands as still as possible for at least two seconds before the jump and then, in a single continuous movement, flexes the hips, knees and ankles (the countermovement) to move into a half-squat position (knee angle approximately 90°) and immediately follows the half-squat with a vertical jump for maximal height to land back on the force platform. The hands remain on the hips throughout the entire movement.

2. After two or three practice trials, two trials are recorded.
3. On a signal from the force platform system operator, the subject steps onto the platform. After the subject has adopted the start position, the system operator starts recording the vertical component of the ground reaction force at 1000 Hz. On another signal from the system operator, the subject performs a jump. When the subject regains a stationary standing position after landing, the system operator stops the recording and signals to the subject to step off the platform. After a 30 s recovery period, a second trial is recorded.
4. The trial with the longer flight time (which is likely to be associated with a higher peak power) is selected for analysis.

Data analysis

1. Data analysis will be described in relation to the example results shown in Table PW10.1 and Figure PW10.1.
2. The force–time graph of the jump should be displayed and the weight W(N) of the subject should be determined by averaging a 0.5 s section of the force–time recording during the period when the subject was standing still before the jump (see Figure PW10.1). Record the weight of the subject in an Excel spreadsheet, as shown in Table PW10.1.
3. Calculate the mass m of the subject where m(kg) $= W/9.81$. Record the subject's mass, as shown in Table PW10.1.
4. The force–time graph should be time-sliced to retain the force–time data from about 0.2 s before the start of the countermovement to just after landing. The time-sliced force–time data should be copied into the first two columns of the Excel spreadsheet, as shown in Table PW10.1. In the example results in Table PW10.1, the period of the time slice is 0.92 s (from 4.3 s to 5.2 s). With a sampling frequency of 1000 Hz, a time period of 0.92 s would require 920 rows in the Excel spreadsheet (920 $\times$ 0.001 s $= 0.92$ s). In the example results in Table PW10.1, the sampling frequency has been reduced from 1000 Hz to 50 Hz, so that the example analysis can be presented on a single page. Consequently, there are 46 rows of data (46 $\times$ 0.02 s $= 0.92$ s) in Table PW10.1. The reduction of the sampling frequency decreases the accuracy of the analysis, but peak power and average power are only reduced by about 4% compared with an analysis based on a sampling frequency of 1000 Hz.
5. The subject's weight should be copied into all of the cells in column 3 of the spreadsheet, as in Table PW10.1.
6. In column 4 of the spreadsheet, the resultant vertical force acting on the centre of gravity (CG) of the subject at each instant in time is calculated by subtracting body weight (column 3) from the vertical component of the ground reaction force (column 2). A negative resultant force indicates downward acceleration of the CG or upward deceleration of the CG. A positive resultant force indicates downward deceleration of the CG or upward acceleration of the CG.
7. In column 5 of the spreadsheet, the impulse of the resultant vertical force in each time interval is calculated by multiplying the average resultant force in the time interval by the length of the time interval. In the first time interval in Table PW10.1 (between 4.3 s and

4.32 s) the resultant force at the start of the time interval is −1.07 N. The resultant force at the end of the time interval is −1.00 N. Consequently, the average resultant force over the time interval is −1.035 N and the impulse of the average resultant force in the time interval is −1.035 N × 0.02 s = −0.0207 N·s.

8. In column 6 of the spreadsheet, the cumulative impulse of the resultant vertical force is calculated by summing the impulses in column 5 from the start to the end of the time slice. At the end of the first time interval the impulse is −0.0207 N·s, i.e. 0 + (−0.02 07) N·s = −0.0207 N·s. At the end of the second time interval (4.32 s to 4.34 s) the cumulative impulse = −0.0207 N·s + (−0.0254) N·s = −0.0461 N·s.

9. In column 7 of the spreadsheet, the cumulative vertical velocity of the CG is calculated by dividing the cumulative impulse data in column 6 by the mass of the subject. As expected, the data in column 7 show that the velocity of the CG was zero (to three decimal places) as the subject was standing still before the jump (4.3 s to 4.44 s). After the start of the coun- termovement (at 4.44 s) the CG accelerated downward (increasing downward velocity) and reached a maximum downward velocity of −1.37 m/s at 4.8 s. This was followed by a period of downward deceleration, in which the downward velocity of the CG was reduced to zero (the lowest point in the countermovement) at approximately 4.93 s. This was followed by a period of upward acceleration of the CG culminating in a maximum upward velocity of 2.85 m/s at 5.14 s and a take-off velocity of 2.65 m/s at 5.18 s (see Figure PW10.1).

10. In column 8 of the spreadsheet, the power output of the body at each instant in time from the start of movement to take-off is calculated by multiplying the ground reac- tion force by the cumulative velocity. For example, at 4.46 s the power output of the body was 762.85 N × −0.01 m/s = −7.63 W. The negative value indicates nega- tive power, i.e. the rate at which the body was losing energy (decrease in the com- bined total of gravitational potential energy, translational kinetic energy and rotational kinetic energy). The body experiences negative power during the whole of the coun- termovement; see Table PW10.1 and Figure PW10.1. The body produces positive power (rate of increase in the combined total of gravitational potential energy, trans- lational kinetic energy and rotational kinetic energy) during the whole of the period of upward propulsion (from the lowest point in the countermovement to take-off). Table PW10.1 shows that peak positive power was 4625.28 W (at 5.1 s); see Figure PW10.1.

11. The average positive power output is the average of the instantaneous power values in the period of upward propulsion. In Table PW10.1, the period of upward propulsion was from approximately 4.93 s to take-off. Consequently, the average power output was approximately 2439.6 W (the average of the instantaneous power values in the period 4.94 s to 5.18 s).

12. Peak positive power (W and W/kg), average positive power (W and W/kg), and propul- sion time (s) are recorded in Table PW10.1.

13. The weight (N), mass (kg), propulsion time (s), peak positive power (W and W/kg) and average positive power (W and W/kg) are recorded for all subjects in Table PW10.2.

Table PW10.1 Analysis of the vertical ground reaction force–time recording of the performance of a countermovement jump (hands on hips) by a young adult male sports science student (sampling frequency of the ground reaction force, 50 Hz).

Name of subject: Brian	Weight (N): 799.05	Mass (kg): 81.45
Peak positive power (W): 4625.28	Average positive power (W): 2439.6	
Peak positive power (W/kg): 56.79	Average positive power (W/kg): 29.95	
Propulsion time (s): 0.25		

Time (s)	GRF (N)	BW (N)	GRF – BW (N)	Impulse (N·s)	Cumulative impulse(N·s)	Cumulative velocity (m/s)	Power (W)
4.3	797.98	799.05	−1.07	0	0	0	0
4.32	798.05	799.05	−1	−0.0207	−0.0207	0	0
4.34	797.51	799.05	−1.54	−0.0254	−0.0461	0	0
4.36	798.78	799.05	−0.27	−0.0181	−0.0642	0	0
4.38	799.35	799.05	0.3	0.0003	−0.0639	0	0
4.4	799.39	799.05	0.34	0.0064	−0.0575	0	0
4.42	799.26	799.05	0.21	0.0055	−0.052	0	0
4.44	799.13	799.05	0.08	0.0029	−0.0491	0	0
4.46	762.85	799.05	−36.2	−0.3612	−0.4103	−0.01	−7.63
4.48	713.89	799.05	−85.16	−1.2136	−1.6239	−0.02	−14.28
4.5	654.35	799.05	−144.7	−2.2986	−3.9225	−0.05	−32.72
4.52	581.66	799.05	−217.39	−3.6209	−7.5434	−0.09	−52.35
4.54	494.14	799.05	−304.91	−5.223	−12.7664	−0.16	−79.06
4.56	382.55	799.05	−416.5	−7.2141	−19.9805	−0.25	−95.64
4.58	302.89	799.05	−496.16	−9.1266	−29.1071	−0.36	−109.04
4.6	259.49	799.05	−539.56	−10.3572	−39.4643	−0.48	−124.56
4.62	258.75	799.05	−540.3	−10.7986	−50.2629	−0.62	−160.43
4.64	320.22	799.05	−478.83	−10.1913	−60.4542	−0.74	−236.96
4.66	328.37	799.05	−470.68	−9.4951	−69.9493	−0.86	−282.4
4.68	372.26	799.05	−426.79	−8.9747	−78.924	−0.97	−361.09
4.7	412.75	799.05	−386.3	−8.1309	−87.0549	−1.07	−441.64
4.72	440.17	799.05	−358.88	−7.4518	−94.5067	−1.16	−510.6
4.74	520.03	799.05	−279.02	−6.379	−100.8857	−1.24	−644.84
4.76	541.43	799.05	−257.62	−5.3664	−106.2521	−1.3	−703.86
4.78	654.22	799.05	−144.83	−4.0245	−110.2766	−1.35	−883.2
4.8	777.3	799.05	−21.75	−1.6658	−111.9424	−1.37	−1064.9
4.82	988.94	799.05	189.89	1.6814	−110.261	−1.35	−1335.07
4.84	1303.28	799.05	504.23	6.9412	−103.3198	−1.27	−1655.17
4.86	1643.57	799.05	844.52	13.4875	−89.8323	−1.1	−1807.93
4.88	1970.25	799.05	1171.2	20.1572	−69.6751	−0.86	−1694.42
4.9	2175.1	799.05	1376.05	25.4725	−44.2026	−0.54	−1174.55
4.92	2233.01	799.05	1433.96	28.1001	−16.1025	−0.2	−446.6
4.94	2180.73	799.05	1381.68	28.1564	12.0539	0.15	327.11
4.96	2095.19	799.05	1296.14	26.7782	38.8321	0.48	1005.69

Table PW10.1 (continued)

Name of subject: Brian   Weight (N): 799.05   Mass (kg): 81.45
Peak positive power (W): 4625.28   Average positive power (W): 2439.6
Peak positive power (W/kg): 56.79   Average positive power (W/kg): 29.95
Propulsion time (s): 0.25

Time (s)	GRF (N)	BW (N)	GRF – BW (N)	Impulse (N·s)	Cumulative impulse(N·s)	Cumulative velocity (m/s)	Power (W)
4.98	2032.53	799.05	1233.48	25.2962	64.1283	0.79	1605.7
5	1971.18	799.05	1172.13	24.0561	88.1844	1.08	2128.87
5.02	1938.57	799.05	1139.52	23.1165	111.3009	1.37	2655.84
5.04	1907.75	799.05	1108.7	22.4822	133.7831	1.64	3128.71
5.06	1889.94	799.05	1090.89	21.9959	155.779	1.91	3609.79
5.08	1887.42	799.05	1088.37	21.7926	177.5716	2.18	4114.58
5.1	1887.87	799.05	1088.82	21.7719	199.3435	2.45	4625.28
5.12	1715.98	799.05	916.93	20.0575	219.401	2.69	4615.99
5.14	1158.97	799.05	359.92	12.7685	232.1695	2.85	3303.06
5.16	210.71	799.05	−588.34	−2.2842	229.8853	2.82	594.2
5.18	0	799.05	−799.05	−13.8739	216.0114	2.65	0
5.2	0	799.05	−799.05	−15.981	200.0304	2.45	0

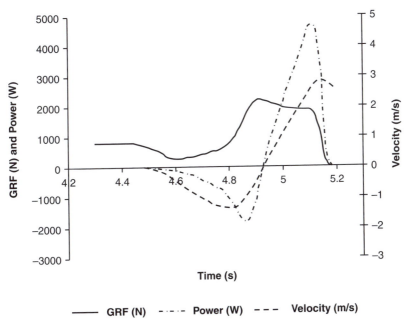

GRF (N)   - · - · - Power (W)   - - - Velocity (m/s)

Figure PW10.1 Vertical ground reaction force–time graph and corresponding vertical velocity–time and vertical power–time graphs of the performance of a countermovement jump (hands on hips) by a young adult male sports science student (data in Table PW10.1).

Table PW10.2 Individual and group results for peak and average power output in a countermovement jump (hands on hips) for 12 young adult male sports science students (sampling frequency of the ground reaction force, 1000 Hz).

Subjects	Weight (N)	Mass (kg)	Propulsion time (s)	Peak power		Average power	
				(W)	(W/kg)	(W)	(W/kg)
1. Brian	799.05	81.45	0.238	4817.81	59.15	2719.07	33.38
2. Leo	694.76	70.82	0.263	3279.73	46.31	1817.93	25.67
3. Sam	849.04	86.55	0.29	3619.15	41.82	2089.87	24.15
4. David	752.72	76.73	0.321	3856.25	50.26	2106.81	27.46
5. Bruce	658.64	67.14	0.235	3878.91	57.77	2235.51	33.3
6. Ieuan	809.72	82.54	0.277	4205.56	50.95	2059.7	24.95
7. Charlie	954.71	97.32	0.296	4304.28	44.23	2415.69	24.82
8. Jack	1083.61	110.46	0.258	3033.12	27.46	1661.11	15.04
9. Chris	877.9	89.49	0.23	4352.34	48.63	2355.05	26.32
10. George	830.81	84.69	0.261	4205.47	49.66	2254.35	26.62
11. Kevin	672.18	68.52	0.286	3479.37	50.78	1899.25	27.72
12. Ben	809.23	82.49	0.301	4282.45	51.91	2100.63	25.47
Mean	816.03	83.18	0.27	3942.87	48.24	2142.91	26.24
Standard deviation	115.66	11.79	0.03	492.93	7.83	271.16	4.46

PRESENTATION OF RESULTS

1. Present your individual force–time analysis as shown in Table PW10.1.
2. Present your individual force–time, velocity–time and power–time graphs as shown in Figure PW10.1.
3. Present your individual and group results as shown in Table PW10.2.

EXAMPLE RESULTS

Example results are shown in Tables PW10.1 and 10.2 and Figure PW10.1. Table PW10.2 shows that the group mean propulsion time was 0.27 s, the group mean peak power was 3942.87 W and 48.24 W/kg and group mean average power was 2142.91 W and 26.24 W/kg. The results for average power are consistent with the example results for average power in stair climbing and running up a slope presented at the end of Practical Worksheet 9, i.e. the shorter the period of maximal effort, the higher the average power output.

Answers to review questions (involving calculations)

CHAPTER 8

6. From Table 8.2:

    1 m/s = 2.2369 mph, i.e. 150 m/s = 150 × 2.2369 mph = 335.5 mph,

    1 mph = 1.609 34 km/h, i.e. 10 mph = 10 × 1.609 34 km/h = 16.0934 km/h,

    1 km/h = 0.277 78 m/s, i.e. 25 km/h = 25 × 0.277 78 m/s = 6.94 m/s.

CHAPTER 9

Linear kinematics

3. **Table 9A.1** Average speed in laps 1 and 2 and in whole race.

Lap	Time (s)	Distance (m)	Average speed (m/s)
1	56.0	400	7.14
2	52.0	400	7.69
Total time (s)	108.0	800	7.41

4. **Table 9A.2** Leg length and stride parameters at 3.5 m/s and 5.5 m/s.

Leg length (m)	Speed (m/s)	Time for 10 strides (s)	Stride rate (strides /s)	Stride length (m/stride)	Relative stride length
0.9	3.5	6.94	1.44	2.43	2.70
0.9	5.5	5.80	1.72	3.20	3.55

5.1a. **Table 9A.3** Distance, time and average speed for winner of women's race in different units.

Distance	Time	Average speed
26.219 miles (m)	2.389 hours (h)	10.974 mph
42.195 kilometres (km)	2.389 hours (h)	17.662 km/h
42 195 metres (m)	8601 seconds (s)	4.905 m/s

5.1b. **Table 9A.4** Distance, time and average speed for winner of men's race in different units.

Distance	Time	Average speed
26.219 miles (m)	2.132 hours (h)	12.298 mph
42.195 kilometres (km)	2.132 hours (h)	19.791 km/h
42 195 metres (m)	7676 seconds (s)	5.497 m/s

5.2 Average speed of the winner of women's race v_w = 4.905 m/s.
Average speed of the winner of men's race v_m = 5.497 m/s.
v_w as a percentage of v_m = 89.23% (4.905 / 5.497 × 100).

5.3 **Table 9A.5** Average time per mile and average time per kilometre for the winner of the women's race and the men's race.

	Distance (miles)	Distance (km)	Winner's time (min)	Per mile (min)	Per km (min)
Women's race	26.219	42.195	143.35	5.47	3.40
Men's race	26.219	42.195	127.93	4.88	3.03

Linear impulse and linear momentum

6. **Table 9A.6** Units and unit abbreviations.

Variable	Unit	Unit symbol
Force	newton	N
Time	second	s
Impulse	newton second	N·s
Mass	kilogram	kg
Velocity	metres per second	m/s or m·s^{-1}
Linear momentum	kilogram metres per second	kg·m/s or kg·m·s^{-1}

7. m = 0.35 kg, v_1 = 0, v_2 = 42 m/s, t = 0.05 s, F = average force exerted on ball.

$$F = \frac{m(v-u)}{t} = \frac{0.35 \times (42-0)}{0.05} = 294 \text{ N}$$

$$= 29.97 \text{ kgf} = 66.07 \text{ lbf.}$$

8. m = 0.06 kg, v_1 = 0, v_2 = 72 m/s, t = 0.0005 s, F = average force exerted on ball.

$$F = \frac{m(v-u)}{t} = \frac{0.06 \times (72-0)}{0.0005} = 8640 \text{ N}$$

$$= 880.73 \text{ kgf} = 1941.66 \text{ lbf} = 0.87 \text{ tons.}$$

9. Impulse $F \cdot t = 159.72$ N·s, $m = 7.26$ kg, $v =$ release velocity of shot.

$F \cdot t = m \cdot v$, i.e.

$$v = \frac{F \cdot t}{m} = \frac{159.72}{7.26} = 22 \text{ m/s.}$$

10. It is necessary to adopt a convention for positive and negative since the vertical component R_V of the braking force (vertical component of the ground reaction force) is in the opposite direction to that of the vertical component of the velocity v_1 of the gymnast on landing. Since it is necessary to calculate R, let upward be positive and downward negative.

R (acting upward) $=$ average magnitude of the ground reaction force during landing,
$W =$ body weight (acting downward),
$v_1 = 6.2$ m/s (downward),
$v_2 = 0$,
$t = 0.2$ s

$F = \dfrac{m(v - u)}{t}$, where F is the resultant upward force acting on the body during landing,

$F = R - W$,

i.e. $R - W = \dfrac{m(v_2 - v_1)}{t} = \dfrac{55 \times (0 - (-6.2))}{0.2} = \dfrac{55 \times 6.2}{0.2} = 1705 \text{ N,}$

i.e. $R = 1705$ N $+ W$.
Since $W = 55$ kgf $= 539.5$ N,
then $R = 1705$ N $+ 539.5$ N $= 2244.5$ N $= 228.8$ kgf $= 504.4$ lbf $= 4.16$ BW.

Vectors

13. $a/c = \sin 40°$, i.e. $a = c \cdot \sin 40° = 20$ cm $\times 0.643 = 12.86$ cm,
    $b/c = \cos 40°$, i.e. $b = c \cdot \cos 40° = 20$ cm $\times 0.766 = 15.32$ cm.

14. $A/F = \cos 40°$, i.e. $A = F \cdot \cos 40° = 200$ N $\times 0.766 = 153.2$ N,
    $B/F = \cos 50°$, i.e. $B = F \cdot \cos 50° = 200$ N $\times 0.643 = 128.6$ N.

15. $T/B = \cos 30°$, i.e. $T = B \cdot \cos 30° = 100$ N $\times 0.866 = 86.6$ N,
    $S/B = \sin 30°$, i.e. $S = B \cdot \sin 30° = 100$ N $\times 0.5 = 50.0$ N.

16. i. Magnitude of F_{XY}:

$F_{XY}^2 = F_X^2 + F_Y^2 = 0.64 + 6.25 = 6.89,$

i.e. $F_{XY} = 2.625$ BW.

Direction of F_{XY} with respect to horizontal: angle α

$\cos \alpha = F_X/F_{XY} = 0.8 / 2.625 = 0.3047$,

i.e. $\alpha = 72.2°$.

16. ii. Magnitude of F_{YZ}:

$F_{YZ}^2 = F_Y^2 + F_Z^2 = 6.25 + 0.16 = 6.41$,

i.e. $F_{YZ} = 2.532$ BW.

Direction of F_{YZ} with respect to horizontal: angle β:

$\cos \beta = F_Z/F_{YZ} = 0.4 / 2.532 = 0.1524$,

i.e. $\beta = 80.9°$.

16. iii. Magnitude of F_{XZ}:

$F_{XZ}^2 = F_X^2 + F_Z^2 = 0.64 + 0.16 = 0.8$,

i.e. $F_{XZ} = 0.894$ BW.

Direction of F_{XZ} with respect to F_Z: angle θ:

$\cos \theta = F_Z/F_{XZ} = 0.4 / 0.894 = 0.4474$,

i.e. $\theta = 63.4°$.

16. iv. Magnitude of F:

$F^2 = F_Y^2 + F_{XZ}^2 = 6.25 + 0.7992 = 7.049$,

i.e. $F = 2.655$ BW.

Direction of F with respect to F_{XZ}: angle δ

$\cos \delta = F_{XZ}/F = 0.894 / 2.655 = 0.3367$

i.e. $\delta = 70.32°$.

17. **Table 9A.7** Magnitude and direction of F_X, F_Y and F_{XY}

	Frame 2	Frame 4
F_X (BW)	−0.58	+0.42
F_Y (BW)	+2.22	+2.7
F_{XY} (BW)	2.29	2.73
F_{XY} (°)	75.3	81.2

18. ii. L_V and L_H: vertical and horizontal components of L,
F_V and F_H: vertical and horizontal components of F,
M_V and M_H: vertical and horizontal components of M.

All the vertical components are upward and therefore positive.
Since horizontal components to the left will counteract horizontal components to the right, it is necessary to regard horizontal components to the left as negative and all horizontal components to the right as positive.

$L_V = L \cdot \sin 70° = 50 \times 0.9396 = 46.98$ N,

$$L_H = L \cdot \cos 70° = 50 \times 0.342 = -17.10 \text{ N},$$
$$F_V = F \cdot \sin 84° = 100 \times 0.9945 = 99.45 \text{ N},$$
$$F_H = F \cdot \cos 84° = 100 \times 0.1045 = -10.45 \text{ N},$$
$$M_V = M \cdot \sin 60° = 56.5 \times 0.866 = 48.93 \text{ N},$$
$$M_H = M \cdot \cos 60° = 56.5 \times 0.5 = 28.25 \text{ N}.$$

Vertical component Q_V of the resultant quadriceps force
$$Q = 46.98 + 99.45 + 48.93 = 195.36 \text{ N}.$$

Horizontal component Q_H of the resultant quadriceps force
$$Q = -17.10 - 10.45 + 28.25 = +0.7 \text{ N}.$$

Resultant quadriceps force $Q = 195.36$ N, at an angle of $89.85°$ (upward and slightly to the right in Figure 9Q.6).

Ground reaction force

20. **Table 9A.8** Analysis of vertical component (F_Y–time) of ground reaction force acting on right foot of subject during contact time in running.

Name of subject:

	Mass (kg)	Weight (N)	
Mass and weight of subject	70	686.7	
Key points on F_Y–time graph	Time (s)	Force (N)	Force (BW)
1. Heel contact (t_1, F_{Y1})	0	0	0
2. Impact force peak (t_2, F_{Y2})	0.0264	1022.4	1.489
3. End of the passive phase (minimum force following impact force peak) (t_3, F_{Y3})	0.0422	649.1	0.945
4. End of absorption phase (t_4, F_{Y4}) (when $F_X = 0$)	0.1217	1384.8	2.017
5. Toe-off (t_5, F_{Y5})	0.2650	0	0
	Time (s)	Proportion of contact time (%)	
6. Contact time $(t_5 - t_1)$	0.2650	100	
7. Time to impact force peak $(t_2 - t_1)$	0.0264	9.96	
8. Duration of passive phase $(t_3 - t_1)$	0.0422	15.92	
9. Duration of absorption phase $(t_4 - t_1)$	0.1217	45.92	
10. Duration of propulsion phase $(t_5 - t_4)$	0.1433	54.08	
	L_R (N/s)	L_R (BW/s)	
Rate of loading (L_R) during impact ($F_{Y2}/(t_2 - t_1)$)	38 727.2	56.40	

Uniformly accelerated motion

21. i. Vertical displacement of the centre of gravity from take-off to maximum height s_f:
Consider vertical motion from take-off to maximum height.

From $v^2 - u^2 = 2a \cdot s$,

where: u = vertical velocity at take-off = 4.2 m/s,
v = vertical velocity at maximum height = 0,
$a = -9.81$ m/s^2,
$s = s_f$ = flight height,

i.e.   flight height $s_f = \dfrac{(v^2 - u^2)}{2a} = \dfrac{(0 - 17.64)}{-19.62} = 0.90$ m.

21. ii. Time from take-off to maximum height t_f:
Consider vertical motion from take-off to maximum height.

From $v = u + a \cdot t$,

where: u = vertical velocity at take-off = 4.2 m/s,
v = vertical velocity at maximum height = 0,
$a = -9.81$ m/s^2,
t = time from take-off to maximum height.

i.e.   time to maximum height $t_f = \dfrac{(v - u)}{a} = \dfrac{(0 - 4.2)}{-9.81} = 0.43$ s.

22. Consider vertical motion from take-off to maximum height.
Step 1: Calculate take-off velocity v_0

Impulse $I = m \cdot v - m \cdot u$,
where: $I = 246$ N $\cdot$ s,
m = mass of jumper = 60 kg,
u = upward velocity at start of propulsion phase = 0,
$v = v_0$,
i.e. $v_0 = I/m = 246/60 = 4.1$ m/s.

Step 2: Calculate flight height s_f

From $v^2 - u^2 = 2a \cdot s$,
where: $u = v_0 = 4.1$ m/s,
v = vertical velocity at maximum height = 0
$a = -9.81$ m/s^2,
$s = s_f$,

i.e. $s_f = \dfrac{(v^2 - u^2)}{2a} = \dfrac{(0 - 16.81)}{-19.62} = 0.86$ m.

23. Step 1: Calculate fall time t_d

From $\quad s = ut + \dfrac{a \cdot t^2}{2}$,

where: $\quad s = $ fall distance $= 150$ m,

$\qquad u = 0$,

$\qquad a = 9.81$ m/s^2,

$\qquad t = t_d$,

i.e. $\quad 150 = 0 + \dfrac{(9.81 \times t_d^2)}{2}$

$\qquad t_d^2 = \dfrac{300}{9.81} = 30.58$

$\qquad t_d = 5.53$ s.

Step 2: Calculate the velocity of the stone on impact with the ground v_d

From $\quad v = u + a \cdot t$,

where: $\quad u = 0$,

$\qquad v = v_d$,

$\qquad a = 9.81$ m/s^2,

$\qquad t = 5.53$ s,

i.e. $\quad v_d = 0 + 9.81 \times 5.53 = 54.25$ m/s.

24. Step 1: Calculate flight time t_f

Flight time t_f can be found in three steps by finding the time from release to maximum height t_1, the vertical displacement from release to maximum height and the time from maximum height to landing t_2. $t_f = t_1 + t_2$. Flight time t_f can also be found in one step using

$$s = ut + \dfrac{a \cdot t^2}{2},$$

where: $\quad s = -2$ m (the landing point is 2 m below the release point),

$\qquad u = $ release velocity $= 10$ m/s,

$\qquad a = -9.81$ m/s^2,

$\qquad t = t_f$,

i.e. $\quad -2 = 10 \times t_f - 4.905 \times t_f^2$

and $\quad 4.905 \times tf^2 - 10 \times tf - 2 = 0.$ 　　　　　　　Eq. 1

This form of equation, $ax^2 + bx + c$, where a, b and c are constants and x is variable, is called a quadratic equation. A quadratic equation can be solved, i.e. the value of x can be found, by using the following formula:

$$x = \dfrac{-b \pm \sqrt{(b^2 - 4ac)}}{2a}.$$

In Equation 1, $a = 4.905$, $b = -10$, $c = -2$,

i.e. $\quad t_f = \dfrac{-(-10) \pm \sqrt{((-10)^2 - 4 \times 4.905 \times (-2))}}{9.81}$

583

$$t_f = \frac{10 \pm \sqrt{(100 + 39.24)}}{9.81} = \frac{10 \pm 11.8}{9.81}.$$

Clearly, the negative alternative for the term 10 ± 11.8 (resulting in -1.8) cannot be correct. Consequently, the positive alternative is taken, i.e. $10 + 11.8 = 21.8$,

i.e. $t_f = \dfrac{21.8}{9.81} = 2.222$ s.

Step 2: Calculate the velocity v_i of the ball at each time interval t_i

Use $\quad v = u + a \cdot t$,

where: $\quad v = v_i = $ velocity at time t_i,

$u = 10$ m/s,

$a = -9.81$ m/s^2,

$t = t_i$.

For example, at $t_i = 0.2$ s,

$v_i = 10 + ((-9.81) \times 0.2) = 10 - 1.962 = 8.038$ m/s.

Similarly, for $t_i = 0.4$ s,

$v_i = 10 + ((-9.81) \times 0.4) = 10 - 3.924 = 6.076$ m/s,

and for $t_i = 2.222$ s (landing),

$v_i = 10 + ((-9.81) \times 2.222) = 10 - 21.799 = -11.799$ m/s.

The velocity data are shown in Table 9Q.1.

Table 9A.9 Displacement and velocity of ball thrown upward with release velocity of 10 m/s from release height of 2 m.

Time into flight (s)	Velocity (m/s)	Displacement (m)
0	10.0	2.0
0.2	8.038	3.804
0.4	6.076	5.215
0.6	4.114	6.234
0.8	2.152	6.860
1.0	0.190	7.095
1.2	-1.772	6.937
1.4	-3.734	6.386
1.6	-5.696	5.443
1.8	-7.658	4.108
2.0	-9.620	2.380
2.2	-11.582	0.260
2.222	-11.799	0.003

Step 3: Calculate the displacement s_i of the ball at each time interval t_i

At any point after release, the displacement of the stone s_i is given by $s_i = s_0 + s_r$ where s_0 is the vertical displacement at release, which is 2 m and s_r is the displacement from the release point.

s_r can be calculated by using $s = ut + \dfrac{a \cdot t^2}{2}$.

For example, at $t_i = 0.2$ s, the displacement of the ball from the release point can be calculated as follows:

s_r = displacement of stone from release point,
$u = 10$ m/s,
$a = -9.81$ m/s^2,
$t_i = 0.2$ s,

i.e. $s_r = (10 \times 0.2) + \dfrac{((-9.81) \times 0.2^2)}{2}$

$= 2 - 0.196 = 1.804$ m.

As $s_i = s_0 + s_r$ then $s_i = 2$ m $+ 1.804$ m $= 3.804$ m.

Similarly, for $t_i = 0.4$ s,

$s_r = (10 \times 0.4) + \dfrac{((-9.81) \times 0.4^2)}{2}$

$= 4 - 0.785 = 3.215$ m.

and $s_i = 2$ m $+ 3.215$ m $= 5.315$ m.

For $t_i = 2.222$ s (landing),

$s_r = (10 \times 2.222) + \dfrac{((-9.81) \times 2.222^2)}{2}$

$= 22.22 - 24.217 = -1.997$ m

and $s_i = 2$ m $+ (-1.997)$ m $= 0.003$ m (i.e. at ground level).

The displacement data are shown in Table 9A.9.

25. Step 1: Calculate the vertical v_v and horizontal v_h components of release velocity v_0

$v_v = v_0 \cdot \sin \alpha$ and $v_h = v_0 \cdot \cos \alpha$ where $v_0 = 12.5$ m/s and $\alpha = 38°$.
i.e. $v_v = 7.69$ m/s and $v_h = 9.85$ m/s.

Step 2: Calculate flight time t_f
Consider vertical motion during flight:

$s = ut + \dfrac{a \cdot t^2}{2}$,

where: $s = -2.1$ m (the landing point is 2.1 m below the release point),
$u = v_v = 7.69$ m/s,
$a = -9.81$ m/s^2,
$t = t_f$,

i.e. $-2.1 = 7.69 \times t_f - 4.905 \times t_f^2$,

i.e. $4.905 \times t_f^2 - 7.69 \times t_f - 2.1 = 0$.

Calculate t_f by application of the formula for solving a quadratic equation.

i.e. $x = \dfrac{-b \pm \sqrt{(b^2 - 4ac)}}{2a}$

585

where: $a = 4.905, b = -7.69, c = -2.1,$

i.e. $t_f = \dfrac{-(-7.69) \pm \sqrt{((-7.69)^2 - 4 \times 4.905 \times (-2.1))}}{9.81}$

$$t_f = \frac{7.69 \pm \sqrt{(59.14 + 41.20)}}{9.81} = \frac{7.69 \pm 10.02}{9.81}.$$

Clearly, the negative alternative for the term 7.69 ± 10.02 (resulting in -2.33) cannot be correct. Consequently the positive alternative is taken, i.e. $7.69 + 10.02 = 17.71,$

i.e. $t_f = \dfrac{17.71}{9.81} = 1.805$ s.

Step 3: Calculate range s_r

Consider horizontal motion during flight:

$$s = ut + \frac{a \cdot t^2}{2},$$

where: $s = s_r,$
$u = v_h = 9.85$ m/s,
$t = 1.805$ s,
$a = 0.$

i.e.   range $s_r = (9.85 \times 1.805) + 0 = 17.78$ m.

Step 4: Calculate maximum height s_m

Consider vertical motion from release to maximum height:

$$s_m = s_0 + s_f,$$

where $s_0 =$ release height $= 2.1$ m

and $s_f =$ vertical displacement between release and maximum height.

From $v^2 - u^2 = 2a \cdot s,$

$$s_f = \frac{(v^2 - u^2)}{2a},$$

where: $s = s_f,$
$u = v_v = 7.69$ m/s,
$v =$ velocity at maximum height $= 0,$
$a = -9.81$ m/s^{2,}

i.e. $s_f = \dfrac{(0 - 7.69^2)}{-19.62} = 3.01$ m,

i.e.   maximum height $s_m = s_0 + s_f = 2.1$ m $+ 3.01$ m $= 5.11$ m.

Step 5: Calculate the impulse responsible for release velocity:

$$I = m{\cdot}v - m{\cdot}u,$$

where: $I =$ impulse,

m = mass of shot = 7.26 kg,

v = release velocity = 12.5 m/s,

u = 0,

i.e.   impulse I = (7.26 × 12.5) − 0 = 90.75 N·s.

CHAPTER 10

Moment of a force and levers

2. In equilibrium,

$$CM = ACM, \text{ i.e. } W_B \cdot d_B = W_A \cdot d_A$$

$$W_B = \frac{(W_A \cdot d_A)}{d_B} = \frac{(45 \text{ kgf} \times 3 \text{ m})}{3.75 \text{ m}} = 36 \text{ kgf.}$$

3. From Equation 10.5,

$$d_2 = \frac{I \times (S_2 - S_1)}{W_S} = \frac{2.5 \text{ m} \times (42 \text{ kgf} - 10 \text{ kgf})}{80 \text{ kgf}} = 1.0 \text{ m};$$

$$\frac{d}{h} = \frac{1.0 \text{ m}}{1.8 \text{ m}} \times 100 = 55.5 \%.$$

4. In equilibrium,

$$CM = ACM, \text{ i.e. } R \cdot d_R = E \cdot d_E$$

$$R = \frac{(E \cdot d_E)}{d_R} = \frac{(20 \text{ kgf} \times 25 \text{ cm})}{7 \text{ cm}} = 71.4 \text{ kgf.}$$

5. In equilibrium,

$$CM = ACM, \text{ i.e. } E \cdot d_E = R \cdot d_R$$

$$E = \frac{(R \cdot d_R)}{d_E} = \frac{(40 \text{ kgf} \times 7 \text{ cm})}{25 \text{ cm}} = 11.2 \text{ kgf.}$$

The minimum force required to lift lid further is $E > 11.2$ kgf.

6. In equilibrium,

$$CM = ACM, \text{ i.e. } A \cdot d_A = W \cdot d_W$$

$$A = \frac{(W \cdot d_W)}{d_A},$$

i.e. A_1 = 16.9 kgf, A_2 = 38.1 kgf, A_3 = 47.8 kgf.

7. In equilibrium,

$CM = ACM$, i.e. $W{\cdot}d_W = F{\cdot}d_F$

$$F = \frac{(W \cdot d_W)}{d_F} = \frac{5 \text{ kgf} \times 2.5 \text{ cm}}{7.5 \text{ cm}} = 1.67 \text{ kgf.}$$

In equilibrium, $J - F - W = 0$,
i.e. $J = F + W = 5 \text{ kgf} + 1.67 \text{ kgf} = 6.67 \text{ kgf.}$

8. In equilibrium,

$CM = ACM$, i.e. $W{\cdot}d_W = F{\cdot}d_F$

$$F = \frac{(W \cdot d_W)}{d_F} = \frac{5 \text{ kgf} \times 4.5 \text{ cm}}{7.5 \text{ cm}} = 3 \text{ kgf.}$$

In equilibrium, horizontal forces:

$J_H - F_H = 0$
$J_H = F_H$
$J_H = F{\cdot}\cos45° = 3 \text{ kgf} \times 0.7071 = 2.12 \text{ kgf.}$

In equilibrium, vertical forces:

$J_V - F_V - W = 0$
$J_V = F_V + W$
$J_V = F{\cdot}\sin45° + W$
$J_V = 3 \text{ kgf} \times 0.7071 + 5 \text{ kgf}$
$J_V = 2.12 \text{ kgf} + 5 \text{ kgf} = 7.12 \text{ kgf.}$

Calculate J:

$J^2 = J_V^2 + J_H^2 = (7.12^2 + 2.12^2)\text{kgf}^2$
$J^2 = 55.19 \text{ kgf}^2$
$J = 7.43 \text{ kgf.}$

If J makes an angle of θ with respect to the horizontal, then:

$\tan\theta = J_V/J_H = 7.12 / 2.12 = 3.358,$
$\theta = 73.4°.$

9. In equilibrium,

$CM = ACM$, i.e. $W{\cdot}d_W = A{\cdot}d_A$

$$A = \frac{(W \cdot d_W)}{d_A} = \frac{60 \text{ kgf} \times 12 \text{ cm}}{7 \text{ cm}} = 102.86 \text{ kgf.}$$

$A_H = A{\cdot}\cos80° = 17.86 \text{ kgf}$
$A_V = A{\cdot}\sin80° = 101.30 \text{ kgf.}$

In equilibrium, horizontal forces:

$$J_H - A_H = 0$$
$$J_H = A_H = 17.86 \text{ kgf.}$$

In equilibrium, vertical forces:

$$J_V - A_V - W = 0$$
$$J_V = A_V + W = 161.3 \text{ kgf}$$

Calculate J:

$$J = \sqrt{(J_V^2 + J_H^2)} = 162.3 \text{ kgf.}$$

If J makes an angle of θ with respect to the horizontal, then

$$\tan\theta = J_V/J_H = 162.3 / 17.86 = 9.087;$$
$$\theta = 83.7°.$$

10. In equilibrium,

$$CM = ACM, \text{ i.e. } L \cdot d_L = W \cdot d_W,$$
$$d_W = d \cdot \cos30° = 20 \text{ cm} \times 0.8660 = 17.32 \text{ cm},$$

$$L = \frac{(W \cdot d_W)}{d_L} = \frac{4.5 \text{ kgf} \times 17.32 \text{ cm}}{4 \text{ cm}} = 19.48 \text{ kgf.}$$

$$L_H = L \cdot \cos47° = 13.28 \text{ kgf,}$$
$$L_V = L \cdot \sin47° = 14.25 \text{ kgf,}$$

In equilibrium, horizontal forces:

$$L_H - T_H = 0,$$
$$T_H = L_H = 13.28 \text{ kgf.}$$

In equilibrium, vertical forces:

$$L_V - T_V - W = 0,$$
$$T_V = L_V - W = 9.75 \text{ kgf.}$$

Calculate T:

$$T = \sqrt{(T_V^2 + T_H^2)} = 16.47 \text{ kgf.}$$

If T makes an angle of θ with respect to the horizontal, then:

$$\tan\theta = T_V/T_H = 9.75 / 13.28 = 0.7342;$$
$$\theta = 36.3°.$$

11. i. Calculate the magnitude of P and L
    In equilibrium, $CM = ACM$ about J:

$$R \cdot d_R = A \cdot d_A + L \cdot d_L + P \cdot d_P$$

$$P \cdot d_P = R \cdot d_R - A \cdot d_A - L \cdot d_L$$
$$P \cdot d_P = R \cdot d_R - A \cdot d_A - 2P \cdot d_L$$
$$P \cdot d_P + 2P \cdot d_L = R \cdot d_R - A \cdot d_A$$
$$P(d_P + 2d_L) = R \cdot d_R - A \cdot d_A$$

$$P = \frac{R \cdot d_R - A \cdot d_A}{d_P + 2d_L} \qquad \text{Eq. 1}$$

where: $d_R = d_3 \cdot \sin 80° = 60$ cm × 0.9848 = 59.09 cm
$\quad\quad d_A = d_2 = 29$ cm
$\quad\quad d_P = d_1 \cdot \sin 20° = 10$ cm × 0.3420 = 3.42 cm
$\quad\quad d_L = d_1 \cdot \sin 55° = 10$ cm × 0.8191 = 8.19 cm.

By substitution into Equation 1,

$$P = \frac{R \cdot d_R - A \cdot d_A}{d_P + 2d_L} = \frac{(35.54 \text{ kgf} \times 59.09 \text{ cm}) - (3.5 \text{ kgf} \times 29 \text{ cm})}{3.42 \text{ cm} + 16.38 \text{ cm}}$$

$$P = \frac{1998.5 \text{ kgf} \cdot \text{cm}}{19.8 \text{ cm}} = 100.94 \text{ kgf.}$$

Therefore, $L = 201.88$ kgf.

ii. Resolve all forces into their horizontal and vertical components:

$\quad\quad R_V = R \cdot \sin 80° = 35.0$ kgf,
$\quad\quad R_H = R \cdot \cos 80° = 6.17$ kgf,
$\quad\quad A = 3.5$ kgf,
$\quad\quad P_V = P \cdot \sin 20° = 34.52$ kgf,
$\quad\quad P_H = P \cdot \cos 20° = 94.85$ kgf,
$\quad\quad L_V = L \cdot \sin 55° = 165.37$ kgf,
$\quad\quad L_H = L \cdot \cos 55° = 115.79$ kgf.

iii. Equate forces
In equilibrium, resultant vertical force = 0, i.e.

$\quad\quad R_V + S_V - A - P_V - L_V = 0$
$\quad\quad S_V = A + P_V + L_V - R_V$
$\quad\quad S_V = 3.5$ kgf + 34.52 kgf + 165.37 kgf − 35 kgf
$\quad\quad S_V = 168.39$ kgf.

In equilibrium: resultant horizontal force = 0, i.e.

$\quad\quad R_H + P_H + L_H - S_H = 0$
$\quad\quad S_H = R_H + P_H + L_H$
$\quad\quad S_H = 6.17$ kgf + 94.85 kgf + 115.79 kgf
$\quad\quad S_H = 216.81$ kgf.

Calculate S:

$$S = \sqrt{(S_V^2 + S_H^2)} = 274.5 \text{ kgf} = 3.92 \text{ BW.}$$

If S makes an angle of θ with respect to the horizontal, then

$$\tan \theta = S_V/S_H = 0.7767$$
$$\theta = 37.8°.$$

Segmental analysis

12. The solution is based on the method shown in Tables 10.3 and 10.4.

Table 10A.1 Coordinates of segment end points and segment centres of gravity of vaulter.

Segment	Coordinates (cm)[1]		Length (cm)[2]	CG_p[3]	CG_S (cm)[4]	CG_O (cm)[5]
	a	b			c	
Upper limb	Shoulder	Wrist				
x	3.1	2.3	−0.8	0.50	−0.4	2.70
y	6.9	2.9	−4.0	0.50	−2.0	4.90
Lower limb	Hip	Ankle				
x	6.9	9.3	2.4	0.436	1.05	7.95
y	6.4	1.5	−4.9	0.436	−2.14	4.26
Trunk, head and neck	Head	Hip*				
x	0.7	6.9	6.2	0.566	3.51	4.21
y	7.7	6.4	−1.3	0.566	−0.74	6.96

[1], x and y coordinates of segment end points a and b; [2], length of segment in the dimension = b − a; [3], position of segmental centre of gravity as a proportion of segment length in direction a to b (from Table 10.2); [4], position of segmental centre of gravity in the dimension in relation to a; [5], coordinates of the position of the centre of gravity of the segment = a + c.

Table 10A.2 Coordinates of segment centres of gravity and whole body centre of gravity (determined by principle of moments) of vaulter.

Segment	Coordinates(cm)[1]		Weight[2]	Weight (N)[3]	Moment x[4] (N·cm)	Moment y[5] (N·cm)
	x	y				
Upper limb	2.70	4.90	0.0577	39.62	106.97	194.14
Lower limb	7.95	4.26	0.1668	114.54	910.59	487.94
Trunk, head and neck	4.21	6.96	0.5510	378.37	1592.94	2633.45
Coordinates of CG [6]	5.28	5.82				
Totals			1.0	686.70	3628.06	3997.61

[1], x and y coordinates of the segmental centres of gravity from Table 10.3 (cm); [2], weight of segments as a proportion of total body weight (from Table 10.2); [3], weight of segments in newtons (total body weight = 70 kgf = 686.7 N); [4], moments of segmental weights about Z axis with respect to X dimension (N·cm); [5], moments of segmental weights about Z axis with respect to Y dimension (N·cm)
[6], Moment of body weight = sum of moments of segments, i.e.:

$$W \cdot x_G = \text{sum of moment X,}$$

where $\quad W = \text{body weight} = 686.7 \text{ N and } x_G = \text{X coordinate of CG,}$

i.e. $\quad x_G = \dfrac{\text{sum of moment X}}{W} = \dfrac{3628.06 \text{ N} \cdot \text{cm}}{686.7 \text{ N}} = 5.28 \text{ cm.}$

Similarly, $\quad y_G = \dfrac{\text{sum of moment Y}}{W} = \dfrac{3997.61 \text{ N} \cdot \text{cm}}{686.7 \text{ N}} = 5.82 \text{ cm,}$

where $\quad y_G = \text{Y coordinate of CG.}$

Angular displacement, angular velocity angular acceleration

14. i. $\theta_C = 125° = 2.181$ rad, $\theta_E = 120° = 2.094$ rad.
   ii. $\omega = (\theta_D - \theta_B)/t = 400°/s = 6.98$ rad/s.
   iii. $\alpha = (\omega_D - \omega_B)/t = 8$ rad/s^2 = 458.4°/s^2.
   iv. $v_B = r \cdot \omega_B = 3.1$ m/s, $v_D = r \cdot \omega_D = 5.5$ m/s.
   v. $a_B = r \cdot \alpha_B = 7.1$ m/s^2, $a_D = r \cdot \alpha_D = 9.3$ m/s^2.

15. From Equation 10.16, $F_C = (m_H \cdot v_H{}^2)/r_H = 3084.5$ N.
   From Equation 10.18, $r_T = (m_H \cdot r_H)/m_T = 0.129$ m.

16. From Equation 10.16, $F_C = (m_C \cdot v_C{}^2)/r_C = 364.5$ N.
   From Equation 10.19, $\tan \theta = F_C/F_V$, where $F_V = $ weight of cyclist and bike $= 686.7$ N;
   $\theta = 27.9°$.

Angular impulse and angular momentum

17. **Table 10A.3**

Variable	Unit	Unit abbreviation
Moment of a force	newton metre	N·m
Time	second	s
Angular impulse	newton metre second	N·m·s
Moment of inertia	kilogram metres squared	kg·m²
Angular velocity	radians per second	rad/s
Angular momentum	kilogram metres squared per second	kg·m²/s

18. i.   Using Pythagoras' theorem, calculate the distances between a_G and the parallel axes through the centres of gravity of each upper limb, each lower limb and the trunk head and neck. Distance scale: 1 cm on the figure ~ 0.132 m.

Table 10A.4 x and y coordinates (cm) of whole body centre of gravity and centres of gravity of each upper limb, each lower limb and trunk, head and neck.

	x	y
Whole body	5.28	5.82
Upper limb	2.70	4.90
Lower limb	7.95	4.26
Trunk, head and neck	4.21	6.96

d_A = distance between a_G and centre of gravity of each upper
limb = 2.74 cm ~ 0.36 m

d_L = distance between a_G and centre of gravity of each lower
limb = 3.09 cm ~ 0.41 m

d_T = distance between a_G and centre of gravity of the trunk, head and
neck = 1.56 cm ~ 0.20 m

ii. Use $I_z = m \cdot k_z^2$ to calculate the moment of inertia of each segment about the
mediolateral axis a_z through its centre of gravity parallel to a_G (columns 1 to 6 of Table
10A.5).

iii. Use the parallel axis theorem to calculate the moment of inertia of each segment
about a_G (columns 7 to 9 of Table 10A.5).

iv. Sum the total moment of inertia about a_G (column 10 of Table 10A.5).

Table 10A.5 Determination of moment of inertia of vaulter about mediolateral axis through centre of gravity.

Mass of segment as percentage of whole body mass (%)	Mass (kg)	Length of segment (m)	k_z (as percentage of segment length; (%)	k_z (m)	I_z (kg·m²)	d (m)	$m \cdot d^2$ (kg·m²)	I_G (kg·m²)	I_0 (kg·m²)
Upper arm, forearm and hand	5.77	4.04	0.54	0.368	0.20	0.1616	0.36	0.5236	0.6852	1.3704
Trunk, head and neck	55.1	38.6	0.50	0.503	0.25	2.4125	0.20	1.5440	3.9565	3.9565
Thigh, shank and foot	16.7	11.7	0.72	0.326	0.23	0.6189	0.41	1.9667	2.5857	5.1713
Total										10.4982

Whole body mass, 70 kg; a_G, mediolateral axis through centre of gravity of vaulter; k_z, radius of gyration of the segment about the mediolateral axis a_z through its centre of gravity; I_z, moment of inertia of the segment about a_z; d, distance from a_G to centre of gravity of segment; I_G (column 9), moment of inertia of segment about a_G; I_0 (column 10) = moment of inertia of both arms, both legs and the trunk head and neck about a_G and the total moment of inertia about a_G.

19. a_{Z1} = 4.3 rad/s, a_{Z5} = 13 rad/s.

CHAPTER 11

2. Mass of ball m = 0.45 kg; linear velocity of ball after kick v = 25 m/s; contact distance
between ball and foot d = 0.3 m.

i. Work done on the ball $W = F \cdot d$, where F = average force exerted on the ball.

$$W = F \cdot d = \frac{m \cdot v^2}{2} = \frac{(0.45 \text{ kg} \times (25 \text{ m/s})^2)}{2} = 140.6 \text{ J}.$$

$$F = \frac{140.6\,\text{J}}{0.3\,\text{m}} = 468.7\text{ N}.$$

ii. Calculate the contact time t between the ball and the kicker's foot.
From Newton's second law of motion,

$$F \cdot t = m \cdot v - m \cdot u,$$

i.e. $F \cdot t = m \cdot v$ (as $u = 0$)

$$t = \frac{m \cdot v}{F} = \frac{(0.45\,\text{kg} \times 25\,\text{m/s})}{468.7\text{ N}} = 0.024\text{ s}.$$

$$\text{Average power of the impact } P_a = \frac{140.6\,\text{J}}{0.024\,\text{s}} = 5858.3\text{ W}.$$

3.   Mass of hammer $m = 2.25$ kg; translational kinetic energy of the hammer at impact $= 7$ J; distance travelled by hammer before coming to rest $d = 0.03$ m.
(i)   Work done on the wall $W = F \cdot d =$ translational kinetic energy $= 7$ J, where $F =$ average force exerted on the wall, i.e. F $= 7$ J/0.03 m $= 233.3$ N.
(ii) Calculate the contact time t of the impact.
From Newton's second law of motion $F \cdot t = m \cdot v - m \cdot u$, where $u = v_i =$ velocity of hammer at impact and $v = 0 =$ velocity of hammer after the impact.

$$\frac{m \cdot v_i^2}{2} = 7\text{ J},$$

i.e. $v_i = \sqrt{\dfrac{14}{2.25}}$ m/s $= 2.49$ m/s.

$$-F \cdot t = - m \cdot v_i$$
$$t = m \cdot v_i / F = (2.25\text{ kg} \times 2.49\text{ m/s})/233.3\text{ N} = 0.024\text{ s}.$$

$$\text{Average power of the impact } P_a = \frac{7\,\text{J}}{0.024\,\text{s}} = 291.7\text{ W}.$$

4.   Mass of box $m = 20$ kg, $\mu = 0.4$, $d = 3$ m.
$F = \mu \cdot R$ where $F =$ friction between box and floor and $R =$ normal reaction $=$ weight of box, i.e. $F = 0.4 \times 20$ kg $\times 9.81$ m/s$^2 = 78.5$ N.
The work W done on the box is the work needed to overcome F, i.e.
$W = F \cdot d = 78.5$ N $\times 3$ m $= 235.5$ J.

5.   Slope $= 15°$, mass of box $m = 20$ kg, weight of box $B = 196.2$ N.
In this situation, the friction F between the box and the slope will be equal to the component of the weight of the box parallel to the slope, i.e.
$F = B \cdot \sin15° = 196.2$ N $\times 0.2588 = 50.78$ N.

6.   Slope $= 15°$, mass of box $m = 20$ kg, weight of box $B = 196.2$ N, $\mu = 0.4$.
i.   In this situation, the friction between the box and the slope $F = \mu \cdot R$, where $R =$ normal reaction force $=$ component of weight of the box perpendicular to the slope $= B \cdot \cos15° = 189.5$ N, i.e. $F = 0.4 \times 189.5$ N $= 75.8$ N.

ii. The work W required to push the box up the slope is the sum of the work required to overcome friction and the increase in the gravitational potential energy of the box, i.e. $W = F \cdot d + m \cdot g \cdot h$, where h = vertical displacement of box = $d \cdot \sin 15° = 1.29$ m, i.e.

$$W = (75.8 \text{ N} \times 5 \text{ m}) + (20 \text{ kg} \times 9.81 \text{ m/s}^2 \times 1.29 \text{ m}) = 379 \text{ J} + 253 \text{ J} = 632 \text{ J}.$$

iii. Average magnitude of S = work/distance = $632 \text{ J}/5 \text{ m} = 126.4$ N.

7. Mass of ball $m = 7.26$ kg.
   i. If the ball falls from a height of 1.5 m and comes to rest 0.04 m below the ground, its total mechanical energy before it is dropped = $m \cdot g \cdot h$, where $h = 1.54$ m, i.e.

   $m \cdot g \cdot h = 109.7$ J.

   The work done by the ground on the ball $F \cdot d = 109.7$ J, where F = average force exerted on the ball and d = distance travelled by the ball before coming to rest after hitting the ground = 0.04 m, i.e. $F = 109.7 \text{ J}/0.04 \text{ m} = 2742.0$ N.
   ii. When $d = 0.01$ m, $m \cdot g \cdot h = 107.54$ J ($h = 1.51$ m) and $F = 107.54 \text{ J}/0.01 \text{ m} = 10754$ N.

8. Mass of the ball $m = 0.25$ kg, $h_1 = 1.2$ m, $h_2 = 0.8$ m.
   i. The total mechanical energy of the ball before it is dropped = $m \cdot g \cdot h_1$ and the total mechanical energy of the ball at the top of its bounce = $m \cdot g \cdot h_2$, i.e. the energy dissipated during the impact is

   $$m \cdot g \cdot h_1 - m \cdot g \cdot h_2 = m \cdot g (h_1 - h_2) = 0.25 \text{ kg} \times 9.81 \text{ m/s}^2 \times 0.4 \text{ m} = 0.98 \text{ J}.$$

   ii. Resilience of the ball is

   $$(m \cdot g \cdot h_2 / m \cdot g \cdot h_1) \times 100 = (h_2/h_1) \times 100 = 66.7\%.$$

9. Mass of the arrow $m = 0.015$ kg, linear velocity $v = 60$ m/s.
   i. $$F \cdot d = \frac{m \cdot v^2}{2},$$

   where F = average force exerted by the bowstring on the arrow and $d = 0.70$ m, i.e.

   $$F \cdot d = \frac{m \cdot v^2}{2} = \frac{(0.015 \text{ kg} \times (60 \text{ m/s})^2)}{2} = 27 \text{ J},$$

   and $F = 27 \text{ J}/0.70 \text{ m} = 38.6$ N.
   ii. Translational kinetic energy of the arrow at impact with the target = 27 J. $F_1 \cdot d_1$ = work done on arrow by target where F_1 = average force exerted by target on arrow and $d_1 = 0.04$ m, i.e. $F_1 \cdot d_1 = 27$ J and $F_1 = 27 \text{ J}/0.04 \text{ m} = 675$ N.

10. Pedal frequency = 50 rev/min, distance moved by a point on the rim of the fly-wheel = 6 m/rev.

    Work rate $P = W/t$ where W = work done against the friction F between the belt and the flywheel in time t.

$W = F \cdot d$, where d = distance moved by a point on the rim of the flywheel in time t.
d/min = 50 rev/min × 6 m/rev = 300 m/min.

$W/\text{min} = P = F \times d/\text{min}$ = 2 kgf × 300 m/min = 19.62 N × 300 m/min = 5886 J/min = 98.1 J/s = 98.1 W.

11. Mass of vaulter = 70 kg, h_1 = 1.1 m, v_1 = 9.1 m/s, v_2 = 1.0 m/s.
    i. Mechanical energy at take-off = $m \cdot g \cdot h_1 + m \cdot v_1^2/2$
    Mechanical energy at maximum height = $m \cdot g \cdot h_2 + m \cdot v_2^2/2$
    If mechanical energy is conserved, then

$$m \cdot g \cdot h_1 + m \cdot v_1^2/2 = m \cdot g \cdot h_2 + m \cdot v_2^2/2,$$
    i.e. $h_2 - h_1 = (v_1^2 - v_2^2)2g = 4.17$ m.

    ii. h_1 + 4.17 m = 5.27 m.

CHAPTER 12

2. $V = 1000$ m³, W_E = 50 kgf, ρ_o = 1.25 kgf/m³, ρ_i = 1.10 kgf/m³.
    The balloon will float if $B = W_E + W_H + W_L$, where B = the buoyancy force, W_E = the weight of the balloon envelope, W_H = the weight of the hot air inside the balloon and W_L = the weight of the load.

$B = V \cdot \rho_o$ = 1000 m³ × 1.25 kgf/m³ = 1250 kgf

W_E = 50 kgf

$W_H = V \cdot \rho_i$ = 1000 m³ × 1.10 kgf/m³ = 1100 kgf

i.e. the maximum load W_L that the balloon can carry and just float is given by

$W_L = B - W_E - W_H$ = 1250 kgf – 50 kgf – 1100 kgf = 100 kgf.

3. ρ_w = 1025 kgf/m³, V = 1.5 m³.
    The weight of the boat W_B is equal to the weight of the water W_W that the boat displaces when it is floating, i.e.

$W_B = W_W = V \cdot \rho_w$ = 1025 kgf/m³ × 1.5 m³ = 1537.5 kgf.

4. v = 3.5 m/s, η = 0.01002 Pa·s, ρ = 1000 kg/m³, A_S = 1.8 m², v/h = 1.75 /s, C_D = 0.2, A_P = 0.06 m², m = 70 kg.
    i. From Equation 12.8, viscous drag $F_V = \eta \cdot A_S \cdot v/h$, i.e.

F_V = 0.010 02 Pa·s × 1.8 m² × 1.75 /s = 0.0316 N.

From Equation 12.9, pressure drag $F_P = C_D \cdot A_P \cdot \rho \cdot v^2/2$, i.e.

$$F_p = \frac{(0.2 \times 0.06 \text{ m}^2 \times 1000 \text{ kg/m}^3 \times (3.5 \text{ m/s})^2)}{2} = 73.5 \text{ N.}$$

ii. Total drag $= F_V + F_P = 0.0316\ N + 73.5\ N = 73.5316\ N$.

From $F = m \cdot a$, the instantaneous acceleration $a = F/m = -73.5316\ N/70\ kg =$ $-1.05\ m/s^2$.

5. $v = 22.35\ m/s, \eta = 0.000\ 18\ Pa \cdot s, \rho = 1.25\ kg/m^3, A_S = 0.152\ m^2, v/h = 2.2\ /s,$
    $C_D = 0.2, A_P = 0.04\ m^2$.
    i. From Equation 12.8, viscous drag $F_V = \eta \cdot A_S \cdot v/h$, i.e.

    $$F_V = 0.000\ 18\ Pa \cdot s \times 0.152\ m^2 \times 2.2\ /s = 0.000\ 060\ N.$$

    From Equation 12.9, pressure drag $F_P = C_D \cdot A_P \cdot \rho \cdot v^2/2$, i.e.

    $$F_P = \frac{(0.2 \times 0.04\ m^2 \times 1.25\ kg/m^3 \times (22.35\ m/s)^2)}{2} = 2.5\ N.$$

    ii. Total drag $= F_V + F_P = 0.000\ 060\ N + 2.5\ N = 2.5\ N$.
    From $F = m \cdot a$, the instantaneous acceleration $a = F/m = -2.5\ N/\ 0.45\ kg =$ $-5.55\ m/s^2$.

6. $\theta = 5°, m = 390\ kg, \mu = 0.03, C_D = 0.45, A = 0.413\ m^2, \rho = 1.25\ kg/m^3$
    The resultant force acting on the sleigh down the slope (positive down) is given by

    $$R = W_P - F - D = m \cdot a\ (\text{Equation 12.10}),$$

    where W_P is the component of the weight of m parallel to the slope, F is the frictional force and D is the drag force.
    Terminal velocity occurs when $R = W_P - F - D = 0$, i.e. when

    $$W \cdot \sin \theta - \mu \cdot W \cdot \cos \theta - C_D \cdot A \cdot \rho \cdot v^2/2 = 0\ (\text{Equation 12.11}) \text{ where}$$

    $W_P = W \cdot \sin\theta = 390\ kg \times 9.81\ m/s^2 \times 0.0871 = 333.45\ N$

    $F = \mu \cdot W \cdot \cos \theta = 0.03 \times 390\ kg \times 9.81\ m/s^2 \times 0.9962 = 114.34\ N$

    $D = C_D \cdot A \cdot \rho \cdot v^2/2 = (0.45 \times 0.413\ m^2 \times 1.25\ kg/m^3 \times v^2)2 = 0.116v^2\ N$, i.e.

    $333.45\ N - 114.34\ N - 0.116v^2\ N = 0$

    $v = \sqrt{(219.11/0.116)} = 43.46\ m/s = 97.2\ mph.$

7. $m = 0.45\ kg, r = 0.11\ m, t = 1\ s$.
    i.   Atmospheric pressure P_A at ground level is approximately $101\ 325\ Pa = 10.13\ N/cm^2$.
    ii. The cross-sectional area of the ball $A = \pi \cdot r^2 = 0.038\ m^2 = 380\ cm^2$.
    iii. If there is no sideways pressure differential on the ball, i.e. if the atmospheric pressure on each side of the ball is the same, the force F on each side of the ball is given by

    $$F = P_A \cdot A = 10.13\ N/cm^2 \times 380\ cm^2 = 3849.4\ N.$$

iv. A pressure differential of 0.1% would result in a force differential

$$F = 0.001 \times 3849.4 \text{ N} = 3.85 \text{ N}.$$

v. The sideways acceleration of the ball $a = F/m = 3.85$ N/0.45 kg $= 8.55$ m/s^2.

vi. The sideways distance s moved by the ball (assuming constant acceleration of 8.55 m/s^2) in one second is given by $s = u{\cdot}t + a{\cdot}t^2/2$ where $u = 0$, $a = 8.55$ m/s^2 and $t = 1$ s, i.e. $s = 4.3$ m.

References

CHAPTER 1

Alberts, B., Johnson, A., Lewis, J., Raff, M., Roberts, K. and Walter, P. (2002) *Molecular Biology of the Cell*, 4th edition. New York: Garland Publishing.

Dempster, W.T. (1965) Mechanisms of shoulder movement, *Archives of Physical Medicine and Rehabilitation* 46(1):49–70.

Elftman, H. (1966) Biomechanics of muscle, *Journal of Bone and Joint Surgery* 48A(2):363–77.

Fleisig, G.S., Barrentine, S.W., Escamilla, F.R. and Andrews, J.R. (1996) Biomechanics of overhand throwing with implications for injuries, *Sports Medicine* 21(6):421–37.

Freeman, W.H. and Bracegirdle, B. (1967) *An Atlas of Histology*. London: Heinemann.

Frost, H.M. (1990) Structural adaptations to mechanical usage (SATMU): 4. mechanical influences on intact fibrous tissues, *The Anatomical Record* 226:433–9.

Frost, H.M. (2003) Bone's mechanostat: a 2003 update, *The Anatomical Record* 275A:1081–101.

Hennig, E.M., Staats, A. and Rosenbaum, D. (1994) Plantar pressure distribution patterns of young children in comparison to adults, *Foot & Ankle* 15(10):35–40.

Janssen, I., Heymsfield, S.B., Wang, Z. and Ross, R. (2000) Skeletal muscle mass and distribution in 468 men and women aged 18–88 yr, *Journal of Applied Physiology* 89:81–88.

Kenyon, C. (1988) The nematode *Caenorhabditis elegans*, *Science* 240:1448–52.

McArdle W.D., Katch, F.I. and Katch, V.L. (2007) *Exercise Physiology: Energy, Nutrition, and Human Performance*, 6th edition. Philadelphia: Lippincott, Williams & Wilkins.

Miller, D.I.(1980) Body segment contributions to sport skill performance: two contrasting approaches, *Research Quarterly for Exercise and Sport* 51:219–33.

Nigg, B.M. (1985) Biomechanics, load analysis, and sports injuries in the lower extremities, *Sports Medicine* 2:367–79.

Standring, S. (ed.) (2008) *Gray's Anatomy*, 40th edition. Edinburgh: Churchill Livingstone.

Taylor, D.C., Dalton, J.D., Seaber, A.V. and Garrett, W.E. (1990) Viscoelastic properties of muscle-tendon units, *American Journal of Sports Medicine* 18:300–8.

Wozniak, M.A. and Chen, C.S. (2009) Mechanotransduction in development: a growing role for contractility, *Nature Reviews: Molecular Cell Biology* 10:34–43.

CHAPTER 2

Briggs, P.J. (2005) The structure and function of the foot in relation to injury, *Current Orthopaedics* 19:85–93.

Standring, S. (ed.) (2008) *Gray's Anatomy*, 40th edition. Edinburgh: Churchill Livingstone.

CHAPTER 3

Akeson, W.H., Frank, C.B., Amiel, D. and Woo, S.L.Y. (1985) Ligament biology and biomechanics, in *Symposium on Sports Medicine: The Knee*, ed. Finerman, G. St Louis: Mosby, pp. 111–15.

Alexander, R.M. (1968) *Animal Mechanics*. London: Sidgwick & Jackson.

Alexander, R.M. (1975) *Biomechanics*. London: Chapman & Hall.

Ascenzi, A. and Bell G.H. (1971) Bone as a mechanical engineering problem, in *The Biochemistry and Physiology of Bone*, ed. Bourne, G.H. New York: Academic Press.

Bailey, D.A., Martin, A.D., Houston, C.S. and Howie, J.L. (1986) Physical activity, nutrition, bone density and osteoporosis, *Australian Journal of Science and Medicine in Sport* 18:3–8.

Bauer, G. (1960) Epidemiology of fracture in aged persons, *Clinical Orthopedics* 17:219–25.

Bergmann, P., Body, J.J., Boonen, S., Boutsen, Y., Devogelaer, J.P., Goemaere, S., Kaufman, J., Reginster, J.Y. and Rozenberg, S. (2011) Loading and skeletal development and maintenance, *Journal of Osteoporosis*, doi:10.4061/2011/786752.

Burr, D.B. (2004) Anatomy and physiology of the mineralized tissues: role in the pathogenesis of osteoarthrosis, *Osteoarthritis and Cartilage* 12(supplement):20–30.

Caine, D., DiFiori, J. and Maffulli, N. (2006) Physeal injuries in children's and youth sports: reasons for concern?, *British Journal of Sports Medicine* 40:749–60.

Caplan, A.I. (1984) Cartilage, *Scientific American* 251:82–90.

Chalmers, J. and Ho, K.C. (1970) Geographical variations in senile osteoporosis, *Journal of Bone and Joint Surgery* 52:667–75.

Combs, J.A. (1994) Hip and pelvis avulsion fractures in adolescents, *The Physician and Sports Medicine* 22:41–4, 4–9.

Cummings, S.R. and Melton, L.J. (2002) Epidemiology and outcomes of osteoporotic fractures, *Lancet* 359(9319):1761–7.

Frost, H.M. (1979) A chondral modeling theory, *Calcified Tissue International* 28:181–200.

Frost, H.M. (1999) Joint anatomy, design, and arthrosis: insights of the Utah paradigm, *The Anatomical Record* 255:162–74.

Frost, H.M. (2004) A 2003 update of bone physiology and Wolff's law for clinicians, *Angle Orthodontist* 74(1):3–15.

Gross, M.L., Flynn, M. and Sonzogni, J.J. (1994) Overworked shoulders: managing injury of the proximal humeral epiphysis, *The Physician and Sports Medicine* 22:81–2, 85–6.

Kemmler, W., Engelke, K., von Stengel, S., Weineck, J., Lauber, D. and Kalender, W.A. (2007) Long-term four-year exercise has a positive effect on menopausal risk factors: the Erlangen Fitness Osteoporosis Prevention Study, *Journal of Strength and Conditioning Research* 21(1):232–9.

Kohrt, M., Bloomfield, S.A., Little, K.D., Nelson, M.E. and Yingling, V.R. (2004) Physical activity and bone health, *Medicine and Science in Sports and Exercise* 36(11):1985–96.

Krueger-Franke, M., Siebert, C.H. and Pfoerringer, W. (1992) Sports-related epiphyseal injuries of the lower extremity: an epidemiological study, *Journal of Sports Medicine and Physical Fitness* 32:106–11.

Larson, R.L. (1973) Physical activity and the growth and development of bone and joint structures, in *Physical Activity: Human Growth and Development*, ed. Rarick, G.L. New York: Academic Press, p. 24.

Larson, R.L. and McMahan, R.O. (1966) The epiphyses and the childhood athlete, *Journal of the American Medical Association* 196:607–12.

Maddalozzo, G.F., Widrick, J.J., Cardinal, B.J., Winters-Stone, K.M., Hoffman, M.A. and Snow, C.M. (2007) The effects of hormone replacement therapy and resistance training on spine bone mineral density in early postmenopausal women, *Bone* 40(5):1244–51.

McArdle W.D., Katch, F.I. and Katch, V.L. (2007) *Exercise Physiology: Energy, Nutrition, and Human Performance*, 6th edition. Philadelphia: Lippincott, Williams & Wilkins.

Nordin, M.N. and Frankel, V.H. (2001) *Basic Biomechanics of the Skeletal System*. Philadelphia: Lippincott, Williams & Wilkins.

Pappas, A.M. (1983) Epiphyseal injuries in sports, *The Physician and Sports Medicine* 11:140–8.

Peterson, H.A. (2001) Physeal injuries and growth arrest, in *Fracture in Children*, ed. Beaty, J.H. and Kasser, J.R. Philadelphia: Lippincott Williams & Wilkins, pp. 91–138.

Radin, E.L. (1984) Biomechanical considerations, in *Osteoarthritis: Diagnosis and Management*, ed. Moskowitz, R.W., Howell, D.S., Goldberg, V.M. and Mankin, H.J. Philadelphia: W.B. Saunders, pp. 71–9.

Seeman, E. (2008) Bone quality: the material and structural basis of bone strength, *Journal of Bone and Mineral Metabolism* 26:1–8.

Smith, E.L. (1982) Exercise for prevention of osteoporosis, *The Physician and Sports Medicine* 10:72–83.

Speer, D.P. and Braun, J.K. (1985) The biomechanical basis of growth plate injuries, *The Physician and Sports Medicine* 13:72–8.

Standring, S. (ed) (2008) *Gray's Anatomy*, 40th edition. Edinburgh: Churchill Livingstone.

Tortora, G.J. and Anagnostakos, N.P. (1984) *Principles of Anatomy and Physiology*. New York: Harper & Row.

Turner, C.H. and Pavalko, F.M. (1998) Mechanotransduction and functional response of the skeleton to physical stress: the mechanisms and mechanics of bone adaptation, *Journal of Orthopaedic Science* 3:346–55.

Wang, Q. and Seeman, E. (2008) Skeletal growth and peak bone strength, *Best Practice & Research Clinical Endocrinology & Metabolism* 22(5):687–700.

CHAPTER 4

Frost, H.M. (1999) Joint anatomy, design, and arthrosis: insights of the Utah paradigm, *The Anatomical Record* 255:162–74.

Grana, W.A., Holder, S. and Schelberg-Karnes, E. (1987) How I manage acute anterior shoulder dislocations, *The Physician and Sports Medicine* 15(4):88–93.

Herbert, R. (1988) The passive mechanical properties of muscles and their adaptations to altered patterns of use, *Australian Journal of Physiotherapy* 34(3):141–9.

Nicholas, J.A. and Marino, M. (1987) The relationship of injuries of the leg, foot and ankle to proximal thigh strength in athletes, *Foot & Ankle* 7(4):218–28.

CHAPTER 5

Alexander, R.M. (1968) *Animal Mechanics*. London: Sidgwick & Jackson.

Alexander, R.M. (1989) Muscles for the job, *New Scientist* 122(1660):50–3.

Alexander, R.M. (1992) *The Human Machine*. London: Natural History Museum Publications.

Andersen, J.L., Schjerling, P. and Saltin, B. (2000) Muscle, genes and athletic performance, *Scientific American* 283(3):48–55.

Anderson, F.C. and Pandy, M.G. (1993) Storage and utilization of elastic strain energy during jumping, *Journal of Biomechanics* 26(12):1413–27.

Beard, D.J., Dodd, C.A.F., Trundle, H.R. and Simpson, A.H.R.W. (1994) Proproception enhancement for anterior cruciate ligament deficiency, *Journal of Bone and Joint Surgery* 76B:654–9.

Burkholder, T.J. and Lieber, R.L. (2001) Sarcomere length operating range of vertebrate muscles during movement, *Journal of Experimental Biology* 204:1529–36.

Edman, K.A.P. (1992) Contractile performance of skeletal muscle fibres, in *Strength and Power in Sport*, ed. Komi, P.V. Oxford: Blackwell Scientific, pp. 96–114.

Elftman, H. (1966) Biomechanics of muscle, *Journal of Bone and Joint Surgery* 48A(2):363–77.

Enoka, R.M. (2008) *Neuromechanics of Human Movement*, 4th edition. Champaign, IL: Human Kinetics.

Freeman, M. and Wyke, B. (1967) Articular reflexes at the ankle joint: an electromyographic study of normal and abnormal reflexes of ankle joint mechanoreceptors upon reflex activity in the leg muscles, *British Journal of Surgery* 54:990–1001.

Gamble, J.G. (1988) *The Musculoskeletal System: Physiological Basics*. New York: Raven Press.

Gandevia, S.C., McClosky, D.I. and Burke, D. (1992) Kinesthetic signals and muscle contraction, *Trends in Neuroscience* 15:62–5.

Garn, S. and Newton, R. (1988) Kinesthetic awareness in subjects with multiple ankle sprains, *Physical Therapy* 68:1667–71.

Gordon, A.M., Huxley, A.F. and Julian, F.J. (1966) The variation in isometric tension with sarcomere length in vertebrate muscle fibres, *Journal of Physiology (London)* 184:170–92.

Gregor, R.J. (1993) Skeletal muscle mechanics and movement, in *Current Issues in Biomechanics*, ed. Grabiner, M.D. Champaign, IL: Human Kinetics, pp. 171–211.

Gregorio, C.C., Granzier, H., Sorimachi, H. and Labeit, S. (1999) Muscle assembly: a titanic achievement?, *Current Opinion in Cell Biology*, 11:18–25.

Grigg, P. (1994) Peripheral neural mechanisms in proprioception. *Journal of Sport Rehabilitation* 3:2–17.

Hall, MG., Ferrell, W.R., Baxendale, R.H. and Hamblen, D.L. (1994) Knee joint proprioception: threshold detection levels in healthy young subjects, *Neuro-Orthopedics* 15:81–90.

Hall, M.G., Ferrell, W.R., Sturrock, D.L., Hamblen, D.L. and Baxendale, R.H. (1995) The effect of the hypermobility syndrome on knee joint proprioception, *British Journal of Rheumatology* 34:121–5.

Huijing, P.A. (1992) Mechanical muscle models, in *Strength and Power in Sport*, ed. Komi, P.V. Oxford: Blackwell Scientific, pp. 130–50.

Huxley, H.E. and Hanson, J. (1954) Changes in the cross striations of muscle during contraction and stretch and their structural interpretation, *Nature* 173:973–7.

Ishikawa, M., Komi, P.V., Grey, M.J., Lepola, V. and Bruggemann, G.-P. (2005) Muscle–tendon interaction and elastic energy usage in human walking, *Journal of Applied Physiology* 99:603–8.

Kandel, E.R., Schwartz, J.H. and Jessel, T.M. (eds) (2000) *Principles of Neural Science*, 4th edition. New York: McGraw-Hill.

Kawakami, Y. and Fukunaga, T. (2006) New insights into human skeletal muscle function, *Exercise and Sport Sciences Reviews* 34(1):16–21.

Kleinrensink, G.J., Stoeckart, R., Meulstee, J., Kaulesar Sukul D.M.K.S., Vleeming, A., Snijders, C.J. and Van Noort, A. (1994) Lowered motor conduction velocity of the peroneal nerve after inversion trauma, *Medicine and Science in Sports and Exercise* 26(7):877–83.

Komi, P.V. (2003). Stretch–shortening cycle, in *Strength and Power in Sport*, ed. Komi, P.V. Oxford: Blackwell Scientific, pp. 184–202.

Komi, P.V. and Bosco, C. (1978) Utilization of stored elastic energy in leg extensor muscles by men and women, *Medicine and Science in Sports* 10(4):261–5.

Lieber, R.L. (1992) *Skeletal Muscle Structure and Function*. Baltimore: Williams & Wilkins.

Lieber, R.L. and Bodine-Fowler, S.C. (1993) Skeletal muscle mechanics: implications for rehabilitation, *Physical Therapy* 73(12):844–56.

Lindstedt, S.L., LaStayo, P.C. and Reich, T.E. (2001) When active muscle lengthen: properties and consequences of eccentric contractions, *News in the Physiological Sciences* 16:256–61.

Matthews, P.B. (1988) Proprioceptors and their contribution to somatosensory mapping: complex messages require complex processing, *Canadian Journal of Physiology and Pharmacology* 66:430–8.

Mynark, R.G. and Koceja, D.M. (2001) Effects of age on the spinal stretch reflex, *Journal of Applied Biomechanics* 17:188–203.

Nishikawa, K.C., Monroy, J.A., Uyeno, T.E., Yeo, S.H., Pai, D.K. and Lindstedt, S.L. (2012) Is titin a 'winding filament'? A new twist on muscle contraction, *Proceedings of the Royal Society B* 279:981–90.

Noth, J. (1992) Motor units, in *Strength and Power in Sport*, ed. Komi, P.V. Oxford: Blackwell Scientific, pp. 21–8.

Roberts, T.D.M. (1995) *Understanding Balance: The Mechanics of Posture and Locomotion.* London: Chapman and Hall.

Roberts, T.J. (2002) The integrated function of muscles and tendons during locomotion. *Comparative Biochemistry and Physiology Part A* 133:1087–99.

Rome, L. (2006) Design and function of superfast muscles: new insights into the physiology of skeletal muscle, *Annual Review of Physiology* 68:22.1–22.29.

Sargeant, A.J. (1994) Human power output and muscle fatigue, *International Journal of Sports Medicine* 15(3):116–21.

Seddon, J.H. (1972) *Surgical Disorders of Peripheral Nerves.* Edinburgh: Churchill Livingstone.

Skinner, H.B., Wyatt, M.P., Stone, M.L., Hodgdon, J.A. and Barrack, R.L. (1986) Exercise-related knee joint laxity, *American Journal of Sports Medicine* 14:30–4.

Spanjaard, M., Reeves, R.D., van Dieën, J.H., Baltzopoulos, V. and Maganaris, C.N. (2006) Gastrocnemius muscle fascicle behavior during stair negotiation in humans, *Journal of Applied Physiology* 102:1618–23.

Standring, S. (ed.) (2008) *Gray's Anatomy*, 40th edition. Edinburgh: Churchill Livingstone.

Steiner, M.E., Grana, W.A., Chillag, K. and Schelberg-Karnes, E. (1986) The effect of exercise on anterior-posterior knee laxity, *American Journal of Sports Medicine* 14:24–9.

Wilkerson, G.B. and Nitz, A.J. (1994) Dynamic ankle stability: mechanical and neuromuscular relationships, *Journal of Sport Rehabilitation* 3:43–57.

CHAPTER 6

Alexander, R.M. (1968) *Animal Mechanics.* London: Sidgwick & Jackson.

Burstein, A.H. and Wright, T.M. (1994) *Fundamentals of Orthopedic Biomechanics.* Baltimore: Williams & Wilkins.

Cavanagh, P.R., Valiant, G.A. and Misevich, K.W. (1984) Biological aspects of modelling shoe/foot interaction during running, in *Sport Shoes and Playing Surfaces*, ed. Frederick, E.C. Champaign, IL: Human Kinetics, pp. 24–46.

Dickenson, R.P., Hutton, W.C. and Stott, J.R.R. (1981) The mechanical properties of bone in osteoporosis, *Journal of Bone and Joint Surgery* 63B(2):233–8.

Evans, F.G. (1971) Biomechanical implications of anatomy, in *Biomechanics*, ed. Cooper, J.M. Chicago: The Athletic Institute, pp. 3–30.

Frost, H.M. (1967) *An Introduction to Biomechanics.* Springfield, IL: Charles C Thomas.

Garrett, W.E., Safran, M.R., Seaber, A.V., Glisson, R.R. and Ribbeck, B.M. (1987) Biomechanical comparison of stimulated and nonstimulated skeletal muscle pulled to failure, *American Journal of Sports Medicine* 15(5):448–54.

Grimston, S.K. and Zernicke, R.F. (1993) Exercise-related stress responses in bone, *Journal of Applied Biomechanics* 9:2–14.

Hoshino, A. and Wallace, A.W. (1987) Impact absorbing properties of the human knee, *Journal of Bone and Joint Surgery* 69B(5):807–11.

Johnson, G.R. (1988) The effectiveness of shock-absorbing insoles during normal walking, *Prosthetics and Orthotics International* 12(1):91–5.

Ker, R.F., Bennett, M.B., Bibby, S.R., Kester, R.C. and Alexander, R.M. (1987) The spring in the arch of the human foot, *Nature* 325(7000):147–9.

Mair, S.D., Seaber, A.V., Glisson, R.R. and Garrett, W.E. (1996) The role of fatigue in susceptibility to acute muscle strain injury, *American Journal of Sports Medicine* 24(2):137–43.

McMahon, T.A. and Greene, P.R. (1978) Fast running tracks, *Scientific American* 239(6): 148–63.

Radin, E.L. and Paul, I.L. (1971) Response of joints to impact loading I: *in vitro* wear, *Arthritis and Rheumatology* 14:356–62.

Radin, E.L., Parker, H.G., Pugh, J.W., Steinberg, R.S., Paul, I.L. and Rose, R.M. (1973) Response of joints to impact loading III: relationship between trabecular microfractures and cartilage degeneration, *Journal of Biomechanics* 6:51–57.

Simon, S.R., Radin, E.L., Paul, I.L and Rose, R.M. (1972) The response of joints to impact loading II: *in vivo* behavior of subchondral bone, *Journal of Biomechanics* 5:267–72.

Taylor, D.C., Dalton, J.D., Seaber, A.V. and Garrett, W.E. (1990) Viscoelastic properties of muscle-tendon units, *American Journal of Sports Medicine* 18:300–8.

Voloshin, A. and Wosk, J. (1981) Influence of artificial shock absorbers on human gait *Clinical Orthopaedics and Related Research* 160:52–6.

Voloshin, A. and Wosk, J. (1982) *In-vivo* study of low back pain and shock absorption in human locomotor system, *Journal of Biomechanics* 15:21–7.

Wosk, J. and Voloshin, A. (1985) Low back pain: conservative treatment with artificial shock absorbers, *Archives of Physical Medicine and Rehabilitation* 66:145–8.

CHAPTER 7

Aagaard, P., Simonsen, E.B., Andersen, J.L., Magnusson, P. and Dyhre-Puolsen, P. (2002) Neural adaptation to resistance training: changes in evoked V-wave and H-reflex responses, *Journal of Applied Physiology* 92:2309–18.

Akeson, W.H., Amiel, D., Mechanic, G.L., Woo, S.L.Y., Harwood, F.L. and Hamer M.L. (1977) Collagen cross linking alterations in joint contractures: changes in the reducible cross-links in periarticular connective tissue collagen after nine weeks of immobilization, *Connective Tissue Research* 5:15–19.

Akima, H., Kano, Y., Enomoto Y., Ishizu, M., Okada, M., Oishi, Y., Katsuta, S. and Kuno, S. (2001) Muscle function in 164 men and women aged 20–84 years, *Medicine and Science in Sports and Exercise* 33:220–26.

Anderson, S.M. and Nilsson, B.E. (1979) Changes in bone mineral content following ligamentous knee injuries, *Medicine and Science in Sports* 11:351–3.

Baker, M.K., Atlantis, E. and Fiatarone-Singh, M.A. (2007) Multi-modal exercise programs for older adults, *Age and Ageing* 36:375–81.

Booth, F.W. (1987) Physiologic and biochemical effects of immobilisation on muscle, *Clinical Orthopaedics and Related Research* 219:15–20.

Brighton, C.T., Katz, M.J., Goll, S.R. and Nicholls, C.E. (1985) Prevention and treatment of sciatic denervation disuse osteoporosis in a rat tibia with capacitatively coupled electrical stimulation, *Bone* 6:87–97.

Burr, D.B. (1997) Muscle strength, bone mass, and age-related bone loss, *Journal of Bone and Mineral Research* 12(10):1547–51.

Capodaglio, P., Eda, M.C, Facioli, M. and Saibene, F. (2007) Long-term strength training for community-dwelling people over 75: impact on muscle function, functional ability and life style, *European Journal of Applied Physiology* 100:535–42.

Carter, D.R., Wong, M. and Orr, T.E. (1991) Musculoskeletal ontogeny, phylogeny, and functional adaptation, *Journal of Biomechanics* 24S1:3–16.

Cohen, L.A. and Cohen, M.L. (1956) Arthrokinetic reflex of the knee, *American Journal of Physiology* 184:433–7.

Cruz-Jentoft, A.J., Baeyens, J.P., Bauer, J.M., Boirie, Y., Cederholm, T., Landi, F., Martin, F.C., Michel, J.P., Rolland, Y., Schneider, S.M., Topinková, E., Vandewoude, M., Zamboni, M. and the European Working Group on Sarcopenia in Older People. (2010) Sarcopenia: European consensus on definition and diagnosis, *Age and Ageing* 39:412–23.

Donaldson, C., Hulley, S., Vogel, J., Hattner, R., Bayers, J. and McMillan, D. (1970) Effect of prolonged bed rest on bone mineral, *Metabolism* 19:1071–84.

Doschak, M.R. and Zernicke, R.F. (2005) Structure, function and adaptation of bone-tendon and bone-ligament complexes, *Journal of Musculoskeletal & Neuronal Interactions* 5(1):35–40.

Duyar, I. (2008) Growth patterns and physical plasticity in adolescent laborers, *Collegium Antropologicum* 32(2):403–12.

Elliott, D.H. (1965) Structure and function of mammalian tendon, *Biological Reviews* 40:392–421.

Enoka, R.M. (1997) Neural adaptations with chronic physical activity, *Journal of Biomechanics* 30(5):447–55.

Eser, P., Frotzler, A., Zehnder, Y., Wick, L., Knecht, H., Denoth, J. and Schiessl, H. (2004) Relationship between the duration of paralysis and bone structure: a PQT study of spinal cord injured individuals, *Bone* 34:869–80.

Ferretti, A., Papandrea, P. and Conteduca, F. (1990) Knee injuries in volleyball, *Sports Medicine* 10(2):132–8.

Forwood, M.R. (2001) Mechanical effects on the skeleton: are there clinical implications?, *Osteoporosis International* 12:77–83.

Frost, H.M. (1973) *Orthopedic Biomechanics*, volume 5. Springfield, IL: Charles C Thomas.

Frost, H.M. (1979) A chondral modeling theory, *Calcified Tissue International* 28:181–200.

Frost, H.M. (1988a) Structural adaptations to mechanical usage: a proposed three-way rule for bone modeling, part I, *Veterinary and Comparative Orthopaedics and Traumatology* 1:7–17.

Frost, H.M. (1988b) Structural adaptations to mechanical usage: a proposed three-way rule for bone modeling, part II, *Veterinary and Comparative Orthopaedics and Traumatology* 2:80–5.

Frost, H.M. (1990) Skeletal structural adaptations to mechanical usage (SATMU), 4: mechanical influences on intact fibrous tissues, *Anatomical Record* 226:433–9.

Frost, H.M. (2003) Bone's mechanostat: a 2003 update, *Anatomical Record* 275A:1081–1101.

Grabiner, M.D. and Enoka, R.M. (1995) Changes in movement capabilities with aging, *Exercise and Sport Sciences Reviews* 23:65–104.

Gross, T.S. and Bain, S.T. (1993) Skeletal adaptation to functional stimuli, in *Current Issues in Biomechanics*, ed. Grabiner, M.D. Champaign, IL: Human Kinetics, pp. 151–69.

Häkkinen, K. (1994) Neuromuscular adaptation during strength training, aging, detraining, and immobilization, *Critical Reviews in Physical and Rehabilitation Medicine* 6(3):161–98.

Hamrick, M.W. (1999) A chondral modeling theory revisited, *Journal of Theoretical Biology* 201(3):201–8.

Heinert, B., Kernozek, T.W., Greany, J. and Fater, D.C.W. (2008) Hip abductor weakness and lower extremity kinematics during running, *Journal of Sport Rehabilitation* 17(3):243–56.

Herzog, W. (2000) Muscle properties and coordination during voluntary movement, *Journal of Sports Sciences* 18:141–52.

Hootman, J.M., Macera, C.A., Ainsworth, B.E., Martin, M., Addy, C.L. and Blair, S.N. (2001) Association among physical activity level, cardiorespiratory fitness, and risk of musculoskeletal injury, *American Journal of Epidemiology* 154(3):251–8.

Johnson, M.E., Mille, M.L., Martinez, K.M., Crombie, G. and Rogers, M.W. (2004) Age-related changes in hip abductor and adductor joint torques, *Archives of Physical Medicine and Rehabilitation* 85(4):593–7.

Jones, B.H., Cowan, D.N. and Knapik, J. (1994) Exercise, training, and injuries, *Sports Medicine* 18(3):202–14.

Jurimae, T. and Jurimae, J. (2001) *Growth, Physical Activity, and Motor Development in Prepubertal Children*. London: Informa HealthCare.

Kamen, G. and Caldwell, G.E. (1996) Physiology and interpretation of the electromyogram, *Journal of Clinical Neurophysiology* 13(5):366–84.

Konradsen, L., Ravn, J.B. and Sørensen, A.I. (1993) Proprioception at the ankle: the effect of anaesthetic blockade of ligament receptors, *Journal of Bone and Joint Surgery* 75B(3):433–6.

Lanyon, L.E. (1981) Adaptive mechanics: the skeleton's response to mechanical stress, in *Mechanical Factors and the Skeleton*, ed. Stokes, I.A. London: John Libbey.

LeBlanc, A.D., Spector, E.R., Evans, H.J. and Sibonga, J.D. (2007) Skeletal responses to space-flight and the bed rest analog: a review, *Journal of Musculoskeletal & Neuronal Interactions* 7:33–47.

Lieber, R.L. (2002) *Skeletal Muscle Structure, Function & Plasticity: The Physiological Basis of Rehabilitation*. Philadelphia: Lippincott Williams & Wilkins.

Magnusson, S.P., Narici, M.V., Maganaris, C.N. and Kjaer, M. (2008) Human tendon behaviour and adaptation, *in vivo, Journal of Physiology* 586(1):71–81.

Malina, R.M., Bouchard, C. and Bar-Or, O. (2004) *Growth, Maturation, and Physical Activity*. Champaign, IL: Human Kinetics.

Micheli, L.J., 1982, Lower extremity injuries: overuse injuries in the recreational adult, in *The Exercising Adult*, ed. Cantu, R.C. Lexington, MA: Collamore.

Moritani, T. (1993) Neuromuscular adaptations during the acquisition of muscle strength, power and motor tasks, *Journal of Biomechanics* 26(Suppl 1):95–107.

Muller, E.A. (1970) Influence of training and of inactivity on muscle strength, *Archives of Physical Medicine and Rehabilitation* 51:449–62.

Myers, T.W. (2001) *Anatomy Trains: Myofascial Meridians for Manual and Movement Therapists*. Edinburgh: Churchill Livingstone.

Narici, M.V. and Maganaris, C.N. (2006) Adaptability of elderly human muscles and tendons to increased loading, *Journal of Anatomy* 208:433–43.

Nigg, B.M., Denoth, J. and Neukomm, P.A. (1981) Quantifying the load on the human body: problems and some possible solutions, in *Biomechanics*, volume VIIB, ed. Morecki, A., Fidelus, K., Kedzior, K. and Wit, I. Baltimore: University Park Press.

Noyes, F.R. (1977) Functional properties of knee ligaments and alterations induced by immobilization, *Clinical Orthopaedics* 123:210–42.

Radin, E.L. (1986) Osteoarthrosis: what is known about prevention, *Clinical Orthopedics and Related Research* 222:6–65.

Redford, J.B. (1987) Orthotics: general principles, *Physical Medicine and Rehabilitation State of the Art Reviews* 1(1):1–10.

Reeves, N.D., Narici, M.V. and Maganaris, C.N. (2006) Myotendinous plasticity to ageing and resistance exercise in humans, *Experimental Physiology* 91(3):483–98.

Roberts, D., Ageberg, E., Andersen, G. and Fridén, T. (2007) Clinical measurements of proprioception, muscle strength and laxity in relation to function in the ACL-injured knee, *Knee Surgery, Sports Traumatology, Arthroscopy* 15:9–16.

Rubin, C.T. (1984) Skeletal strain and the functional significance of bone architecture, *Calcified Tissue International* 36:S11–S18.

Salenius, P. and Vankka, E. (1975) Development of the tibiofemoral angle of children at different ages, *Journal of Bone and Joint Surgery* 57A:259–61.

Schiessl, H., Frost, H.M. and Jee, W.S.S. (1998) Estrogen and bone-muscle strength and mass relationships, *Bone* 22(1):1–6.

Schoenau, E. and Frost, H.M. (2003) The 'muscle-bone unit' in children and adolescents, *Calcified Tissue International* 70: 405–7.

Schultz, A.B., Alexander, N.B. and Ashton-Miller, J.A. (1992) Biomechanical analyses of rising from a chair, *Journal of Biomechanics* 25:1383–991.

Seynnes, O.R., Maganaris, C.N., de Boer, M.D., di Prampero, P.E. and Narici, M.V. (2008) Early structural adaptations to unloading in the human calf muscles, *Acta Physiologica* 193(3): 265–74.

Sharma, P. and Maffulli, N. (2006) Biology of tendon injury: healing, modeling and remodeling, *Journal of Musculoskeletal & Neuronal Interactions* 6(2):181–90.

Sievänen, H. (2010) Immobilization and bone structure in humans, *Archives of Biochemistry and Biophysics* 503: 146–52.

Taber, L.A. (1995) Biomechanics of growth, remodeling, and morphogenesis, *Applied Mechanical Reviews* 48(8):487–545.

Tyler, T.F., Nicholas, S.J., Campbell, R.J. and McHugh, M.P. (2001) The association of hip strength and flexibility with the incidence of adductor muscle strains in professional ice hockey players, *American Journal of Sports Medicine* 29:124–8.

Wackerhage, H. and Rennie, M.J. (2006) How nutrition and exercise maintain the human muscu-loskeletal mass, *Journal of Anatomy* 208:451–8.

Watkins, J. and Peabody, P. (1996) Sports injuries in children and adolescents treated at a sports injury clinic, *Journal of Sports Medicine and Physical Fitness* 36(1):43–8.

Wearing, S.C., Hennig, E.M., Byrne, N.M., Steele, J.R. and Hills, A.P. (2006) The impact of child-hood obesity on musculoskeletal form, *Obesity Reviews* 7:209–18.

Williams, P. and Goldspink, G. (1973) The effect of immobilization on the longitudinal growth of striated muscle fibers, *Journal of Anatomy* 116:45–55.

Williams, P. and Goldspink, G. (1978) Changes in sarcomere length and physiological properties in immobilized muscle, *Journal of Anatomy* 127:459–68.

Wolff, J. (1988) *The Law of Bone Remodeling*, translated by Maquet, P. and Furlong, R. New York: Springer.

Zernicke, R.F. and Loitz, B.J. (1992) Exercise-related adaptations in connective tissue, in *Strength and Power in Sport*, ed. Komi, P.V. Oxford, UK: Blackwell Scientific.

CHAPTER 8

Rowett, R. (2004) *How Many? A Dictionary of Units of Measurement*. Available online at www.unc.edu/~rowlett/units/sipm.html

Watkins, J. (2008) Developmental biodynamics: the development of coordination, in *Paediatric Exercise Science and Medicine*, 2nd edition, ed. Armstrong, N., and van Mechelen, W. Oxford: Oxford University Press.

CHAPTER 9

Alexander, R.M. (1992) *The Human Machine*. London: Natural History Museum Publications.

Asken, M.J. and Schwartz, R.C. (1998) Heading the ball in soccer, *The Physician and Sports Medicine* 26(11):37–42, 44.

Baumann, W. (1976) Kinematic and dynamic characteristics of the sprint start, in *Biomechanics*, volume VB, ed. Komi, P.V. Baltimore: University Park Press, pp. 194–9.

Castle, F. (1969) *Five-figure Logarithmic and Other Tables*. London: Macmillan.

Cavanagh, P.R. and Lafortune, M.A. (1980) Ground reaction forces in distance running, *Journal of Biomechanics* 13:397–406.

Cavanagh, P.R. and Williams, K.W. (1982) The effect of stride length variation on oxygen uptake in distance running, *Medicine and Science in Sports and Exercise* 14:30–5.

Cavanagh, P.R., Pollock, M.L. and Landa, J. (1977) A biomechanical comparison of elite and good distance runners, *Annals of New York Academy of Sciences* 301:328–45.

Cavanagh, P.R., Valiant, G.A. and Misevich. K.W. (1984) Biological aspects of modelling shoe/foot interaction during running, in *Sport Shoes and Playing Surfaces*, ed. Frederick, E.C. Champaign, IL: Human Kinetics, pp. 24–46.

Cutnell, J.D. and Johnson, K.W. (1995) *Physics*, 3rd edition. New York: Wiley, p. 315.

Czerniecki, J. M. (1988) Foot and ankle biomechanics in walking and running: a review, *American Journal of Physical Medicine and Rehabilitation* 67(6):246–52.

Dagg, A.I. (1977) *Running, Walking and Jumping: The Science of Locomotion*. London: Wykeham Publications.

Daish, C.B. (1972) *The Physics of Ball Games*. London: The English University Press.

Davies, C.T.M. (1980) Effects of wind assistance and resistance on the forward motion of a runner, *Journal of Applied Physiology* 48(4):702–9.

Elert, G. (ed.) *The Physics Factbook*. Available online at http://hypertextbook.com/facts/2000/KatherineMalfucci.shtml

Elliot, B.C. and Blanksby, B.A. (1979) Optimal stride length considerations for male and female recreational runners, *British Journal of Sports Medicine* 13:15–18.

Filippone, A. (2005) *Aerodynamic Database: Drag Coefficients*. Available online at http://aerodyn.org/Drag/tables.html

Hay, J.G. (2002) Cycle rate, length, and speed of progression in human locomotion, *Journal of Applied Biomechanics* 18:257–70.

Hay, J.G., Miller, J.A. and Canterna, R.W. (1986) The techniques of elite male long jumpers, *Journal of Biomechanics* 19(10):855–66.

Heinert, L.D., Serfass, R.C., Stull, G.A. (1988) Effect of stride length variation on oxygen uptake during level and positive grade treadmill running, *Research Quarterly for Exercise and Sport* 59:127–30.

IAAF (1984) *Track and Field Athletics: A Basic Coaching Manual*. London: International Amateur Athletic Federation.

Jones, A.M. and Whipp, B.J. (2002) Bioenergetic constraints on tactical decision making in middle distance running, *British Journal of Sports Medicine* 36:102–4.

Kerr, B.A., Beauchamp, L. and Fisher, B. (1983) Foot-strike patterns in distance running, in *Biomechanical Aspects of Sports Shoes and Playing Surfaces*, ed. Nigg, B.M. and Kerr, B.A. Calgary: University Printing, pp. 34–45.

Kubaha, K., Fiala, D. and Lomas, K. J. (2003) Predicting human geometry-related factors for detailed radiation analysis in indoor spaces, *VIII International IBPSA Conference, Eindhoven, Netherlands*, pp. 681–8. Available online at www.ibpsa.org/proceedings/BS2003/BS03_0681_688.pdf

Kyrolainen, H., Belli, A. and Komi, P.V. (2001) Biomechanical factors affecting running economy, *Medicine and Science in Sports and Exercise* 33(8):1330–7.

Lees, A., Fowler, N. and Derby, D. (1993) A biomechanical analysis of the last stride, touch-down and take-off characteristics of the women's long jump, *Journal of Sports Sciences* 11:303–14.

Lees, A., Graham-Smith, P. and Fowler, N. (1994) A biomechanical analysis of the last stride, touch-down and take-off characteristics of the men's long jump, *Journal of Applied Biomechanics* 10:61–78.

Lichtenberg, D.B. and Wills, J.G. (1978) Maximising the range of the shot put, *American Journal of Physics* 46(5):546–9.

Linthorne, N.P. (1994) The effect of wind on 100 m sprint times, *Journal of Applied Biomechanics* 10(2):110–31.

Linthorne, N.P. (2001) Optimum release angle in the shot put, *Journal of Sports Sciences* 19:359–72.

Linthorne, N.P., Guzman, M.S. and Bridgett, L.A. (2005) Optimal take-off angle in the long jump, *Journal of Sports Sciences* 23(7):703–12.

Matheras, A.V. (1998) Shot-put: optimum angles of release, *Track & Field Coaches Review* 72(2):24–6.

Mero, A. and Komi, P.V. (1986) Force-, EMG-, and elasticity-velocity relationship at submaximal, maximal and supramaximal running speeds in sprinters, *European Journal of Applied Physiology* 55:553–61.

Moravec, P.J., Ruzicka, P., Susanka, P., Dostal, E., Kodejs, M. and Nosek, M. (1988) The 1987 International Athletic Foundation/IAAF Scientific Project Report: time analysis of the 100 metres events at the II World Championships in Athletics, *New Studies in Athletics* 3:61–96.

Murase, Y., Hoshikawa, T., Yasuda, N., Ikegami, Y. and Matsui, H. (1976) Analysis of changes in progressive speed during 100-meter dash, in *Biomechanics*, volume VB, ed. Komi, P.V. Baltimore: University Park Press, pp. 200–7.

Mureika, J.R. (2001) A realistic quasi-physical model of the 100 m dash, *Canadian Journal of Physics* 79:697–713.

Nigg, B.M., Denoth, J., Kerr, B., Luethi, S., Smith, D. and Stacoff, A. (1984) Load, sports shoes and playing surfaces, in *Sport Shoes and Playing Surfaces*, ed. Frederick, E.C. Champaign, IL: Human Kinetics, pp. 1–23.

Orendurff, M.S., Segal, A.D., Klute, G.K., Berge, J.S., Rohr, E.S. and Kadel, N.J. (2004) The effect of walking speed on center of mass displacement, *Journal of Rehabilitation Research & Development* 41(6A):829–34.

Roberts, T.D.M. (1995) *Understanding Balance: The Mechanics of Posture and Locomotion*. London: Chapman & Hall.

Serway, R.A. and Jewett, J.W. (2004) *Physics for Scientists and Engineers*. Fort Worth: Harcourt College Publishers.

Susanka, P. and Stepanek, J. (1988) Biomechanical analysis of the shot put, in *Scientific Report on the Second IAAF World Championships in Athletics*. Monaco: IAAF pp. 1–77.

Tsirakos, D.K., Bartlett. R.M. and Kollias, I.A. (1995) A comparative study of the release and temporal characteristics of shot put, *Journal of Human Movement Studies* 28:227–42.

Wagner, G. (1998) The 100-meter dash: theory and experiment, *The Physics Teacher* 36(3):144–6.

Ward-Smith, A.J. (1985) The influence on long jump performance of the aerodynamic drag experienced during the approach and aerial phases, *Journal of Biomechanical Engineering* 107:336–40.

Watkins, J. (2000) The effect of body configuration on the locus of the whole-body centre of gravity, *Journal of Sports Sciences* 18(1):10.

Watt, D.G.D. and Jones, G.M. (1971) Muscular control of loading from unexpected falls in man, *Journal of Physiology* 219:729–37.

Weyand, P.G., Sternlight, D.B., Bellizzi, M.J. and Wright, S. (2000) Faster top running speeds are achieved with greater ground reaction forces not more rapid leg movements, *Journal of Applied Physiology* 89:1991–9.

Williams, K.R. and Cavanagh, P.R. (1987) Relationship between distance running mechanics, running economy, and performance, *Journal of Applied Physiology* 63(3):1236–45.

Winter, D.A. (1990) *Biomechanics and Motor Control of Human Movement*, 2nd edition. New York: John Wiley.

CHAPTER 10

Chow, J.W. (1999) Knee joint forces during isokinetic knee extensions: a case study, *Clinical Biomechanics* 14:329–38.

Clauser, C., McConnville, C. and Young, J. (1969) Weight, volume and centre of mass segments of the human body, AMRL-TR-69-70. Wright-Patterson Air Force Base, Ohio. Available online at www.dtic.mil/dtic/tr/fulltext/u2/710622.pdf

Dapena, J. (1984) The pattern of hammer speed during a hammer throw and influence of gravity on its fluctuations, *Journal of Biomechanics* 17(8):553–9.

Dempster, W.T. (1955) Space requirements of the seated operator, WADC Technical Report 55-

159. Wright-Patterson Air Force Base, Ohio. Available online at www.smpp.northwestern.edu/savedLiterature/DempsterEtAl.1955.pdf

Dempster, W.T. (1965) Mechanisms of shoulder movement, *Archives of Physical Medicine and Rehabilitation* 46(1):49–70.

Dyson, G. (1977) *The Mechanics of Athletics*. London: Hodder & Stoughton.

Frohlich, C. (1979) Do springboard divers violate angular momentum conservation?, *American Journal of Physics* 47(7):583–92.

Frohlich, C. (1980) The physics of somersaulting and twisting, *Scientific American* 242(3):112–18,120.

Hamill, J., Ricard, M.D. and Golden, D.M. (1986) Angular momentum in multiple rotation nontwisting platform dives, *International Journal of Sport Biomechanics* 2:78–87.

Hanavan, E.P. (1964) A mathematical model of the human body, AMRL Technical Report 64-102, Wright-Patterson Air Force base, Ohio. Available online at www.dtic.mil/cgi-bin/GetTRDoc?AD=AD0608463

Hatze, H. (1980) A mathematical model for the computational determination of parameter values of anthropomorphic segments, *Journal of Biomechanics* 13:833–43.

Hay, J.G. (1973) The center of gravity of the human body, in *Kinesiology III*, ed. Widule, C. Washington DC: American Alliance for Health, Physical Education and Recreation, pp. 20–44.

Hay. J.G. (1974) Moment of inertia of the human body, in *Kinesiology IV*. Washington DC: American Alliance for Health, Physical Education and Recreation, pp. 43–52.

Lees, A., Fowler, N. and Derby, D. (1993) A biomechanical analysis of the last stride, touch-down and take-off characteristics of the women's long jump, *Journal of Sports Sciences* 11:303–14.

Lieber, R.L. (1992) *Skeletal Muscle Structure and Function*. Baltimore: Williams & Wilkins.

Linthorne, N.P., Guzman, M.S. and Bridgett, L.A. (2005) Optimal take-off angle in the long jump, *Journal of Sports Sciences* 23(7):703–12.

McDonald, D. (1960) How does a cat fall on its feet?, *New Scientist* 7:1647–9.

Ninio, F. (1993) Acceleration in uniform circular motion, *American Journal of Physics* 61(11):1052.

Plagenhoef, S., Evans, F.G. and Abdelnour, T. (1983) Anatomical data for analysing human motion, *Research Quarterly for Exercise and Sport* 54(2):169–78.

Santschi, W.R., DuBois, J. and Omoto, C. (1963) Moments of inertia and centers of gravity of the living human body, AMRL Technical Documentary Report 63-36, Wright-Patterson Air Force Base, Ohio. Available online at www.dtic.mil/cgi-bin/GetTRDoc?AD=AD0410451

Spriging, E.J., Burko, D.B., Watson, G. and Laverty, W.H. (1987) An evaluation of three segmental methods used to predict the location of the total body CG for human airborne movements, *Journal of Human Movement Studies* 13:57–68.

Van Eijden, T.M.G.J., De Boer, W. and Weijs, W.A. (1985) The orientation of the distal part of the quadriceps femoris muscle as a function of the knee flexion-extension angle, *Journal of Biomechanics* 18(10):803–9.

Wallace, D.A., Salem, G.J., Salinas, R. and Powers, C.M. (2002) Patellofemoral joint kinetics while squatting with and without an external load, *Journal of Orthopaedic & Sports Physical Therapy* 32(4):141–8.

Weyand, P.G., Sternlight, D.B., Bellizzi, M.J. and Wright, S. (2000) Faster top running speeds are achieved with greater ground reaction forces not more rapid leg movements, *Journal of Applied Physiology* 89:1991–9.

Whitsett, C.E. (1963) Some dynamic response characteristics of weightless man, AMRL Technical Report 63-18, Wright-Patterson Air Force base, Ohio. Available online at www.dtic.mil/cgi-bin/GetTRDoc?AD=AD0412451

Wikipedia (2005) *Velodrome*. Available online at http://en.wikipedia.org/wiki/Velodrome

Winter, D.A. (1990) *Biomechanics and Motor Control of Human Movement*. New York: John Wiley.

Yeadon, M.R. (1990) The simulation of aerial movement. II. A mathematical inertia model of the human body, *Journal of Biomechanics* 23:67–74.

Yeadon, M.R. (1993a) The biomechanics of twisting somersaults part I: rigid body motions, *Journal of Sports Sciences* 11:187–98.

Yeadon, M.R. (1993b) The biomechanics of twisting somersaults part II: contact twist, *Journal of Sports Sciences* 11:199–208.

Yeadon, M.R. (1993c) The biomechanics of twisting somersaults part III: aerial twist, *Journal of Sports Sciences* 11:209–18.

Yeadon, M. R. (1993d) The biomechanics of twisting somersaults part IV: partitioning performances using the tilt angle, *Journal of Sports Sciences* 11:219–25.

Yeadon, M.R. (1997) The biomechanics of the human in flight, *American Journal of Sports Medicine* 25(4):575–80.

CHAPTER 11

Bogdanis, G.C. and Yeadon, M.R. (1994) The biomechanics of pole vaulting, *Athletics Coach* 28(4):20–4.

Brancazio, P.J. (1984) *Sport Science: Physical Laws and Optimum Performance*. New York: Simon and Schuster.

Canavan, P.K. and Vescovi, J.D. (2004) Evaluation of power prediction equations: peak vertical jumping power in women, *Medicine and Science in Sports and Exercise* 36(9):1589–93.

Davies, C.T.M. and Rennie, R. (1968) Human power output, *Nature* 217:770–1.

Frost, H.M. (1967) *An Introduction to Biomechanics*. Springfield, IL: Charles C Thomas.

Kyle, C.R. and Caiozzo, V.J. (1985) A comparison of the effect of external loading upon power output in stair climbing and running up a ramp, *European Journal of Applied Physiology* 54:99–103.

McArdle, W.D., Katch, F.I. and Katch, V.L. (1991) *Exercise Physiology: Energy, Nutrition, and Human Performance*, 3rd edition. Philadelphia: Lea & Febiger.

Margaria, R. Aghemo, P. and Rovelli, E. (1966) Measurement of muscular power (anaerobic) in man, *Journal of Applied Physiology* 21:1662–4.

Pierrynowski, M.R., Winter, D.A. and Norman, R.W. (1980) Transfers of mechanical energy within the total body and mechanical efficiency during treadmill walking, *Ergonomics* 23(2):147–56.

Plagenhoef, S., Evans, F.G. and Abdelnour, T. (1983) Anatomical data for analysing human motion, *Research Quarterly for Exercise and Sport* 54(2):169–78.

Winter, D.A. (1979) A new definition of mechanical work in human movement, *Journal of Applied Physiology* 47:79–83.

Winter, D.A. (1990) *Biomechanics and Motor Control of Human Movement.* New York: John Wiley.

CHAPTER 12

Alexander, R.M. (1968) *Animal Mechanics.* London: Sidgwick & Jackson.

Armenti, A. (1984) How can a downhill skier move faster than a sky diver?, *The Physics Teacher* 22(2):109–11.

Barthels, K. (1977) Swimming biomechanics: resistance and propulsion, *Swimming Technique* 14(3):66–70.

Brancazio, P.J. (1984) *Sport Science: Physical Laws and Optimum Performance.* New York: Simon and Schuster.

Brown, R.M. and Counsilman, J.E. (1971) The role of lift in propelling the swimmer, in *Selected Topics in Biomechanics*, ed. Cooper, J.M. Chicago: The Athletic Institute, pp. 179–90.

Clugston, M.J. (1998) *The Penguin Dictionary of Science.* London: Penguin.

Corlett, G. (1980) *Swimming Teaching, Theory and Practice.* London: Kaye & Ward.

Costill, D.L., Maglischo, E.W. and Richardson, A.B. (1992) *Handbook of Sports Medicine and Science in Swimming.* Oxford: Blackwell Science.

Counsilman, J.E. and Counsilman, B.E. (1994) *The New Science of Swimming.* Englewood Cliffs, NJ: Prentice Hall.

Daish, C.B. (1972) *The Physics of Ball Games.* London: The English University Press.

Filippone, A. (2004) Aerodynamic database: drag coefficients. Available online at www.if.ufrj.br/~carlos/palestras/futebol/dragData/Aerodynamic%20Drag%20Data.htm

Fuchs, V. (ed.) (1985) *Oxford Illustrated Encyclopedia Volume 1: The Physical World.* Oxford: Oxford University Press.

Gagnon, M. and Montpetit, R. (1981) Technological development for the measurement of the center of volume in the human body, *Journal of Biomechanics* 14(4):235–41.

Gardner, M. (1993) Bernoulli's principle, *The Physics Teacher* 31(5):304.

Kyle, C.R. (1979) Reduction in wind resistance and power output of racing cyclists and runners travelling in groups, *Ergonomics* 22(4):387–97.

Malina, R.M. and Bouchard, C. (1991) *Growth, Maturation, and Physical Activity.* Champaign IL: Human Kinetics.

McArdle, W.D., Katch, F.I. and Katch, V.L. (1994) *Essentials of Exercise Physiology.* Philadelphia: Lea & Febiger.

NASA (1999) *Flight Testing Newton's Laws*. Available online at www.nasa.gov/pdf/563411main_
  FTNL_Student_Manual.pdf

Pickard, G.L. and Emery, W.J. (1990) *Descriptive Physical Oceanography: An Introduction*. London:
  Butterworth-Heinemann.

Pugh, L.G.C.E. (1971) The influence of wind resistance on walking and running and the mechanical efficiency of work against horizontal or vertical forces, *Journal of Physiology* (London)
  213:255–76.

Wagner, G. and Wood, R. (1996) Skydiver survives depth plunge, *The Physics Teacher* 34(12):543–5.

Whiting, H.T.A. (1963) Variations in floating ability with age in the male, *Research Quarterly*
  31(1):84–91.

Whiting, H.T.A. (1965) Variations in floating ability with age in the female, *Research Quarterly*
  36(2):216–18.

Wright, J. (2005) Shape effects on drag. Available online at www.grc.nasa.gov/WWW/Wright/
  airplane/shaped.html

Index